ATLAS OF
VASCULAR ANATOMY

An Angiographic Approach

Illustrations by

José Falcetti
Director, Center for Medical Arts, Hospital das Clinicas
Faculdade de Medicina da Universidade de São Paulo
Functional Neurosurgery
São Paulo, SP, Brazil

With Contributions by

Carlos Jader Feldman, M.D.
Chief, Department of Radiology
Hospital Hernesto Dornelles
Porto Alegre, RS, Brazil
—Vascular Anatomy of the Lower Genital Tract

Luiz Maria Yordi, M.D.
Chief, Department of Hemodynamic and Cardiovascular Radiology
Hospital São Francisco
Porto Alegre, RS, Brazil
—The Heart and Coronary Arteries
—The Heart Venous Circulation

Ronie L. Piske, M.D.
Interventional Neuroradiologist, Med–Imagem
Hospital Beneficência
Poruguesa, São Paulo, SP, Brazil
—Arteries of the Head and Neck
—Veins of the Head and Neck

Francisco J.B. Sampaio, M.D., Ph. D.
Professor of Anatomy and Urology
Head, Department of Anatomy
State University of Rio de Janeiro
Brazil
—Kidney Arterial Vascularization
—Kidney Venous Drainage
—Lymphatic Drainage of the Kidney
—Periprostatic Venous Plexus

ATLAS OF VASCULAR ANATOMY

An Angiographic Approach

Renan Uflacker, M.D.

Professor of Radiology
Department of Radiology
Medical University of South Carolina
Charleston, South Carolina

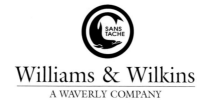

Williams & Wilkins
A WAVERLY COMPANY

BALTIMORE • PHILADELPHIA • LONDON • PARIS • BANGKOK
BUENOS AIRES • HONG KONG • MUNICH • SYDNEY • TOKYO • WROCLAW

Editor: Charles W. Mitchell
Associate Managing Editor: Grace E. Miller
Production Coordinator: Barbara J. Felton
Designer: Wilma E. Rosenberger
Ilustration Planner: Wayne Hubbel, Lorraine Wrzosek, Ray Lowman
Compositor: Donna M. Smith
Printer/Binder: Everbest
Digitized Illustrations: Prestige Color, Inc.

Copyright © 1997
Williams & Wilkins
351 West Camden Street
Baltimore, MD 21201-2435 USA

Accurate indications, adverse reactions, and dosage schedules for drugs are provided in this book, but it is possible that they may change. The reader is urger to review the package information data of the manufacturers of the medications mentioned.

Printed in Hong Kong

Library of Congress Cataloging-in-Publication Data

Atlas of vascular anatomy: an angiographic approach / edited by Renan Uflacker; illustrations by José Falcetti; with contributions by Carlos Jader Feldman... [et al.].
    p. cm.
Includes bibliographical references and index.
ISBN 0-683-18110-6
    1. Blood-vessels—Atlases. 2. Angiography—Atlases. I. Uflacker, Renan. II. Feldman, Carlos Jader. [DNLM: 1. Blood Vessels—anatomy & histology—atlases. 2. Angiography—atlases. WG 17 A88468 1997]
QM191.A87   1997
611'.13—DC20
DNLM/DLC
for Library of Congress   96-32248
                                        CIP

The Publishers have made every effort to trace the copyright holders for borrowed material. If they have inadvertently overlooked any, they will be pleased to make the necessary arrangements at the first opportunity.

97 98 99 00
2 3 4 5 6 7 8 9 10

To purchase additional copies of this book, call our customer service department at (800) 638-0672, or fax orders to (800) 447-8438. For other book services, including chapter reprints and large quantity sales, ask for the Special Sales department.

Canadian customers should call (800) 268-4178, or fax (905) 470-6780. For all other calls originating outside the United States, please call (410) 528-4223 or fax us at (410) 528-8550.

Visit Williams & Wilkins on the Internet http://www.wwilkins.com or contact our customer service department at http://custserv@wwilkins.com. Williams & Wilkins customer service representatives are available from 8:45 am to 6:00 pm, EST, Monday through Friday, for either telephone or Internet access.

PREFACE

The development of imaging techniques to study and demonstrate the human vascular anatomy has been increasingly important for the modern understanding and management of most vascular diseases. The use of angiograms as roadmaps for vascular surgery and interventional procedures is currently the best way to demonstrate the vascular anatomy. New several, different and modern imaging modalities including ultrasound, computed tomography, magnetic resonance imaging, and magnetic resonance angiography have been developed to evaluate vascular diseases with unprecedented and unparalleled noninvasive means of assessing patients. Although further improvement in these techniques may obviate the need for the more invasive diagnostic angiography, the angiographic perception of the vessels is hitherto the gold standard to learn vascular anatomy.

The knowledge of the vascular anatomy is essential for the performance, understanding, and interpretation of diagnostic and interventional vascular procedures, as well as performing surgical procedures. The analysis of angiographic pictures, correlated to the anatomic conventional illustrations is still the best way to understand normal vascular anatomy and to perceive minute anatomical variations without cadavers dissection.

The idea of producing an *Atlas of Vascular Anatomy* was triggered by the need to have available a high-quality book with illustrations and correlation with normal angiograms. *The Atlas of Vascular Anatomy* is intended to provide a response to clinical anatomic challenges that abound in many aspects of vascular surgery and vascular radiology practice. The basic aim is to provide photographs of real angiographic cases and fine art color illustrations for the study of the details and spatial disposition of anatomic vascular structures, as well as some of the variations encountered.

The format was designed to facilitate the use of the book, minimizing page turning by the assignment of individual topics to opposing pages, followed by a sequence of correlated illustrations. The descriptive text was kept to the minimum necessary for the understanding of the subjects and preceding the actual illustrations.

The edition of the *Atlas of Vascular Anatomy: An Angiographic Approach* is intended to be a quick and practical reference of vascular anatomy for those involved with anatomy, diagnosis and treatment of vascular diseases. Vascular and Interventional Radiologists, Surgeons, Cardiologists, Medical Students as well as Residents and Fellows in Radiology and Surgery compounds the target population of the book.

All the vascular territories are covered and correlation with function and other critical anatomical structures related to the clinical and surgical application of vascular anatomy is presented when pertinent.

I hope that the major effort on the part of the editor of the book and the contributing authors will fill a niche in our field of work. I would like to thank and share with the readers the continuing support and enthusiasm with this project from the Publisher's senior staff, who made possible the commissioning of the art work from an amazing medical artist, Jose Falcetti, who frequently exceeded the requirements of the color pictures only for the sake of quality and perfection.

Renan Uflacker, M.D.
Editor

CONTENTS

1

THE FETAL CIRCULATION

The fetal blood reaches the placenta through the two umbilical arteries and returns to the fetus by the two umbilical veins early in the fetal life. Later, the right umbilical vein disappears and the left persists as the single returning vessel. The fetal blood receives oxygen and nutrients by close contact with maternal blood in the placenta. The umbilical vein (persistent left umbilical vein) enters the abdomen at the umbilicus and runs along the edge of the falciform ligament to the hepatic visceral surface-sending branches to the left hepatic lobe, joining the left branch of the portal vein. At the opposite side of this anastomoses arises the Ductus Venosus who joins the Inferior Vena Cava conveying the oxygen-rich blood coming from the maternal placenta. The fetal portal vein is small, and the right and left branches function as branches of the ductus venosus, carrying oxygenated blood to the liver. At the inferior vena cava, the oxygenated blood mixes with a small amount of blood poor in oxygen from the caudal portion of the fetus. The blood from the inferior vena cava together with the blood from the ductus venosus enters the right atrium and hits the interatrial membrane and is directed through the foramen ovale into the left atrium, guided by the inferior vena cava's valve. At the left atrium the oxygen-rich blood mixes with a small amount of nonoxygenated blood from the pulmonary vein. From the left atrium, the blood enters the left ventricle and subsequently the aorta. A small portion of oxygenated blood, instead of crossing the foramen ovale, joins the blood flow from the superior vena cava and, after passing through the right atrium, enters the right ventricle of the heart. The inflow from the superior vena cava plus the small amount of blood from the umbilical vein is diverted to the pulmonary artery, supplying the lungs. Most of this blood flow, however, is shunted through the ductus arteriosus directly into the descending aorta, joining the blood stream ejected from the left ventricle. Most of the oxygenated blood ejected from the left ventricle reaches the heart and brain circulation providing a higher oxygen content to these organs as opposed to structures less sensitive to hypoxia in the abdomen and extremities. The blood in the descending aorta is poorer in oxygen and is partly distributed to the lower limbs and viscera of the abdomen and pelvis, but most of it returns to the placenta via the umbilical arteries, branches of the internal iliac arteries (Fig. 1.1).

After birth, the ductus venosus closes rapidly, and after obliteration, it is transformed into the ligamentum venosum, connecting with the ligamentum teres (round ligament), where lies the occluded umbilical vein. The round ligament reaches the umbilicus, as well as the lateral umbilical ligaments, remnants of the umbilical arteries, reaching the internal iliac arteries. After closure of the ductus venosus and umbilical vein, the liver is supplied by oxygenated blood from the abdominal aorta through the celiac trunk and from the portal vein.

With the first respiration, the resistance of the pulmonary vascular bed reduces markedly, and the pressure changes cause a redistribution of pressures and flow between the right and left atrium in a way that no blood passes through the Foramen Ovale, with subsequent closure of the foramen ovale within the first year of life in most of the individuals, at first by apposition and later fusion of the interatrial septa. In adults, the fossa ovalis indicates the locale of the foramen. The ductus arteriosus closes by muscular contraction and is obliterated by intimal proliferation. The connective tissue, remnant of the ductus arteriosus, is called ligamentum arteriosum.

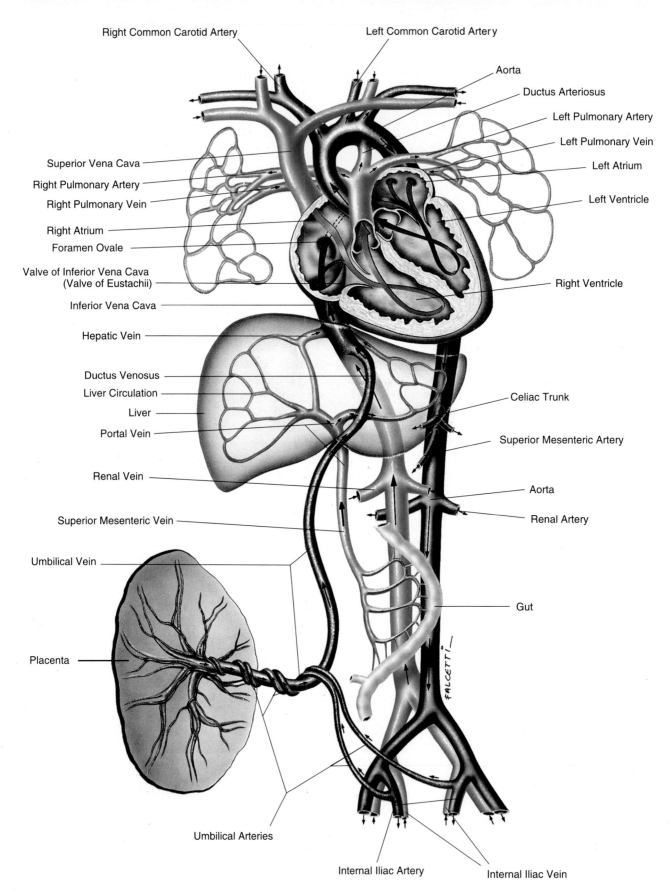

Right Common Carotid Artery

Left Common Carotid Artery

Aorta

Ductus Arteriosus

Left Pulmonary Artery

Left Pulmonary Vein

Left Atrium

Left Ventricle

Superior Vena Cava

Right Pulmonary Artery

Right Pulmonary Vein

Right Atrium

Foramen Ovale

Valve of Inferior Vena Cava
(Valve of Eustachii)

Inferior Vena Cava

Right Ventricle

Hepatic Vein

Ductus Venosus

Liver Circulation

Liver

Portal Vein

Celiac Trunk

Superior Mesenteric Artery

Renal Vein

Aorta

Renal Artery

Superior Mesenteric Vein

Umbilical Vein

Gut

Placenta

FALCETTI

Umbilical Arteries

Internal Iliac Artery

Internal Iliac Vein

Figure 1.1. Fetal circulation. The fetus receives oxygenated blood from the placenta through the umbilical vein. Part of the received blood passes through the hepatic sinusoids while most of the incoming blood passes through the ductus venosus directly into the inferior vena cava. At the inferior vena cava, the oxygen-rich blood from the placenta mixes with the blood from the caudal portions of the fetus. The mixed blood stream enters the right atrium and crosses the interatrial membrane through the foramen ovale into the left atrium. At the left atrium, the blood is mixed again with poorly oxygenated blood from the pulmonary veins and passes through the left ventricle to the aorta. The blood from the superior vena cava and a small amount of blood from the inferior vena cava are diverted into the pulmonary artery, where the blood is shunted into the descending thoracic aorta through the ductus arteriosus. The resultant mixed blood goes into the abdominal aorta, to the visceral and lower extremities circulation, eventually reaching the placenta through the umbilical arteries, for oxygenation.

2

ARTERIES OF THE HEAD AND NECK

The arterial vascularization of the head and neck originates from the three main arteries at the aortic arch (Fig. 2.1). In two thirds of the population, the brachiocephalic trunk is the first vessel that originates from the aortic arch; the left carotid artery is the second; and the left subclavian artery is the third. The right common carotid begins at the bifurcation of the brachiocephalic trunk and the right vertebral artery originates from the right subclavian artery, also a branch of the brachiocephalic trunk. The left common carotid artery arises directly from the aortic arch, while the left vertebral artery originates from the left subclavian artery.

In one third of people, three most common variations may be encountered: 1) the left common carotid artery either has a common origin with the brachiocephalic trunk or originates from the proximal portion of this trunk (most common variation); 2) the left vertebral artery originates directly from the aortic arch between the left common carotid artery and left subclavian artery; 3) aberrant origin of the right subclavian artery from the aortic arch distal to the left subclavian artery.

COMMON CAROTID ARTERY

The common carotid artery has a thoracic part and a cervical portion. It is enclosed within the carotid sheath, together with the vagus nerve and the jugular vein. The common carotid artery ascends from the arch of the aorta, in front of the trachea, to the cervical portion, where they incline laterally to both sides of the trachea (Figs. 2.1, 2.2). The left common carotid artery is usually longer than the right common carotid artery, and in individuals with short necks, the bifurcation of both common carotids is higher.

The common carotid arteries usually have no branches either in the thoracic portion or the cervical part, but it may give origin to the vertebral, the superior thyroid or its laryngeal branch, the ascending pharyngeal, the inferior thyroid, or the occipital artery. At the level of the upper border of the thyroid cartilage, the common carotid arteries bifurcate into the external and internal carotid arteries (Figs. 2.3, 2.4). At the division, the vessel dilates and is called the carotid sinus, which usually involves only the origin of the internal carotid artery. The carotid sinus contains a large number of sensory nerve endings, from the glossopharyngeal nerve, acting as a baroreceptor mechanism exercising control over the intracranial pressure. The carotid body lies behind the level of the bifurcation of the common carotid artery and has a chemoreceptor function.

EXTERNAL CAROTID ARTERY

The external carotid artery arises medial and anterior to the internal carotid artery (Figs. 2.5, 2.6). Occasionally it may arise laterally to the internal carotid artery, particularly in older individuals.

Branches (Figs. 2.3, 2.7)

> *Anterior Branches*
> > Superior thyroid artery
> > Lingual artery
> > Facial artery
> *Posterior Branches*
> > Ascending pharyngeal artery
> > Occipital artery
> > Posterior auricular
> > Terminal branches
> > Superficial temporal artery
> > Internal maxillary artery

Superior Thyroid Artery

This artery arises from the external carotid artery, as the first anterior branch, just below the level of the greater cornu of the hyoid bone and divides into terminal branches at the apex of the lobe of the thyroid gland. It may arise from the common carotid artery.

Branches

Anterior branch or superior marginal arcade (anastomose with the opposite artery through the isthmus)
Posterior branch or posterior glandular arcade (anastomose with the inferior thyroid artery)
Lateral branch or lateral glandular arcade (not constant)
Hyoid branch (anastomose the thyrolaryngeal system inferiorly with the linguofacial system superiorly)

Sternocleidomastoid artery
Superior laryngeal artery (anastomose with the opposite artery and the inferior laryngeal artery)
Cricothyroid artery (anastomose with the opposite artery)

Lingual Artery (Figs 2.8, 2.9)

It is the second branch of the external carotid artery and main feeder of the tongue muscles of the floor of the mouth and the sublingual gland. It arises from the anteromedial aspect of the proximal external carotid artery, between the origin of the superior thyroid artery and the facial artery. Occasionally, it may have a common origin with the facial artery constituting the linguofacial trunk (Fig. 2.3). This artery runs obliquely upwards and medially, curving downwards and forwards forming a loop. It runs horizontally forward and finally ascends sharp cranially coursing under the surface of the tongue as far as its tip.

The lingual artery may be divided in three parts. The first part is in the carotid triangle. The second part of the lingual artery traverses the upper border of the hyoid bone, deep to the hyoglossal and the lower part of the submandibular gland. The hyoglossal separates the artery from the hypoglossal nerve and its vena comitans. The third part of the artery is also called arteria profunda linguae. It runs close to the tongue and is accompanied by the lingual nerve. At the tip of the tongue, it anastomoses with the contralateral artery.

Branches

Suprahyoid branch (small, anastomoses with the contralateral artery)
Dorsal artery of the tongue (largest branch supplying the tongue)
Sublingual artery (supplies the sublingual gland and neighboring muscles and mucous membrane of the mouth and gums. Anastomoses with the submental artery arising from the facial artery. A medial mandibular branch supplies the anterolateral surface of the body of the mandible. Depending on the hemodynamic balance of the region, the lingual artery, through its anastomotic branches, can take over the supply of the gland and the mandible, and occasionally part of the submental territory [Figs. 2.9, 2.10]).

Facial Artery (Figs. 2.5, 2.10, 2.11)

Originates from the anterior aspect of the external carotid artery, as the third branch, still in the carotid triangle, just above the lingual artery and the greater cornu of the hyoid bone. Runs medial to the ramus of the mandible causing a groove on the posterior border of the submandibular gland. It turns downwards and forwards reaching the lower border of the mandible, and becoming superficial and subcutaneous. At this point, the main facial trunk can have two different courses, a more posterolateral or jugal course, or a more anteromedial or labial course (Fig. 2.11). The facial artery turns cranially to the side of the nose, ending at the medial palpebral commissure, supplying the lachrymal sac and anastomosing with the dorsal nasal branch of the ophthalmic artery.

The facial artery supplies the muscles and tissues of the face, the submandibular gland, the tonsil and the soft palate. The branches may be separated in cervical and facial groups. There are abundant anastomoses of the facial artery, not only with the contralateral branches of the vessel at the opposite side, but also in the neck, with the sublingual branch of the lingual artery, and with the palatine branch of the maxillary, and in the face with the mental branch of the inferior alveolar artery, the transverse facial branch of the superficial temporal artery, the infraorbital branch of the maxillary and the dorsal nasal branch of the ophthalmic artery. The territory vascularized by the facial artery is in hemodynamic equilibrium with the adjacent arteries that may be part of the facial territory (Figs. 2.9, 2.10, 2.12, 2.13).

Branches

Cervical Branches (Figs 2.11, 2.14)
Ascending palatine artery (arises close to the origin of the facial. Runs upwards at the side of the pharynx, in the pillar). Divides in two branches: 1) to the muscle levator veli palatine and soft palate (Fig. 2.15), where it anastomoses with a branch of the descending palatine artery; 2) the other branch penetrates the superior constrictor and supplies the tonsils and the auditory tube. (Anastomoses with the tonsillar, accessory meningeal and ascending pharyngeal artery and with its counterpart on the other side). The ascending palatine artery or artery of the soft palate may arise directly from the external carotid artery (Fig. 2.14), from the ascending pharyngeal artery (Fig. 2.15) or from the accessory meningeal artery.
Tonsillar artery (supplies the tonsil and root of the tongue)
Glandular branches (three or four branches supplying the submandibular salivary gland, lymph nodes and neighboring muscles and skin) (Fig. 2.11).
Submental artery (largest cervical branch. Supplies the musculocutaneous region of the mandible and chin, and anastomoses with the sublingual branch of the lingual artery and mylohyoid of the inferior alveolar artery. Divides in superficial and deep branches) (Figs. 2.9, 2.10). The submental artery replaces sometimes the entire facial trunk, when it is hypoplastic.

Facial Branches (Figs. 2.9—2.13)

Inferior labial artery (arises at the angle of the mouth. Runs near the edge of the lower lip between the muscle and mucous membrane. Anastomose with the contralateral artery and the mental branch of the submental artery).

Superior labial artery (courses along the edge of the upper lip, between the muscle and mucous membrane). Anastomoses with the contralateral artery. Gives off a septal branch to the lower and frontal part of the nasal septum, and an alar branch to the ala of the nose.

Lateral nasal branch (also called the angular artery; ascends along the side of the nose. Supplies the alar artery and the nasal arcade at the dorsum of the nose, anastomosing with the contralateral artery, the septal and alar branches of the superior labial artery, and with the dorsal nasal ramus of the ophthalmic artery and the infraorbital branch of the maxillary artery).

Inferior masseteric artery (arises from the facial artery after it has passed under the mandible. It anastomoses with the middle and superior masseteric arteries).

Jugal trunk. It includes two different functional units.

1. The bucomasseteric system or buccal branch. It anastomoses with the facial artery and with the maxillary artery in the upper part of the pterygopalatine fossa. It supplies the deep muscle-mucosal structures and constitutes the preferential collateral pathway between both systems.

2. The posterior jugal artery, which pursues a superficial course connecting the lower border of the mandible with the external orifice of the infraorbital canal, where it anastomoses with the infraorbital artery, the superior alveolar artery and the anterior and middle jugal branches.

Middle mental artery (arises midway up the lateral surface of the body of the mandible).

Anterior jugal artery (supplies the anterior part of the jugal area and anastomoses with the posterior and middle jugal arteries).

Internal Maxillary Artery (Fig. 2.7)

It is the larger terminal branch of the external carotid artery, arises behind the neck of the mandible and it is proximately embedded in the parotid gland, subsequently passes close to the lower head of the lateral pterygoid muscle and distally enters to the deep of the pterygopalatine fossa between the two heads of that muscle. It may be divide into three segments: mandibular, pterygoid, and pterygopalatine.

Mandibular Segment (Behind the neck of the mandible)

Branches of the Mandibular Segment

Deep auricular artery (small, may be a branch of the anterior tympanic artery. Supplies the outer aspect of the tympanic membrane and temporomandibular joint)

Anterior tympanic artery (supplies the medial aspect of the tympanic membrane. Anastomose with the posterior tympanic branch of the stylomastoid artery)

Middle meningeal artery (the largest meningeal artery) (Figs. 2.16, 2.17, 2.18). Enters the cranial cavity through the foramen spinosum of the sphenoid bone. Runs forward and laterally in a temporal bone groove. Vascularizes large areas of the supratentorial meninges and anastomoses with other meningeal branches and with the ophthalmic artery. It may give origin to the ophthalmic artery or to its glandular and muscular branches (meningolacrimal artery) (Fig. 2.19).

Frontal branch (anterior)

Parieto-occipital branch (posterior)

Petrosquamosal trunk

Accessory meningeal artery (Fig. 2.18) (May be a branch of the maxillary artery (Fig. 2.19) or the middle meningeal artery (Fig. 2.16). Enters the cranium through the foramen ovale. It has an extracranial branch that goes to the cavum at the pharyngotympanic tube level and another intracranial branch anastomosing with branches of the internal carotid, ophthalmic artery, and middle meningeal artery)

Inferior alveolar (dental) artery (Figs 2.12, 2.16). (Arises from the proximal portion of the internal maxillary artery and follows a descending direction. It enters the mandibular canal at the internal surface of the mandible together with the nerve and inferior alveolar vein. Anastomoses with the submental artery, branch of the facial artery; originates the mylohyoid branch)

Pterygoid Segment (Superficial or Deep to the Lateral Pterygoid Muscle in the Temporal Fossa)

Branches of the Pterygoid Segment

Deep temporal branches (Figs. 2.16, 2.20) (anterior, middle and posterior. They supply the temporal muscle. These vessels distinguish themselves by the straight of their course and by the fact that their course is not altered at the base of the skull. The anterior branch anastomoses with the lachrymal artery, through the zygomatic bone and sphenoid bone)

Pterygoid branches (supply the pterygoid muscle)

Masseteric arteries (Figs. 2.16, 2.12) (supply the masseter a muscle of mastication. This muscle is supplied by four groups of vessels: superior, middle, inferior, and deep masseteric arteries)

Buccal artery (Fig. 2.16) (runs along the buccal nerve, to the buccinator muscle and anastomoses with branches of the facial and infraorbital arteries. This branch constitutes the most important connection between the maxillary and facial systems. It arises from the distal part of the maxillary artery and descends vertically posterior to the maxillary tuberosity)

Pterygopalatine Segment

This segment enters the pterygopalatine fossa and terminates by dividing into several branches denominated accordingly to the direction they exit from the fossa.

Branches of the pterygopalatine segment (Figs. 2.12, 2.16)

Superior alveolar (dental) artery (Originates as the maxillary artery enters the pterygopalatine fossa. Gives several branches, some to the alveolar canals, and others to the alveolar process to supply the gums)

Infraorbital artery (Fig. 2.16). (This artery is the most anterior branch of the maxillary artery. It defines the superior boundary of the maxillary sinus and corresponds to the most inferior part of the orbit. It enters the inferior orbital fissure and emerges with the infraorbital nerve on the face through the infraorbital foramen. On the face, there are anastomoses with terminal branches of the facial artery, dorsal nasal branch of the ophthalmic artery, transverse facial and buccal arteries)

Greater palatine artery (Fig. 2.16) (runs through the greater palatine canal and gives off two or three lesser palatine arteries to the soft palate and tonsil. Anastomoses with the ascending palatine artery and branches of the sphenopalatine artery)

Pharyngeal branch (It is very small and distributes to the mucosa of the nose, pharynx, sphenoidal air sinus and auditory tube)

Artery of the pterygoid canal (a branch of the greater palatine artery. Feeder of the upper pharynx, the auditory tube, and tympanic cavity)

Sphenopalatine artery (Fig. 2.16) (the real terminal part of the maxillary artery. Passes into the nose at the posterior part of the superior meatus. The branches are the posterior lateral nasal branches, with anastomoses with the ethmoidal arteries and the nasal branches of the greater palatine artery. The sphenopalatine artery ends on the nasal septum as the posterior septal branches and anastomoses with the ethmoidal arteries, the terminal ascending branch of the greater palatine artery and the septal branch of the superior labial artery)

Ascending Pharyngeal Artery (Figs. 2.15, 2.21, 2.22)

This artery arises close to the origin of the external carotid and ascends vertically in between the internal carotid and the side of the pharynx, to the base of the skull. It has two divisions, one is anterior and the other posterior, also called neuro-meningea.

The anterior division gives origin to pharyngeal branches (superior, middle, inferior) (Fig. 2.15) and to the inferior tympanic artery (Fig. 2.21), which may be a single independent branch. The posterior division gives origin, distally, to a jugular branch (enters the jugular foramen and feeds the IX, X, and XI nerves) and a branch called hypoglossal nerve branch (enters the hypoglossal canal and feeds the hypoglossal nerve, reaching the meninges of the posterior fossa) (Fig. 2.15). The hypoglossal branch may give origin to the odontoid arcade, which vascularize the meninges close to the odontoid process.

The two branches of the posterior division anastomose with the clival branches (Fig. 2.18) of the meningohypophyseal trunk from the internal carotid artery (Fig. 2.22). Another branch of the posterior division is the musculospinal artery, oriented downwards and posteriorly, supplying the XI nerve and the superior sympathetic ganglion. The ascending pharyngeal artery may arise from the external carotid artery, from a common trunk with the occipital artery (Fig. 2.23) or from the internal carotid artery (Fig. 2.24). It has anastomoses with the vertebral artery at the 2nd and 3rd cervical levels (Figs. 2.15, 2.22) and with the internal carotid artery (Fig. 2.21).

Occipital Artery (Figs. 2.23, 2.25)

The occipital artery is a posterior branch of the external carotid artery (Fig. 2.3). It arises at the level of the facial artery in the opposite direction. The artery runs backwards and upwards crossing the internal carotid artery, the internal jugular vein, and the hypoglossal, vagus, and accessory nerves. The distal artery reaches the space between the transverse process of the atlas and mastoid process of the temporal bone. It then runs in the occipital groove on the temporal bone, where it is medial to the mastoid process and attachment of the sternocleidomastoid and other muscles. Distally it turns upwards and divides in several smaller branches.

Branches

Sternocleidomastoid branches (lower and upper branches, supply the muscle)

Mastoid branch (usually small and sometimes absent; enters through the mastoid foramen to feed the mastoid air cells and dura mater at the level of the cerebellopontine angle. Anastomoses with the middle meningeal artery)

Auricular branch (supplies the back of the auricle and anastomoses with the posterior auricular artery)

Muscular branches. There are several unnamed muscular branches, the most important of them follows a pattern determined by the intervertebral spaces. For each posterior space, a parasagittal branch gives rise to a posterior anastomotic radicular branch and a lateral branch. There are anastomoses with the vertebral artery in the first three cervical intervertebral spaces (Fig. 2.25).

Meningeal branches. Two branches supply the meninges of the posterior cranial fossa: 1) the artery of the falx cerebelli (Fig. 2.23). This artery arises from the anastomoses in the first cervical space; 2) mastoid branch.

Posterior Auricular Artery

This is a small artery, that arises directly from the posterior aspect of the external carotid artery (Fig. 2.3). It supplies muscles, the parotid gland, and has three main branches. It has a hemodynamic equilibrium with the occipital and temporal superficial arteries (Fig. 2.20)

Branches

Stylomastoid artery (Fig. 2.27). Enters the stylomastoid foramen, supplies the tympanic cavity, the mastoid antrum, the mastoid air cells, and the semicircular canals. In youngsters, the posterior tympanic artery forms a vascular circle surrounding the tympanic membrane.

Auricular branch (supplies the auricularis posterior)

Occipital branch (anastomoses with the occipital artery)

Superficial Temporal Artery (Fig. 2.5)

This is one of the terminal branches of the external carotid artery. It arises close to the parotid gland, behind the neck of the mandible and has an anterior and a posterior branches (Fig. 2.20). Supplies the parotid gland, the temporomandibular joint, the masseter, the auricula, and the skin and scalp.

Branches

Transverse facial artery (Fig. 2.27). Arises from the parent artery inside the parotid gland. It divides into numerous branches to the parotid gland and duct, the masseter and the skin. Anastomoses with the facial, masseteric, buccal, lachrymal and infraorbital arteries.

Anterior auricular branch (supplies the lobule, the anterior part of the auricle and the external acoustic meatus)

Zygomatico-orbital artery (occasionally it is a branch of the middle temporal artery. Supplies the orbicular muscles and anastomoses with branches of the ophthalmic artery, lachrymal and palpebral arteries)

Middle temporal artery (anastomoses with the deep temporal branches of the maxillary artery)

Frontal (anterior) branch (runs upwards and forwards over the frontal bone. It is tortuous. Anastomoses with the contralateral artery)

Parietal (posterior) branch (runs upwards and backwards on the side of the head. Anastomoses with the posterior auricular and occipital arteries)

INTERNAL CAROTID ARTERY

The internal carotid artery originates from the bifurcation of the common carotid artery, in general at the level of the fourth cervical vertebra, or the superior border of the thyroid cartilage, in adults. It usually lies posterior and lateral to the external carotid artery (Figs. 2.1, 2.2). It may, however, have a course anterior and medial to the external carotid artery. In about half of the cases, the internal carotid artery presents a fusiform dilatation near the origin, called carotid sinus. Beyond the carotid sinus the caliber of the internal carotid artery is uniform (Fig. 2.26).

The internal carotid artery has three main segments: cervical, petrous and intracranial segments.

Cervical Segment

At the cervical segment, the internal carotid artery is almost vertical, from the origin to the carotid canal at the base of the skull. It is closely connected to the jugular vein and to the vagus nerve, which lies behind and in between these two vessels, forming a neurovascular bundle. It has two parts, one lower part localized at the sternocleidomastoid region and an upper part localized at the retrostyloid region. Elongation, loops, and tortuosity are common in older patients and are accentuated by flexion of the neck and straightened by extension of the neck.

Petrous Segment

There is a vertical and a horizontal portion of the petrous segment. The vertical portion passes inside the petrous bone for about 1 cm and then turns anteriorly and medially. The horizontal portion passes forward and medially within the petrous bone to emerge near the apex of the bone.

Intracranial Segment

The intracranial portion of the internal carotid artery may be divided in three segments, the precavernous segment, the cavernous segment, and the supraclinoid segments.

The precavernous segment courses upward, forward, and medially from the apex of the petrous temporal bone to the point where it is related to the lower and posterior aspect of the sella turcica, before entering the cavernous sinus. It is also called ganglionar segment because it is in contact with the gasser ganglion, located laterally to the internal carotid.

The cavernous segment lies within the cavernous sinus and ascends a short distance lateral to the lower and posterior, aspects of the sella. At the carotid sulcus, it passes anteriorly on the lower and lateral aspects of the sella, and then curves upward, medial to the anterior clinoid process. Within the cavernous sinus the sixth (VI) nerve lies on the lateral aspect of the artery. The third (III), the fourth (IV), the ophthalmic (V) and the maxillary nerves are closely related to the lateral wall of the cavernous sinus.

The supraclinoid segment courses upward, after crossing the dura, medial to the anterior clinoid process, posteriorly, and laterally to its point of bifurcation. The optic nerve lies medial to the lower part of this segment (Fig. 2.27).

Branches

> *Mandibular artery*
> *Caroticotympanic branch*
> *Meningohypophyseal trunk*
> > Basal tentorial branch
> > Inferior hypophyseal artery
> > Clivus branches
> *Inferolateral trunk*
> > Marginal tentorial branch
> > Branches to the Gasserian ganglion, IV, V and VI nerves and wall of cavernous sinus.
> > Branches to the orbit
> > Superior hypophyseal branches
> > Ophthalmic artery
> > Posterior communicating artery
> > Anterior choroidal artery
> > Anterior cerebral artery (terminal branch of internal carotid artery)
> > Middle cerebral artery (terminal branch of internal carotid artery)

Mandibular Artery

It arises from the petrous segment either in the foramen lacerum or in the horizontal portion at the carotid canal.

Caroticotympanic Branch

Arises from the posterior distal vertical petrous segment of the internal carotid artery. This small branch penetrates the tympanic cavity and anastomoses with the inferior tympanic branch of the ascending pharyngeal artery (Fig. 2.21), anterior tympanic branch of the maxillary artery, and stylomastoid artery.

Meningohypophyseal Trunk (Figs 2.27, 2.28, 2.29)

The branches of the meningohypophyseal trunk arise from the posterior aspect of the internal carotid artery. The tentorial branch, inferior hypophyseal artery, and clival branches arise from the dorsal main stem.

Branches

Basal tentorial branch (Fig. 2.28). Enters the tentorium anterior to the apex of the petrous bone and continues in the tentorium near the tentorium attachment to the petrous bone (tentorial basal),

supplying the adjacent tentorium, or at the free edge of the tentorium (Marginal of Tentorium).

Clivus branches (Fig. 2.27). Supply the dura of the dorsum sellae and clivus. Anastomose with the contralateral corresponding arteries.

Inferior hypophyseal artery (Figs. 2.27—2.29). Supplies the posterior lobe of the gland.

Inferolateral Trunk (Fig. 2.27)

The inferolateral trunk arises more anteriorly from the lateral and inferior aspects of the internal carotid artery. It passes downward and laterally over the lateral aspect of the sixth nerve and further downward through, lateral or under the fifth nerve. It also gives branches to the gasserian ganglion, the fourth, fifth, and sixth nerves and the wall of the cavernous sinus. The main vessel supplies the dura in the floor of the middle fossa and anastomoses with branches of the middle meningeal artery and accessory meningeal artery, while other small branches go anteriorly and through the superior orbital fissure or directly through the greater wing of the sphenoid to the orbit, where they anastomose with branches of the Ophthalmic Artery.

Superior Hypophyseal Branches

These are branches of the internal carotid artery at the level of the supraclinoid segment or Posterior Communicating Artery. They supply the pituitary stalk and the anterior lobe of the pituitary gland.

Ophthalmic Artery

The ophthalmic artery (Fig. 2.13) arises immediately above the superior limit of the cavernous sinus. It is the first major branch of the internal carotid artery. In 83% of the cases the origin of the ophthalmic artery is in the subdural space at the level where the internal carotid artery exits the cavernous sinus, penetrating the dura (Fig. 2.2). In 6.5% it may be slightly distal to this site by 1 mm or so. In 7.5% of the cases it may be extradural, arising from the intracavernous portion of the internal carotid artery (Fig. 2.29). In 2% of the cases it arises from the internal carotid artery, at the level it penetrates the dura.

Other Origins and Anastomoses of the Ophthalmic Artery

The anomalous origins of the ophthalmic artery depend on the embryological development established by this artery with the adjacent vessels, throughout the fetal life. One of the several possible embryonic arrangements becomes prominent and replaces the blood flow to the ophthalmic artery bed. The collateral blood supply to the orbit is adequate to prevent permanent blindness after occlusion of the internal carotid and ophthalmic artery in about 90% of the cases.

Functionally and embryologically there are 2 groups of ophthalmic arteries. One that supplies the optic nerve and the eye, originary from the anterior cerebral artery and internal carotid artery (dorsal ophthalmic artery). The other group supplies the other orbital structures, such as muscles, eye lids, lachrymal gland, meninges, and is originated from the stapedial system, also given origin to the middle meningeal artery and internal maxillary artery (ventral ophthalmic artery). From this alternate embryological development two anatomic arrangements may develop and one or two groups of ophthalmic branches may originate in different places.

From the Middle Meningeal Artery (Fig. 2.19). This is the most common anomalous origin of the Ophthalmic Artery, in about 1% of the cases. Due to embryological regression of the dorsal ophthalmic artery, part or all the ophthalmic artery originates from the middle meningeal artery.

From the Intracavernous Segment of Internal Carotid Artery (Fig. 2.29). Anomalous development of anastomosis between the ophthalmic artery and the internal carotid artery through the superior orbital fissure. Due to regression of the meningolachrymal segment and dorsal ophthalmic artery.

From Ascending Pharyngeal Artery. Is called the Pharyngo-meningo-lachrymal artery.

Course of the Ophthalmic Artery (Fig. 2.13)
    Intracranial Course
    Intracanalicular Course
    Intraorbital Course

Intracranial and Intracanalicular Course: May be subdivided in 5 different parts
    1. Short Limb
    2. Angle A (90 to 135º)
    3. Long Limb
    4. Angle B (90 to 210º)
    5. Distal Part (up to the apex of the orbit)

Intraorbital Course. Runs inferolaterally to the optic nerve until it crosses over or under the optic nerve to proceed medially. It may be subdivided in 3 parts (Fig. 2.18).
    1. *First Part.* The angle (120º to 135º) (between the 1st and 2nd part)
    2. *Second Part* (crosses over (82.6%) or under (17.4%) the optic nerve). The bend (between the 2nd and 3rd part)
    3. *Third Part.* Medial to the optic nerve

Terminal Segment of the Ophthalmic Artery

The ophthalmic artery terminates at the superomedial angle of the orbital opening.

Branches of the Ophthalmic Artery

There are three groups of branches from the Ophthalmic Artery.

Ocular Group
Central retinal artery
Anterior ciliary (medial and lateral posterior ciliary and anterior ciliary arteries)
Choroid plexus of the eyeball (supplied by the Ciliary Arteries)

Orbital Group
Lachrymal Artery
Muscular Arteries
Orbital Periosteum and Areolar tissue Arteries

Extraorbital Group
Posterior Ethmoidal Artery
Anterior Ethmoidal Artery
Supraorbital Artery
Medial Palpebral Artery
Dorsal Nasal Artery (Terminal Branches)
Supratrochlear Artery (Terminal Branches)

Posterior Communicating Artery

In humans a large posterior communicating artery joins the posterior cerebral artery to the internal carotid artery, representing an embryological caudal division of the carotid system. Late in the fetal life the posterior communicating artery involutes and the posterior cerebral artery shifts the dependence from the carotid to the basilar system. The posterior communicating artery runs backwards from the internal carotid artery (Fig. 2.30) above the oculomotor nerve and anastomoses with the posterior cerebral artery (Fig. 2.1). The caliber of the posterior communicating artery varies indirectly with the increased dependence of the ipsilateral posterior cerebral artery on the basilar artery (Fig. 2.31). It is frequently larger on one side than on the other. The posterior half of the posterior communicating artery gives off several small central branches that perforate the posterior perforated substance and supply the medial surface of the thalamus and the walls of the third ventricle. A slight dilatation of the junction of the posterior communicating artery and the internal carotid artery may occur, if it is less than 3 mm in size and it is referred as infundibulum, if it is larger it is considered an aneurysm. The posterior communicating artery and the carotid arteries makes the posterior portion of the circle of Willis.

Anterior Choroidal Artery

The anterior choroidal artery usually originates from the posterior aspect of the internal carotid artery 2 to 4 mm above the origin of the posterior communicating artery and about 5 mm before the internal carotid bifurcation (Figs. 2.22 and 2.30). It may, however, arise from the posterior communicating artery, from the middle cerebral trunk or before the posterior communicating artery (Fig. 2.32). This artery courses posteroinferiorly and medially immediately below the optic tract. It then passes posteriorly and laterally and crosses the optic tract from the medial to the lateral side. This portion of the vessel is within the crural cistern near the medial and posterior surface of the uncus. Continues laterally across the wing of the ambient cistern to enter the choroidal fissure and joins the choroidal plexus within the supracornual cleft at or just posterior to the knee of the temporal bone (Fig. 2.33).

Two segments are recognized: the cisternal segment and the plexal segment.

The cisternal segment has three to ten branches. The proximal branches are small perforating vessels that supply the posterior two thirds of the optic tract, perforating substance and globus pallidus and genu of the internal capsule (Fig. 2.37). Lateral and inferiorly directed branches supply part of the piriform cortex and uncus of the temporal lobe (Fig. 2.32). Medially directed branches enter the midbrain to supply part of the middle third of the cerebral peduncle which contains the corticospinal fibers. A distal group of branches supplies the inferior half of the posterior limb of the internal capsule, retrolenticular fibers of the internal capsule and the hilum of the lateral geniculate body. These distal branches anastomose with tributaries from the lateral choroidal branch of the posterior cerebral artery.

The plexal segment begins where this vessel enters the supracornual recess of the temporal horn, and supply the plexus only in the temporal horn, but may occasionally supply the entire plexus in the temporal horn and atrium (Fig. 2.40). The size and extension of distribution is in equilibrium with the posterior choroidal branches of the homolateral posterior cerebral artery. A few branches of the posterior choroidal artery may arise from the anterior choroidal artery which will be bigger (Fig. 2.34). Branches of the posterior cerebral artery may arise from the anterior choroidal artery and feed that territory (Figs. 2.34, 2.35)

Anterior Cerebral Artery

The anterior cerebral artery complex is composed of the anterior cerebral artery, the anterior communicating artery, the pericallosal artery and its orbital, frontopolar, and callosomarginal branches. The horizontal portion of the anterior cerebral artery arises anteriorly as the smaller of the two terminal branches of the internal carotid artery (Fig. 2.36). It courses anteriorly and medially to the interhemispheric fissure, passing over the optic nerve and chiasm and below the medial olfactory stria with a slightly posterior convex curve. In the interhemispheric fissure it is joined by the opposite anterior cerebral artery through the anterior communicating artery (Figs. 2.1 and 2.2). The anterior cerebral artery may be hypoplastic and in that case the contralateral anterior cerebral artery supplies both pericallosal arteries through the anterior communicating artery. The horizontal segment or segment A1 may be duplicated by a fenestration of the artery.

The anterior cerebral artery gives origin to two groups of small arteries: an inferior and a superior. The small inferior group of branches supplies the superior surface of the optic nerve and chiasm and the Superior group is formed by the medial striate arteries, including the artery of Heubner. There are 5 to 10 small arteries that supply the anterior hypothalamus, the septum pellucidum, the medial portion of the anterior commissure, the pillars of the fornix and the anterior inferior part of the striatum. The recurrent artery of Heubner (Fig. 2.36) originates from the horizontal segment of the anterior cerebral artery, or from the initial portion of the segment A2, close to the anterior communicating artery. It has a parallel course to the horizontal segment in anterior perforated substance, feeding a variable extension of the base nuclei. When fully developed, it may reach the territory of the middle cerebral artery receiving a few branches from the middle cerebral artery, being therefore known as the accessory middle cerebral artery.

Anterior Communicating Artery (Fig. 2.1)

The anterior communicating artery is very short (1 to 2 mm in length) and communicates both anterior cerebral arteries in the interhemispheric fissure (Fig. 2.36). It completes the anterior portion of the Circle of Willis. The anterior communicating artery is usually single but may be duplicated or triplicated. It may be found hypoplastic or very wide simulating an aneurysm.

Several small branches may arise from the anterior communicating artery, to the infundibulum, chiasm, and preoptic areas of the hypothalamus. Occasionally, the anterior middle cerebral artery or median artery of the corpus callosum may be encountered.

Pericallosal Artery

It is the portion of the major anterior cerebral artery complex distal to the anterior communicating artery. It ascends in front of the lamina terminalis, between the two hemispheres along the longitudinal fissure, making a curve around the genu of the corpus callosum in the pericallosal cistern (Figs. 2.2, 2.36 and 2.37).

Segments

Infracallosal Segment. Ascends in front of the lamina terminalis to the level of the genu of the corpus callosum.

Precallosal Segment. Curved portion of the artery around the genu of the corpus callosum.

Supracallosal Segment. Lies in the pericallosal cistern and passes backward toward the splenium generally following the upper surface of the corpus callosum.

The posterior length of the pericallosal artery depends on the size of the callosomarginal artery and the posterior pericallosal branch of the posterior cerebral artery. Sometimes the posterior pericallosal branch may be the terminal portion of the pericallosal artery and, therefore, not originate from the posterior cerebral artery. Several large cortical branches arise from the convexity of the pericallosal artery to supply the white matter of the medial part of the orbital gyri, the gyrus rectus, the olfactory bulb and tract, the medial surface, and a strip of the lateral surface of the frontal and parietal lobes. Multiple small branches arising from the concavity of the pericallosal artery are found, to supply the corpus callosum, septum pellucidum and columns of the fornix (Fig. 2.2). The distribution pattern of the anterior cerebral artery is variable and sometimes it is not possible to identify precisely one isolated artery from its origin, but from the topography of distribution.

Branches of the Pericallosal Artery (Fig. 2.37)

Orbital Artery (Frontobasilar Artery). First branch of the pericallosal artery. Usually arises from the infracallosal segment of the pericallosal artery or from a common trunk that also gives rise to the frontopolar artery. The forward course of the Orbital artery lies in the medial or inferior surface of the frontal lobe, and supplies the medial basal region of the frontal lobe, including the gyrus rectus, the medial part of the medial gyri and the olfactory bulb and tract

Frontopolar Artery. Usually the second branch of the pericallosal artery, arising from the infracallosal segment. It may arise as a common trunk with the frontobasilar artery or from the callosomarginal artery. This artery passes in an anterior direction along the medial surface of the brain hemisphere describing a gentle curve in direction of the frontal pole to supply the anterior portion of the medial and lateral surfaces of the superior frontal gyrus.

Callosomarginal Artery. It may be a single vessel or a group of several ascending vessels arising from the pericallosal artery. This artery runs over the cingulate gyrus at the cingulate sulcus. When this branch is a single trunk it follows a course roughly parallel to that of the pericallosal artery. The branches of the callosomarginal artery ascend on the medial surface of the hemisphere and continue to the lateral convexity for about 2 cm, supplying premotor, motor and sensory areas.

Branches

Anterior Internal Frontal Artery
Middle Internal Frontal Artery
Posterior Internal Frontal Artery
Paracentral Artery

Cortical Branches of the Anterior Cerebral Artery

Eight territories of vascular supply are identified, regarding the cortical branches of the anterior cerebral artery (Fig. 2.2).

Orbitofrontal (OF)
Frontopolar (FPol)
Anterior internal frontal (AIF)
Middle internal frontal (MIF)
Posterior internal frontal (PIF)
Paracentral (PC)
Superior internal parietal (SIP)
Inferior internal parietal (IIP)

The distribution of the cortical branches of the anterior cerebral artery is related to the anatomy of the medial surface of the cerebral hemisphere. The medial surface supplied by the Anterior Cerebral Artery is compartmentalized by several named sulci or fissures.

The sulci and fissures are subfrontal sulcus (frontopolar artery); cingulate sulcus (callosomarginal artery); marginal limb of the cingulate sulcus (paracentral artery and/or SIP artery); paracentral sulcus (posterior internal frontal artery); central sulcus (paracentral artery branch); subparietal sulci; and parieto-occipital fissure.

The subfrontal sulcus is constant and located at the inferior limit of the superior frontal gyrus. The gyrus rectus lies beneath the subfrontal sulcus. Superior to the subfrontal sulcus is the large superior frontal gyrus, which is subdivided by many inconstant and unnamed sulci. The paracentral sulcus marks the posterior limit of the superior frontal gyrus and the limit between it and the paracentral lobule. The paracentral lobule is variable in size and is divided from above by the central sulcus, which extends from the lateral surface of the hemisphere. The marginal limit of the cingulate sulcus separates the paracentral lobule from the precuneus, or quadrilateral lobe, which is bounded inferiorly by the subparietal sulcus and posteriorly by the parieto-occipital fissure.

The cortical arteries arise from either the pericallosal artery or a marginal trunk of the pericallosal artery. The size of the pericallosal artery varies inversely with that of the callosomarginal trunk. The cortical arteries are named according to their territories of supply.

Orbitofrontal Artery (OF) (Fig. 2.33)

This is the first cortical branch of the anterior cerebral artery. Arises independently from the pericallosal artery, in the majority of the cases. It may share a common origin with the frontopolar artery or is a branch of a callosomarginal trunk together with two or more other cortical branches. The OF artery supplies the gyrus rectus and the medial half of the inferior surface of the frontal lobe. There are anastomoses with the orbitofrontal branch of the middle cerebral artery in the area of the H-shaped sulcus. In lateral views of angiograms this branch projects at the level or underneath the level of the ophthalmic artery.

Frontopolar Artery (FPol)

Arises from the pericallosal artery or callosomarginal trunk in opposition to the knee of the corpus callosum and runs anteriorly in and along the subfrontal sulcus. The origin may be in common with the OF artery as well as with the anterior and middle internal frontal arteries is less than half of the cases. A single artery is the rule, with two major branches. It supplies the inferior portion of the superior frontal gyrus.

Anterior Internal Frontal Artery (AIF)

Arises directly from the pericallosal artery in 40% of the cases. May share a common origin with any other cortical branch, except the internal parietal artery. May have a common origin with the FPol and middle internal frontal arteries. In three fourths of the cerebral hemisphere presents as a single artery dividing in two or more branches. Supplies the anterior third of the internal surface of the superior frontal gyrus.

Middle Internal Frontal Artery (MIF)

Originates, most commonly from the pericallosal artery. Less frequently arises from the callosomarginal trunk, in combination with the other internal frontal arteries. Supplies the middle third of the internal surface of the superior frontal gyrus.

Posterior Internal Frontal Artery (PIF)

It is a branch of the calloso marginal trunk in more than 50% of the cases, most often in combination with the MIF and paracentral arteries. In the remaining cases it is a branch of the pericallosal artery. Before leaving the medial surface of the hemisphere the PIF artery gives off a branch that lies in the paracentral sulcus. Supplies the posterior third of the medial aspect of the superior frontal gyrus.

Paracentral Artery (PC)

May be small in caliber but is always present. In about 50% of the cases it arises from the pericallosal artery. May originate from a common trunk with the PIF, the superior internal parietal artery or both. Courses in the marginal limb of the cingulate sulcus but may occasionally run in the paracentral sulcus. Supplies the paracentral lobule and sends a branch from the medial surface of the brain in the central sulcus.

Superior Internal Parietal Artery (SIP)

This is usually the largest cortical branch of the anterior cerebral artery. Arises directly from the pericallosal artery in about 75% of the cases. In the remaining 25% of the cases shares the origin with the posterior internal frontal, paracentral or inferior internal parietal arteries. Runs in the marginal limb of the cingulate sulcus. Supplies the upper two thirds of the precuneus. This territory extends posteriorly to include approximately 80% of the precuneus, where the artery anastomoses with the parieto-occipital branches of the posterior cerebral artery.

Inferior Internal Parietal Artery (IIP)

This is the last cortical branch of the anterior cerebral artery and arises at the point before the pericallosal artery courses around the splenium of the corpus callosum. May be multiple and supplies the inferior third of the precuneus and extends posteriorly as far as the SIP artery.

Middle Cerebral Artery (Figs. 2.1 and 2.38)

The middle cerebral artery originates from the division of the internal carotid artery. The middle cerebral artery is about 20% larger than the anterior cerebral artery (Fig. 2.27) and is located below the medial part of the anterior perforated substance at the medial end of the lateral cerebral fissure. An accessory middle cerebral artery may be found in about 3% of the cases, below the bifurcation of the internal carotid artery. More rarely the accessory middle cerebral artery may originate from the anterior cerebral artery and its embryologic origin is likely to be related to the artery of Heubner. The anterior choroidal artery may rarely arise from the middle cerebral artery.

The middle cerebral artery has been divided in three segments: horizontal, sylvian, and cortical. The horizontal segment (Fig. 2.1) supplies the basal ganglia, the orbital surface of the frontal lobe, and the temporal pole. The sylvian segment supplies the insula. The cortical branches supply the lateral convexities of the cerebrum.

Horizontal Segment of the Middle Cerebral Artery

The horizontal segment or segment M1 of the middle cerebral artery begins at the internal carotid bifurcation, runs laterally in the lateral cerebral fissure, and terminates entering the Sylvian fissure. The horizontal segment is not always horizontal and may course downwards or upwards before entering the Sylvian fissure. The junction between the end of the horizontal segment and the beginning of the insular segment is known as the "knee" of the middle cerebral artery. The horizontal segment of the middle cerebral artery bifurcates or trifurcates near the island of Reil (Fig. 2.27) in most patients. Earlier division, however, is not uncommon (Fig. 2.36).

The segment M1 presents three main groups of branches.

Lenticulostriate branches (Figs. 2.27 and 2.33)
Orbitofrontal branch
Anterior temporal arteries

Lenticulostriate Branches (Fig. 2.39)

These six to twelve branches usually arise from the posterosuperior aspect of the horizontal segment of the middle cerebral artery, entering the anterior perforated substance. They may be divided in a lateral and a medial group arising from the proximal segments for M1 and A1. Occasionally they arise from an early branch of the middle cerebral artery. The lenticulostriate arteries supply most of the head of the caudate nucleus, most of the putamen, the lateral one third of the globus pallidus and the superior half of the anterior limb of the internal capsule. The recurrent artery of Heubner is one of the larger medial striate arteries. Rarely, the recurrent artery of Heubner may give origin to orbital branches, supplying portions of the frontal lobe.

Orbitofrontal Branch

Arises from the anterior surface of the horizontal segment of the middle cerebral artery and passes forward, upward and laterally to supply the inferior and lateral surface of the frontal lobe. The size of this artery is inversely proportional to the size of the frontopolar branch of the pericallosal artery.

Anterior Temporal Arteries

Arises from the anterior surface of the horizontal segment, opposite to the lenticulostriate arteries, and courses over the temporal lobe. It may have a common trunk with the orbitofrontal artery or the posterior temporal artery.

It usually has two branches. A small branch that passes downward and anteriorly to supply the pole and a recurrent branch that runs laterally and posteriorly in the Sylvian fissure or in the lateral aspect of the temporal lobe. The caliber of these branches is in equilibrium with the posterior temporal artery.

Sylvian Segment of the Middle Cerebral Artery

The insula is a triangular area of cerebral cortex lying in the floor of the Sylvian fissure and hidden by the operculum (Fig. 2.38), outlined by branches of the middle cerebral artery (ascending branches or ascending frontal artery complex) before they exit through the Sylvian fissure to supply the cortex over the cerebral convexity. The term ascending frontal artery complex includes the operculofrontal or candelabra group and the arteries of the central sulcus. The arteries in the insula are triangular when viewed laterally. The inferior point of the triangle is formed by the horizontal segment of the middle cerebral artery, the anterior superior point is formed by the most anterior artery in the insula as it begins to loop inferiorly to leave the Sylvian fissure, and the posterior superior point is formed by the most posterior artery as it begins to loop inferiorly to leave the insula. The posterior superior point is also called the Sylvian

point. The superior border of the triangle is drawn by connecting the arteries in the superior limiting sulcus before they loop inferiorly to leave the Sylvian fissure.

In frontal projection the insular branches of the middle cerebral artery curve gently outward until they reach the superior limiting sulcus (Fig. 2.27 and 2.33). The anterior portion of the insula is more medially located than the posterior portion.

The candelabra group may bifurcate or trifurcate symmetrically in the proximal part of its course, suggesting the form of a candelabrum. These arteries supply the Broca's area. The posterior branches always supply the premotor area and may supply accessory to the motor strip.

The arteries of the central sulcus are one or two in number, with an accessory artery to the motor strip in about 50% of the cases, from the operculofrontal branch. The arteries in the central sulcus may arise as a separate part of the ascending frontal complex or from another trunk in the Sylvian fissure. When passing through the Sylvius fissure the several branches of the middle cerebral artery feed the insula cortex.

Cortical Branches of the Middle Cerebral Artery (Figs. 2.28, 2.33, 2.40, 2.41 and 2.42)

The middle cerebral artery supplies the entire superficial lateral surface of the cerebral hemisphere in the frontal, temporal, parietal and occipital lobes. Twelve branches of the middle cerebral artery may be identified. These branches arise separately from the trunk of the middle cerebral artery or from one of the two or three principal trunks in a bifurcation or trifurcating divisional pattern.

Branches

Orbitofrontal Artery
Prefrontal Artery
Precentral Artery
Central Arteries
Anterior Parietal Artery
Posterior Parietal Artery
Angular Artery (Terminal Artery)
Temporo-occipital Artery
Posterior Temporal Artery
Middle Temporal Artery
Anterior Temporal Artery
Temporal Polar Artery

Orbitofrontal Artery

Arises directly from the horizontal segment of the middle cerebral artery or from a common trunk with the prefrontal artery. When the middle cerebral artery bifurcates or trifurcates early, the orbitofrontal artery originates from the more anterior trunk of the middle cerebral artery. Supplies the orbital aspect of the middle and inferior frontal gyri and sometimes the inferior part of the pars orbitalis of the inferior frontal gyrus.

Prefrontal Artery

Constitutes the anterior part of the operculofrontal or candelabra group. Supplies the lateral aspect of the frontal lobe anterior to the Sylvian triangle, including the pars marginalis of the inferior frontal gyrus, the pars orbitalis and pars opercularis of the inferior frontal gyrus. It may have a common origin with the orbitofrontal artery or the precentral artery. It emerges from the Sylvian fissure at the level of the pars orbitalis of the inferior frontal gyrus. In lateral angiograms it has an inclined path anterior and superior beyond the anterior portion of the Sylvius fissure. Divides in two trunks which further divides in four to six branches supplying the middle and inferior frontal gyri.

Precentral Artery

When the middle cerebral artery bifurcates, the precentral artery arises from the anterior trunk. When the middle cerebral artery trifurcates it arises from the anterior or middle trunk. The precentral and prefrontal arteries may originate from a single trunk. It emerges from the Sylvian fissure at or behind the pars opercularis of the inferior frontal gyrus and has an almost vertical course. It is the most vertical branch of the middle cerebral artery. The two major branches usually follow the course of the precentral sulcus. It supplies the pars opercularis of the inferior frontal gyrus, the posterior part of the middle frontal gyrus and the inferior two thirds of the precentral gyrus.

Central Arteries

The central arteries have variable origin, dependent of the division pattern of the middle cerebral artery. When the middle cerebral artery is a single vessel it may originate from a common trunk with the anterior parietal artery. When the middle cerebral artery bifurcates it arises from the anterior trunk. When the middle cerebral artery trifurcates it arises from the middle trunk. The central artery may be single in 66.6% of the cases and in 33.3% two arteries are encountered. Runs near the Rolandic fissure as two branches encircling the operculum. Supplies the precentral and postcentral gyri, and runs with a slight posterior superior inclined course after emerging from the fissure.

Parietal Arteries

There are two parietal arteries: the anterior and posterior. The anterior parietal artery has a variable origin. It may arise with the central artery or with the posterior parietal artery. Emerges from the posterior third of the Sylvian fissure at the base of the ascending parietal gyrus to pass upward and posterior in the postcentral sulcus. Supplies the ascending parietal gyrus, the upper portion of the central sulcus and the anterior part of the first two parietal gyri. The posterior parietal artery is the most posterior of the ascending branches of the middle cerebral artery. Varies in size and site of origin. It may originate from the anterior or posterior trunk of a bifurcated middle cerebral artery. If the middle cerebral artery trifurcates it arises from the middle trunk. It emerges from the Sylvian fissure at the level of the parietal operculum and passes backward and upward in the posterior part of the parietal lobe. Supplies the posterior part of the first and second parietal gyri and the supramarginal gyrus.

Angular Artery

It is the terminal and largest branch of the middle cerebral artery. Its origin is from the posterior trunk of the middle cerebral artery when it bifurcates, and when it trifurcates the angular artery arises from the middle or posterior trunk. Emerges at the end of the Sylvian fissure running over the superior temporal gyrus. This is the most horizontal branch of the middle cerebral artery in lateral angiograms and the most posterior branch of the Sylvian fissure in a Towne view of angiography. It supplies the posterior part of the superior temporal gyrus, the supramarginal gyrus, the angular gyrus and the first two occipital gyri.

Temporo-occipital Artery

The temporo-occipital artery may have a common origin with the angular artery and may be sometimes considered a branch of the angular artery. The size of this artery is inversely proportional to the size of the posterior temporal artery. Supplies the area posterior to and above the area usually supplied by the posterior temporal artery. It has a posterior and inferior bend after arising from the Sylvius fissure.

Posterior Temporal Artery

The posterior temporal artery arises from the posterior trunk of the middle cerebral artery, if a bifurcation or trifurcation is present. It is a single branch in most of the cases and leaves the Sylvian fissure through the posterior part, crossing the external surface of the superior temporal gyrus. Runs through the superior temporal sulcus, crossing the middle temporal gyrus and terminating opposite the preoccipital fissure. Supplies the middle and posterior part of the superior temporal gyrus, the posterior third of the middle temporal gyrus and the posterior extremity of the inferior temporal gyrus.

Middle Temporal Artery

It is frequently a small artery. Leaves the Sylvian fissure opposite or slightly behind the pars opercularis of the inferior frontal gyrus. The direction is similar to that of the posterior temporal artery. Supplies the temporal gyri anterior to the territory of supply of the posterior temporal artery.

Anterior Temporal Artery

Supplies the remainder of the anterior portion of the temporal lobe. The vessel outlines the temporal operculum. Descends posteriorly over the temporal gyri, immediately behind the temporal polar artery to terminate at the level of the middle temporal sulcus. It may originate from the segment M1.

Temporal Polar Artery

This is a relatively constant vessel that passes forward to the anterior and inferior aspects of the tip of the temporal lobe to supply the anterior portions of the superior, middle and inferior temporal gyri.

Posterior Cerebral Artery (Figs. 2.1 and 2.2)

The posterior cerebral artery generally receives the blood supply from the basilar artery. They are located above the tentorium, and originally (embryologically) derive the blood supply from the internal carotid artery. The posterior cerebral artery shifts its origin from the carotid to the basilar system in the final stages of embryonic development and the ultimate origin is from the basilar artery bifurcation at the interpeduncular fossa. But this pattern is not constant and in some cases the embryonic pattern persists. In 10.4% of the cases the fetal type (Fig. 2.32) persists on the right side, while 9.5% persists on the left side, and it is bilateral in 7.7% of the cases. In the fetal type the posterior cerebral artery originates from the internal carotid artery.

The posterior cerebral artery has a communication with the internal carotid artery through the posterior communicating artery and with the basilar artery through the communicating basilar segment or P1 (Fig. 2.31). The caliber of these arteries are inversely proportional among them, varying from agenesis (Figs. 2.43 and 2.44) to a size equal to the posterior cerebral artery. Both may have the same size and the same importance in the flow into the posterior cerebral artery.

The posterior cerebral artery courses posteriorly in the perimesencephalic cisterns to encircle the midbrain. Terminal cortical branches supply the occipital poles, the medial and inferior portions of the occipital lobes, and the medial portions of the temporal lobes. The proximal trunk of the posterior cerebral artery is divided into peduncular, ambient and quadrigeminal segments, corresponding to the cisterns through which the vessel passes (Fig. 2.45).

Peduncular Segment

This is the proximal segment of the posterior cerebral artery, which arises from the basilar artery and it is closely related to the anteromedial portion of the peduncle of the midbrain. The posterior communicating artery connects to the midportion of the peduncular segment. The proximal portion of the peduncular segment is closely related to the oculomotor nerve. The peduncular segment is usually horizontal, but when the basilar artery is short with a low bifurcation the peduncular segments are directed upwards in a V like configuration. With elongation of the basilar artery, the peduncular segments pass anteriorly and inferiorly to reach the surface of the peduncles. Asymmetry is common in more than 50% of the cases.

Ambient Segment

It is the second cisternal segment of the Posterior Cerebral Artery. It courses posteriorly in the hippocampal fissure between the midbrain and the hippocampal gyrus. It parallels the basal vein, which lies superior, and to the throclear nerve, at the free edge of the tentorium. The superior cerebellar artery is inferior to the ambient segment. The relationship of this segment with the free margin of the tentorium varies. With low origin of the posterior cerebral artery the ambient segment cross the line of the tentorial margin from below. With high origin, the ambient segment courses posteriorly in the hippocampal fissure above the tentorium.

Quadrigeminal Segment

It is the continuation of the posterior cerebral artery within the lateral aspect of the quadrigeminal cistern. At this level the quadrigeminal segments approach each other and then continue posteriorly beneath the splenium of the corpus callosum to terminate in cortical branches.

Branches (Figs. 2.45, 2.46 and 2.47)

Mesencephalic and Thalamic Branches
    Mesencephalic Branches
        Interpeduncular Perforating Branches
        Tiny Peduncular Branches
        Circumflex Mesencephalic Branches
    Thalamic Branches (Fig. 2.46 B)
        Anterior Thalamoperforating Arteries
        Posterior Thalamoperforating Arteries
            Interpeduncular Thalamoperforating Branches
        Thalamogeniculate Perforating Branches
Posterior Choroidal Branches (Figs. 2.47 and 2.34)
    Medial Posterior Choroidal Artery
    Lateral Posterior Choroidal Artery
Hippocampal Branches
Meningeal Branches
Posterior Pericallosal Artery
Cortical Branches
    Anterior Temporal Artery
    Posterior Temporal Artery
    Parieto-Occipital Artery
    Calcarine Artery

Mesencephalic and Thalamic Branches

Mesencephalic Branches

The interpeduncular perforating branches arise from the initial posterior surface of the posterior cerebral artery. There are three to six perforating branches which penetrate the rostral floor of the interpeduncular fossa through the posterior perforated substance. Supply the oculomotor and trochlear nuclei, the paramedian mesencephalic reticular formation, the pretectum, and the rostroedian floor of the IV ventricle.

The tiny peduncular branches arise from the posterior cerebral artery and penetrate the cerebral peduncle. They supply the corticospinal and corticobulbar pathways as well as the substantia nigra, red nuclei, and other structures of the tegmentum (oculomotor nerve).

The circumflex mesencephalic branches are a group of several small vessels of variable length, arising from the peduncular segment of the posterior cerebral artery that passes around the midbrain. Supply small perforating branches to the cerebral peduncle and substantia nigra, but also the posterior tegmental structures.

Thalamic Branches

The so called thalamoperforating arteries are divided into an anterior and a posterior group.

The anterior thalamoperforating arteries are a group of 7 to 10 arteries, arising from the lateral aspect of the posterior communicating artery. They supply the posterior chiasm, optic tract, posterior hypothalamus, and part of the cerebral peduncle.

The posterior thalamoperforating arteries consist of two groups of arteries.

The interpeduncular thalamoperforating branches originate from the proximal peduncular segment of the posterior cerebral artery. Penetrate the thalamus via the paramedian aspect of the posterior perforate substance.

The thalamogeniculate perforating branches arise from the ambient segment of the posterior cerebral artery. Three to six small arteries that penetrates the base of the thalamus and the geniculate bodies.

Posterior Choroidal Branches

Posterior Medial Choroidal Artery

It usually arises from the proximal segment of the posterior cerebral artery. Runs parallel to the posterior cerebral artery and is interposed between that artery and the midbrain to which gives small branches. Enters the lateral portion of the quadrigeminal cistern, supplying the quadrigeminal plate and the pineal gland. Approaches the midline and courses forward in the roof of the III ventricle adjacent to the internal cerebral vein. Multiple small branches of this artery reach the level of the foramen of Monro and supply the choroid plexus of the III ventricle. Supplies also the dorsal medial nucleus of the thalamus.

Posterior Lateral Choroidal Artery

Originates from the ambient segment of the posterior cerebral artery. Variations in origin are common. May be a single trunk in more than 50% of the cases and multiple trunks in the rest. The anterior branch supplies the anterior portion of the choroid plexus of the temporal horn of the ventricles, while the posterior branch supplies the choroid plexus of the trigone and lateral ventricle. The lateral choroidal artery also supplies the crus, comissure, body and part of the anterior columns of the fornix and thalamus. The size of this vessel is usually inversely proportional to the size of the anterior choroidal artery. There is anastomoses between branches of this artery with branches of postero-medial and anterior choroidal arteries.

Hippocampal Branches

The arteries to the hippocampus originate from the trunk of the posterior cerebral artery near the origin of the lateral choroidal arteries. They are 1 to 4 in each side.

Meningeal Branches

The meningeal branches are small and arise from the peduncular segment of the posterior cerebral artery. They course around the midbrain and supply the midline strip of the inferior surface of the tentorium opposite to the junction of the falx cerebri with the tentorium.

Posterior Pericallosal Artery (Fig. 2.46B)

Usually arises at the level of the quadrigeminal cistern from the parieto-occipital branch of the posterior cerebral artery. It may also arise from the Posterior cerebral artery or from the lateral choroidal artery or from the posterior temporal artery. It is usually a plexus of small arteries, rather than a single vessel. This artery passes around the splenium running anteriorly within the supracallosal cistern and anastomosing with the distal branches of the anterior pericallosal artery.

Cortical Branches (Figs. 2.34A and 2.46)

There are 4 main cortical branches of the posterior cerebral artery.

Anterior Temporal Artery

Arises as a single trunk or as multiple branches from the proximal ambient segment of the posterior cerebral artery. Runs lateral and anterior under the hippocampal gyrus supplying the inferior aspect of the anterior portion of the temporal lobe. There are anastomoses with the anterior temporal branches of the middle cerebral artery

Posterior Temporal Artery

Arises from the midambient segment of the posterior cerebral artery as a single trunk in 80% of the cases. May give origin to an anterior temporal branch. Courses posteriorly and laterally along the hippocampal gyrus. Several small branches originate from this artery along the inferior surface of the posterior temporal lobe and adjacent occipital lobe. The distal vessels may anastomose with branches of the calcarine artery in the posterior third of the calcarine fissure. Supplies the primary visual cortex in 22.5% of the cases.

Parieto-Occipital Artery

May arise independently from the posterior cerebral artery at the level of the ambient cistern. It may also originate with the calcarine artery from the bifurcation of the posterior cerebral trunk in the proximal third of the calcarine fissure. This artery originates from the quadrigeminal segment in 22% and more distally in 40% of the cases. It arises as single trunk in 95% of the cases. Branches include lateral posterior choroidal arteries, branches to the hippocampus, pulvinar, and medial and lateral geniculate bodies. Supplies the visual cortex as accessory in 35% of the cases. The main trunk of the parieto-occipital artery usually divides into a number of cortical branches that supply the medial portion of the parieto-occipital lobe, precuneus and deep into the parieto-occipital fissure. On the lateral view of the arteriogram the parieto-occipital branches course posteriorly and superiorly as the uppermost of the three posterior cortical branches of the posterior cerebral artery. In the frontal projection the proximal parieto-occipital artery is usually the most medial of the three posterior cortical branches as it surrounds the medial face of the parieto-occipital lobe.

Calcarine Artery

Arises at the bifurcation of the main posterior cerebral trunk in the rostral third of the calcarine sulcus. At its origin, this artery lies just lateral to the parieto-occipital branch. After this it follows a winding posterior course deep in the calcarine fissure. The origin of the calcarine artery is variable as well as the number of trunks. One in 40% and two in 60% of the cases. Supplies part of the visual cortex.

VERTEBRAL ARTERY (FIGS. 2.1 AND 2.2)

The vertebral artery, in more than 80% of the cases, originates at the upper posterior aspect of the first segment of the subclavian artery as the most proximal and largest branch of this artery (Fig. 2.48). The most common variation in origin is related to a more proximal location. On the left the vertebral artery originates from the arch between the left common carotid and left subclavian arteries in about 2.4% to 5.8% of the cases. In that case the vertebral artery enters the foramen of the transverse process of the fifth cervical vertebra, instead of the sixth cervical vertebra as usual. Other variations like origin of the left vertebral artery distal to the left subclavian artery or from the left common carotid artery or external carotid artery are extremely rare. The right vertebral artery originating from the right common carotid artery or the aortic arch is found in less than 1% of the cases. A bifid origin of the vertebral artery is also very uncommon. The size of the vertebral arteries is variable but the left dominant artery is more common.

Segments of the Vertebral Artery

The first segment of the vertebral artery extends from the origin to its point of entrance into the foramen of the transverse process (usually) of the sixth cervical vertebra (in 87.5% of the cases). It is directed upwards and posteriorly at the extravertebral segment. It is surrounded by the cervical sympathetic nerve plexus and is related anteriorly to the vertebral and jugular vein and the inferior thyroid artery. The inferior thyroid artery (Fig. 2.49) and costocervical trunk may rarely originate from the beginning of the vertebral artery.

The second segment courses cranially through the foramina of the transverse processes until it reaches the transverse process of the axis. The artery is in close contact medially with the uncinate process of the vertebral body and posteriorly with the ventral rami of the cervical nerves. In this segment it is surrounded by the vertebral venous plexus.

The third segment extends from its exit at the axis to its entrance into the spinal canal. After leaving the transverse foramen of axis, it courses laterally and posteriorly to pass through the transverse foramen of the atlas. After passing the transverse foramen of the atlas the artery runs posteromedially at the horizontal groove on the upper surface of the posterior arch of the atlas. When it approaches the midline, it turns cephalad and perforates the posterior atlanto-occipital membrane to enter the vertebral canal. At this level, the persistence of the embryonic proatlantal intersegmental artery may result in a rare but exuberant communication between the internal or external carotid arteries and the vertebral artery. The occipital artery may occasionally arise as a branch of the third segment of the vertebral artery.

The fourth segment of the vertebral artery perforates the dura and runs anteromedially through the foramen magnum. At this level the artery lies in front of the medulla oblongata and joins the contralateral vertebral artery forming the basilar artery. In 0.2% the vertebral artery fails to join the basilar artery on one side and thus terminates in the posterior inferior cerebellar artery (Fig. 2.50).

Branches

> *Muscular Branches*
> *Meningeal Branches*
> *Spinal Branches*
> *Radicular Branches*
> *Proatlantal Intersegmental Artery*
> *Posterior Inferior Cerebellar Artery*

Muscular Branches

In every cervical space the vertebral artery sends a radicular branch, following the ventral (anteriorly) and dorsal (posteriorly) nervous roots, and muscular branches creating an anastomotic network with muscular branches from the deep cervical artery, occipital artery (posteriorly), ascending cervical artery and ascending pharyngeal artery (anteriorly). The anastomoses create a longitudinal vascular axis by the connection of the three vertical axis (anteriorly created by the ascending cervical artery and ascending pharyngeal artery, in the center by the vertebral artery, and posteriorly by the deep cervical artery and occipital artery). Together with the muscular and radicular branches, some branches give origin to the adjacent meninge. Some of the radiculary branches give origin to the radiculo-medullary (anterior or posterior).

Meningeal Branches

Posterior Meningeal Branch

Arises above the level of the arch of the atlas just below the foramen magnum. Supplies the medial portion of the dura of the posterior fossa, as well as the falx cerebeli (Fig. 2.50). It may extend cephalad to supply the tentorium and the falx cerebri. It may rarely arise as a branch from the posterior inferior cerebellar artery. It may arise from the posterior division of the ascending pharyngeal artery (neuro-meningeal trunk) (Fig. 2.15) or from the occipital artery (Fig. 2.23).

Anterior Meningeal Branch

Originates from the distal part of the second segment of the vertebral artery. It runs medially and cephalad to enter the spinal canal to supply the medulla at the level of the foramen magnum.

Arterial Arch of the Odontoid (Figs. 2.15, 2.22, 2.43)

Each one of the vertebral arteries feeds the posterior meninge of the odontoid process through an arterial arch. The arterial arch of the odontoid may originate or have anastomoses with the ascending pharyngeal artery.

Spinal Branches

Anterior Spinal Artery (Fig. 2.1)

Near the junction with each other to form the basilar artery there is the origin of the a branch, from each vertebral artery, caudally and medially oriented. These branches join at the midline and generally fuse about 2 cm from the origin forming the anterior spinal artery. The anterior spinal artery extends the length of the spinal cord, in close relationship with the anterior median fissure, presenting various sizes according to the segment observed.

Postero-lateral Spinal Arteries

The posterior spinal arteries may originate from the posterior inferior cerebellar artery or from the intradural portion of the vertebral artery. They run caudally along the posterolateral aspect of the medulla and spinal cord.

Radicular Branches

Several small and posterior radicular branches enter the spinal canal via the neural foramina anastomosing with the spinal arteries. There are one to six arteries anteriorly and zero to eight posteriorly.

Proatlantal Intersegmental Artery

This is the rare embryonic primitive cervical segmental artery that persists into the adult life. When it is present the proximal segment of the vertebral artery may be atretic. It usually joins the internal or external carotid arteries to the distal vertebral artery

Posterior Inferior Cerebellar Artery (Fig. 2.50)

The posterior inferior cerebellar artery (PICA) is the largest and most distal branch of the vertebral artery. Most of the time (57%), the PICA originates above the foramen magnum, while in only 4% it is identified at the level of the foramen magnum and in 18% it was found below. It is occasionally absent (up to 20%) and the PICA territory is supplied by the anterior inferior cerebellar artery (AICA) (Fig. 2.31). Anastomoses between the two arteries are common. A single stem may take place of both the AICA and PICA (Fig. 2.44).

There are many variations in the course of the PICA and it is divided in several segments. The segmental division is intimately related to the adjacent structures that it supplies, including the medulla, the inferior portion of the fourth ventricle, the inferior vermis, the tonsils, and the inferior aspect of the cerebellar hemispheres—anterior medullary segment, lateral medullary segment, posterior medullary segment, supratonsillar segment and branches.

Anterior Medullary Segment

The PICA courses posteriorly within the medullary cistern and turns around the lower end of the olive of the medulla oblongata, adjacent to the biventral lobule. This is the anterior medullary segment. It is also called proximal cisternal segment.

Lateral Medullary Segment

The PICA continues posteriorly in the cerebellomedullary fissure around the lateral aspect of the medulla and it is called the lateral medullary segment, and correspond to the caudal loop.

Posterior Medullary Segment

When the PICA reaches the posterior margin of the medulla oblongata, it ascends behind the roots of the ninth and tenth cranial nerves to the anterior aspect of the superior pole of the tonsil behind the posterior medullary velum. It is called the posterior medullary segment. It is also known as medullary segment.

Supratonsillar Segment

The PICA continues in the posterior course over the superior pole of the tonsil as the supratonsillar segment. It is also known as cranial loop or choroid arch.

Branches

Perforating Branches

There are multiple small arterial branches that arise from the anterior, lateral, and posterior medullary segments of the PICA to supply the posterolateral aspect of the medulla. When the PICA is hypoplastic or absent these bulbar branches originate from the vertebral artery. A small branch of the PICA may extend upward lateral to the tonsil to supply the dentate nucleus of the cerebellum.

Terminal Branches

In most cases the PICA bifurcates a short distance distal to the apex of the cranial loop into two main terminal branches: the tonsillohemispheric (lateral) and the vermis (medial) branches.

Tonsillohemispheric Branches

Descend along the posterior margin of the medial aspect of the tonsil and divide into tonsillar branches, extending anteriorly, and hemispheric branches coursing downward and posterolaterally. Currently there are anastomoses between the Hemispheric branches and the AICA or superior cerebellar artery. When there are no hemispheric branches from the PICA the hemispheric branches may arise from the AICA or the superior cerebellar artery.

Vermis Branches

These branches pass at the inferior aspect of the inferior vermis in the sulcus valleculae between the inferior vermis and the cerebellar hemisphere. At this point these branches form a loop of inferior and lateral convexity. In some cases all the vermis branches arise from a single PICA.

Meningeal Branches

A posterior meningeal branch is occasionally seem arising from the PICA, instead of from the vertebral artery.

BASILAR ARTERY (FIGS. 2.1 AND 2.2)

The basilar artery is formed by the junction of the two vertebral arteries at the level of the pontomedullary sulcus. It follows an ascending course along the shallow groove in close contact with the anterior aspect of the pons. This artery is found within the prepontine cistern posteriorly to the clivus. The distal part of the artery usually bends posteriorly and divides in the two posterior cerebral arteries just after passing in between the two oculomotor nerves. Sometimes the course of the basilar artery is tortuous and deviated from the midline.

Branches

> *Pontine Branches*
> > Median Branches
> > Transverse Branches
> *Anterior Inferior Cerebellar Artery (AICA)*
> *Superior Cerebellar Artery (SCA)*
> *Pontine Branches (Fig. 2.31)*

The basilar branches to the pons and midbrain are small arteries that arise from the lateral and posterior sides of the main vessel. They may be divided in median or paramedian branches and transverse or circumferential branches.

Median Branches

Small and numerous arteries that originate from the posterior part of the basilar artery, entering the pons at the median groove. These arteries penetrate the pons deeply, reaching the floor of the fourth ventricle.

Transverse Branches

There are usually four to six pairs of these arteries. The transverse branches arise from the lateral aspect of the basilar artery and encircle the anterior and lateral borders of the brain stem. These arteries originate several small perforating branches that penetrate the pons at right angle with the parent vessel.

Anterior Inferior Cerebellar Artery (AICA) (Fig. 2.44)

The AICA originates from the proximal or middle third of the basilar artery. The artery is divided in main trunk, recurrent limb, and is further divided in two major branches, the lateral branch and medial branch. The internal auditory artery is in general a proximal branch of the AICA. The size of the AICA is inversely proportional to the size of the PICA. When one is absent or hypoplastic the other ipsilateral artery is larger and replaces blood flow to the normally nourished territory.

The main trunk of the AICA courses laterally and downward, in contact with either the dorsal or the ventral aspects of the abducens nerve. Within the cerebellopontine angle cistern the proximal arterial trunk usually lies ventral and medial to the roots of the facial, intermediate and acoustic nerves. These nerves are very close together and may be considered as a unit regarding the relation with the AICA. The main trunk of the AICA supplies small branches to the pons, to the lateral aspect of the pons from the middle third down to the upper part of the medulla.

The recurrent limb of the AICA arises from the area of the internal acoustic meatus and courses medially to reach the cerebellopontine angle and extends to reach the cerebellum dorsally.

The lateral branch courses laterally and turns around the flocculus running within the horizontal fissure between the superior and inferior semilunar lobules of the cerebellum. This artery sends hemispheric branches to the superior and inferior semilunar lobules and the distal hemispheric branches anastomoses with branches of the superior cerebellar artery and PICA.

The medial branch of the AICA courses medially and downwards to the medial and anterior border of the cerebellum, supplying the biventral lobule. This branch also anastomoses with the PICA.

The internal auditory artery originates from the proximal segment of the AICA in 95% of the cases or may arise from the basilar artery above the origin of the AICA. This artery supplies the structures within the meatus of the auditory canal including the nerve roots and internal ear.

Superior Cerebellar Artery (SCA)

This artery originates from the basilar artery, proximal to the origin of the posterior cerebral artery. It may also arise from the posterior cerebral artery. The proximal trunks of the SCA runs posteriorly in the perimesencephalic cisterns encircling the upper pons and lower mesencephalon. It supplies portions of the midbrain, the superior surface of the cerebellar hemisphere, the superior vermis, and the cerebellar nucleus.

The proximal trunk (perimesencephalic) or cisternal segment of the SCA is divided in 3 segments. anterior pontine, ambient and quadrigeminal segments. It has cortical and perforating branches.

Anterior Pontine Segment

This is the proximal portion of the SCA, it courses laterally on the anterior surface of the pons in an arcu-

ate curve. It lies inferiorly to the emerging roots of the oculomotor nerve, separating it from the proximal segment of the posterior cerebral artery. This segment may duplicate (Fig. 2.43) or triplicate and give of the marginal and superior vermis branches.

Ambient Segment

This is the second portion of the SCA, beginning at the lateral border of the pons and turning posteriorly over the brachium pontis or middle cerebellar peduncle. It courses posteriorly in the infratentorial portion of the ambient cistern. This segment parallels the course of the trochlear nerve.

Quadrigeminal Segment

This is the distal segment of the SCA which lies within the lateral aspects of the quadrigeminal cistern. At this point the arteries approach each other near the midline, giving off anastomotic branches.

Cortical Branches

Lateral (marginal) Branch. The marginal branch is the first largest branch of the SCA, originating at the second portion of the SCA within the ambient cistern, or more rarely from the anterior pontine segment. This artery reaches the anterolateral margin of the cerebellum running posterolaterally in the region of the horizontal fissure. It demarcates the superior and inferior cerebellar lobes. The hemispheric branches originate from the marginal branch of the SCA.

Hemispheric Branches. There are two or three of these branches arising distally to the origin of the marginal branch from the ambient or second segment of the SCA when the artery runs around the posterior surface of the brain stem. These branches course upwards reaching the superior surface of the cerebellum where they distribute radially in direction of the horizontal fissure. They supply the dentate nucleus, and at the cortical territory they supply the medial portion of the quadrigeminal and superior semilunar lobules and the superior half of the vermis.

Superior Vermis Branch (Fig. 2.45). This is the terminal branch of the SCA originated at the third or quadrigeminal segment. There are one or two vermis branches on each side. Anastomoses may be found in between these branches, when they get closer within the quadrigeminal cistern, and between these branches and the inferior vermis branches from the PICA They run over the vermis close to the midline.

Perforating Branches. Many small branches originate from the main trunk of the SCA perforating the brain stem. These branches are more common in the interpeduncular and quadrigeminal regions. The branches to the pons and mesencephalon originate from the anterior pontine segment of the SCA. The few branches arising from the ambient segment of the SCA are also perforating, and supply the lateral portion of the brain stem. The inferior colliculae are supplied by the small branches that arise from the quadrigeminal region of the SCA. Several larger branches arising from the distal ambient segment of the SCA supply the dentate nucleus and course down the superior cerebellar peduncle.

COLLATERAL CIRCULATION

After occlusion of the cerebral vessels the blood supply to the affected area of the brain may be replaced adequately if the collateral circulation is well developed. Collateral flow to the brain may occur from extracranial sources, from the external carotid artery, to the internal carotid artery or from intracranial sources by anastomoses in the subarachnoid space and the leptomeninge. Intracranial subarachnoid collateralization occurs through the circle of Willis, in the terminal branches of the cerebral arteries, and in embryonic connections between the basilar and carotid arteries.

The most common intracranial collateral pathway is the circle of Willis, anteriorly made of the A_1 segment of the anterior cerebral arteries, the supraclinoid segment of the internal carotid arteries and the anterior communicating artery. Laterally it is made by the posterior communicating arteries and posteriorly by the P1 segment of the posterior cerebral arteries. When one of the major arteries of the circle of Willis is occluded, the blood flows from the normal pressure to the low pressure territory, minimizing ischemic problems. Unfortunately the circle of Willis is incomplete or abnormal in a large percentage of cases.

When the circle of Willis is incomplete and the internal carotid is occluded, the extracranial arteries may supply blood to the intracranial circulation. Normal antegrade flow through the external carotid artery, and through the anastomoses, retrograde flow at the ophthalmic artery may recanalize the flow at the distal internal carotid artery. Additional flow may be supplied through the rete mirabile from the meningeal arteries to the cortical arteries on the surface of the brain. When the vertebral arteries system is occluded, in the event of hypoplasia of the posterior communicating arteries, muscular branches of the vertebral arteries may develop and recanalize the distal vertebral arteries.

There are supratentorial cortical anastomoses between the cortical branches of the anterior, middle, and posterior cerebral arteries at the surface of the brain. Similarly, in the infratentorial territory, on the surface of the cerebellum there are cortical anastomoses between the cortical branches of the posterior inferior, anterior inferior, and superior cerebellar arteries. The deep penetrating medullary arteries

that arise from this network do not anastomose with one another, therefore, occlusions of these vessels results in infarction.

CIRCLE OF WILLIS (CIRCULUS ARTERIOSUS OF WILLIS) (FIG. 2.1)

Most of the brain is supplied by the two internal carotid Arteries and the central anastomosis between them, called the circle of Willis, connects the internal carotid arteries to the vertebrobasilar system, that supplies the remainder brain. The circle of Willis is more polygonal than circular. It is located in the cisterna interpeduncularis, surrounding the optic chiasm, the neural infundibular stem of the hypophysis gland and other neural structures in the interpeduncular fossa. Anteriorly the anterior cerebral arteries are joined by the anterior communicating artery. Posteriorly the basilar artery divides and originates the two cerebral arteries and each artery is joined to the ipsilateral internal carotid by a posterior communication artery. The description above, however, refers only to a minority of cases. The vessels of the circle of Willis vary in caliber, and are often maldeveloped or even absent. In about 60% of the cases the circle shows some variation or anomaly. Cerebral and communicating arteries, anterior and posterior, may be absent, hypoplastic, double or triple. It is found, however, in about 90% of the cases some form of complete circular arterial channel between the internal carotid arteries, the posterior cerebral arteries and the anterior cerebral arteries, but in most cases one vessel is sufficiently small or narrowed to reduce the collateralization capability. The greatest variation in length is found in the anterior communicating artery and in diameter in the posterior communicating artery. The hemodynamic balance is usually disturbed by variation in the caliber of the communicating arteries, often associated with variations in size of the first segments of the anterior and posterior cerebral arteries extending from their origins to their junctions with the corresponding communicating arteries. The first segment of the posterior cerebral arteries is particularly variable, where it might be reduced or absent. When the posterior cerebral artery is connected to an ipsilateral large posterior communicating artery it is often filled from the internal carotid artery. Anteriorly, hypoplasia or absence of the first segment of the anterior cerebral artery is more frequent than anomalies in the anterior communicating artery.

EMBRYONIC COMMUNICATIONS

The most common embryonic communication between the internal carotid artery and the basilar artery is the persistent trigeminal artery (Fig. 2.30).

This embryonic vessel communicates with the pre-cavenous segment of the internal carotid artery with the basilar artery. The persistent hypoglossal artery connects the cervical portion of the internal carotid artery with the proximal extremity of the basilar artery after passing through the hypoglossal canal. The proatlantal intersegmental artery communicates the internal carotid artery or occipital with the vertebral artery, through the 1st (Type I) or 2nd cervical spaces (Type II).

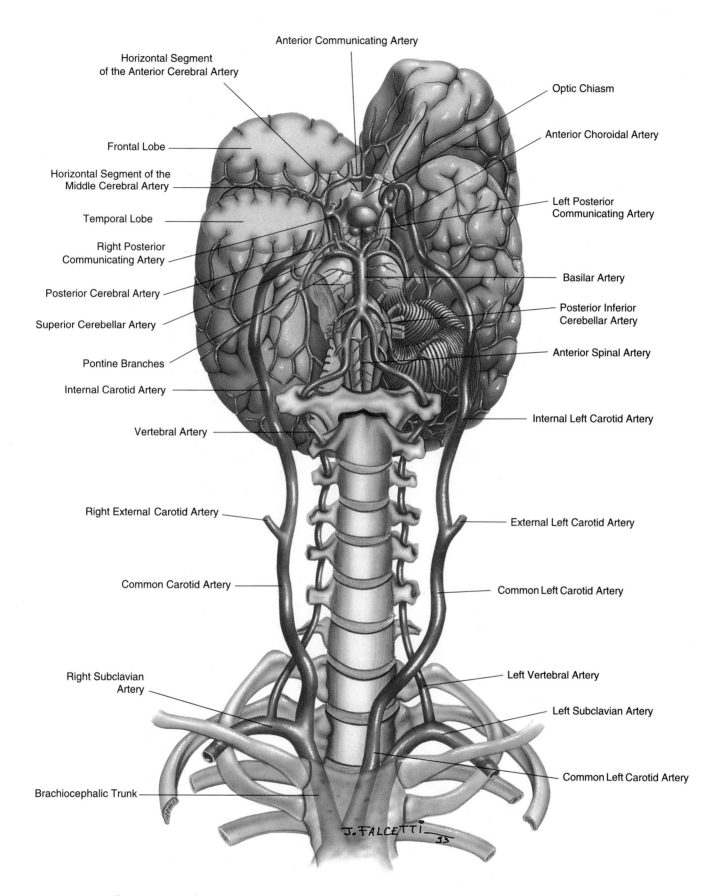

Anterior Communicating Artery

Horizontal Segment
of the Anterior Cerebral Artery

Optic Chiasm

Anterior Choroidal Artery

Frontal Lobe

Horizontal Segment of the
Middle Cerebral Artery

Left Posterior
Communicating Artery

Temporal Lobe

Right Posterior
Communicating Artery

Basilar Artery

Posterior Cerebral Artery

Posterior Inferior
Cerebellar Artery

Superior Cerebellar Artery

Pontine Branches

Anterior Spinal Artery

Internal Carotid Artery

Vertebral Artery

Internal Left Carotid Artery

Right External Carotid Artery

External Left Carotid Artery

Common Carotid Artery

Common Left Carotid Artery

Right Subclavian
Artery

Left Vertebral Artery

Left Subclavian Artery

Common Left Carotid Artery

Brachiocephalic Trunk

Figure 2.1. Frontal view of a schematic drawing of the carotid arteries, vertebral arteries and intracranial vessels
and the relationships with the brain.

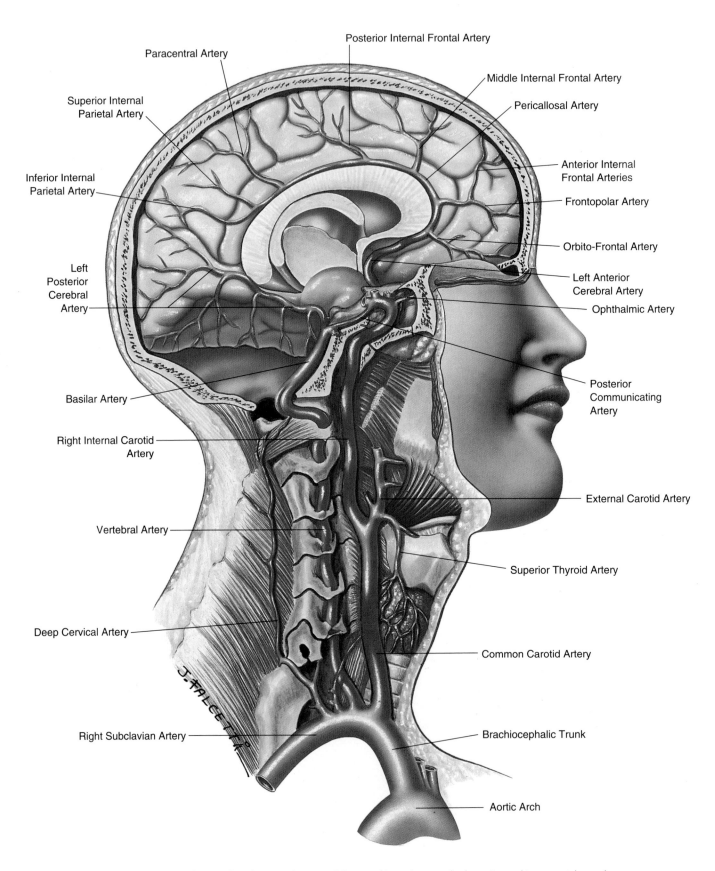

Figure 2.2. Lateral view of a schematic drawing of the carotíd arteries, vertebral arteries and intracranial vessels and the relationships in the neck and brain.

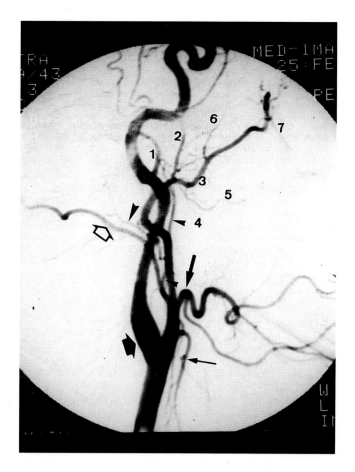

Figure 2.3. Common carotid artery. Lateral view. Carotid sinus (large short arrow). Branches of the external carotid: occipital artery (open arrow). Ascending pharyngeal artery (small arrowheads) with origin in the occipital artery. Posterior auricular artery (large arrowhead). Superior thyroidal artery (small arrow). Linguo-facial trunk (large arrow). **1.** Superficial temporal artery. **2.** Middle meningeal artery. **3.** Internal maxillary artery. **4.** Inferior alveolar artery. **5.** Transverse facial artery. **6.** Middle deep temporal artery. **7.** Descending palatine artery.

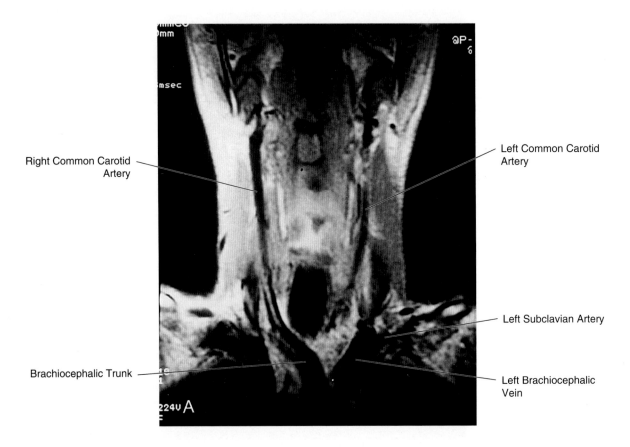

Figure 2.4.   A–D. Frontal view of the MRI of the neck showing the carotid arteries and the vertebral arteries and the relationships of these vessels with the soft tissues in the neck. **E and F.** Lateral view of the MRI of the neck showing the carotid artery in the neck.

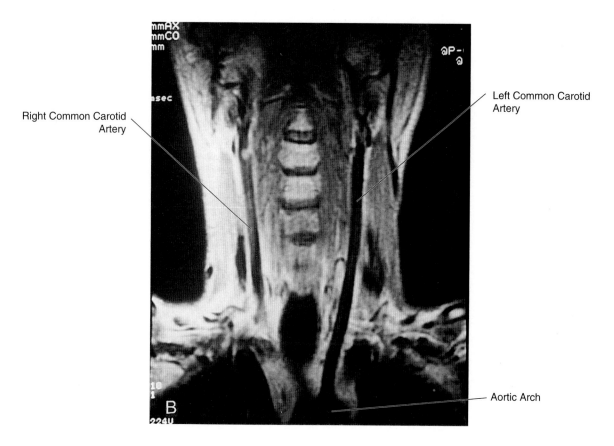

Right Common Carotid
Artery

Left Common Carotid
Artery

Aortic Arch

Figure 2.4. *Continued*

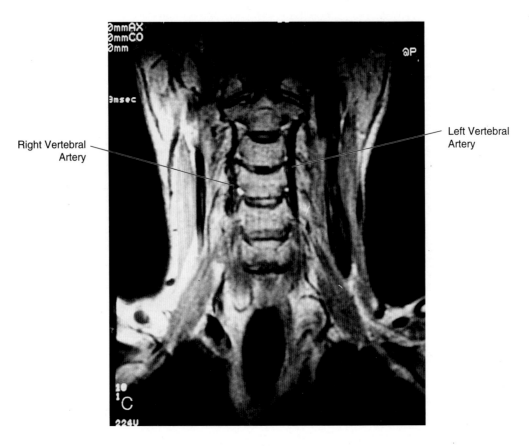

Right Vertebral Artery

Left Vertebral Artery

Figure 2.4. *Continued*

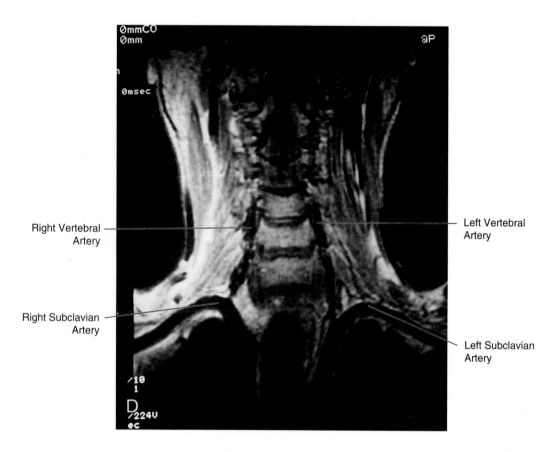

Right Vertebral Artery

Left Vertebral Artery

Right Subclavian Artery

Left Subclavian Artery

Figure 2.4. *Continued*

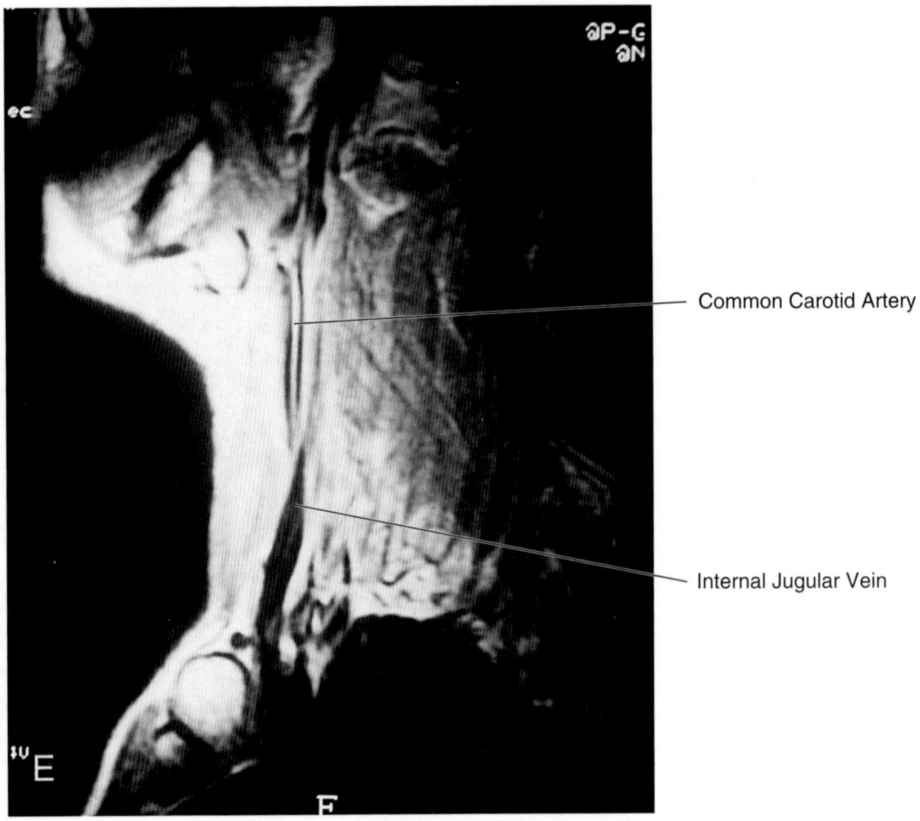

Figure 2.4. *Continued*

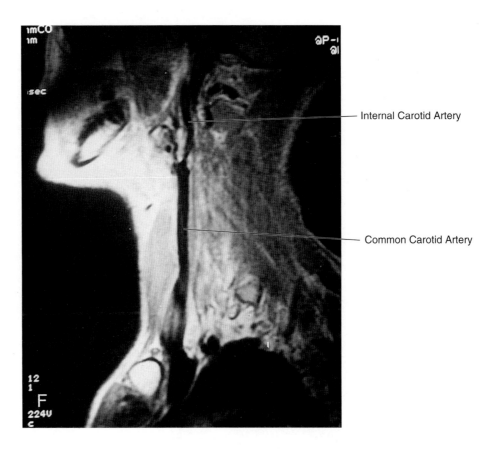

Internal Carotid Artery

Common Carotid Artery

Figure 2.4. *Continued*

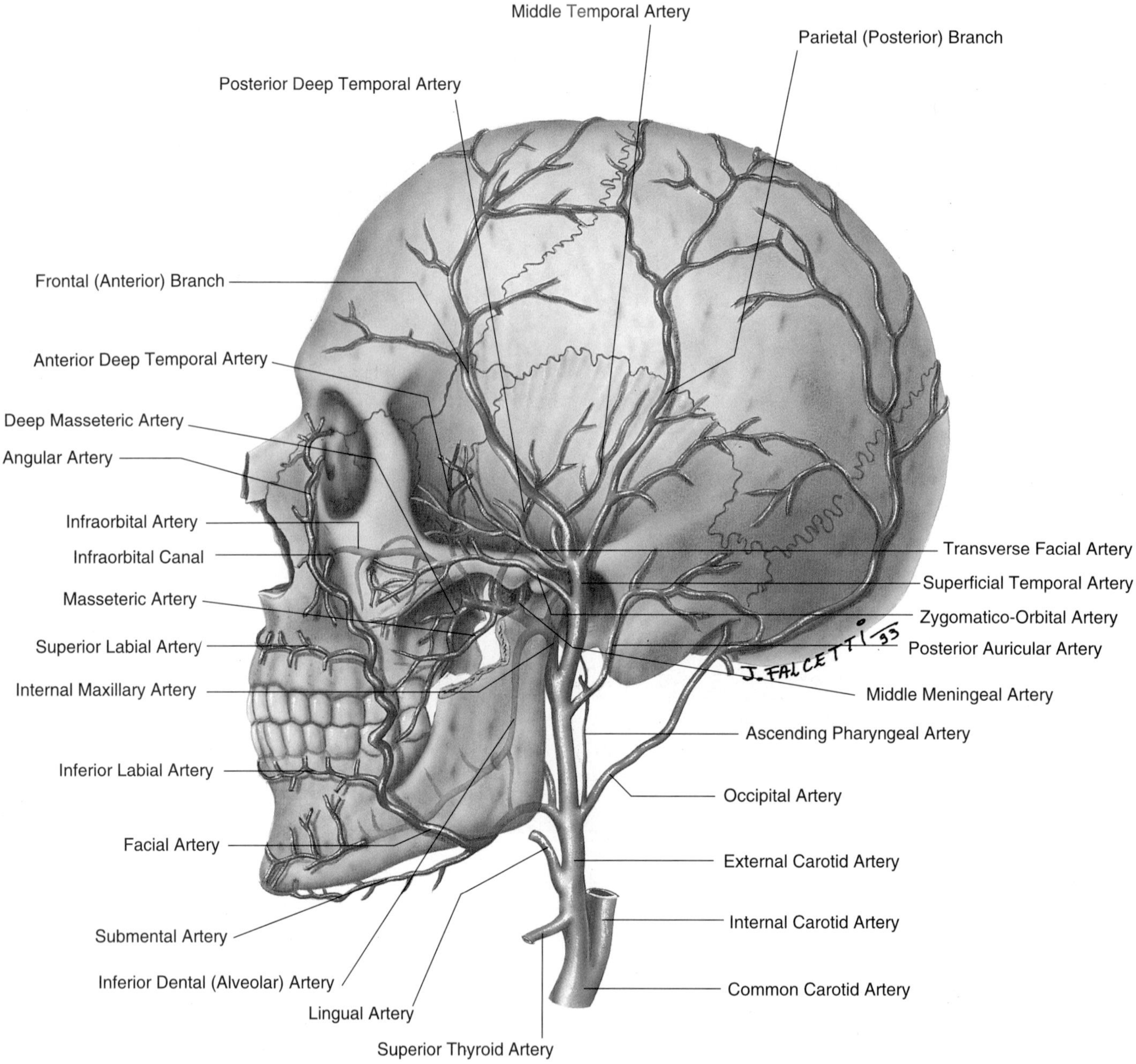

Middle Temporal Artery

Parietal (Posterior) Branch

Posterior Deep Temporal Artery

Frontal (Anterior) Branch

Anterior Deep Temporal Artery

Deep Masseteric Artery

Angular Artery

Infraorbital Artery

Infraorbital Canal

Masseteric Artery

Superior Labial Artery

Internal Maxillary Artery

Inferior Labial Artery

Facial Artery

Submental Artery

Inferior Dental (Alveolar) Artery

Lingual Artery

Superior Thyroid Artery

Transverse Facial Artery

Superficial Temporal Artery

Zygomatico-Orbital Artery

Posterior Auricular Artery

Middle Meningeal Artery

Ascending Pharyngeal Artery

Occipital Artery

External Carotid Artery

Internal Carotid Artery

Common Carotid Artery

J. FALCETTI '93

Figure 2.5. Schematic drawing of the relationships with the skull of the external carotid artery and branches, in the lateral view.

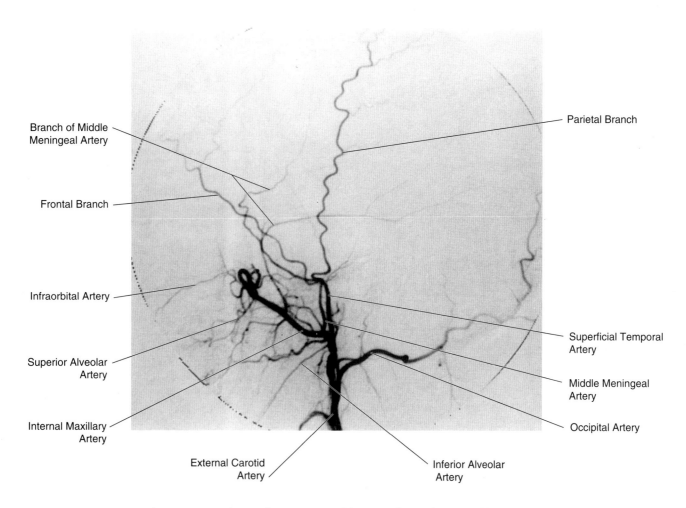

Branch of Middle
Meningeal Artery

Frontal Branch

Infraorbital Artery

Superior Alveolar
Artery

Internal Maxillary
Artery

External Carotid
Artery

Inferior Alveolar
Artery

Parietal Branch

Superficial Temporal
Artery

Middle Meningeal
Artery

Occipital Artery

Figure 2.6. Lateral view of an angiogram of the external carotid artery and branches.

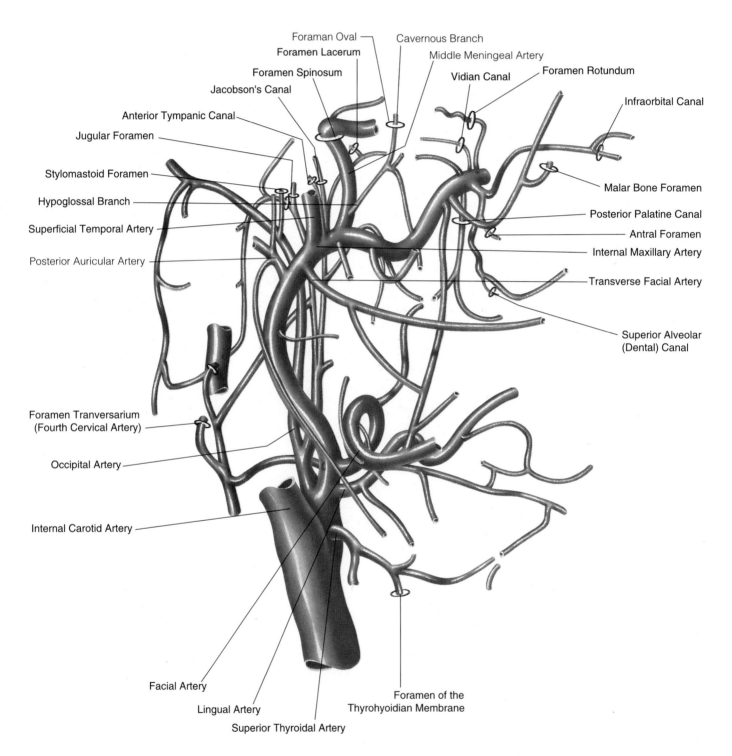

Foraman Oval
Foramen Lacerum
Cavernous Branch
Middle Meningeal Artery
Foramen Spinosum
Vidian Canal
Foramen Rotundum
Jacobson's Canal
Infraorbital Canal
Anterior Tympanic Canal
Jugular Foramen
Stylomastoid Foramen
Malar Bone Foramen
Hypoglossal Branch
Posterior Palatine Canal
Superficial Temporal Artery
Antral Foramen
Internal Maxillary Artery
Posterior Auricular Artery
Transverse Facial Artery
Superior Alveolar
(Dental) Canal
Foramen Tranversarium
(Fourth Cervical Artery)
Occipital Artery
Internal Carotid Artery
Facial Artery
Lingual Artery
Foramen of the
Thyrohyoidian Membrane
Superior Thyroidal Artery

Figure 2.7. Schematic drawing of the multiple branches of the external carotid artery and relationships with the foramens.

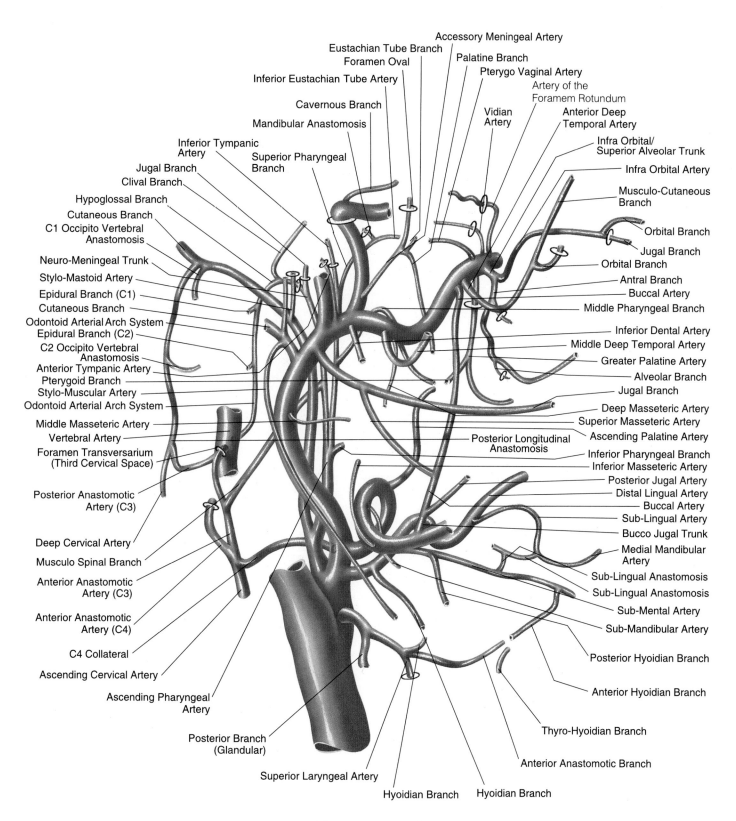

Figure 2.7. *Continued*

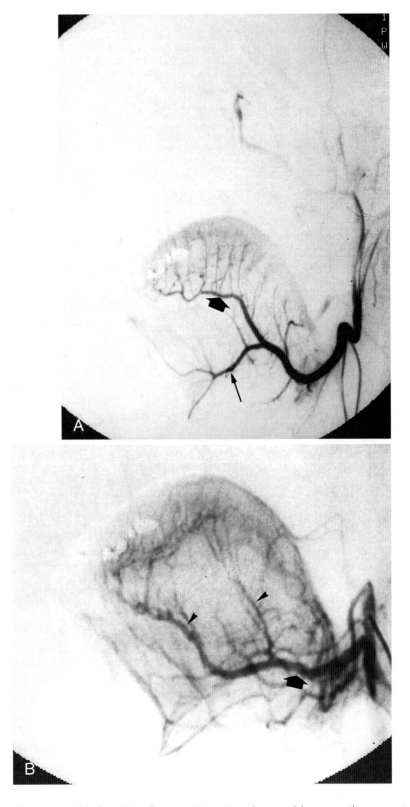

Figure 2.8. Lingual artery, arterial phase (A) and venous (B). A. Dorsal artery of the tongue (large arrow) and multiple muscular branches. Sublingual artery (long arrow). **B.** Two dorsal lingual veins (arrow heads) draining into the lingual vein (large arrow).

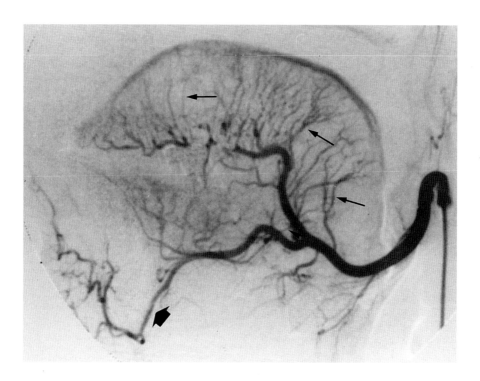

Figure 2.9. Lingual Artery, lateral view. Note the typical muscular branches (arrows). The mental artery is large (short large arrow) and originates from the lingual artery.

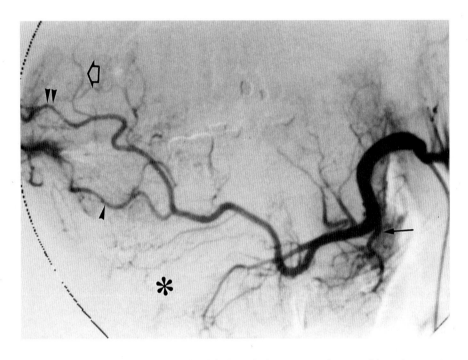

Figure 2.10. Facial artery, lateral view. Glandular branch (long arrow). The mental branch is missing (*).
Inferior labial artery (arrow head) and superior labial artery (double arrow head). Distal facial artery
is hypoplastic (open arrow).

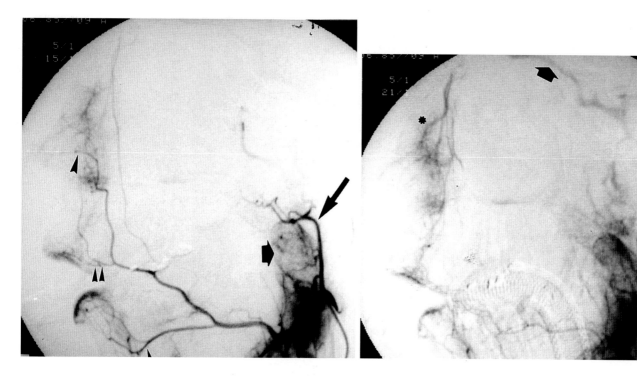

Figure 2.11. Lateral view of the facial artery, arterial phase (A) and venous (B). A. Ascending palatine artery arising from the facial artery (large arrow). Dense stain of palatine tonsil (wide arrow) and branches to the submandibular gland (large open arrow). Submental artery (*). Inferior labial artery (small arrow head) and superior labial artery (double arrow head). Alar artery (large arrow head). **B.** Venous phase. Nasal veins and orbitary veins (*) draining to the superior ophthalmic vein (large arrow). The lips and jugal area drain to the retromandibular vein (arrow).

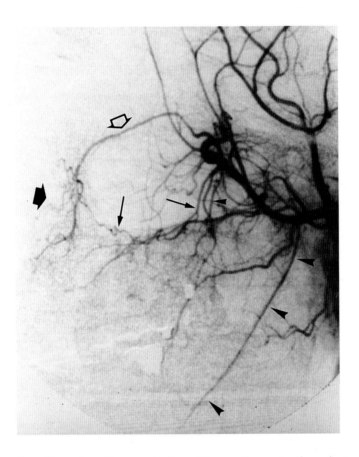

Figure 2.12. Internal maxillary artery. Cutaneous territory of the maxillary region (large short arrow) is supplied by the infraorbital artery (open arrow). Inferior alveolar artery (large arrowheads). Superior alveolar artery (small arrowhead). Descending palatine artery (arrows).

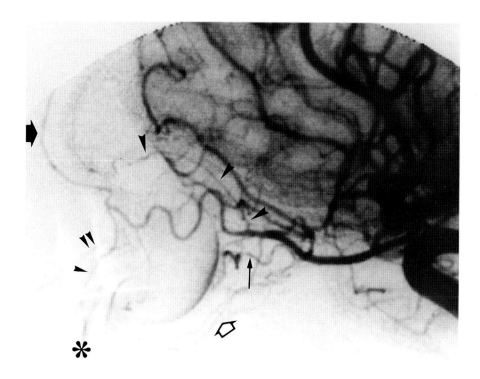

Figure 2.13. Internal carotid artery, lateral view. Angular artery (small arrowhead), vascularizes the high territory of the superior maxillary region (*). Frontal branch of the ophthalmic artery (large arrow). Central artery of the retina (small arrow) and choroid plexus blush of the eyeball. Anterior ethmoidal artery (large arrowheads). Inferior muscular branches (open arrow). Dorsal nasal artery (double arrowhead).

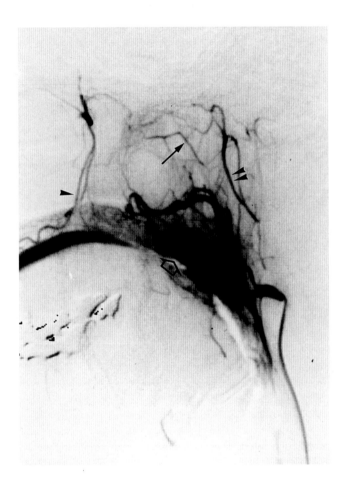

Figure 2.14. Artery of the soft palate (ascending palatine artery), lateral view. Dense blush of the soft palate (open arrow). Anastomoses of the ascending palatine artery (arrowhead) with the ascending pharyngeal artery (double arrowhead) and accessory meningeal artery (arrow).

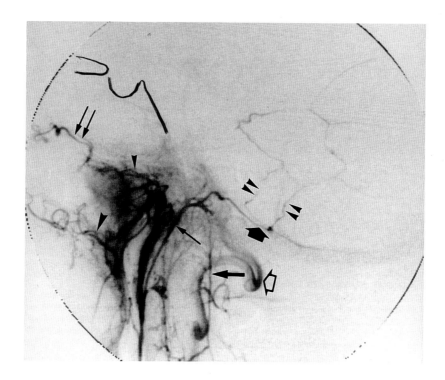

Figure 2.15. Ascending pharyngeal artery. Lateral view. The superior pharyngeal branch (small arrowhead), gives origin to the soft palate artery (large arrowhead), it has anastomosis with the pterigo-vaginal artery (double arrow). Posterior branch (small arrow) gives origin to the meningeal artery of the cerebellar fossa (large arrow) and branches around the sigmoid sinus (double small arrowheads). The arterial arch of the odontoid (large arrow), and the anastomosis with the vertebral artery (large open arrow) at the level of the 1st and 2nd cervical spaces are seen.

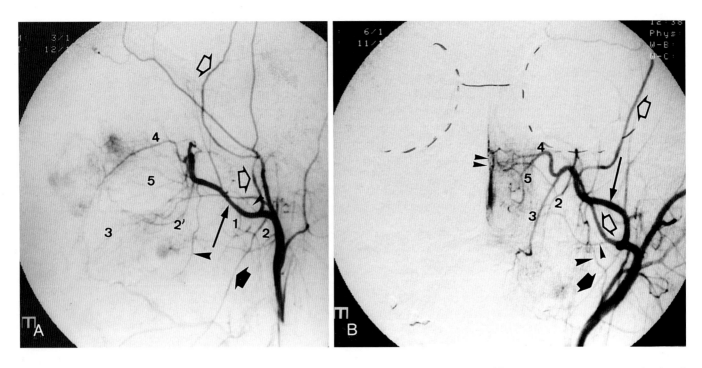

Figure 2.16. Lateral view of the distal external carotid artery (A) and frontal view (B). Branches of the internal maxillary artery (long arrow). Inferior alveolar artery (large arrow). Middle meningeal artery (open arrows). Accessory meningeal artery (small arrowhead) arising from the middle meningeal artery. Deep masseteric artery (1). Middle masseteric artery (2). Descending bucal artery (large arrowhead). Superior alveolar artery (2′). Descending palatine artery (3). Infraorbitary artery (4), with septal branches (double arrowhead in B). Sphenopalatine artery and branches (5).

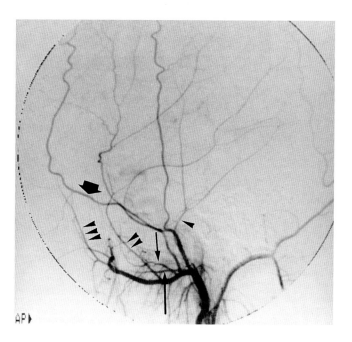

Figure 2.17. Branches of the external carotid artery: Deep temporal arteries; posterior (small arrow head), middle (double arrow heads) and anterior (triple arrow heads). Zygomatic-orbital artery of the temporal artery; superficial (large arrow). Accessory meningeal artery (small arrow) with direct origin from the internal maxillary artery. Transverse artery of the face (long arrow). Note the tortuous aspect of the superficial temporal artery and straight pattern of the middle meningeal artery.

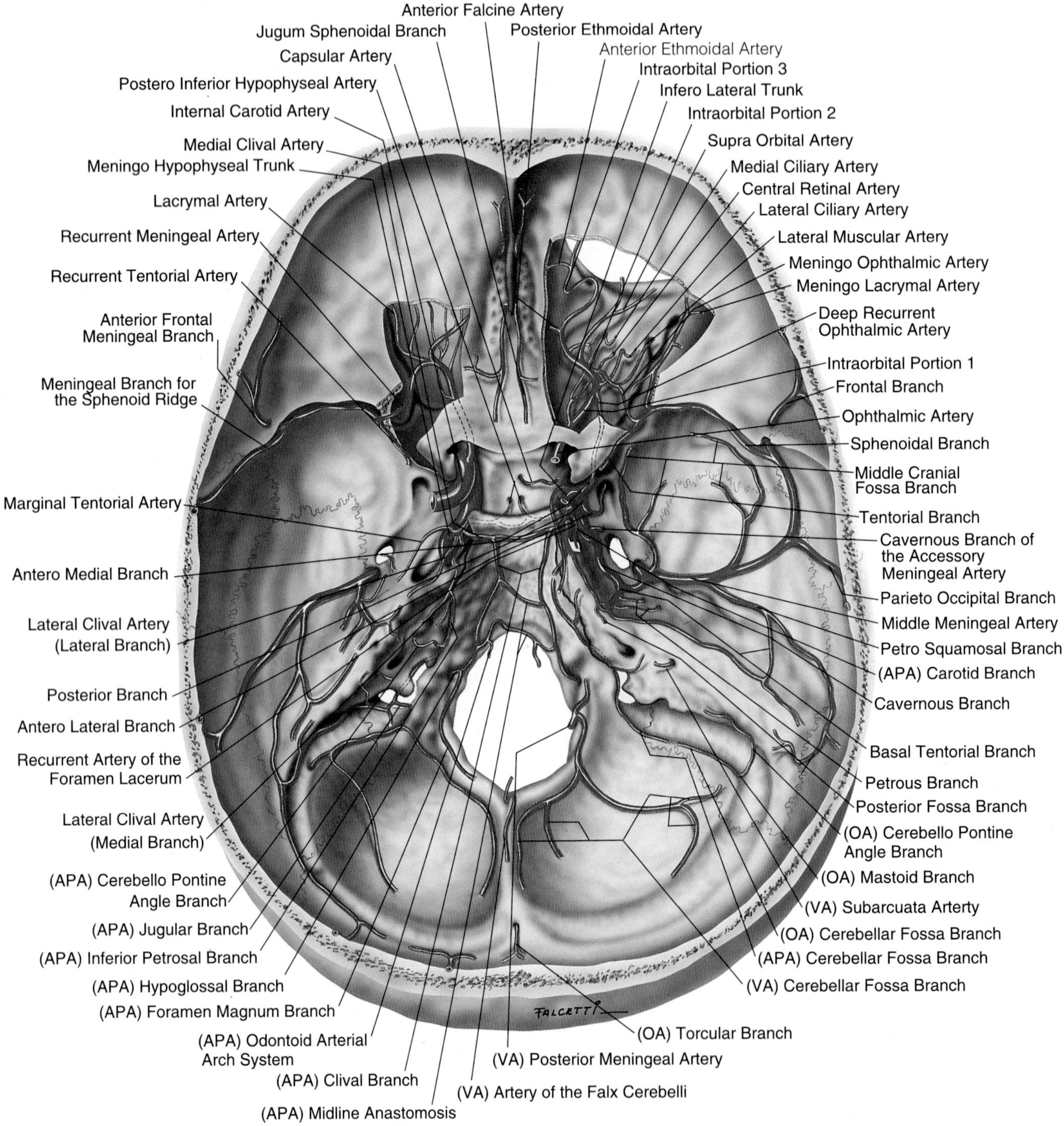

Anterior Falcine Artery
Jugum Sphenoidal Branch
Posterior Ethmoidal Artery
Capsular Artery
Anterior Ethmoidal Artery
Postero Inferior Hypophyseal Artery
Intraorbital Portion 3
Internal Carotid Artery
Infero Lateral Trunk
Medial Clival Artery
Intraorbital Portion 2
Meningo Hypophyseal Trunk
Supra Orbital Artery
Medial Ciliary Artery
Lacrymal Artery
Central Retinal Artery
Lateral Ciliary Artery
Recurrent Meningeal Artery
Lateral Muscular Artery
Recurrent Tentorial Artery
Meningo Ophthalmic Artery
Meningo Lacrymal Artery
Anterior Frontal
Meningeal Branch
Deep Recurrent
Ophthalmic Artery
Meningeal Branch for
the Sphenoid Ridge
Intraorbital Portion 1
Frontal Branch
Ophthalmic Artery
Sphenoidal Branch
Middle Cranial
Fossa Branch
Marginal Tentorial Artery
Tentorial Branch
Cavernous Branch of
the Accessory
Meningeal Artery
Antero Medial Branch
Parieto Occipital Branch
Lateral Clival Artery
(Lateral Branch)
Middle Meningeal Artery
Petro Squamosal Branch
(APA) Carotid Branch
Posterior Branch
Cavernous Branch
Antero Lateral Branch
Recurrent Artery of the
Foramen Lacerum
Basal Tentorial Branch
Lateral Clival Artery
(Medial Branch)
Petrous Branch
Posterior Fossa Branch
(OA) Cerebello Pontine
Angle Branch
(APA) Cerebello Pontine
Angle Branch
(OA) Mastoid Branch
(APA) Jugular Branch
(VA) Subarcuata Arterty
(APA) Inferior Petrosal Branch
(OA) Cerebellar Fossa Branch
(APA) Hypoglossal Branch
(APA) Cerebellar Fossa Branch
(APA) Foramen Magnum Branch
(VA) Cerebellar Fossa Branch
(APA) Odontoid Arterial
Arch System
(OA) Torcular Branch
(VA) Posterior Meningeal Artery
(APA) Clival Branch
(VA) Artery of the Falx Cerebelli
(APA) Midline Anastomosis

Figure 2.18. Schematic drawing of the base of the skull in axial view with the relationships of the branches of the external carotid arteries and some branches of the internal carotid arteries.

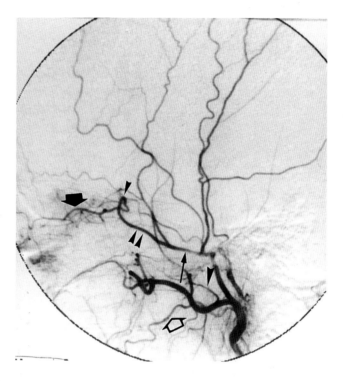

Figure 2.19. Distal external carotid artery in lateral view. The ophthalmic artery (large arrow) originates from the middle meningeal artery, surrounding the optic nerve (small arrow head). The accessory meningeal artery (large arrow head) has the origin at the internal maxillary artery. Frontal branch of the middle meningeal artery with the meningo-lacrimal (double arrow head) artery reaching the orbit through the superior orbitary fissure. Transverse artery of the face (large open arrow).

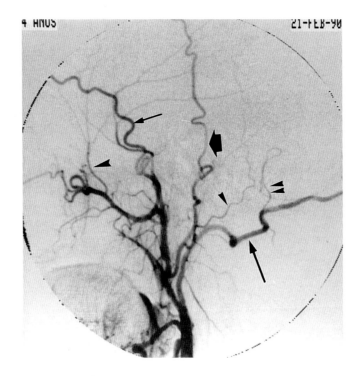

Figure 2.20. External carotid artery. Double origin of the superficial temporal artery. Frontal branch (small arrow). Parietal branch (large arrow) originating from the external carotid artery as a common trunk with the posterior auricular artery (small arrow head). Single deep temporal artery with three branches (large arrow head). Occipital artery (long arrow) and the meningeal branch (double arrow head).

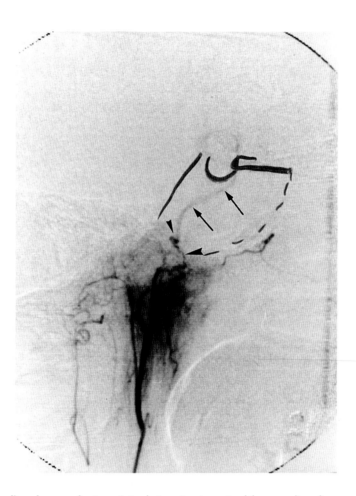

Figure 2.21. Ascending pharyngeal artery. Lateral view. Anastomosis of the ascending pharyngeal artery with the internal carotid artery. Inferior tympanic artery (large arrow head) originated from the anterior branch of the ascending pharyngeal artery and anastomosed with the caroticotympanic artery (small arrow head), branch of the petrous segment of the internal carotid artery (arrows). This anastomosis is called "aberrant segment of the internal carotid artery," in case of agenesis of the cervical segment of the internal carotid artery.

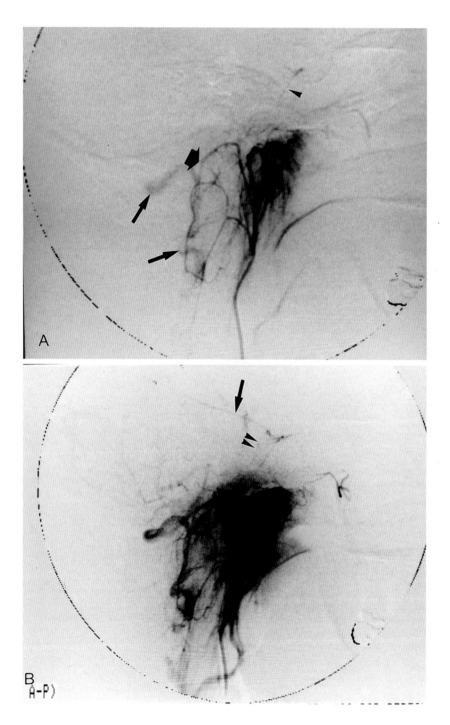

Figure 2.22. Ascending pharyngeal artery. A. Early phase arteriogram. Anterior branch (large arrow head) fills the recurrent artery of the foramen lacerum (branch of the C4 segment of the internal carotid artery) (small arrow head) via carotid branch. The posterior branch and arterial arch of the odontoid (large arrow) shows anastomosis with the vertebral artery (large arrows). **B.** Late phase arteriogram. The clival artery is visualized (double arrow head) and is branch of the hypoglossal artery. Anastomoses with the meningohypophyseal trunk and the artery of the free margin of the tentorium (arrow).

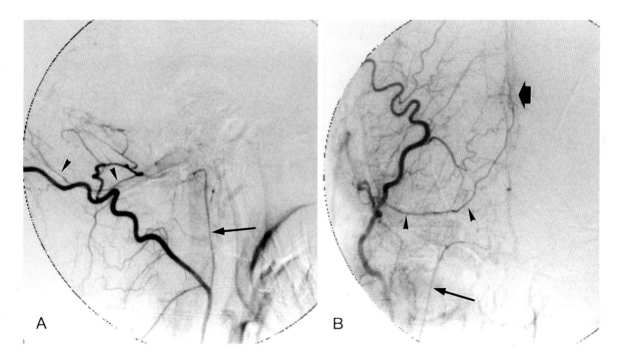

Figure 2.23. Occipital artery. A. Lateral view of the occipital artery. Note the meningeal branch of the cerebellar fossa (arrow heads in A and B) reaching the torcula Herophili (large arrow in B). **B.** Towne view of the occipital artery. Posterior branch of the ascending pharyngeal artery (long arrow in A and B) originated from the occipital artery.

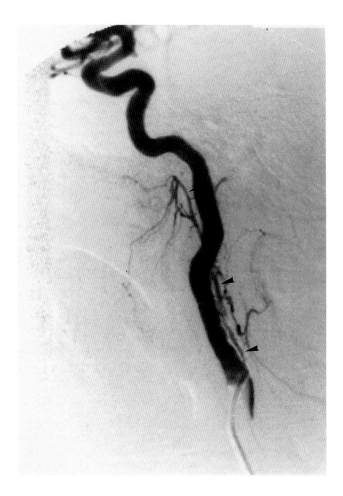

Figure 2.24. Ascending pharyngeal artery (arrow heads) with origin at the internal carotid artery.

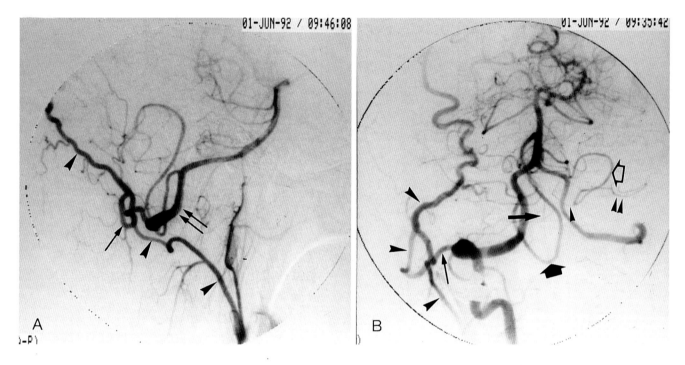

Figure 2.25. Occipital artery, lateral view. A. Occipital artery (arrow heads) with wide anastomosis at the level of the 1st cervical space (arrow) with the vertebral artery (double arrow). **B.** Right vertebral artery, frontal view. The anastomosis (small arrow) with the occipital artery (large arrow heads) is visualized. Left posterior inferior cerebellar artery (PICA) (open arrow) originates from the anterior inferior cerebellar artery (AICA), with vermian branches (small arrow head) and hemispheric branch (double small arrow head). Anterior spinal artery (large arrow).

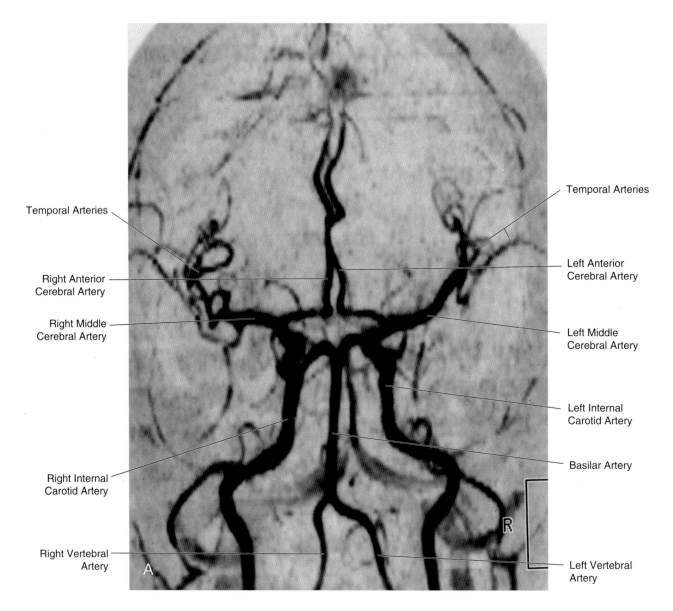

Figure 2.26. **A.** Frontal view of an MRI of the intracranial vessels. **B.** Lateral view of an MRI of the intracranial vessels.

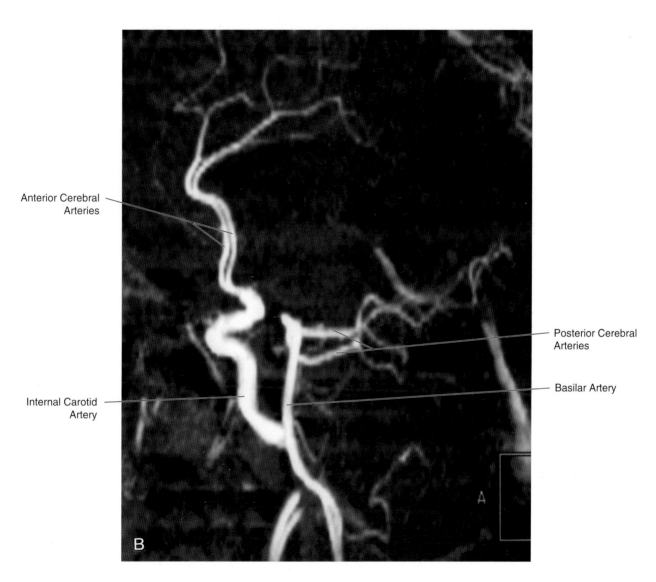

Figure 2.26. *Continued*

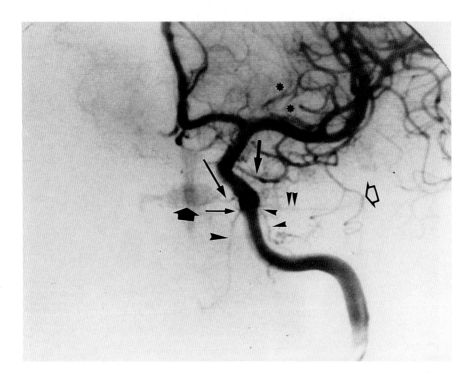

Figure 2.27. Left internal carotid artery, anterior view. Hypophysis blush is normal (large short arrow). Meningo-hypophyseal trunk (small arrow) with meningeal branch - Clival Artery (large arrowhead) and postero-inferior hypophyseal artery (long arrow). Infero-lateral trunk (small arrow head) with a basal tentorial branch (double arrow head) and ophthalmic artery (long thick arrow). Temporo-polar branch (open arrow) of the middle cerebral artery. Note the inverted "S" shape of the lenticulostriate branches (*).

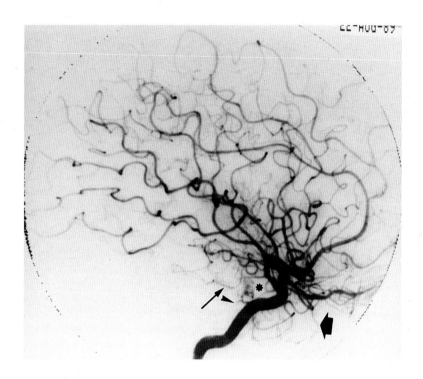

Figure 2.28. Left internal carotid artery, lateral view - Meningo-hypophyseal trunk with the clival branches (arrow head) and artery of the free margin of the tentorium (arrow). Note hypophysis blush (*). The branches of the middle cerebral artery arise separately from the origin, without dominance of one trunk. Note the temporo-polar branches (large short arrow) of the middle cerebral artery.

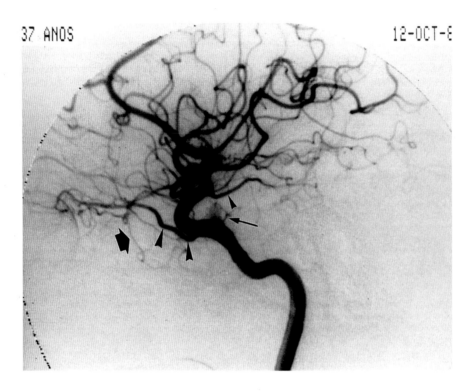

Figure 2.29. Internal carotid artery. Intracavernosal origin of the ophthalmic artery (large arrow heads). Meningo-
hypophyseal trunk and hypophysis gland blush (small arrow). Posterior communicating artery, anterior
choroidal artery and small perforating branches of the distal internal carotid artery (small
arrow head). Temporo-polar branch of the middle cerebral artery (large arrow).

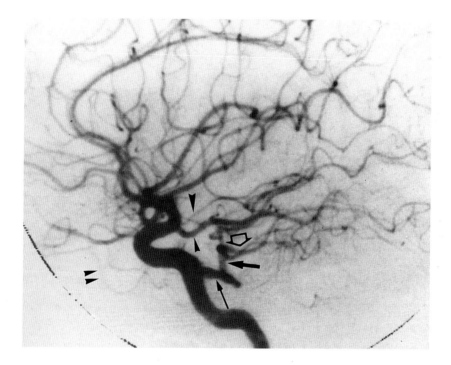

Figure 2.30. Left internal carotid artery, lateral view. Persistent trigeminal artery (arrow) communicating with the superior third of the basilar artery (thick arrow). Posterior communicating artery (small arrow head) fetal type, and anterior choroidal artery (large arrow head). Open arrow denotes the superior cerebellar arteries. Temporo-polar Branches of the middle cerebral artery (double arrow head).

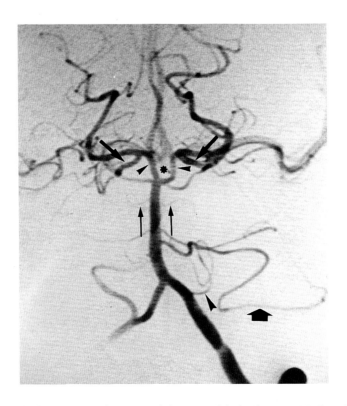

Figure 2.31. Left vertebral artery. Frontal view. Low bifurcation of the basilar artery (*) after origin of the superior cerebellar arteries. Segment P1 (arrow heads), Posterior communicating artery (large arrows). On the left side, there are 2 AICAs, one vascularizing the hemispheric territory of the PICA (large arrow). Left hypoplastic PICA (large arrow head). Two pontine arteries are visible (small arrows).

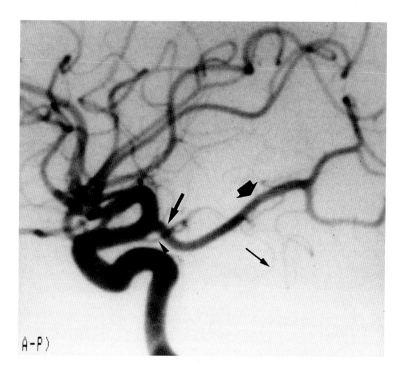

Figure 2.32. Internal carotid artery. Lateral view. Anterior choroidal artery (arrow head), arising below the posterior communicating artery (large arrow). Curved uncal artery (small arrow). The posterior cerebral artery (large short arrow) is of the fetal type, arising from the internal carotid artery, with the same diameter of the posterior communicating artery.

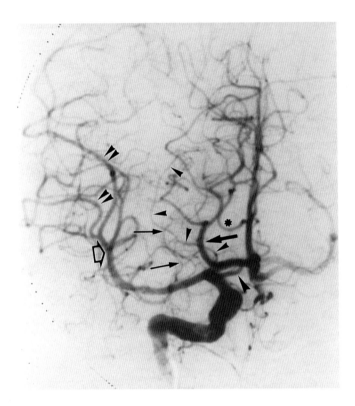

Figure 2.33. Right internal carotid artery. Towne view. Anterior choroidal arteries (small arrow heads) crossing the posterior cerebral artery (large arrow) and more distally the lenticulostriate branches (small arrows). The posterior communicating artery (large arrow heads) has a more medial path than the anterior choroidal artery. Orbitofrontal artery of the anterior cerebral artery (*). Note the bifurcation of the middle cerebral artery inside the fissure of Sylvius (large arrow). The branches of the middle cerebral artery arise earlier from the fissure of Sylvius (double arrow heads).

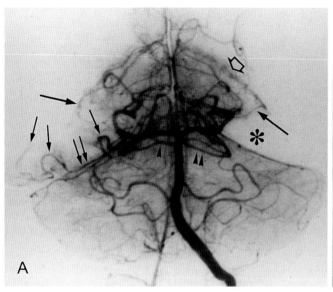
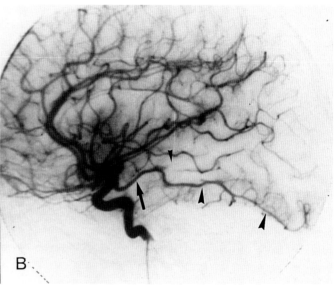

Figure 2.34. Temporal branches of the posterior cerebral artery originated from the anterior choroidal artery in A and B. A. Left vertebral artery. Waters projection. Right temporal branches (large arrow). Note the loops of the temporal branches inside the temporal sulci (small arrows) and the straight segments on top of the gyri (double small arrows). Note also the parallel path to the hemispheric branches (marginal artery) of the superior cerebellar artery, separated by the tentorium cerebelli. On the left there are no temporal branches of the posterior cerebral artery (*). The superior cerebellar artery is duplicated on the left (double small arrow head) and bifurcated on the right (arrow head). Postero-lateral choroidal artery (large arrow) and choroidal blush of the ventricular carrefour (open arrow). Note that on the left the postero-lateral Choroidal Artery is larger. **B.** Left internal carotid artery, same subject. Anterior choroidal artery is large and originates the temporal branches (medial aspect of the temporal lobe) of the posterior cerebral artery. (large arrow heads). The plexal branch of the anterior choroidal artery (small arrow head) is hypoplastic and has hemodynamic balance with the large posterior choroidal branch of the posterior cerebral artery (see in A).

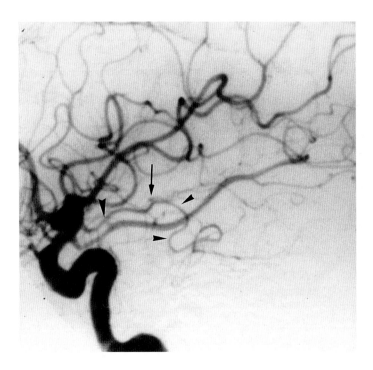

Figure 2.35. Internal carotid artery, lateral view. Anterior choroidal artery (large arrow head) originating a temporal branch (small arrow heads). Ponto-coroideal (arrow).

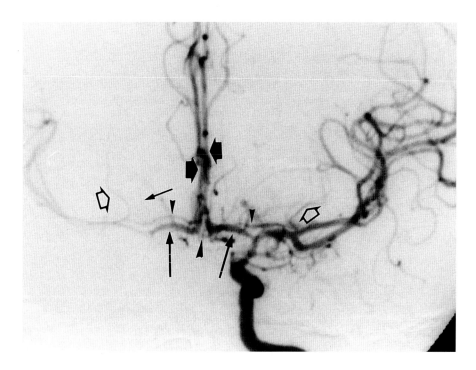

Figure 2.36. Left internal carotid injection in frontal view. Segments A1 (long arrows), A2 (large arrows) and the anterior communicating artery (large arrow head). The recurrent artery of Heubner is visible in both sides (small arrow heads), with large branches to the basal nuclei (large open arrows). On the right a medial lenticulostriate artery (small arrow head) arises from the A1 segment. The left middle cerebral artery shows an early bifurcation in the segment M1.

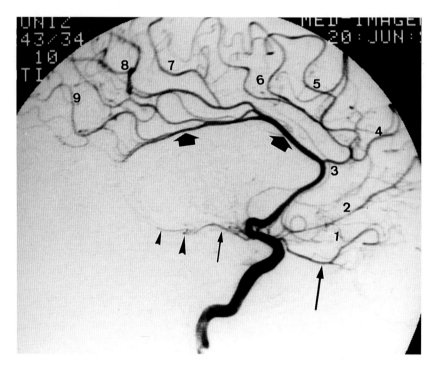

Figure 2.37. Internal carotid artery, lateral view. Occlusion of the middle cerebral artery. Anterior choroidal artery (small arrow) with superior deep branches. Ponto choroidal (large arrow head) and plexal branches (small arrow head). Pericallosal artery and branches: 1. Orbitofrontal artery (frontobasilar artery). Overlaps the ophthalmic artery (large arrow). 2. Frontopolar artery. 3. Common trunk of the internal frontal arteries, anterior (4), middle (5) and posterior (6). 7. Paracentral artery. 8. Superior internal parietal artery. 9. Inferior internal parietal artery. In this case there is no callosomarginal artery. The large short arrows denote the pericallosal artery.

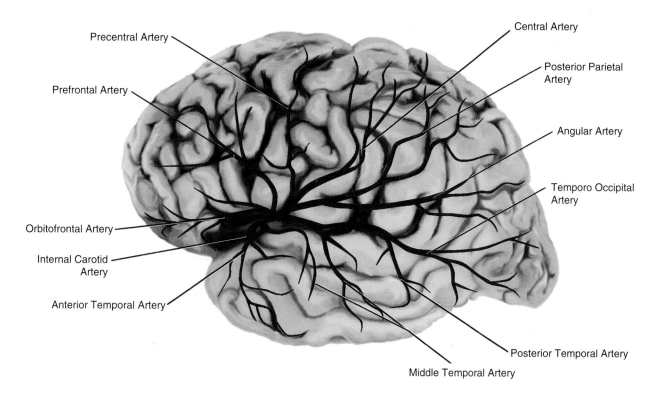

Precentral Artery

Prefrontal Artery

Orbitofrontal Artery

Internal Carotid
Artery

Anterior Temporal Artery

Central Artery

Posterior Parietal
Artery

Angular Artery

Temporo Occipital
Artery

Posterior Temporal Artery

Middle Temporal Artery

Figure 2.38. Schematic drawing showing the distribution of the peripheral branches of the middle cerebral artery
and territories.

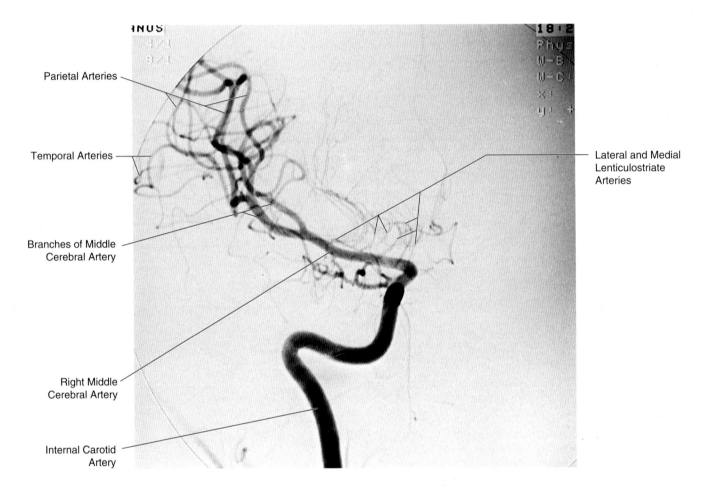

Figure 2.39. Frontal view of injection in the right internal carotid artery, showing the lenticulostriate branches and the bifurcation of the middle cerebral artery. Note that the segment A1 of the anterior cerebral artery is hypoplastic.

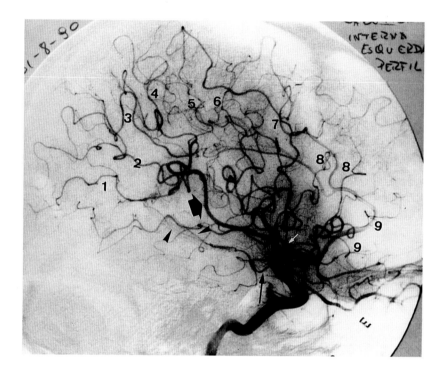

Figure 2.40. Left internal carotid artery. Anterior choroidal artery (small arrow) with the plexal branches (arrow heads). Posterior division of the middle cerebral artery with a single trunk (large arrow) up to the outlet of the fissure, where gives origin to the temporo-occipital (1), angular (2), superior parietal (4) and inferior (3) arteries. The post central artery (5) originates from the parietal trunk (3,4) while the central (6) originates from the division of the middle cerebral artery (white arrow). Pre central (7) and pre frontal (8) arteries. Orbito frontal artery (9).

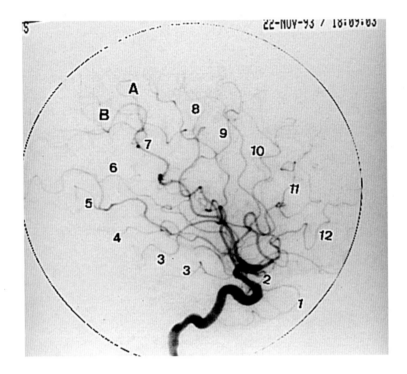

Figure 2.41. Internal carotid artery. Lateral view. Branches of the middle cerebral artery. 1. Temporal polar artery. 2. Anterior temporal artery. 3. Middle temporal artery. 4. Posterior temporal artery. 5. temporo-occipital artery. 6. Angular artery (small size). 7. Posterior parietal artery. 8. Anterior parietal artery. 9. Central artery. 10. Precentral artery. 11. Prefrontal artery. 12. Orbitofrontal artery.

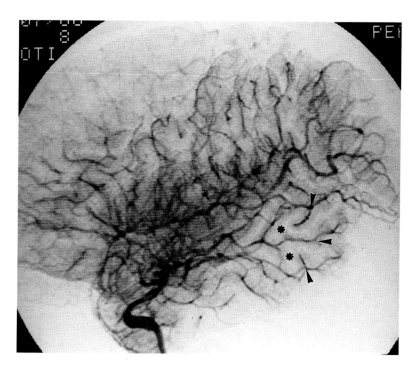

Figure 2.42. Late phase of an angiogram of the internal carotid artery. Lateral View. Capillary blush is more intense in the sulci (small arrow heads) allowing to delineate the cortical gyrus (*) best visualized in the temporal lobe.

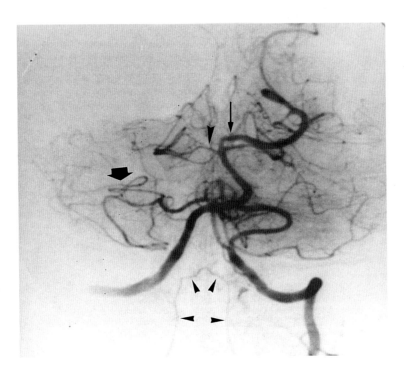

Figure 2.43. Left vertebral artery, anterior view. Arterial arch of the odontoid (small arrow heads). Double superior right cerebellar artery (large arrow head). The P1 segment is hypoplastic and the left (arrow) is normal. Right PICA with high intradural origin giving origin to the distal third of the AICA (large short arrow).

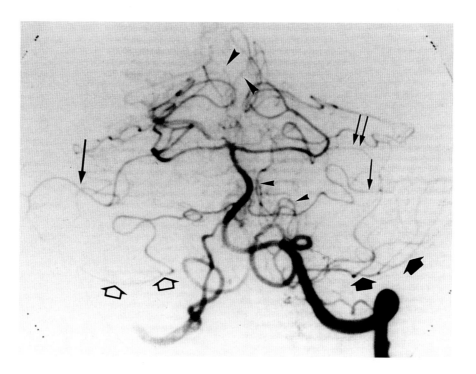

Figure 2.44. Left vertebral artery, anterior view. Hemodynamic balance: Left PICA is normal with vermian branches (small arrow heads) and hemispheric branches (large short arrows). Left AICA has a large hemispheric branch (small arrow) and a small marginal branch of the left superior cerebellar artery (double arrow). Right PICA originates vermian branches only. Right AICA originates the hemispheric branches of the PICA (open arrows) and has a hypoplastic hemispheric branch, and a large marginal branch of the superior cerebellar artery (large arrow). Vermian branches of the superior cerebellar artery (large arrowheads). There is hypoplasia of the distal basilar artery and segments P1.

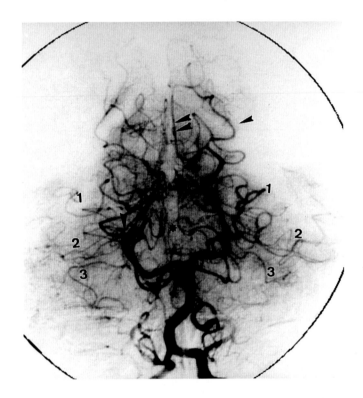

Figure 2.45. Vertebral artery. Towne view. Asymmetric posterior cerebral arteries. The right posterior cerebral artery
shows an early bifurcation (large arrow head). Note posterior temporal branch (1), middle (2), and anterior (3).
Calcarine artery (small arrow head) and parieto-occipital artery (double arrow head). Vermian branches of
the posterior superior cerebellar arteries (*).

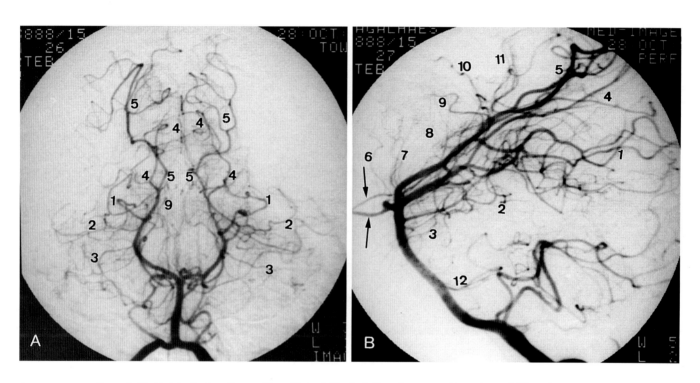

Figure 2.46. Vertebral artery. Towne (A) and lateral (B). A. 1. Posterior temporal branch, 2. Middle and 3. Anterior. 4. Calcarine artery. 5. Parieto-occipital artery. **B.** Posterior communicating arteries (arrows). 6. Anterior thalamoperforating arteries. 7. Middle. 8. Posterior. 9. Postero-medial choroidal artery. 10. Postero-lateral choroidal artery. 11. Posterior pericallosal artery. 12. AICA (Anterior inferior cerebellar artery).

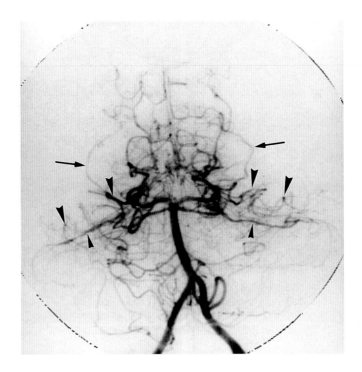

Figure 2.47. Anterior view of the vertebral artery. Temporal branches of the posterior cerebral artery (large arrow heads) over the tentorium. Marginal branches of the superior cerebellar arteries (small arrow heads) under the tentorium. Typical aspect of the postero-lateral choroidal arteries (arrows).

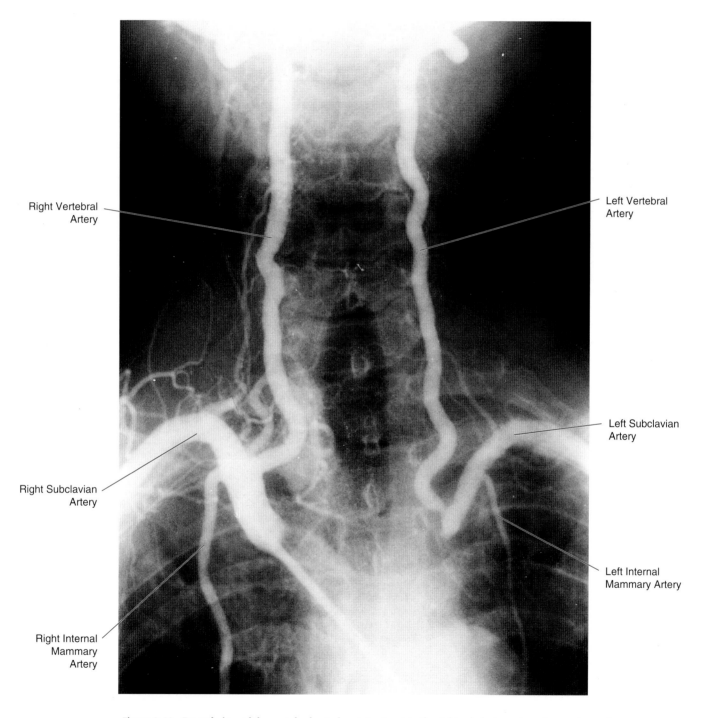

Right Vertebral
Artery

Left Vertebral
Artery

Left Subclavian
Artery

Right Subclavian
Artery

Left Internal
Mammary Artery

Right Internal
Mammary
Artery

Figure 2.48. Frontal view of the vertebral arteries. Injection into the right subclavian artery shows retrograde filling of the left vertebral artery due to occlusion of the left subclavian artery.

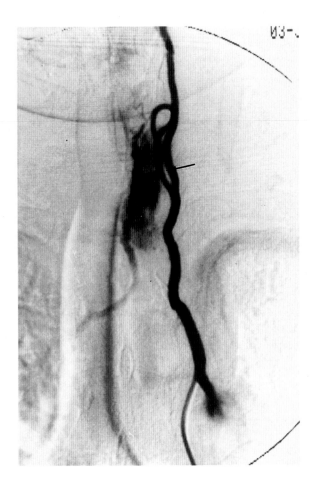

Figure 2.49. Left vertebral artery, frontal view. Inferior thyroid artery (arrow) originated from the vertebral artery. The thyroid gland blush is normal.

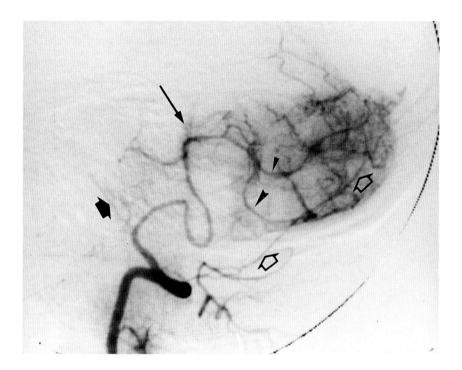

Figure 2.50. Lateral view of the vertebral artery. Hypoplasia of the vertebral artery (large short arrow) distally to the origin of the PICA. Vermian branches (small arrow head) and hemispheric branches (large arrow head) of the PICA. Blush of the choroidal plexus of the IV ventricle (long arrow). Artery of the cerebellar falx (open arrows) with a typical pattern projecting more anteriorly than the hemispheric branches of the PICA.

3

VEINS OF THE HEAD AND NECK

EXTERNAL VEINS OF THE HEAD AND FACE

The superficial veins of the head and neck vary in number and position. The most common pattern of venous distribution is the following (Fig. 3.1).

Supratrochlear Vein

The supratrochlear vein originates in the anterior part of the head resulting from the junction of a scalp venous network, which is connected to the tributaries of the frontal superficial temporal vein (Fig. 3.2). The supratrochlear veins descend close and parallel to the middle line and reach the surface of the nose, where they are joined by the nasal arch and subsequently joined by the supraorbital vein. These veins may anastomose and separate subsequently to form the facial veins. The supratrochlear veins diverge laterally and form the facial vein near the medial canthus of the eye lids.

Supraorbital Vein

This vein originates near the zygomatic process of the frontal bone and runs medially above the orbit until it reaches the supratrochlear vein to form the facial vein near the medial canthus. A branch through the supraorbital notch anastomose with the superior ophthalmic vein (Figs. 3.3, 3.4).

Facial Vein

The facial vein is formed by the junction of the supratrochlear and supraorbital veins. It descends obliquely near the side of the nose (also called angular vein in this level), turning posterolateral under the orbit, passing downwards and backwards behind the facial artery, until it reaches the mandible angle, where it is joined by the retromandibular vein (Figs. 3.3, 3.4). The facial vein joins the internal jugular vein near the greater horn of the hyoid bone. The facial vein is connected to the cavernous sinus by the superior ophthalmic vein (Figs. 3.3, 3.4) or its supraorbital tributary, or by the deep facial vein to the pterygoid plexus and hence to the cavernous sinus. The main tributaries in the face are the superior ophthalmic vein (Figs. 3.3, 3.4), the deep facial vein from the pterygoid venous plexus, inferior palpebral vein, superior and inferior labial veins. The main tributaries below the mandible are the submental, tonsillar, external palatine (peritonsillar), and submandibular veins. The vena comitans of the hypoglossal nerve and the pharyngeal and superior thyroid veins are also tributaries at the level below the mandible.

Superficial Temporal Vein (Figs. 3.2, 3.4)

This vein originates in the scalp venous network. This venous network is drained by the supratrochlear, supraorbital, posterior auricular, and occipital veins. Anterior and posterior tributaries join above the zygoma to form the superficial temporal vein and are joined by the middle temporal vein. It joins the maxillary vein forming the retromandibular vein. Main tributaries are the parotid veins, temporomandibular joint rami, anterior auricular veins, transverse facial vein, and orbital veins.

Pterygoid Venous Plexus

Main tributaries are the sphenopalatine, deep temporal, pterygoid, masseteric, buccal, dental, greater palatine, middle meningeal veins, and branches from the inferior ophthalmic artery. The plexus connects with the facial vein through the deep facial vein and with the cavernous sinus through the sphenoidal emissary foramen, foramen ovale, and foramen lacerum (Figs. 3.4, 3.5, 3.6).

Maxillary Vein

It is a short vein that accompanies the first part of the maxillary artery. It represents the confluence of veins from the pterygoid plexus with the superficial temporal vein to form the retromandibular vein (Figs. 3.3, 3.4).

Retromandibular Vein

This vein is within the parotid gland, between the external carotid artery and superficially the facial nerve. It has an anterior branch forward that joins the facial vein and a posterior branch backwards that forms the external jugular vein after joining the posterior auricular vein.

Posterior Auricular Vein

The posterior auricular vein is formed in the parieto-occipital network and drains also the occipital and superficial temporal veins. It has a descent path behind the auricle and joins the posterior division of the retromandibular vein. It receives tributaries from the auricle and stylomastoid vein.

Occipital Vein

The occipital vein originates in the posterior venous network in the scalp and joins the deep cervical and vertebral veins, through anastomoses. It is a tributary of the internal jugular vein.

VEINS OF THE NECK

The veins of the neck may be superficial and deep, but they are not entirely separable and are connected by anastomoses at various levels (Fig. 3.1).

External Jugular Vein

The external jugular vein drains mainly the scalp and face but also some deeper tissues.

It results from the union of the posterior division of the retromandibular and posterior auricular veins near the angle of the mandible. It descends superficially, covered by the platysma, superficial fascia, and skin. It ends in the subclavian vein. Main tributaries are the posterior external cervical vein, transverse cervical, suprascapular and anterior jugular veins.

Posterior External Jugular Vein

The posterior external jugular vein is originated in the occipital scalp and drains the skin and muscles. It joins the middle part of the external jugular.

Anterior Jugular Vein

The anterior jugular vein starts near the hyoid bone from the junction of the superficial submandibular veins. It has a descendent direction parallel to the midline. Distally it turns lateral, deep and joins the end of the external jugular vein. It receives the laryngeal veins and a small thyroid vein. The anterior jugular vein is usually connected to the contralateral, distally by the jugular arch, receiving thyroid tributaries. Both veins may be replaced by a midline trunk.

Internal Jugular Vein

The internal jugular vein drains most of the blood from the skull, brain, and superficial and deep parts of the face and neck. It begins at the jugular foramen at the cranial base, in continuation with the sigmoid sinus. The vein is dilated at the beginning and is called the superior bulb. The vein descends along the neck in the carotid sheath, reaching the subclavian vein posteriorly to the sternal end of the clavicle, forming the brachiocephalic vein. At the end, the vein is dilated at the level of the valve and is called inferior bulb (Fig. 3.7). The internal jugular vein is directly anterior and lateral to the carotid artery. The landmark to locate the distal portion of the internal jugular vein is the apex of the bifurcation of the two heads of the sternocleidomastoid muscle (Fig. 3.8). The triangle formed by the two heads of the sternocleidomastoid muscle exposes the jugular vein for percutaneous puncture. The knowledge of this anatomic relationship is important for the internal jugular vein puncture and catheterization. Main tributaries of the internal jugular vein are the inferior petrosal sinus, facial, lingual, pharyngeal, superior and middle thyroid veins (Fig. 3.9). On the left, the thoracic duct opens near the union of the left subclavian vein and internal jugular vein. The right lymphatic duct ends at the same site on the right.

Inferior Petrosal Sinus

The inferior petrosal sinus leaves the skull through the anterior part of the jugular foramen and joins the superior jugular bulb (Figs. 3.10, 3.11).

Lingual Veins

There are two main lingual veins (see Fig. 2.8B). The dorsal lingual vein drains the dorsum and sides of the tongue and joins the lingual vein, which follows the lingual artery. It is a tributary of the internal jugular vein.

The deep lingual vein begins at the tip of the tongue and runs posteriorly along the inferior surface of the tongue. At the base of the tongue it is joined by the sublingual vein from the salivary gland, forming the vena comitans nerve hypoglossi until it joins the facial, internal jugular, or the lingual veins.

Pharyngeal Veins

The pharyngeal veins begin at the pharyngeal plexus external to the pharynx. These veins receive meningeal veins and a vein from the pterygoid canal. The pharyngeal veins end in the internal jugular vein, but sometimes may end in the facial, lingual, or superior thyroid veins.

Superior Thyroid Vein

The superior thyroid vein corresponds to the branches of the superior thyroid artery. It is formed by deep and superficial tributaries. It is joined by the superior laryngeal and cricothyroid veins. It is a tributary of the internal jugular vein or facial vein (Figs. 3.7, 3.9).

Middle Thyroid Vein

The middle thyroid vein drains the inferior part of the thyroid gland and receives some veins from the larynx and trachea. It crosses anterior to the common carotid artery and is a tributary of the distal part of the internal jugular vein (Figs. 3.7, 3.9).

Inferior Thyroid Veins

The inferior thyroid veins drain caudally the thyroid gland, arising from the venous network that communicates with the middle and superior thyroid veins. These veins form a plexus in front of the trachea, and from this plexus, the left vein arises and joins the left brachiocephalic vein, while the right descends to the right and joins the right brachiocephalic vein in the junction with the superior vena cava. Frequently, a common trunk opens in the vena cava or brachiocephalic vein (Figs. 3.7, 3.9).

Vertebral Vein

The vertebral vein is formed from numerous small tributaries from the internal vertebral plexuses, which arise from the vertebral canal above the posterior arch of the atlas. There are anastomoses with small veins from the muscles, and they form a vein that enters the foramen in the transverse process of the atlas and descends as a plexus around the vertebral artery. This plexus ends as a vein in the vertebral vein, which emerges from the transverse foramen of the sixth cervical vertebra, descends posterior to the artery, and opens in the posterior aspect of the brachiocephalic vein. Main tributaries are branches from the occipital vein, muscular veins, veins from the internal and external vertebral plexus, and also the anterior vertebral and deep cervical veins. Sometimes the first intercostal vein opens in the vertebral vein.

Anterior Vertebral Vein

The anterior vertebral vein arises from a plexus around the transverse processes of the upper cervical vertebra. It runs downwards parallel to the ascending cervical artery and joins the terminal vertebral vein.

Deep Cervical Vein

The deep cervical vein begins in the suboccipital region by communicating branches from the occipital vein and small veins from the deep muscles at the posterior aspect of the neck. It receives tributaries form the plexuses around the cervical vertebras. It ends in the lower part of the vertebral veins.

CRANIAL AND INTRACRANIAL VEINS AND DURAL VENOUS SINUSES

Diploic and Meningeal Veins

Diploic Veins (Fig. 3.1)

These veins run through channels in the diploë of some of the cranial bones, and present no valves. The diploic veins are large and present dilatation at intervals. The walls of these veins are thin and are only endothelium surrounded by elastic tissue. There are anastomoses of these veins with the meningeal veins, dural sinuses, and pericranial veins. The main diploic veins are frontal diploic vein; anterior temporal (parietal) diploic vein; posterior temporal (parietal) diploic vein; occipital diploic vein; numerous small diploic veins tributaries of the superior sagittal sinus.

Meningeal Veins

The meningeal veins are formed by venous plexus in the dura mater and join efferent veins in the outer dural layer, which subsequently connect to the superior sagittal sinus, other cranial sinus and diploic veins.

Supratentorial Venous System
(Fig. 3.11)

The supratentorial venous system is commonly divided in two groups, the superficial system of veins and the deep system of veins. The knowledge of these two different systems is important for the evaluation of venous occlusion, in the superficial group, through the abnormal filling sequence and flow pattern, and the evaluation of ventricular size and mass effect, in the deep system through displacement.

Superficial System of Veins
(Figs. 3.5, 3.6, 3.10, 3.12, 3.13, 3.14)

Above the Sylvian fissure, the lateral convexity of the brain is drained by the anterior frontal, central and parietal veins. These veins also receive venous drainage from the medial surface of the brain from the interhemispheric fissure, just before when they enter the superior sagittal sinus (SSS). The largest vein draining into the SSS is known as the vein of Trolard (Fig. 3.13), usually in the parietal region, above the Sylvian fissure.

The superficial middle cerebral vein (Fig. 3.6) drains the lateral aspect of the brain close to the Sylvian fissure. The superficial middle cerebral vein drains posteriorly into the transverse sinus but may also drain anteriorly into the deep middle cerebral vein.

The superficial portions of the brain, under the Sylvian fissure and the inferior aspect of the temporal and occipital lobes, drain directly into the transverse sinus. The largest lateral vein under the Sylvian fissure is called vein of Labbé (Fig. 3.12).

Deep System of Veins

The deep system of veins of the brain is formed by the internal cerebral veins, the basal veins of Rosenthal, and the thalamic veins. The site of drainage of this system is the Great Vein of Galen and subsequently into the straight sinus.

The two internal cerebral veins (Figs. 3.10, 3.14) run about 2 mm off the midline in a parallel manner, being useful to diagnose midline displacement. The internal cerebral veins drain the deep white matter around the frontal horns and the body of the lateral ventricles via medial and lateral subependymal veins.

The thalamostriate (subependymal) veins (Figs. 3.15, 3.16) outline the inferolateral wall of the body of the lateral ventricle. Seen from a frontal view, the distance from the superolateral corner of the thalamostriate veins and the internal cerebral vein corresponds to the width of the body of the lateral ventricles and should not be wider than 2 cm in normal subjects. Seen from a lateral view, the thalamostriate vein drains anteroinferiorly in a sulcus between the head of the caudate nucleus and the thalamus. The angle made by the thalamostriate vein as it drains into the internal cerebral vein is called the venous angle. A false venous angle is likely to occur when the thalamostriate vein is absent or small (Fig. 3.17). In this situation, the thalamostriate vein is replaced by a vein 0.5 to 1 cm posterior to it. The anterior septal veins are medial subependymal veins that drain the white matter around the frontal horns of the ventricles and genu of the corpus callosum. On a lateral view, the septal veins look like an anterior extension of the internal cerebral veins (Fig. 3.15). The body and atrium of the lateral ventricles are drained by other medial and lateral subependymal veins (Fig. 3.16). The medullary veins (Fig. 3.15) are small and drain into the subependymal veins. When detectable they are seen along the superior surface of the lateral ventricle.

The basal veins of Rosenthal (Fig. 3.18) are formed in the medial portion of the lateral cerebral fissures after receiving the deep middle cerebral veins, which are lateral branches from the insulae, the superior branches from the anterior perforated substances, anterior branches from the under surface of the frontal lobes, and medial branches from the interhemispheric fissures. The basal veins of Rosenthal leave the lateral cerebral fissures and course around the superior aspect of the uncus and pass posteriorly in the perimesencephalic cisterns to drain into the Great Vein of Galen. The basal veins also drain the inferior portion of the ventricles through the inferior ventricular veins (Fig. 3.25), the thalamus and the hippocampus, while circling the mesencephalon. The basal veins of Rosenthal usually drain posteriorly into the Great Vein of Galen, but when the mesencephalic portion of the vein does not segment properly, it may drain anteriorly into the sphenoparietal sinus or the superior petrosal sinus, and inferiorly into the lateral mesencephalic vein or anterior pontomesencephalic vein, or medially into the contralateral basal vein of Rosenthal through the posterior communicating vein (Fig. 3.5).

The Great Vein of Galen receives the internal cerebral veins, the basal veins of Rosenthal, the pericallosal veins, and the veins that drain the superior aspect of the posterior fossa. The Great Vein of Galen courses beneath the splenium of the corpus callosum and then communicates to the straight sinus. The posterior pericallosal vein indicates the position of the splenium of the corpus callosum.

Dural Sinuses (Fig. 3.10)

The superior sagittal sinus (SSS) is long and has a triangular shape and is located within the dura at its junction with the falx cerebri, about the midline projection. The SSS is connected laterally with the venous lacunae into which the arachnoid granulations drain. The SSS usually extends from the foramen cecum to the torcula herophili. In some cases, it is not formed anteriorly to the coronal suture. The frontal vein runs in the posterior direction, parallel to the midline, in the absence of the anterior SSS. The torcula herophili is the great connection of the venous drainage of the brain within the cranium. It receives the SSS, the straight sinus, and the occipital sinus (Fig. 3.19), and drains into the transverse sinus. One common variation is the diversion of the SSS into the right transverse sinus, while the straight sinus drains into the left transverse sinus.

The cavernous sinus (Figs. 3.5, 3.10, 3.20) constitutes the lateral border of the sella turcica and contains the oculomotor, trochlear, ophthalmic, and abducens nerves, as well as the internal carotid artery within it. Anteriorly, the superior and inferior ophthalmic veins drain into the cavernous sinus, connecting the facial vein via the angular vein to the cavernous sinus. Anterolaterally, the cavernous sinus receives the sphenoparietal sinus. The superficial Sylvian veins and the uncal veins (Fig. 3.5) occasionally drain into the cavernous sinus. The cavernous sinus drains posteriorly into the superior petrosal sinus (Fig. 3.20), which is located at the attachment of the falx to the petrous pyramid, connecting the cavernous sinus with the transverse/sigmoid sinuses. Posteroinferiorly, the cavernous sinus drains into the inferior petrosal sinus, which runs along the lower border of the pyramids towards the ventromedial part of the jugular foramen and enters the internal jugular vein, immediately below the skull base, passing through the pars nervosa of the jugular foramen (Figs. 3.11, 3.21). Inferiorly, the cavernous sinus drains into the pterygoid plexus through the foramina of Vesalius (venosum), ovale, rotundum, and lacerum (Fig. 3.22).

Right and left cavernous sinuses are interconnected by additional sinuses (Figs. 3.21, 3.22). The sinus intercavernous (sive coronarius) anterior is located between the anterior surface of the anterior pituitary lobe and the anterior sella margin, in or directly below the diaphragma sellae. It can be found in 76 to 85% of the cases. The sinus intercavernous (sive coronarius) posterior in most cases is larger than the anterior intercavernous sinus. It runs behind the posterior pituitary lobe, and in front of the posterior clinoid plate, and is observed in about 32% of the cases. The sinus intercavernous inferior is located in front of the sulcus, which delineates the border between anterior and posterior lobe of the pituitary. The sinus may be a single channel, often, however, it consists of multiple channels, with a diameter of 1 mm or less. The basilar plexus is a complex venous plexus spread on the clivus. It extends down to the foramen magnum with the surrounding marginal sinus and continues as internal and external vertebral venous plexus. Varying anastomoses with the cavernous sinus can be observed.

The venous drainage of the pituitary gland is complex (Fig. 3.23). Blood leaves the anterior lobe of the pituitary by numerous small hypophyseal veins. They empty into lateral adenohypophyseal veins, which converge into the confluent pituitary veins on the surface of the gland. These then course laterally to join the ipsilateral cavernous sinuses (Fig. 3.23). The cavernous sinuses are immediately lateral to the pituitary fossa.

Sequence of Venous Drainage

The angiographic sequence of venous drainage is constant. The evaluation of the sequence of venous drainage is important to detect venous occlusion or early venous drainage.

The superficial venous system fills sequentially from anterior to posterior with filling of the frontal and middle cerebral veins first. The parietal veins almost always fill after the frontal vein; then, the occipital veins and the vein of Labbé are filled. The last superficial vein to be filled is the vein of Trolard.

The deep venous system starts to fill later than the superficial venous system, and opacification lasts longer, due to slower blood flow. The thalamostriate veins, the internal cerebral veins, and the basal veins of Rosenthal usually fill at about the same time as the parietal veins. The last deep vein to fill is the septal vein.

Posterior Fossa Venous System (Figs. 3.20, 3.24, 3.25)

The superficial vessels of the posterior fossa may be used for the perception of the outline of the anterior border of the brain stem, cerebellopontine angles, vermis, and cerebellar hemispheres.

From a lateral point of view, the anterior margin of the pons and mesencephalon is outlined by the anterior pontomesencephalic vein, the superior vermis by both the superior vermian artery and vein, and the inferior surface of the cerebellar vermis by both the inferior vermian artery and vein. The brain stem can be separated from the vermis and cerebellar hemispheres by the precentral cerebellar vein superiorly and by the posterior medullary segment of the PICA inferiorly.

From an anteroposterior point of view, the antero-lateral surface of the midbrain is outlined by the posterior mesencephalic vein, while a rougher outline is provided by the superior cerebellar arteries. The anterior surface of the pons and its relationship to the cerebellopontine angles is outlined by the transverse pontine veins and the petrosal sinuses. The midline can be roughly approximated by studying the PICAs.

There are three major groups of veins in the posterior fossa, and they are identified accordingly to the direction of the flow.

The superior group drains into the great vein of Galen.

The anterior group drains into the petrosal sinus.

The posterior group drains into the torcula herophili and transverse sinus.

Superior Group

The precentral cerebellar vein (Figs. 3.25) originates in the precentral cerebellar fissure. It divides the posterior fossa into an anterior and a posterior compartment.

The posterior mesencephalic veins drain the posterior perforated substance and the cerebral peduncles. These veins are close to the cerebral peduncles and on a frontal view outline it. The posterior mesencephalic veins are more directly oriented to the Great Vein of Galen than to the basal veins of Rosenthal.

The superior vermian veins drain the superior aspect of the vermis and adjacent cerebellum. These veins outline the superior surface of the vermis.

Anterior Group

The anterior pontomesencephalic vein (Fig. 3.25) drains the interpeduncular fossa and the anterior surfaces of the pons and cerebellum. It outlines the anterior surface of the pons and is located posteriorly to the basilar artery. The anterior pontomesencephalic vein usually drains into the petrosal veins through the transverse pontine veins.

The petrosal veins (Fig. 3.20) are located in the cerebellopontine angles close to the porus acusticus. The petrosal veins receive tributaries from various directions and displays an irradiated shape. Main tributaries are transverse pontine veins (medial branches form the pons), superior hemispheric veins, veins of the greater horizontal fissure, and inferior hemispheric veins (lateral branches from the cerebellar hemispheres), brachial veins (superomedial branches from the wings of the precentral cerebellar fissure), and inferior branches from the hemispheric veins of the lateral recess (inferomedial branches from the cerebellar pontine fissure).

Posterior Group

The inferior vermian veins are formed by the superior and inferior retrotonsillar tributaries. They outline the inferior surface of the vermis.

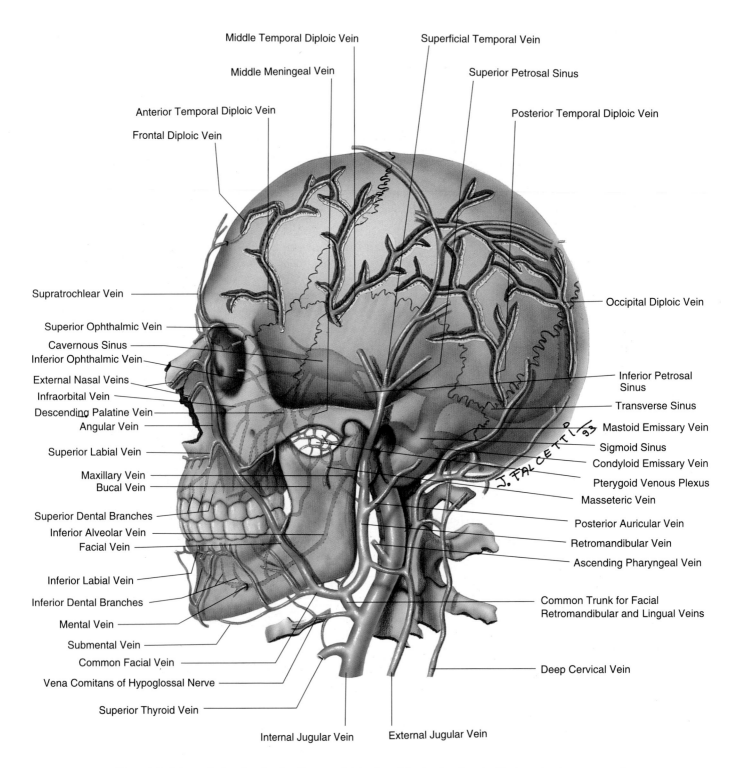

Middle Temporal Diploic Vein

Middle Meningeal Vein

Anterior Temporal Diploic Vein

Frontal Diploic Vein

Superficial Temporal Vein

Superior Petrosal Sinus

Posterior Temporal Diploic Vein

Supratrochlear Vein

Superior Ophthalmic Vein

Cavernous Sinus

Inferior Ophthalmic Vein

External Nasal Veins

Infraorbital Vein

Descending Palatine Vein

Angular Vein

Superior Labial Vein

Maxillary Vein

Bucal Vein

Superior Dental Branches

Inferior Alveolar Vein

Facial Vein

Inferior Labial Vein

Inferior Dental Branches

Mental Vein

Submental Vein

Common Facial Vein

Vena Comitans of Hypoglossal Nerve

Superior Thyroid Vein

Occipital Diploic Vein

Inferior Petrosal Sinus

Transverse Sinus

Mastoid Emissary Vein

Sigmoid Sinus

Condyloid Emissary Vein

Pterygoid Venous Plexus

Masseteric Vein

Posterior Auricular Vein

Retromandibular Vein

Ascending Pharyngeal Vein

Common Trunk for Facial Retromandibular and Lingual Veins

Deep Cervical Vein

J. FALCETTI 93

Internal Jugular Vein

External Jugular Vein

Figure 3.1. Schematic drawing showing the superficial veins of the head and neck. The bone has been removed for better visualization of the diploic veins.

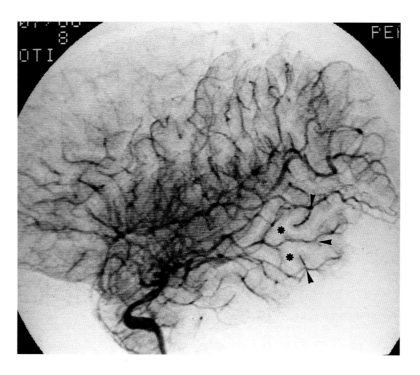

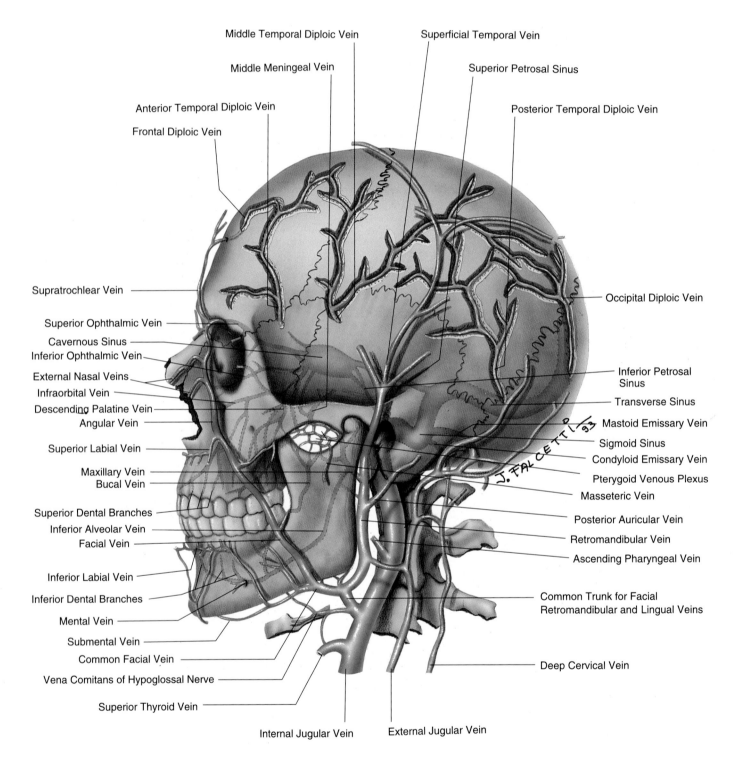

Figure 3.1. Schematic drawing showing the superficial veins of the head and neck. The bone has been removed for better visualization of the diploic veins.

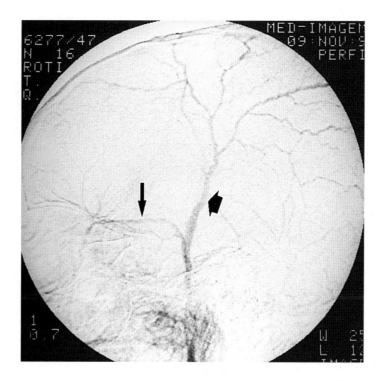

Figure 3.2. Veins of the scalp. Late phase of the external carotid injection. Lateral view. Superficial temporal vein (large short arrow) parietal branch. Frontal branch of the superficial temporal vein (zygomatico-orbitary vein) (arrow).

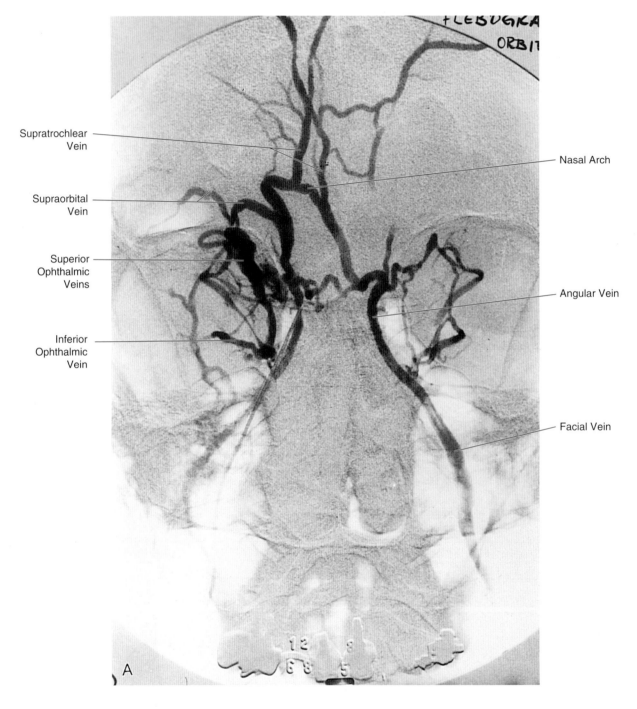

Figure 3.3. A, Frontal view of an orbital venogram showing the facial vein, the supratrochlear vein, and the superior ophthalmic vein. **B,** Lateral view of the same orbital venogram showing the superior and inferior ophthalmic vein, as well as the cavernous sinus.

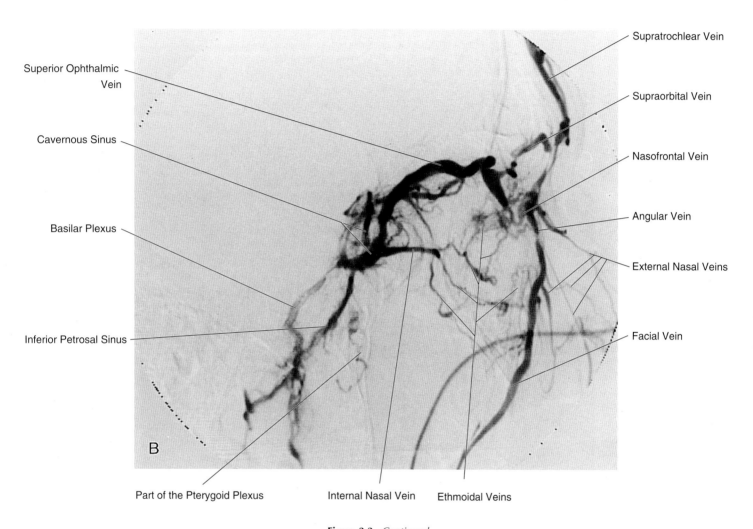

Figure 3.3. *Continued*

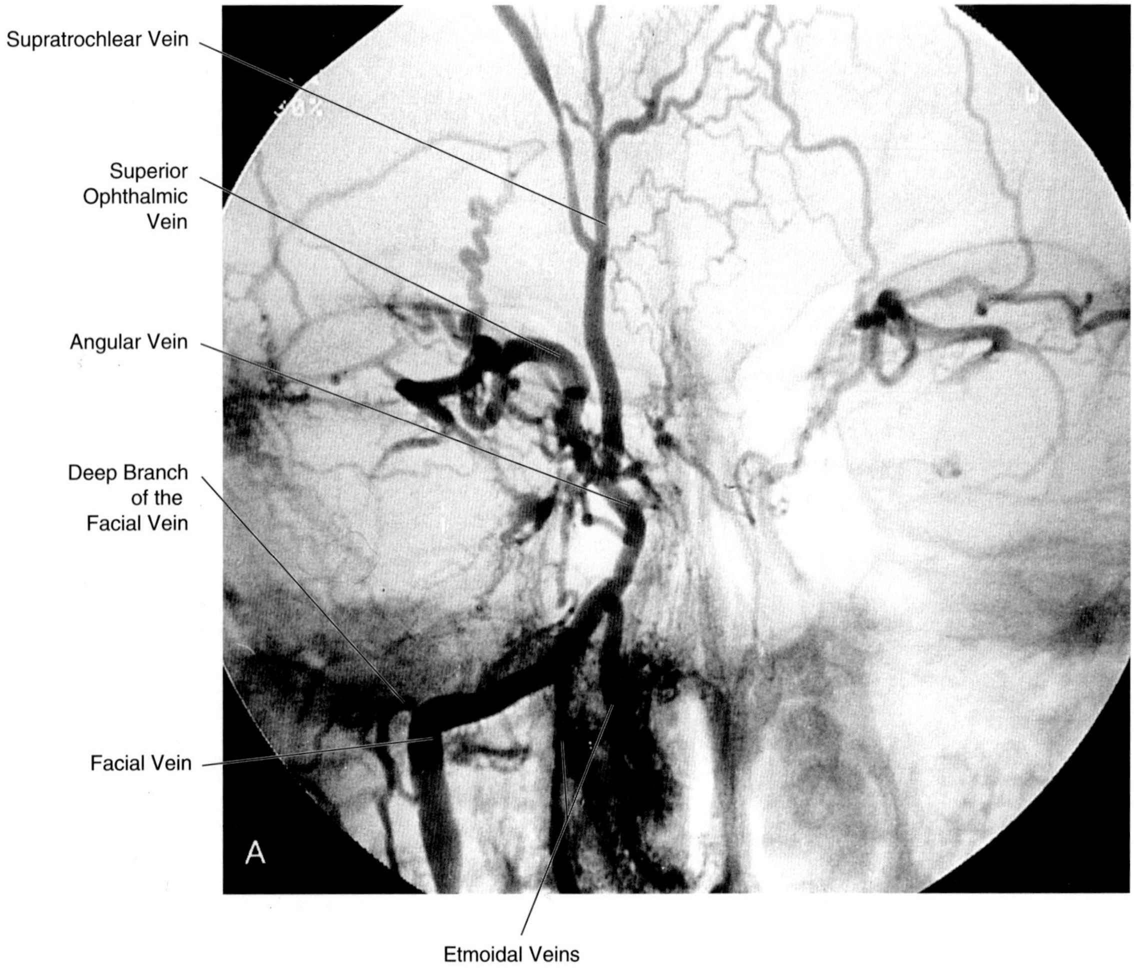

Supratrochlear Vein

Superior
Ophthalmic
Vein

Angular Vein

Deep Branch
of the
Facial Vein

Facial Vein

A

Etmoidal Veins

Figure 3.4. A, Frontal view of an orbital venogram showing mostly the right side. **B**, Lateral view of the orbital venogram, showing the facial vein, the superior ophthalmic vein and the internal maxillary vein.

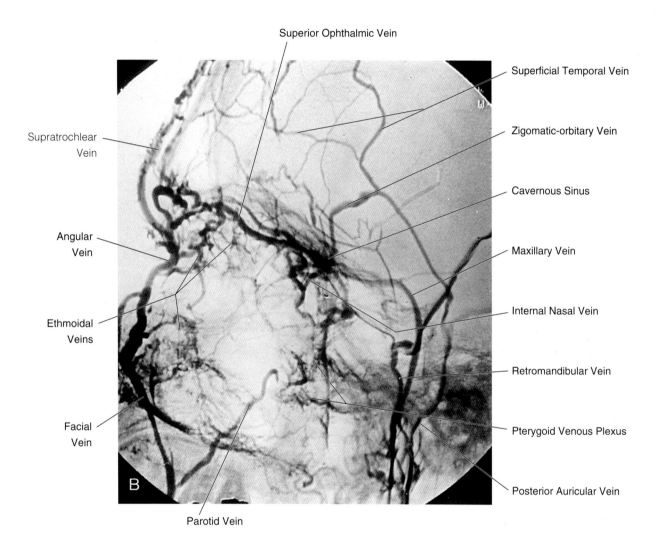

Figure 3.4. *Continued*

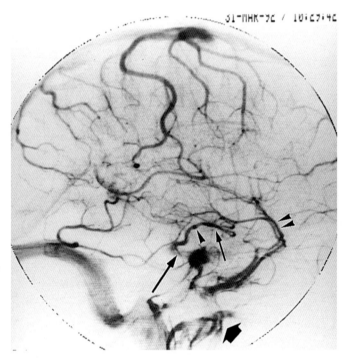

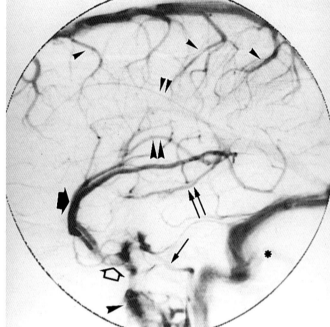

Figure 3.5. Venous phase of internal carotid arteriography. Lateral view. There is no dominance of the cortical venous groups. The superior group veins are larger than usual. The basal vein of Rosenthal in not complete. The first portion is visualized (arrow), draining inferiorly through an uncal vein (arrow head), into a tentorial sinus (large arrow) and, anteriorly, into the cavernous sinus. The superficial Sylvian vein (double arrow head) does not reach the cavernous sinus, draining instead to the pterygoid plexus (large short arrow).

Figure 3.6. Venous system of the brain. Late phase of an injection into the left internal carotid artery. Lateral view. The cortical venous drainage is dominantly done from the superficial Sylvian vein (large short arrow), draining to the cavernous sinus (open arrow) and to the pterygoid plexus (large arrow head) through the bone by a large vein. Veins of the superior group with smaller diameter (arrow heads). Inferior sagittal sinus (double arrow head). Basal vein of Rosenthal (double arrow). Retromastoid emissary vein (*). Inferior petrosal sinus (arrow). Internal cerebral vein (double large arrow head) higher than the usual.

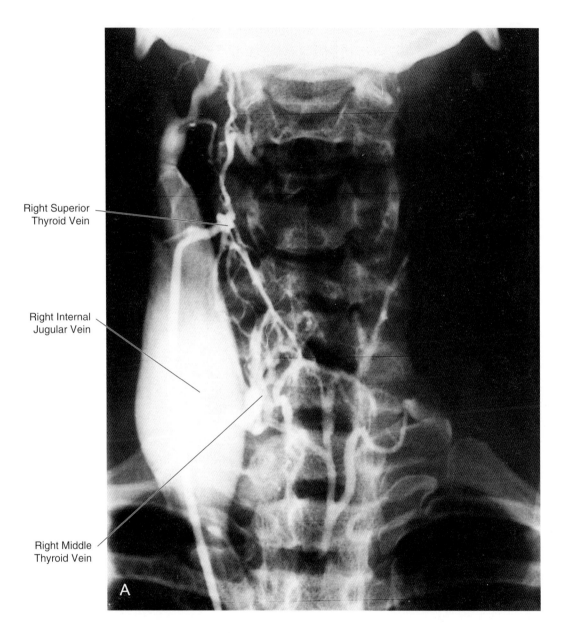

Right Superior
Thyroid Vein

Right Internal
Jugular Vein

Right Middle
Thyroid Vein

A

Figure 3.7. **A**, Venogram of the right internal jugular vein shows the dilatation of the inferior bulb. Note the
tributary selectively catheterized, superior thyroid vein. **B**, Venogram of the left internal jugular vein.
Note the superior thyroid vein, tributary of the internal jugular vein.

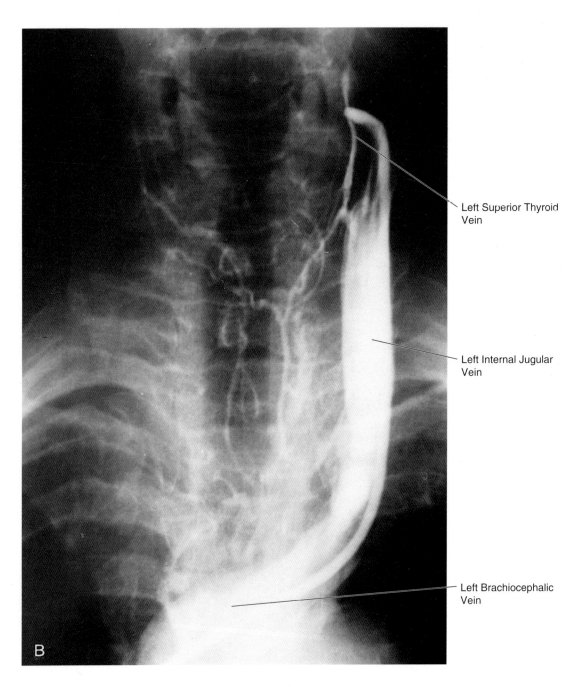

Left Superior Thyroid
Vein

Left Internal Jugular
Vein

Left Brachiocephalic
Vein

Figure 3.7. *Continued*

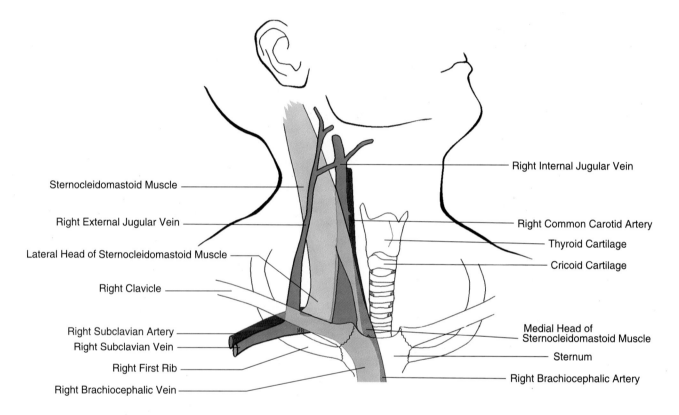

Figure 3.8. Internal jugular vein and subclavian vein anatomy at the level of the neck. Anterolateral view.
Note the triangle formed by the medial and lateral heads of the sternocleidomastoid muscle showing
as a window for puncture and catheterization of the internal jugular vein. The internal jugular
vein is lateral and anterior to the common carotid artery.

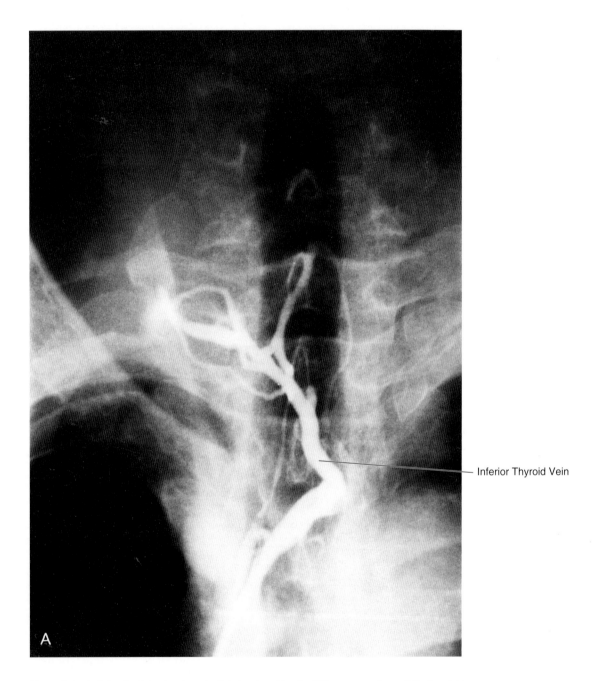

Inferior Thyroid Vein

Figure 3.9. **A**, Selective injection into the inferior thyroid vein, filling retrograde partially the right middle thyroid vein. **B**, Selective injection into the left superior thyroid vein. Note filling of the middle thyroid vein and the inferior thyroid vein.

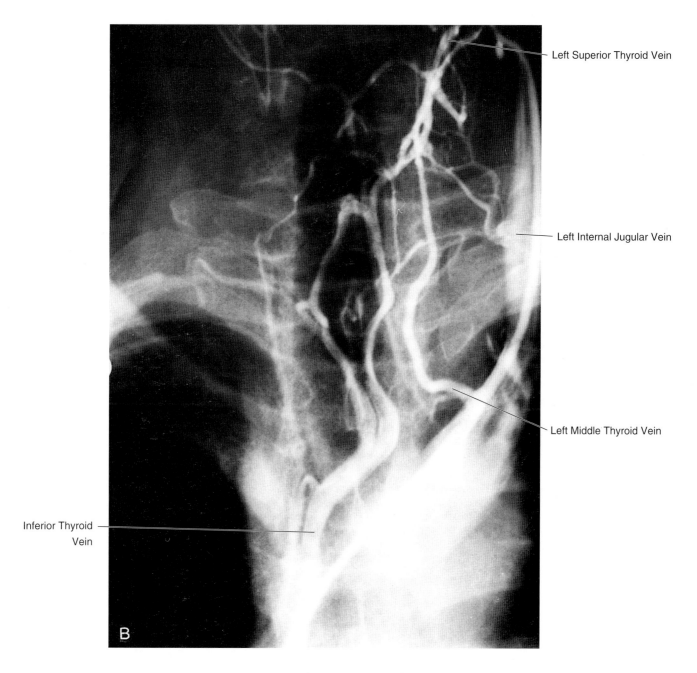

Left Superior Thyroid Vein

Left Internal Jugular Vein

Left Middle Thyroid Vein

Inferior Thyroid
Vein

Figure 3.9. *Continued*

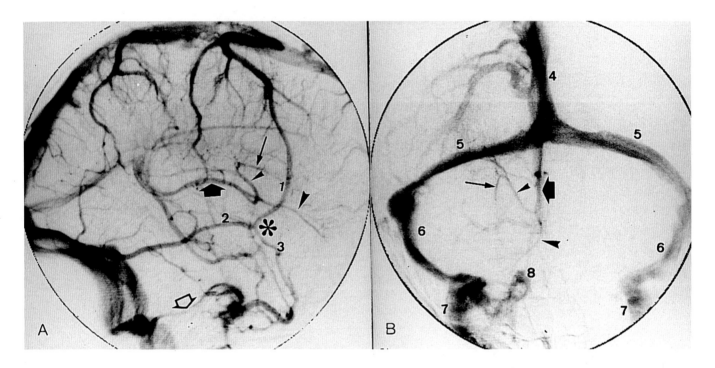

Figure 3.10. Late phase of injection of the internal carotid artery. Lateral view (A) and anterior view (B). Internal cerebral vein (large short arrow). Septal vein (large arrow head). Inferior thalamostriate vein (small arrow head). Longitudinal caudate vein (arrow). A, Anastomosis between the frontal vein (1), temporal vein (2), and superficial Sylvian vein (3). Inferior petrosal sinus (open arrow). B, Superior sagittal sinus (4), lateral sinus (transverse sinus) (5), sigmoid sinus (6), internal jugular veins (7), cavernous sinus (8).

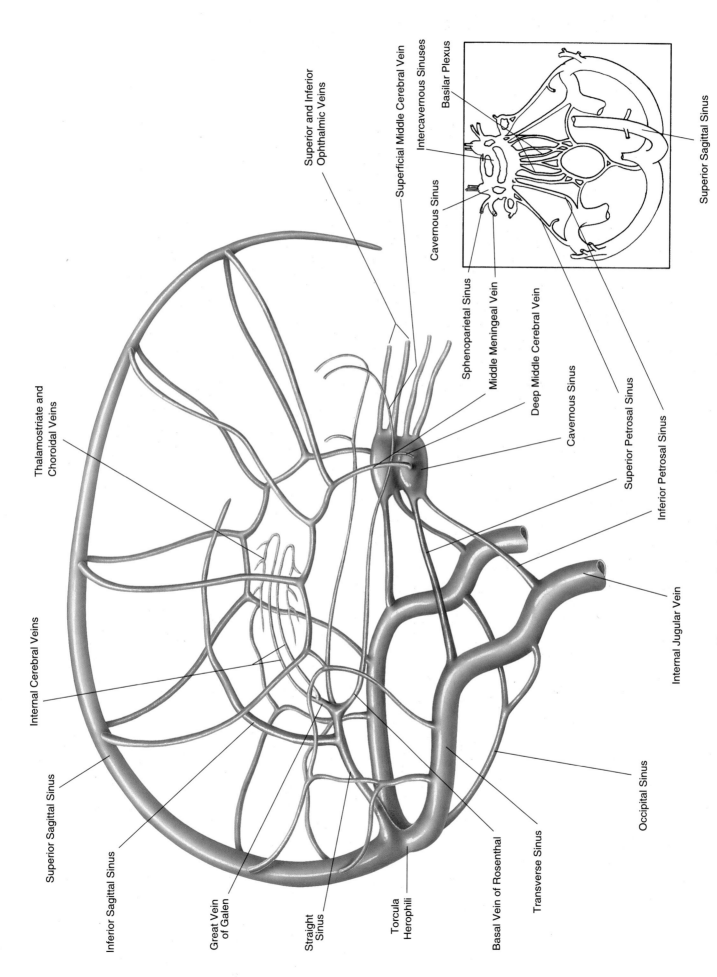

Superior and Inferior Ophthalmic Veins

Superficial Middle Cerebral Vein

Intercavernous Sinuses

Basilar Plexus

Superior Sagittal Sinus

Cavernous Sinus

Sphenoparietal Sinus

Middle Meningeal Vein

Deep Middle Cerebral Vein

Cavernous Sinus

Superior Petrosal Sinus

Inferior Petrosal Sinus

Internal Jugular Vein

Thalamostriate and Choroidal Veins

Internal Cerebral Veins

Superior Sagittal Sinus

Inferior Sagittal Sinus

Great Vein of Galen

Straight Sinus

Torcula Herophili

Basal Vein of Rosenthal

Transverse Sinus

Occipital Sinus

Figure 3.11. Schematic drawing of the intracranial venous system.

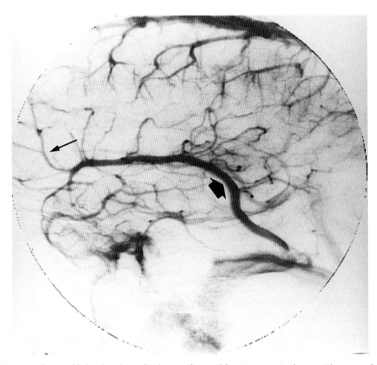

Figure 3.12. Late phase of injection into the internal carotid artery. Lateral view. The superficial venous drainage is dominantly done by a vena of Labbé (large short arrow). Note veins of the frontal lobe draining into the vena of Labbé.

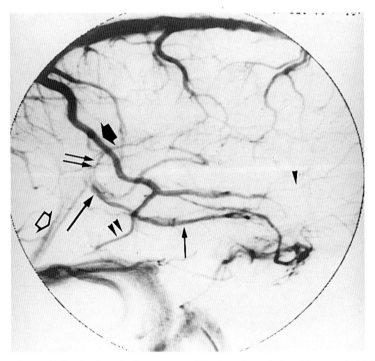

Figure 3.13. Late phase of injection into the internal carotid artery. Lateral view. The superficial brain drainage is predominantly by a vein of the Trolard type (large short arrow) with tributaries from the frontal lobe (arrow head) and temporal (double arrow head). The basal vein of Rosenthal is complete (short arrow). Posterior pericallosal vein (double arrow). Vein of Galen (long arrow). Straight sinus (open arrow).

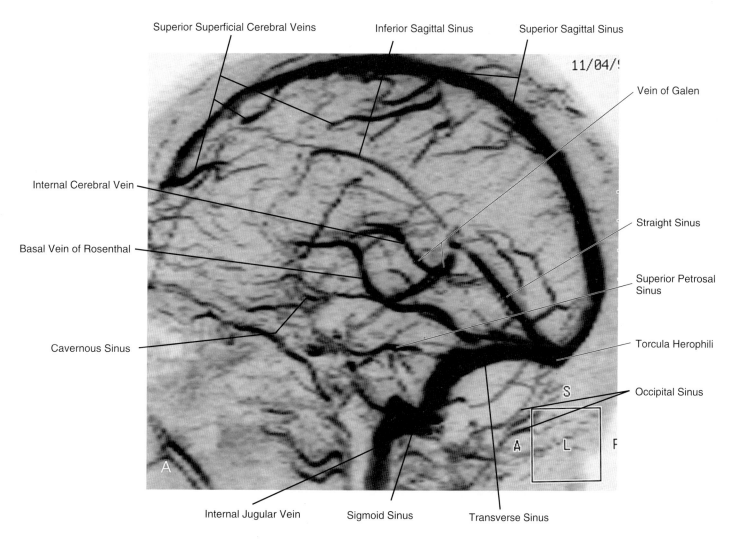

Figure 3.14. A, Lateral view of MRI of the veins of the head. **B**, Frontal view of the MRI of the veins of the head.

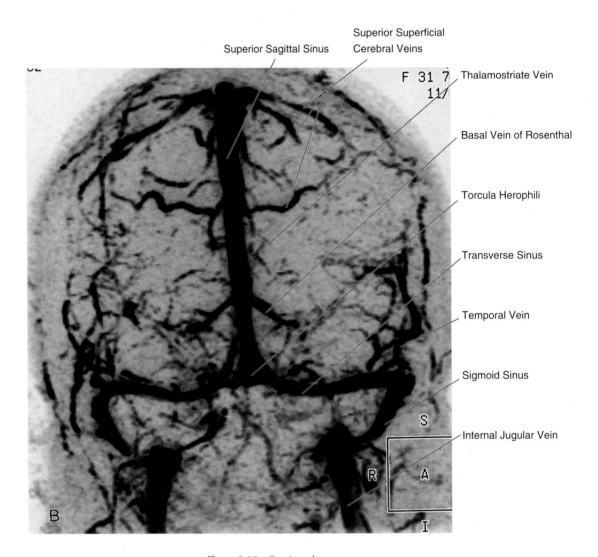

Figure 3.14. *Continued*

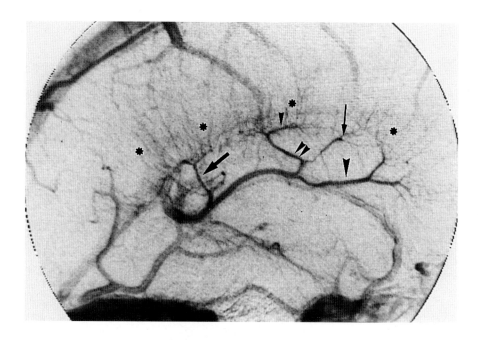

Figure 3.15. Medullary veins (*,*). Septal vein with two tributaries (large arrow head). Posterior caudal vein (small arrow head) and anterior caudal vein (arrow) draining into the thalamostriate vein (double arrow head). Middle atrial vein (large arrow).

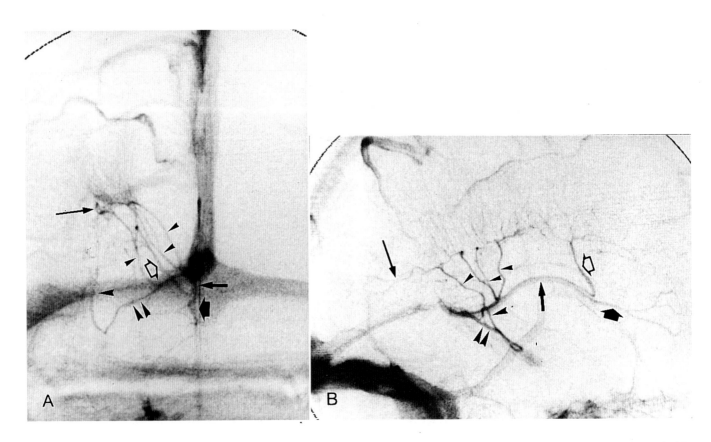

Figure 3.16. Late phase of injection at the internal carotid artery. Frontal view (A) and lateral view (B). Deep venous system. Septal vein (large short arrow). Thalamostriate vein (open arrow). Internal cerebral vein (large arrow). Vein of the occipital horn (long arrow). Lateral atrial vein (large arrow head) draining into the basal vein of Rosenthal (double arrow head). There are three medial atrial veins (small arrow heads), the most anterior one is more medial in the frontal view, the most posterior one is more lateral in the frontal view.

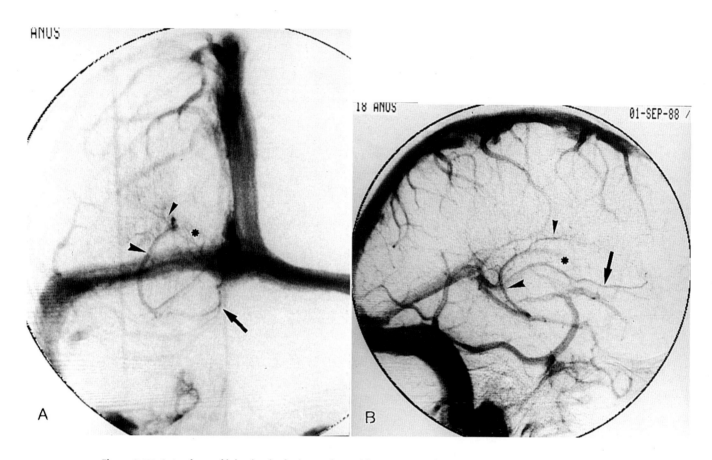

Figure 3.17. Late phase of injection in the internal carotid artery. Frontal view (A) and lateral view (B). The anterior and posterior longitudinal caudal veins (arrow head) drain to the inferior ventricular vein (large arrow head) with typical curved pattern. Absence of the thalamostriate vein (*). Septal vein (arrow).

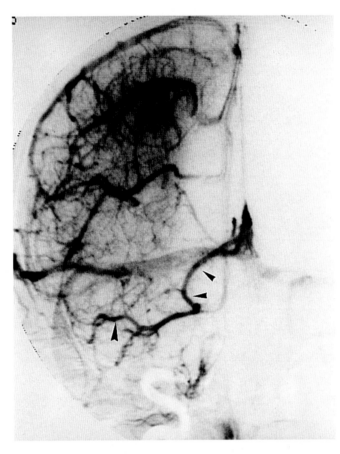

Figure 3.18. Late phase of injection in the internal carotid artery. Towne view. Typical presentation of the basal vein of Rosenthal. Deep Sylvian vein (large arrow head). Typical curve of the vein around the cerebral trunk (small arrow heads).

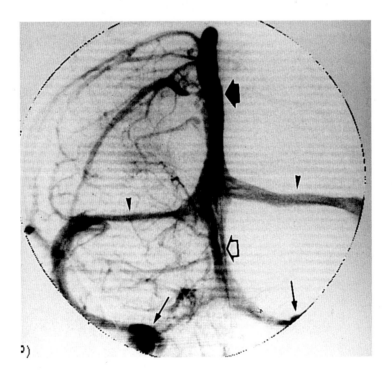

Figure 3.19. Venous system of the brain. Late phase of an injection into the right internal carotid artery. Anterior view. Occipital sinus (open arrow) draining to the internal jugular veins (arrows). Transverse sinus (arrow heads), the left is larger and higher than the right. Superior sagittal sinus (large arrow).

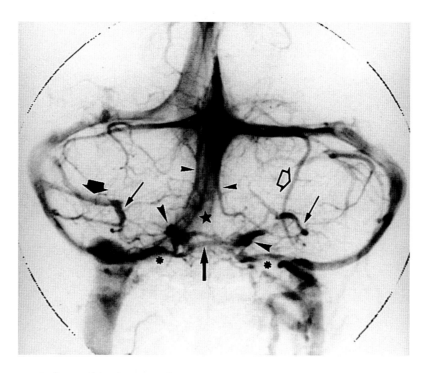

Figure 3.20. Vertebral artery injection. Late phase. Towne projection. Petrous veins (small arrows), draining to the superior petrous sinus on the right (large short arrow), cavernous sinus (large arrow head), intercavernous sinus (large arrow). Inferior vermian veins (small arrow heads). Inferior hemispheric veins (open arrow). Inferior petrosal sinus (*). Occipital sinus (★).

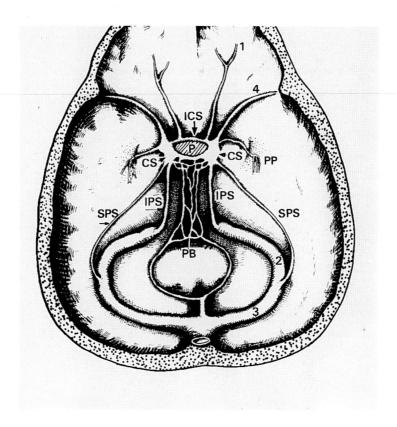

Figure 3.21. Schematic drawing of the anatomic relationships of the cavernous and inferior petrosal sinuses in axial view. The inferior petrosal sinus drains into the internal jugular vein. The superior petrosal sinus drains into the sinus sigmoid. 1. Ophthalmic vein. 2. Sinus sigmoid. 3. Sinus transversus. 4. Sinus sphenoparietalis. P, pituitary gland. CS, cavernous sinus. ICS, intercavernous sinus. IPS, inferior petrosal sinus. SPS, superior petrosal sinus. PP, pterygoid plexus. PB, plexus basilaris.

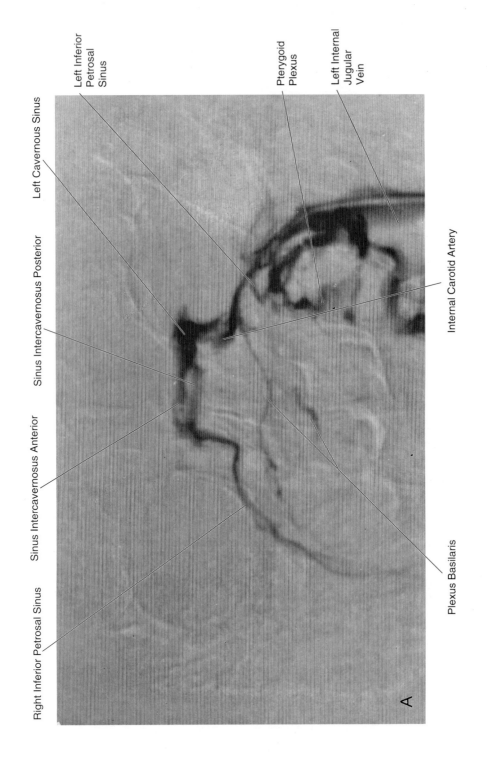

Left Inferior Petrosal Sinus

Left Cavernous Sinus

Sinus Intercavernosus Posterior

Sinus Intercavernosus Anterior

Right Inferior Petrosal Sinus

Pterygoid Plexus

Left Internal Jugular Vein

Internal Carotid Artery

Plexus Basilaris

A

Figure 3.22. Selective injection into the inferior petrosal sinuses showing retrograde filling of the intercavernous sinuses and pterygoid plexus. A, Frontal view. B, Lateral view. C, Towne view.

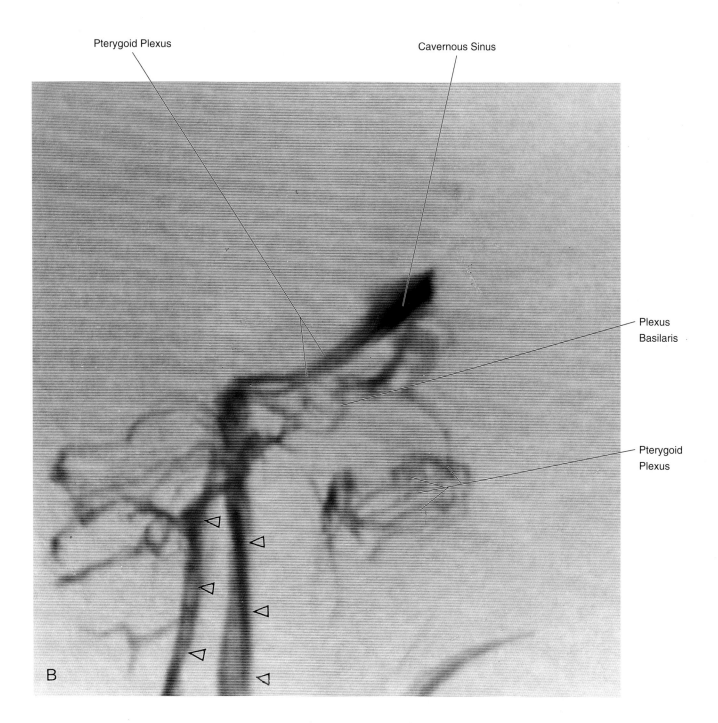

Figure 3.22. *Continued*

Right Sinus Cavernosus   Sinus Intercavernosus   Left Sinus Cavernosus

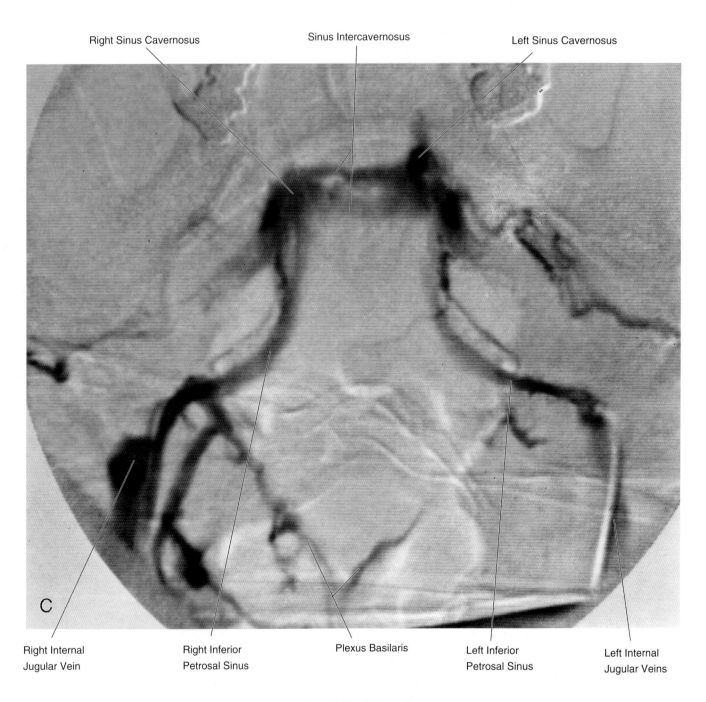

C

Right Internal
Jugular Vein

Right Inferior
Petrosal Sinus

Plexus Basilaris

Left Inferior
Petrosal Sinus

Left Internal
Jugular Veins

Figure 3.22. *Continued*

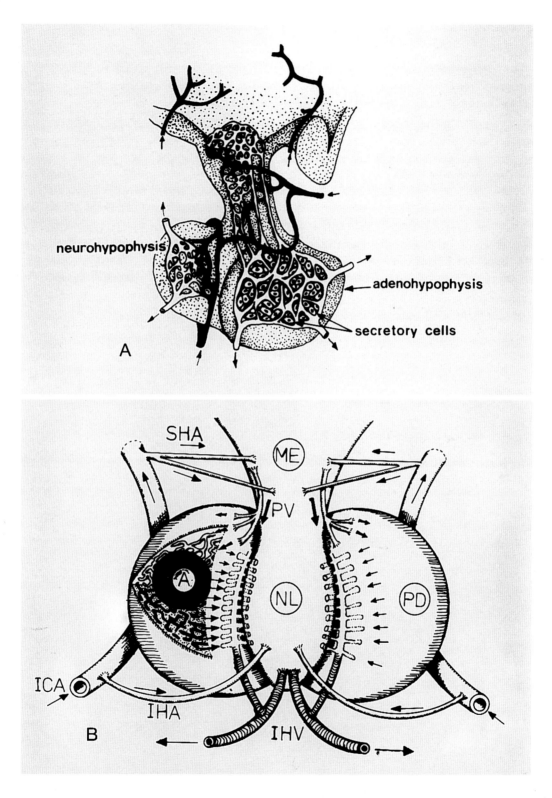

Figure 3.23. Schematic representation of the pituitary blood supply. Blood enters the median eminence (ME) through superior hypophyseal arteries (SHA) and the neural lobe (NL) through inferior hypophyseal arteries (IHA), which originate from the internal carotid arteries (ICA). The blood from the SHA passes through the primary capillary plexus of the pars distalis (PD). The inferior hypophyseal veins (IHV) drain both the neuro- and adenohypophysis to the left and right cavernous sinuses, respectively.

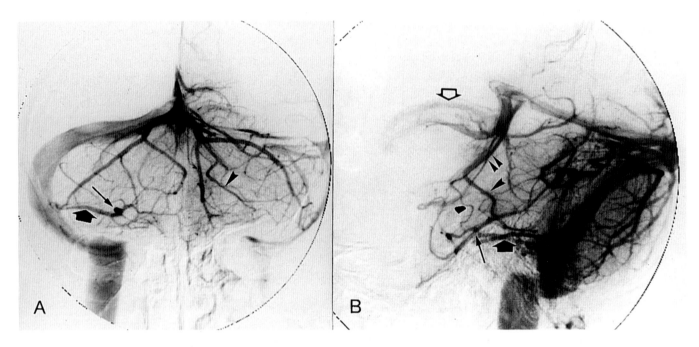

Figure 3.24. Late phase of injection in the vertebral artery. Anterior view (A) and lateral view (B). Petrosal vein (arrow). Superior petrosal sinus (large short arrow). Latero mesencephalic vein (large arrow head). Choroidal vein (open arrow). Posterior mesencephalic vein (double small arrow head).

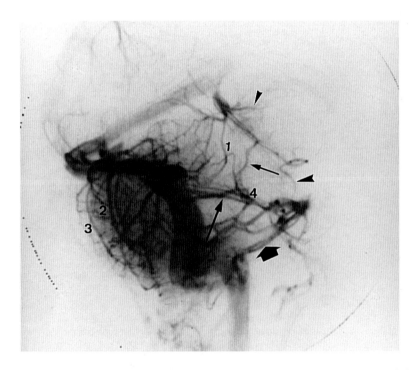

Figure 3.25. Late phase of injection in the vertebral artery. Lateral view. Anterior pontomesencephalic vein (large arrow head). Posterior thalamic vein (small arrow head). Lateromesencephalic vein (arrow). Vein of the cerebellar pre central fissure (1). Inferior vermian vein (2). Hemispheric veins (3). Petrosal veins (4). Superior petrosal sinus (long arrow). Inferior petrosal sinus (large short arrow).

4

LYMPHATIC SYSTEM OF THE HEAD AND NECK

The lymph nodes of the head and neck have a terminal group and a number of intermediary groups. The terminal group is associated with the carotid sheath and is called the deep cervical group. All the lymph vessels of the head and neck drain into this group, directly or indirectly. The efferents from the deep cervical lymph nodes comprise what is called the jugular trunk (Fig. 4.1).

DEEP CERVICAL LYMPH NODES

These are the nodes located along the carotid sheath. They are divided in superior and inferior groups.

Upper Deep Cervical Lymph Nodes

These lymph nodes drain in the upper part of the internal jugular vein. Efferents from this group pass to the lower deep cervical group and direct to the jugular trunk. The jugulodigastric group of nodes is related to the drainage of the tongue.

Lower Deep Cervical Lymph Nodes

These lymph nodes are partly deep to the lower sternocleidomastoid and extend into the subclavian triangle. The jugulo-omohyoid lymph node of this group drains the tongue. The efferents from the lower deep cervical lymph nodes join the jugular trunk.

LYMPHATIC DRAINAGE OF THE SUPERFICIAL TISSUES OF THE HEAD AND NECK

There are several groups concerned with the drainage of the superficial tissues of the head and neck. Most of the superficial tissues are drained by vessels that drain into the neighboring groups of node and whose efferents drain into the deep cervical lymph nodes.

The regional groups are as follows: (Fig. 4.1)

In the head
  Occipital Lymph Nodes
  Retroauricular (Mastoid) Lymph Nodes
  Parotid Lymph Nodes
  Buccal (Facial) Lymph Nodes
In the neck
  Submandibular Lymph Nodes
  Submental Lymph Nodes
  Anterior Cervical Lymph Nodes
  Superficial Cervical Lymph Nodes

Lymphatic Drainage of the Scalp and Ear (Fig. 4.2)

The lymphatic vessels from the forehead, the temporal region, and the upper half of the lateral surface of the auricle and the anterior wall of the external acoustic meatus drain through the superficial parotid lymph nodes. These nodes are located in front of the tragus or on the fascia of the parotid gland and also drain the lymph from the eyelids and the skin over the zygomatic bone. The efferents drain into the upper deep cervical lymph nodes.

The posterior aspect of the auricle and the scalp on the lateral aspect of the skull drain to the upper deep cervical lymph nodes and some part of it to the retroauricular group.

The retroauricular lymph nodes are superficial to the sternocleidomastoid attachment on the mastoid. The efferents drain into the upper deep cervical lymph nodes.

The lobule of the auricle, the inferior meatus and the skin over the angle of the mandible are drained by vessels that go to the superficial cervical lymph nodes or to the upper deep cervical lymph nodes.

The superficial cervical lymph nodes are located along the external jugular vein, superficial to the sternocleidomastoid. Some of the efferents of this group may join the upper deep cervical lymph nodes and some join the lower deep cervical lymph nodes.

The occipital region is drained partly to the occipital group of lymph nodes and partly by a trunk along the posterior border of the sternocleidomastoid reaching the lower deep cervical lymph nodes.

113

Lymphatic Drainage of the Face (Fig. 4.2)

There is a lymphatic plexus in the face, including the frontal scalp, the superior and inferior eyelids and conjunctiva, the caruncula lacrimalis that drains part to the superficial parotid lymph nodes and to the deep parotid lymph nodes. The more medial lymphatics follow the course of the facial vein and terminate in the submandibular group of lymph nodes.

The submandibular group of lymph nodes are located under the deep cervical fascia in the region of the submandibular gland. They receive afferents from the submental, buccal, and lingual group of lymph nodes. The efferents drain into the upper and lower deep cervical lymph nodes.

The external nose, cheek and upper lip, and lateral part of the lower lip drain to the submandibular nodes.

The central part of the lower lip, the floor of the mouth and the tip of the tongue drain to the Submental Group of Lymph Nodes. This group of lymph nodes is located on the mylohyoid between the anterior bellies of the two digastric. Receive afferents from both sides. Efferents go to the Submandibular and Jugulo-omohyoid Nodes.

Lymphatic Drainage of the Superficial Tissues of the Neck

Many of the vessels draining the superficial tissues of the neck go to the upper or lower deep cervical lymph nodes. Some of these vessels drain into the superficial cervical and occipital lymph nodes.

LYMPHATIC DRAINAGE OF THE DEEPER TISSUES OF THE NECK

The deeper tissues of the head and neck drain to the deep cervical lymph nodes either directly, or indirectly through one of the mentioned groups. There are additional groups of lymph nodes concerned with the drainage of the deeper tissues, including the retropharyngeal lymph nodes, paratracheal lymph nodes, lingual lymph nodes, infrahyoid lymph nodes, prelaryngeal and pretracheal lymph nodes.

Lymphatic Drainage of the Nasal Cavity, Nasopharynx, and Middle Ear

The lymphatic drainage of the anterior nasal cavity is through the vessels that drain the skin over the nose to the submandibular nodes. The remaining nasal cavity, paranasal tissues, nasopharynx and pharyngeal end of the auditory tube drain to the upper deep cervical nodes, directly or through the retropharyngeal lymph nodes.

Lymphatic Drainage of the Larynx, Trachea, and Thyroid Gland

There is an upper and a lower group of lymph vessels at the larynx, divided by the vocal fold. The two systems anastomose on the posterior wall.

There is a dense lymphatic network in the walls of the trachea. The cervical part is drained to the pretracheal and paratracheal nodes, or directly to the nodes of the Lower Deep Cervical Group.

The thyroid gland is drained mainly to the tracheal plexus. Laterally, the gland is drained to the deep cervical lymph nodes. Some vessels may enter the thoracic duct directly.

Lymphatic Drainage of the Mouth, Teeth, Tonsil, and Tongue

The lymphatic vessels of the mouth drain to the submandibular lymph nodes, upper deep cervical, and retropharyngeal lymph nodes.

The teeth drain to the submandibular and deep cervical lymph nodes. The tonsil lymph vessels drain into the upper deep cervical lymph nodes. The tongue has a widely distributed lymphatic drainage, but drains mainly to the anterior or middle submandibular lymph nodes, but also to the jugulo-omohyoid lymph node and jugulodigastric lymph nodes.

Lymphatic Drainage of the Pharynx and Cervical Esophagus

The pharynx and cervical esophagus drain to the deep cervical nodes directly or indirectly through the retropharyngeal and paratracheal nodes. From the epiglottis, the lymph vessels drain to the infrahyoid nodes.

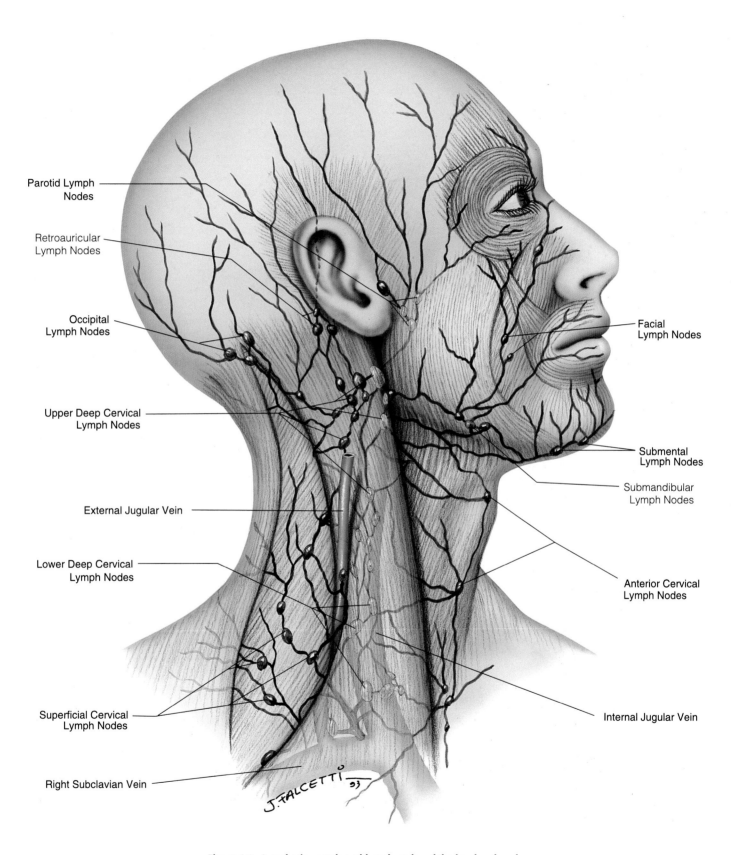

Parotid Lymph Nodes

Retroauricular Lymph Nodes

Occipital Lymph Nodes

Upper Deep Cervical Lymph Nodes

External Jugular Vein

Lower Deep Cervical Lymph Nodes

Superficial Cervical Lymph Nodes

Right Subclavian Vein

Facial Lymph Nodes

Submental Lymph Nodes

Submandibular Lymph Nodes

Anterior Cervical Lymph Nodes

Internal Jugular Vein

Figure 4.1. Lymphatic vessels and lymph nodes of the head and neck.

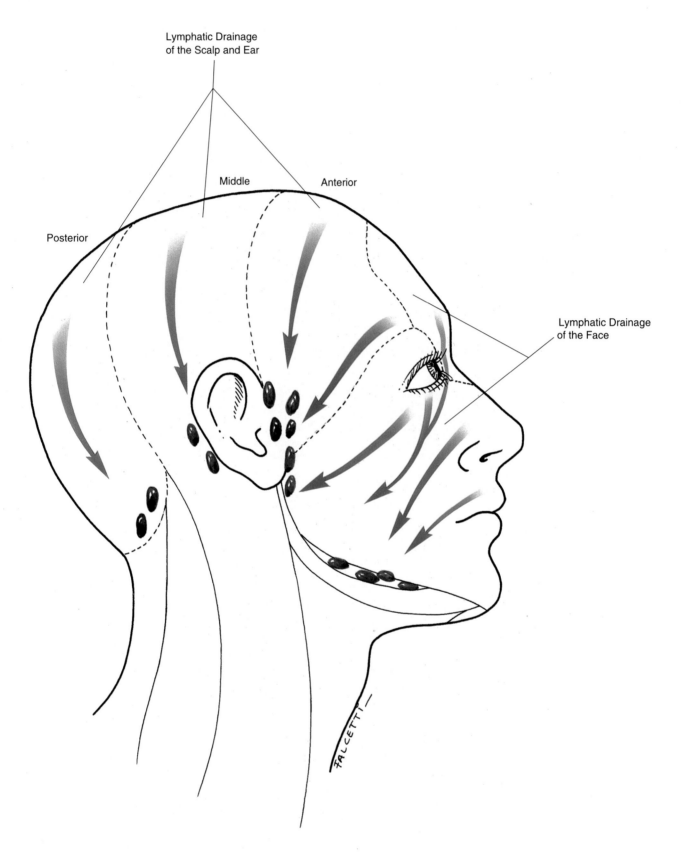

Figure 4.2. Main lymphatic drainage zones of the scalp and ear and of the face and frontal scalp.

5

ARTERIES OF THE SPINAL CORD AND SPINE

The arterial supply of the cervical spinal cord arises from several branches from the subclavian artery (Figs. 5.1, 5.2), vertebral artery (Fig. 5.3), deep cervical artery (Fig. 5.4), ascending cervical artery, while the thoracolumbar segment is vascularized by branches of the thoracoabdominal aorta through the intercostal and lumbar arteries, and occasionally from the iliac and sacral arteries as well. The spinal cord has two almost independent arterial systems, or longitudinal anastomotic chains, one anterior and two posterior.

In the upper cervical region, the anterior spinal artery originates from the junction of the intradural segment of the vertebral arteries, just below the basilar artery (Fig. 5.5). In all other segments, the arteries cross through the intervertebral foramina to reach the intrathecal level. These are called segmental arteries (intercostal and lumbar arteries). The segmental artery divides into an anterior branch (along the costal groove) and a posterior branch to the spine. The posterior branch originates the muscular branches and the medial radiculomedullary artery. The radicular artery further bifurcates into two branches, the dorsal and ventral vertebral branches and continues as the radicular artery and gives off a ganglionic branch and divides into an anterior spinal radicular artery and a posterior spinal radicular artery, following each anterior and posterior nerve root. In some preferential levels, these arteries are larger and constitute the anterior and posterior radiculomedullary arteries, proceeding as direct connections within the radicular artery and the longitudinal anterior and posterior anastomotic chains on the spinal cord surface (Fig. 5.6).

The anterior spinal artery is located in the midline on the ventral aspect of the cord lying in the groove of the anterior median fissure of the spinal cord. It is formed by the union of two branches from the terminal portion of the vertebral artery at the level of the foramen magnum. The anterior spinal artery descends as a single trunk (Fig. 5.7) in the entire length of the ventral aspect of the medulla spinalis to the conus medullaris. It is reinforced by a succession of small spinal rami at the cervical level from the vertebral arteries and by larger branches from the ascending cervical artery a the level C4-C6. Most of the tributaries in the lower two thirds of the cervical spinal cord are derived from the deep cervical artery at the level C6-T1. The superior intercostal artery may also send a branch to the spinal arteries. The anterior spinal artery continues downwards being reinforced by branches from the thoracic and abdominal aorta down to the conus medullaris, continuing along the cauda equina ending as a fine artery at the filum terminale. In that level, there are anastomoses with branches from the iliolumbar artery. The anterior radicular arteries joining the anterior spinal artery varies considerably in size, number, and location. The total varies from 3 to 15 with an average of 7. The cervical region of the spinal cord receives an average of three arteries, the thoracic region has an average of three to four, and the lumbar region has an average of one. The position of the great anterior radicular artery, also called artery of Adamkiewicz, varies from T8 to L3 (Figs. 5.8, 5.9, 5.10), being often the only ventral feeder to the lower thoracic and lumbosacral cord (Fig. 5.11). The size of the anterior spinal artery usually tapers gradually from the lower part of the cervical region down to the middle or lower thoracic region, also narrowing in the upper thoracic region in some cases. At the point of anastomoses with the artery of Adamkiewicz, an enlargement of the anterior spinal artery, usually occurs, remaining constant in size down to the lower end of sacral region, being reduced at that point to a tiny vessel, after giving off communicating branches, called rami cruciantes, to the posterior spinal arteries. This tiny artery may have an anastomoses with branches of the iliolumbar artery.

The posterolateral spinal artery arise from the posterior rami of the vertebral artery, but occasionally from the posterior inferior cerebellar artery (PICA). They run along the dorsolateral surface of the spinal cord, posterior but near to the entrance of the posterior nerve roots, receiving additional supply from the posterior radicular arteries. There are free anastomoses between the posterior radicular arteries, as well as with the corresponding vessels on the opposite side, forming an arterial network between the two posterior spinal arteries. Some branches pass over the lateral surface of the spinal cord and make tiny anastomotic connections with branches from the anterior spinal artery. The posterior spinal arteries are usually distinct vessels, but they are smaller than those of the anterior aspect. At the lower end of the spinal cord, the posterior spinal arteries communicate with the anterior spinal artery via the rami cruciantes (Fig. 5.9).

The knowledge of the pelvic vasculature to the spinal cord and femoral and sciatic nerves is important for embolization procedures. The inferior and superior lateral sacral arteries, which are branches of the posterior division of the internal iliac artery, give off spinal arteries that enter the spinal canal via the anterior sacral foramina. The inferior gluteal artery, which is usually a branch of the anterior division of the internal iliac artery, supplies the sciatic nerve via the sciatic artery. The sciatic artery is a small vessel that comes off of the descending branch of the inferior gluteal artery. The iliolumbar artery, another branch of the posterior division of the internal iliac artery, supplies the region of the femoral nerve as it passes over the iliac wing via an iliac branch that perforates the iliacus muscle.

There is the arterial pial plexus made by circumferential branches from the anterior and posterior spinal arteries, forming the pial arterial network. Small branches from the pial arterial plexus penetrate into the substance of the spinal cord to supply the adjacent white and gray matter (Fig. 5.6).

The nutrient vessels of the spinal cord are divided into a central and a peripheral arterial system. The central system derives from the anterior spinal artery, and the blood flow becomes centrifugal. In the peripheral system, the blood comes from the posterior spinal arteries and the pial arterial plexus, and the blood has a centripetal flow.

The gray matter of the spinal cord has a dense capillary network, best developed within the anterior and lateral gray horns, whereas the white matter is poorly supplied and the capillaries form wide meshes extended longitudinally along the nerve fibers.

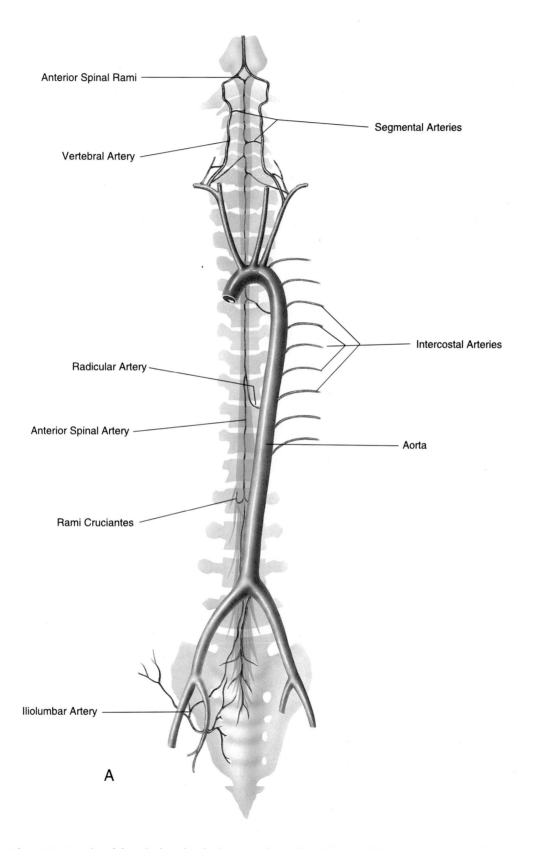

Anterior Spinal Rami

Segmental Arteries

Vertebral Artery

Intercostal Arteries

Radicular Artery

Anterior Spinal Artery

Aorta

Rami Cruciantes

Iliolumbar Artery

A

Figure 5.1. Arteries of the spinal cord and spine. A, Relationships of the spinal feeders with the vertebral levels and the aorta and branches in an anteroposterior view. **B**, Relationships of the spinal feeders with the vertebral levels and the aorta in a lateral view.

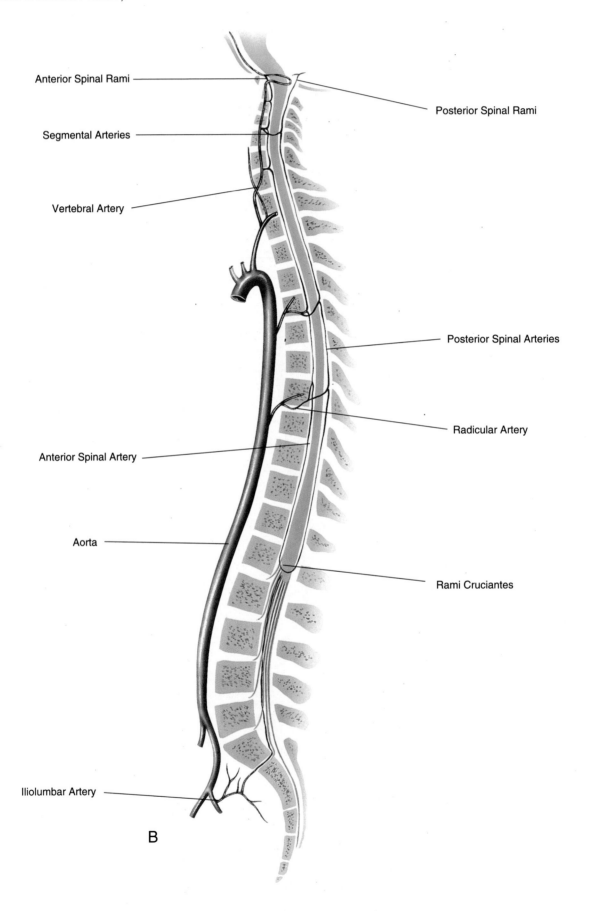

Anterior Spinal Rami

Posterior Spinal Rami

Segmental Arteries

Vertebral Artery

Posterior Spinal Arteries

Radicular Artery

Anterior Spinal Artery

Aorta

Rami Cruciantes

Iliolumbar Artery

B

Figure 5.1. *Continued*

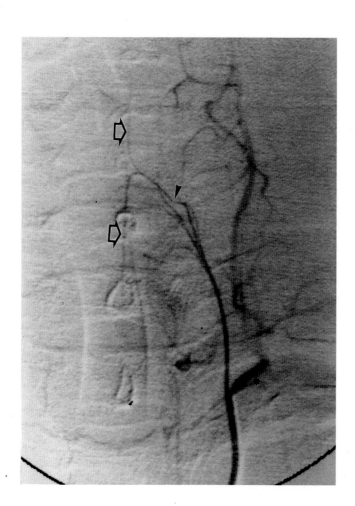

Figure 5.2. Low anterior cervical spinal artery (open arrows) originated directly from the left subclavian artery (*).
Note narrowing of the radiculomedullary artery when entering at the dura mater (arrow head).

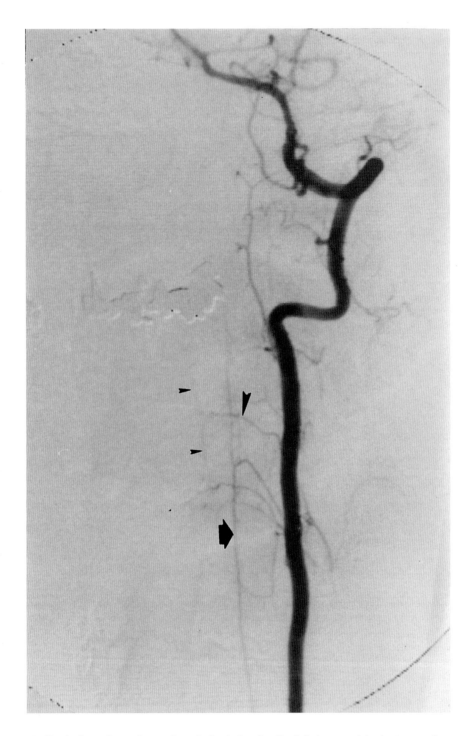

Figure 5.3. Cervical anterior and posterior spinal arteries visualized during a vertebral artery angiogram. The anterior spinal artery is small (small arrow head) and the radiculomedullary artery originates in the left vertebral artery (arrow head). The left posterior spinal artery (arrow) is larger and is also connected to the left vertebral artery. Multiple muscular arteries are observed.

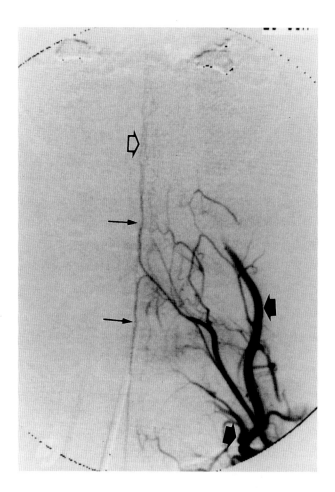

Figure 5.4. Cervical anterior spinal artery (cervical enlargement) (arrows), arising from the deep cervical artery (large short arrows). The ascending branch is duplicated (open arrow).

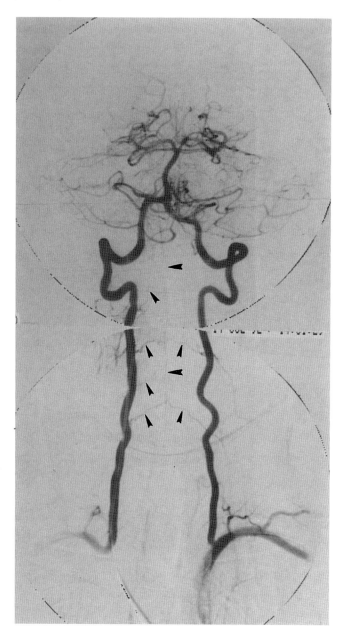

Figure 5.5. Anteroposterior view of an angiogram of both vertebral arteries showing the anterior spinal artery (large arrow heads) and the connections with the vertebral system just below the basilar artery and with the radiculomedullary arteries (small arrow heads).

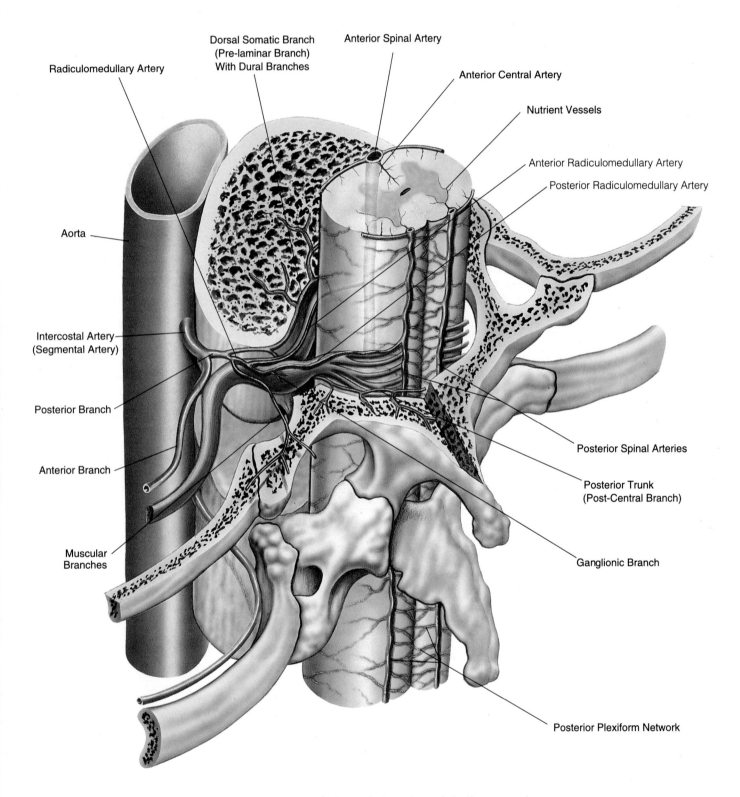

Figure 5.6. Radiculomedullary, spinal arteries, and plexiform network.

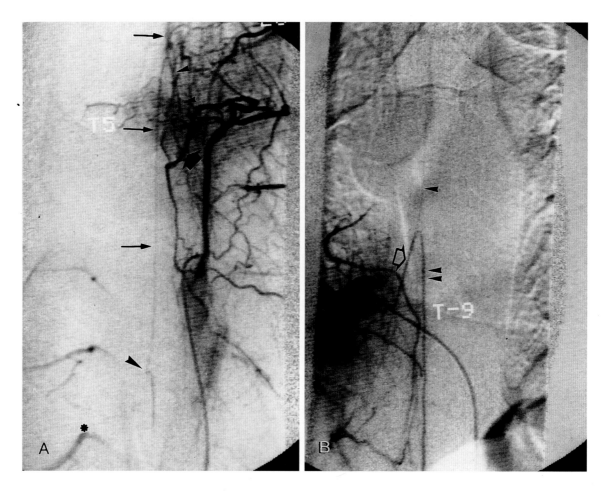

Figure 5.7. A, Injection at the 5th right posterior intercostal showing the anterior radicular artery (arrow) at the high thoracic region anastomosed with the anterior spinal artery (Adamkiewicz artery) (large arrow head). 9th right posterior intercostal artery (*). Note the ascending direction of the radicular artery (small arrow heads), different from the descending direction of the muscular branch (large short arrow). **B**, Injection at the 9th right posterior intercostal artery. Anterior radiculomedullary artery (Adamkiewicz) (open arrow), with the descending branch (double arrow heads) and ascending branch (arrow head). A and B show the continuous anterior spinal axis at the thoracic region.

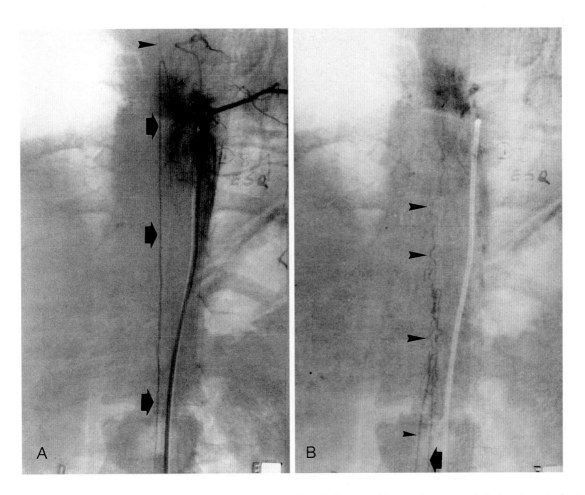

Figure 5.8. 8th left intercostal artery. Anterior view. The anterior spinal artery is well visualized at the thoracolumbar segment (Adamkiewicz). Arterial phase (A) and venous (B). **A,** Anterior radiculomedullary artery (small arrow head) with typical ascending curve. Anterior ascending spinal branch (large arrow head) and descending branch, larger and longer (large arrows). **B,** Anterior spinal vein with the typical tortuous aspect, all along the thoracolumbar medulla (large arrow heads). Typical straight aspect of a radiculomedullary vein following a nerve root exiting the dura mater (small arrow head). Vein of the filum terminalis (large arrow).

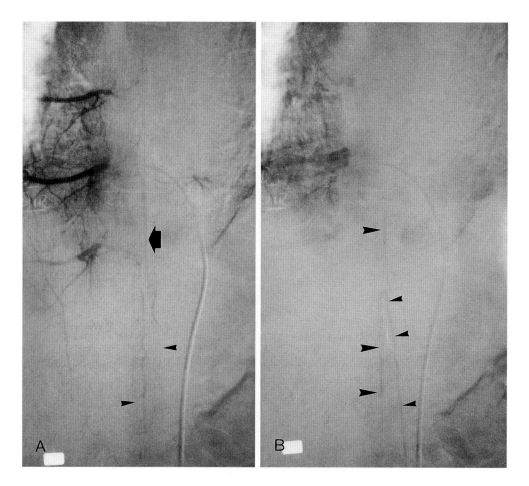

Figure 5.9. 9th right intercostal artery. Anteroposterior view. Anterior spinal artery in the thoracolumbar segment. **A**, Arterial phase. Anterior spinal artery (large arrow) at the level of the cone fills the arterial network of the medullar cone (small arrow heads). Note a capillary blush at that level. **B**, Venous phase. The anterior spinal vein is single and large (large arrow heads) with a descending radicular vein long and straight, progressively leaving the midline, following a nerve root (small arrow heads).

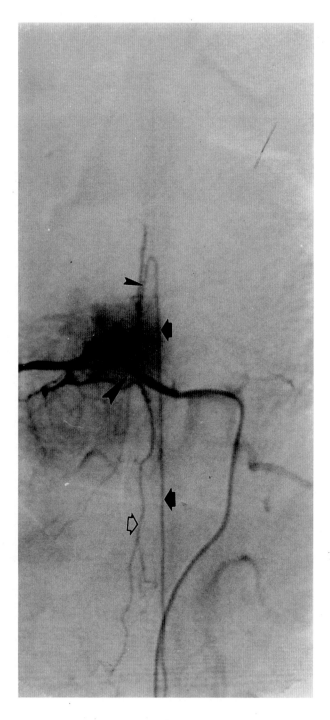

Figure 5.10. 8th right intercostal artery (large arrow head). Anterior view. The anterior spinal artery is well visualized at the thoracolumbar segment (Adamkiewicz). Anterior radiculomedullary artery (small arrow head) with typical ascending curve. The anterior ascending spinal branch is not well visualized, but the descending branch, larger and longer, is well opacified (large arrows).

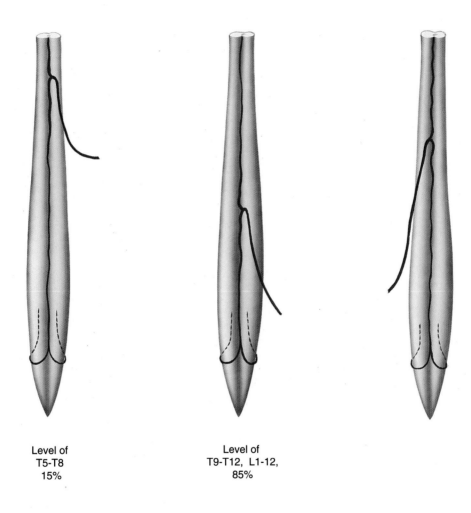

Level of
T5-T8
15%

Level of
T9-T12, L1-12,
85%

Left 75%

Right 25%

Figure 5.11. Different possible levels of origin of the anterior spinal artery (Adamkiewicz).

6

VEINS OF THE SPINAL CORD AND SPINE

VEINS OF THE SPINE

Inside and outside of the vertebral canal, along the entire length of the spinal cord, there are a number of venous plexuses, with free anastomoses with each other, connected with the intervertebral veins. Two groups of venous plexuses are found on the outside of the vertebral canal. The anterior group and the posterior group: the anterior group lies in front of the vertebral bodies and receives venous tributaries from other vertebral bodies and communicates with the basivertebral and intervertebral veins. It is most developed in the cervical region. The posterior group forms a network of venous plexuses mainly inside the spinal canal. There are three communicating valveless venous networks bearing a constant relationship to the vertebral bodies and intervertebral discs (Fig. 6.1). They are the intraosseous vertebral veins, the epidural venous plexus, and the paravertebral veins.

Intraosseous Vertebral Veins

These veins drain the body of each vertebra. They empty into a venous sinus (the basivertebral vein) at the nutrient foramen of each vertebral body posteriorly (Fig. 6.2). This vein connects at each level with the second network, the epidural plexus.

Epidural Venous Plexus

This plexus is composed of two vertical channels, which are the anterior internal vertebral veins that course the length of the spinal canal circling around the backs of the vertebral bodies and intervertebral discs, between the dura mater and bone. Both the left and right anterior internal vertebral veins have a medial and a lateral component. The lateral component is a single channel, whereas the medial component has a variable configuration and is a rather irregular group of vessels. The medial anterior internal vertebral veins are located close to the lateral anterior internal vertebral veins at all levels of the lumbar spine, except at the level L5-S1. At this level, the medial anterior internal vertebral veins leave the lateral anterior internal vertebral veins and lie close to the midline. The anterior internal vertebral veins are

medial to the pedicles and bulge laterally as they cross the intervertebral disc spaces. The anterior internal vertebral veins communicate with the basivertebral veins through the nutrient foramina. There are segmental connections between the epidural venous plexus and the paravertebral veins at every level. At every intervertebral level, there are two connecting veins on each side, named supra- and infrapedicular veins (Figs. 6.2, 6.3, 6.4, 6.5).

There is also the posterior internal vertebral venous plexus, which is small and rudimentary, anastomosed to the anterior internal vertebral venous plexus through the lateral transverse branches. It is located on each side in front of the vertebral arches and ligamenta flava, having anastomoses with the posterior external plexuses by veins passing through and between the ligaments.

The internal venous plexuses form venous rings near each vertebra, connected to the intervertebral veins draining to the ascending lumbar veins at the lumbar spine level. The intervertebral veins are thought to be valveless with occasional reversal of flow, explaining how pelvic neoplasms may metastasize to vertebral bodies during increased intraabdominal pressure or postural alterations.

The anterior group of venous plexus is most developed in the cervical region (Fig. 6.6). Around the foramen magnum, the epidural plexus form a dense network connecting with the vertebral veins, occipital and sigmoid sinuses, basilar plexus, venous plexus of the hypoglossal canal, and the condylar emissary vein.

Paravertebral Veins

The paravertebral veins change names as they course along the spine. They are called vertebral veins, in the neck, azygos and hemiazygos veins in the thorax (Fig. 6.7), ascending lumbar veins in the abdomen (Fig. 6.3), and internal iliac veins in the pelvis. The presacral veins that join the internal iliac veins reaching the epidural veins through the sacral foramina are analogous to the infra- and suprapedicular veins. The paravertebral veins system connects with the vena cava and tributaries at any level (Figs. 6.1, 6.3, 6.4).

VEINS OF THE SPINAL CORD

The veins of the spinal cord are small and form a tortuous and delicate venous plexus. There are two main spinal cord venous systems: intrinsic venous system and extrinsic venous system.

Intrinsic Venous System

It is formed by three systems.
1. Network of venous capillaries largely anastomosed in an axial plane, linking sulcal and axial veins. Although with ventral and dorsal predominance in the thoracolumbar and thoracic regions, this network is spread in almost equal territories.
2. Vertical anastomoses (vertical), following the white or gray matter tracts.
3. Transmedullary anastomotic veins.

Extrinsic Venous System

It is formed by three recognized segments.
1. Pial network
2. Longitudinal collectors
3. Radicular veins

Pial Network

The pial network collects the intrinsic venous perforators. It is a large anastomotic system surrounding the surface of the cord.

Longitudinal Collectors

Longitudinal collectors are represented by two systems. Lateral main intersegmental bridges link two adjacent radial collectors. Two main longitudinal collectors are located dorsal and ventral to the cord. One single collector system is seen on the midline at the cervical and lumbar levels; however, at the thoracic portion, the longitudinal system may be triplicate.

Radicular Veins

These veins almost never follow the arterial contributors when exiting the spine. The venous drainage is equally distributed between dorsal and ventral veins. A large vein is usually seen at the thoracolumbar enlargement. In 60% of cases, the radicular veins follow the nerve roots and exit the dura at the same level of the companion nervous structure. In 40% of cases, a distinct exit hole can be found.

The spinal venous system drains into the epidural venous plexus through the radicular veins, joining the venous drainage of the bony structures of the spinal canal. Near the foramen magnum, the epidural venous plexus is connected to the inferior cerebellar veins or the inferior petrosal sinuses.

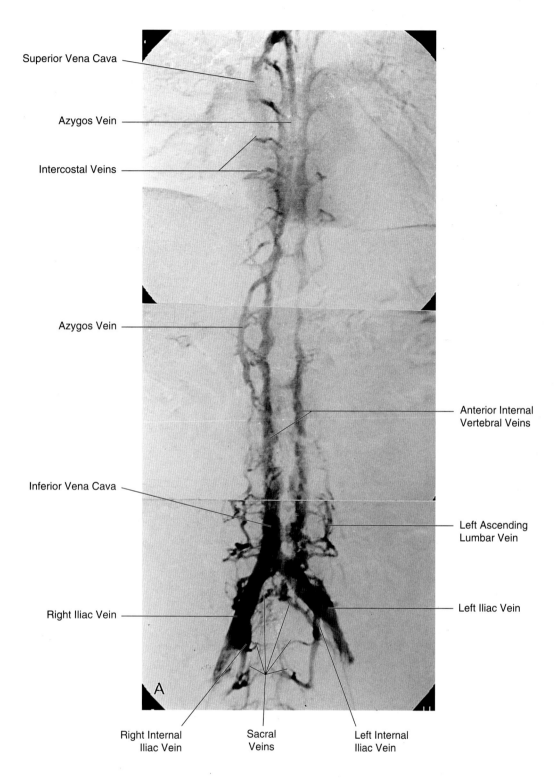

Superior Vena Cava

Azygos Vein

Intercostal Veins

Azygos Vein

Anterior Internal
Vertebral Veins

Inferior Vena Cava

Left Ascending
Lumbar Vein

Left Iliac Vein

Right Iliac Vein

Right Internal
Iliac Vein

Sacral
Veins

Left Internal
Iliac Vein

A

Figure 6.1. A, Anterior view of an angiogram of the spinal venous network, showing the three levels of spinal venous drainage: sacral, lumbar, and thoracic. The iliac veins are partially opacified as well as the inferior vena cava. The ascending lumbar veins are not totally opacified. The ascending flow of contrast is through the epidural plexus. The suprapedicular and infrapedicular veins are visible in almost all the extension of the spine. The azygos vein is also identified. **B**, Lateral view of the epidural angiogram showing the anterior internal vertebral venous plexus and very faintly the posterior internal and external venous plexus. The inferior vena cava is only partially visualized due to the pathologic narrowing. The azygos vein is also depicted from its origin. Note the communication of the iliac venous system with the perivertebral venous plexus through the sacral veins, explaining the role of the vertebral veins in the spread of metastases, accordingly to Batson.

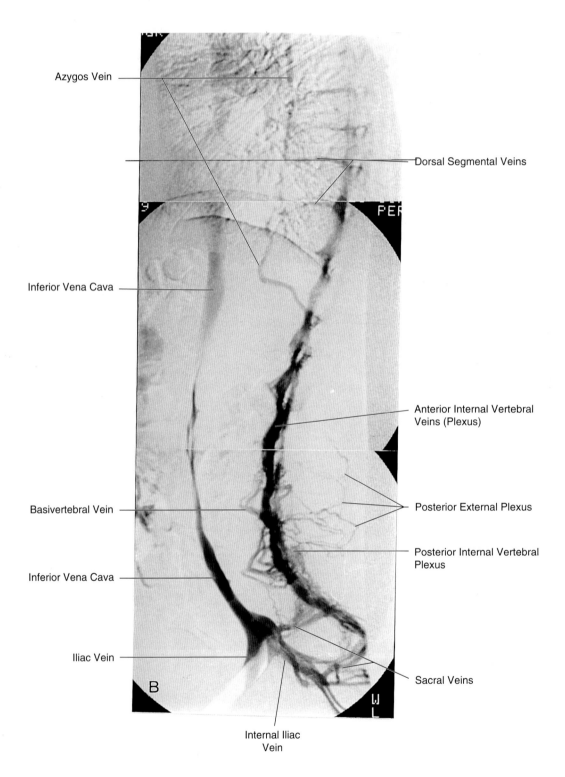

Azygos Vein

Dorsal Segmental Veins

Inferior Vena Cava

Anterior Internal Vertebral
Veins (Plexus)

Posterior External Plexus

Basivertebral Vein

Posterior Internal Vertebral
Plexus

Inferior Vena Cava

Iliac Vein

Sacral Veins

Internal Iliac
Vein

Figure 6.1. *Continued*

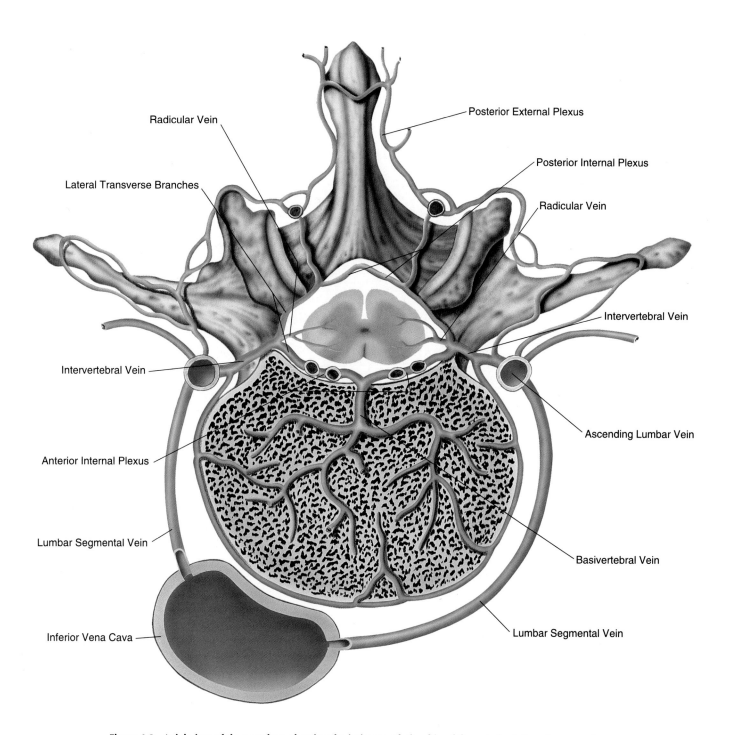

Figure 6.2. Axial view of the vertebrae showing the intimate relationship of the anterior internal venous plexus to the posterior aspect of the vertebrae. Four vertical channels are seen end-on connected by the lateral transverse branches.

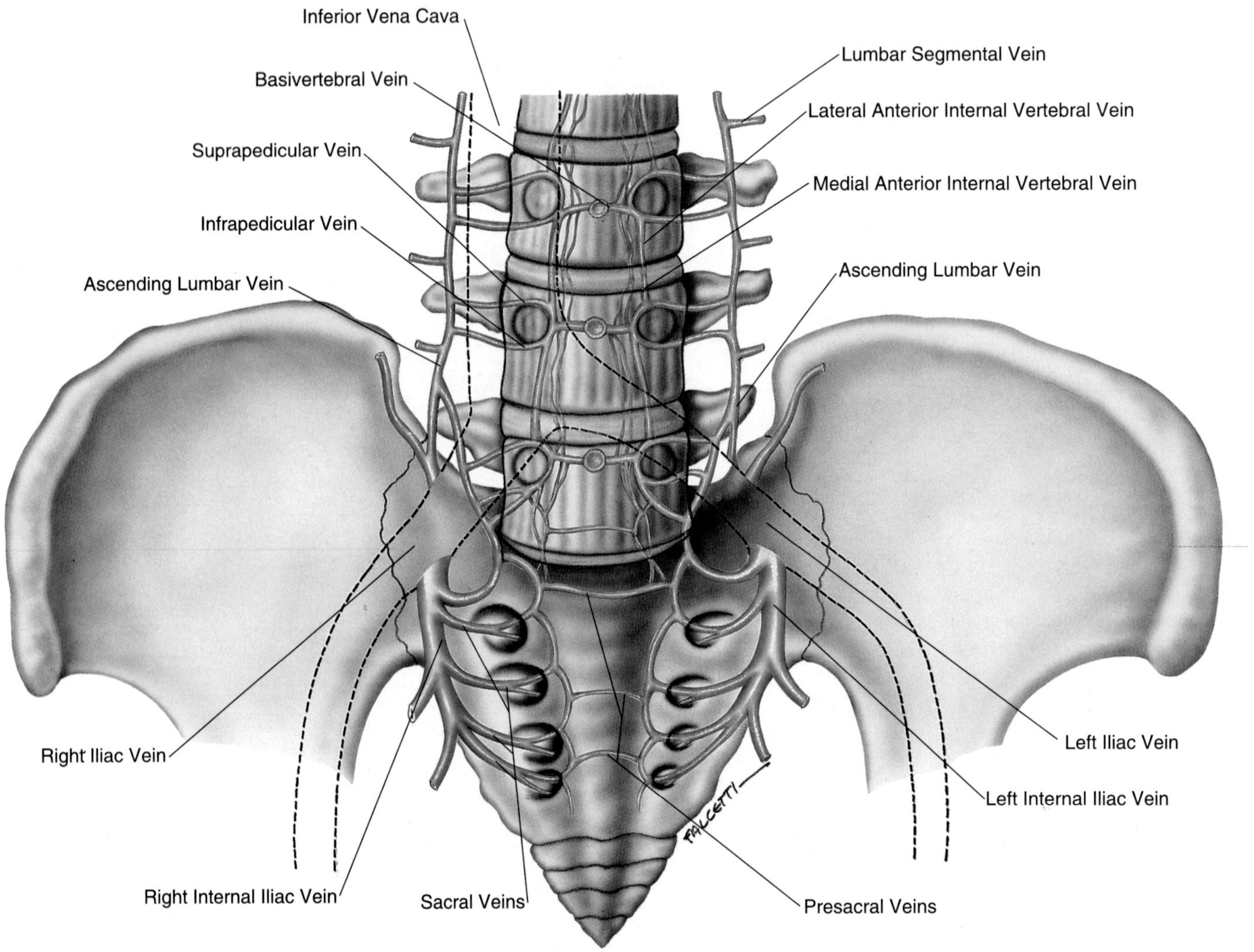

Figure 6.3. Anterior view of the epidural plexus and connections with the paravertebral veins.

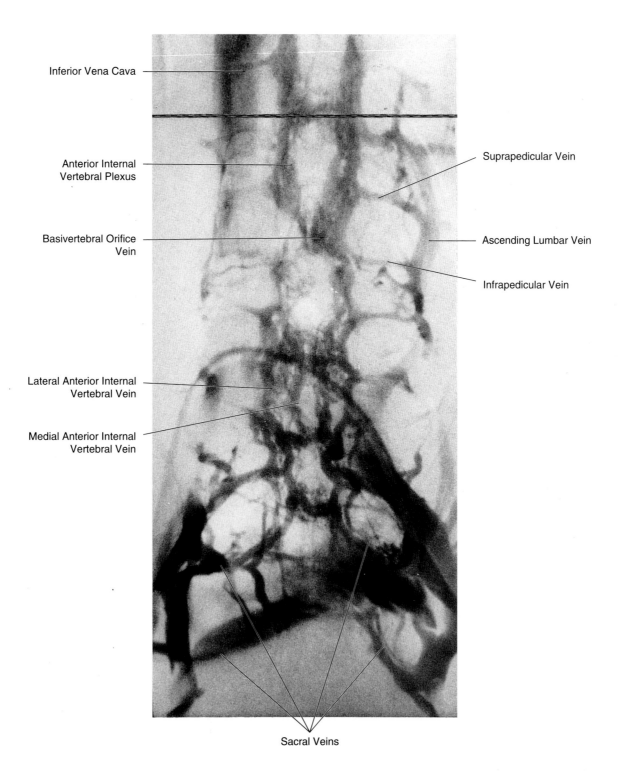

Inferior Vena Cava

Anterior Internal
Vertebral Plexus

Basivertebral Orifice
Vein

Lateral Anterior Internal
Vertebral Vein

Medial Anterior Internal
Vertebral Vein

Suprapedicular Vein

Ascending Lumbar Vein

Infrapedicular Vein

Sacral Veins

Figure 6.4. Epidural venogram. The medial anterior internal vertebral veins are plexiform with multiple irregular
venous channels, and the lateral anterior internal vertebral veins are larger single vessels. At L5-SI level,
they leave the lateral aspect and come closer to the midline.

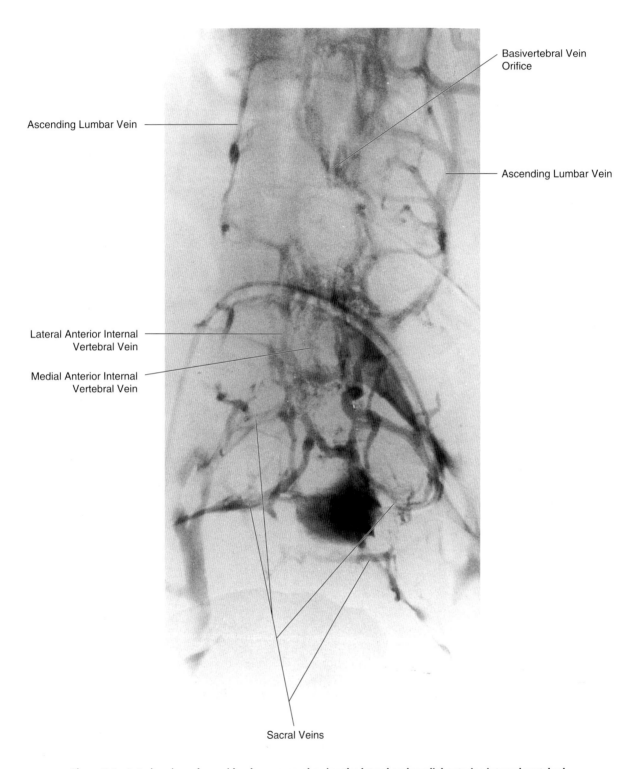

Basivertebral Vein
Orifice

Ascending Lumbar Vein

Ascending Lumbar Vein

Lateral Anterior Internal
Vertebral Vein

Medial Anterior Internal
Vertebral Vein

Sacral Veins

Figure 6.5. Anterior view of an epidural venogram showing the lateral and medial anterior internal vertebral veins. Note the filling defect at the level L4-L5 due to a disc herniation.

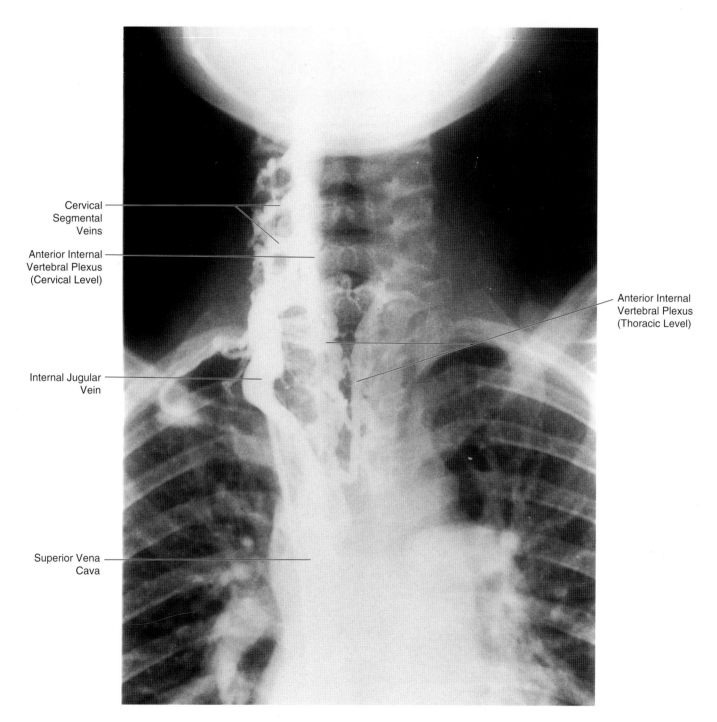

Cervical Segmental Veins

Anterior Internal Vertebral Plexus (Cervical Level)

Anterior Internal Vertebral Plexus (Thoracic Level)

Internal Jugular Vein

Superior Vena Cava

Figure 6.6. Cervical venogram in anterior view. The anterior group of venous plexuses are more developed in the cervical region than in the lumbar region. From C7 level up, spinal canal is broader and the anterior internal vertebral veins are not defined. From C7 level down, the anterior internal vertebral veins can be observed.

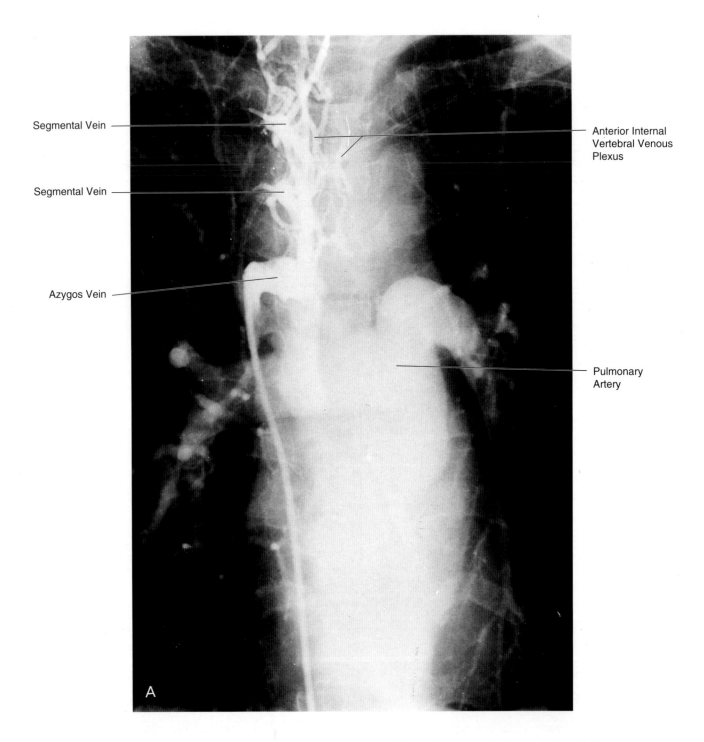

Segmental Vein

Segmental Vein

Azygos Vein

Anterior Internal
Vertebral Venous
Plexus

Pulmonary
Artery

A

Figure 6.7. A, Angiogram of the azygos vein showing retrograde filling of the paravertebral veins and partial filling of the anterior internal vertebral veins. **B**, Lateral view of the azygogram showing the segmental veins and part of the anterior internal vertebral plexus.

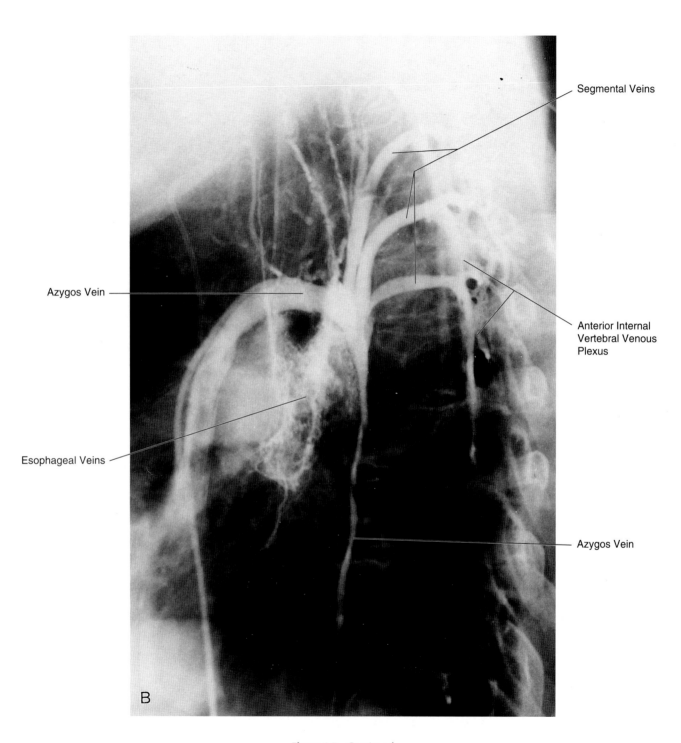

Segmental Veins

Azygos Vein

Anterior Internal
Vertebral Venous
Plexus

Esophageal Veins

Azygos Vein

B

Figure 6.7. *Continued*

7

THORACIC AORTA AND ARTERIES OF THE TRUNK

THORACIC AORTA

The thoracic aorta is conventionally divided in three segments: the ascending aorta, the aortic arch, and the descending aorta, which is subsequently divided in thoracic and abdominal segments (Fig. 7.1).

The ascending aorta arises from the left ventricle of the heart, where it is closed by the aortic valve. It is about 5 cm in length (Fig. 7.2). The aorta courses an anterior ascending tract to the right side of the chest, curving backwards and crossing the mediastinum in the segment called the aortic arch, to the posterior mediastinum and to the left of the vertebral column (Fig. 7.3). The descending aorta approaches the median plane and terminates in front of the column, where it crosses the diaphragm at the aortic hiatus, where begins the abdominal aorta (Fig. 7.4).

The walls of the thoracic and abdominal aorta are supplied by the vasa vasorum. The vasa vasorum system is formed by small nutrient vessels to the walls of other larger vessels. These are the vessel's vessels, which deliver blood to a capillary network within the large arterial wall. However, only part of the vessel wall is supplied by the vasa vasorum. The part of the wall that is fed by the filtration of nutrients through the vascular endothelium is called the physiologic intima. There is a "critical deepness" of vascularization, which varies accordingly to the different arteries and species. At the thoracic aorta, the avascular zone is of about 500 μm in thickness, whereas the avascular zone of the abdominal aorta is of about 700 μm. The tunica intima and the internal third of the tunica media receive nutrients directly from the blood within the lumen of the main artery by diffusion, while the two external thirds of the tunica media and the tunica adventitia are fed by arterial blood from the vasa vasorum (Figs. 7.5, 7.6).

The vasa vasorum arises from the intercostal arteries at the thoracic aorta and from the lumbar arteries at the abdominal aorta. The vasa vasorum originates at the level of the tunica adventitia with a diameter of about 350 μm. The initial trunk has a ventral direc-

tion with a length of about 4 mm. Still at the tunica adventitia, the vasa vasorum trunk with a diameter of about 150 μm divides in two secondary branches of equal diameter. These branches run parallel to the main axis of the aorta in an opposite cranial and caudal direction. From these branches, a network of smaller branches is found with a lateral and ventral distribution, and with several contralateral anastomoses, forming vascular arcades on the aortic wall. The vascular disposition of the vasa vasorum follows a reticular distribution with a polygonal appearance. From the reticular vasa vasorum network originates a rich anastomotic plexus with arterioles of 1st order with a diameter of 200 μm to 100 μm. The microcirculation of the vasa vasorum is formed by the vessels bellow 200 μm in diameter (Fig. 7.5).

Microcirculation of the Aorta

Arterioles of 1st order - between 200 μm and 100 μm
Arterioles of 2nd order - between 100 μm and 30 μm
Precapillaries or terminal - between 30 μm and 10 μm
Capillaries - between 3 μm and 10 μm
Postcapillaries venules - between 10 μm and 30 μm
Venules of 2nd order - between 30 μm and 100 μm
Venules of 1st order - between 100 μm and 200 μm

The arterioles of 2nd order with a diameter of 100 μm and 30 μm are also called arcuate arterioles. These vessels extend for sectors of the aortic circle varying from 90° to 220°, but with an average size of 120°. The precapillaries or terminal arterioles originate from the arcuate arterioles and distribute to the junction of the medium and external third of the tunica media. The distal portion of the terminal branches do not reach the internal third of the tunica media and spread as a tree with a flat top (Figs. 7.5, 7.6).

The arterial vasa vasorum is followed by the venous vasa vasorum with inverted direction of flow. Morphologically, two venous structures correspond to the arterial structure, at the precapillaries and arcuate arterioles.

143

SEGMENTS OF THE THORACIC AORTA

Ascending Aorta

At the origin of the ascending aorta, just after the cusps of the aortic valve, there are three dilatations called aortic sinuses. The coronary arteries orifices are located high up in the aortic sinuses or even above them (Figs. 7.2, 7.7, 7.8, 7.9).

Branches

Coronary arteries are described in the Chapter 13.

Aortic Arch (Fig. 7.10)

There are three branches at the aortic arch.

Branches

Brachiocephalic trunk (innominate artery) and right common carotid artery
Left common carotid artery
Left subclavian artery

Variations of the Aortic Arch

Right aortic arch
Double aortic arch
Cervical aortic arch

Brachiocephalic Trunk

It is the first and largest branch of the aortic arch. This trunk arises from the superior-posterior aspect of the aortic arch. It ascends posterolaterally to the right. At first anteriorly to the trachea, it gradually moves to the right. From it bifurcation originates the two terminal branches, the right subclavian and right common carotid arteries. Occasional branches are the arteria thyroidea ima, thymic artery, and bronchial artery. The right vertebral artery originates from the right subclavian artery.

The right subclavian artery has been described at the arterial supply of the upper limb section. The right common carotid artery is the principal terminal branch of the brachiocephalic artery.

The principal arteries of the head and neck are the common carotid arteries. These arteries ascend in the neck up to the level of the upper border of the thyroid cartilage, where they divide into two main branches, the external and internal carotid arteries. At the division of the vessel, there is a dilatation known as carotid sinus. At the bifurcation, there are terminal nerve fibers, a baroreceptor, and a chemoreceptor called carotid body. The common carotid arteries differ in length and place of origin. Whereas the right carotid artery originates from the brachiocephalic trunk, the left carotid artery arises directly from the arch of the aorta.

Left Common Carotid Artery (Fig. 7.10)

It is the second branch of the arch of the aorta, arising immediately behind and to the left of the brachiocephalic trunk, presenting a thoracic and cervical portion. The artery courses in upward direction, originally in front of the trachea and progressively inclining to the left side.

Left Subclavian Artery (Fig. 7.10)

It is the third branch of the arch of the aorta, arising after and behind the left common carotid artery. It is described in Chapter 15. The left vertebral artery originates from the left subclavian artery.

Variations of the Branches of Aortic Arch

65% Usual pattern (Figs. 7.10, 7.11)
27% Left common carotid artery shares the brachiocephalic trunk with the right subclavian and right common carotid artery (Fig. 7.12)
2.5% The four large arteries branched separately. Independent origin of all vessels (Fig. 7.13)
5.0% Variety of patterns. Right subclavian artery with origin at the distal aortic arch (Fig. 7.14). Common carotid trunk and right subclavian originated from the posterolateral wall of the aortic arch (Fig. 7.15). Left common carotid originating together with the brachiocephalic trunk and the right common carotid originating from the aortic arch (Fig. 7.16).
1.2% Symmetrical right and left brachiocephalic trunk
    Common carotid trunk giving off the left subclavian artery
    Common carotid trunk
    Left and right brachiocephalic arteries
    Single arch vessel
    Left brachiocephalic artery

When there is a right aortic arch, the arrangement of the three branches is reversed; there is a left brachiocephalic trunk, and the right common carotid artery and right subclavian artery arise independently.

Descending Thoracic Aorta

Pericardial Branches

These are small vessels arising from the descending aorta, supplying the posterior aspect of the pericardium.

Bronchial Arteries

The right bronchial artery usually arises together with a right intercostal artery, the third posterior intercostal artery, but other intercostal arteries may arise from that trunk. This common trunk is called intercostobronchial trunk and originates from the right lateral, anterolateral, or dorsal aspect of the descending aorta (Figs. 7.17, 7.18). The left bronchial arteries arise directly from the anterior aspect of the descending aorta, either as single arteries (Fig. 7.19) or as common bronchial trunks, giving branches to both sides (Fig. 7.20) and usually came off perpendicularly to the aortic wall (Fig. 7.21). The site of origin may range from the level T_4 to T_9, but about 90% of the bronchial arteries arise at the level of T_5 and T_6.

Bronchial arteries vascularize mainly the bronchi and the peribronchial connective tissue, but also supply parts of the trachea, the esophagus, the prevertebral muscles, the vagus nerve, the visceral pleura, and the parietal leaf of the pericardium. They supply paratracheal, carinal, hilar, and intrapulmonary lymph nodes and vasa vasorum of the aorta and pulmonary arteries and veins. The peripheral bronchial artery includes various components, including arterioles, capillaries, and venous plexuses. There is a dense vascular network around the bronchi, which is an arteriolar network terminating in bronchial capillaries and numerous bronchial venous plexuses with a characteristic irregular shape and course. The vascular components of this circulation exist either in the bronchial wall or in the peribronchial connective tissue. These microvascular structures are observed along the entire length of the bronchial tree as far distally as the terminal bronchioles, with a progressive decrease in caliber and number. The connective tissue around the pulmonary arteries contains the same vascular network as that in the bronchial wall.

The bronchial arteries, in addition of the vascular system around the bronchi, are also observed with direct communications of the bronchial venous plexuses with the surrounding alveolar capillaries through small venules. There is also nutrition of the visceral pleura by the bronchial arteries (Fig. 10.15).

The distribution of the main bronchial arteries has been described by several authors.

According to Caldwell's description, in 90% of the cases the bronchial artery anatomy is one of four types.

Type I: Two bronchial arteries on the left and one intercostal bronchial trunk (ICBT) on the right (40.6%)

Type II: One bronchial artery on the left and one ICBT on the right (21.3%)

Type III: Two bronchial arteries on the left and two on the right, one of which is an ICBT (20.6%)

Type IV: One bronchial artery on the left and two on the right, one of which is an ICBT (9.7%)

There is no mention of a Common Bronchial Trunk in the Caldwell's classification.

According to Botenga's classification, ten different patterns of bronchial arteries are encountered.

Type I: One intercostobronchial trunk on the right and two bronchial arteries on the left (27.7%)

Type II: One intercostobronchial trunk on the right and one bronchial artery on the left (17.0%)

Type III: One intercostobronchial trunk on the right, one bronchial artery on the left and one common bronchial trunk with one artery to the right and one to the left (17.0%)

Type IV: One intercostobronchial trunk and one bronchial artery on the right and two bronchial arteries on the left (10.7%)

Type V: Two bronchial arteries on the right and one bronchial artery on the left (8.5%)

Type VI: One intercostobronchial trunk on the right and one common bronchial trunk with one artery to the right and one to the left (8.5%)

Type VII: One common bronchial trunk (4.3%)

Type VIII: One intercostobronchial trunk, plus one bronchial artery on the right, and three bronchial arteries on the left (2.1%)

Type IX: One intercostobronchial trunk plus two bronchial arteries on the right and one bronchial artery on the left (2.1%)

Type X: One common bronchial trunk, with one artery to the right and to the left, and one bronchial artery to the left (2.1%)

According to Uflacker's description of the bronchial arteries anatomy, ten different patterns may be encountered, including common bronchial trunks (Fig. 7.23).

Pattern I: One ICBT on the right and a bronchial artery on the left (30.5%)

Pattern II: One ICBT on the right and a common trunk with a bronchial artery on the right and one on the left (25.0%)

Pattern III: One ICBT on the right and two bronchial arteries on the left (12.5%)

Pattern IV: One ICBT on the right, one bronchial artery on the right, and one on the left (11.1%)

Pattern V: One ICBT on the right, one common bronchial trunk, and one left bronchial artery (8.3%)

Pattern VI: One ICBT on the right, one bronchial artery on the left, and one common bronchial trunk in caudal position (4.2%)

Pattern VII: Only one common bronchial trunk (2.8%)

Pattern VIII: One ICBT on the right, giving origin to a left bronchial artery, and one bronchial artery on the left (2.8%)

Pattern IX: Two common bronchial trunks giving origin to bronchial arteries on the right and on the left (1.4%)

Pattern X: One ICBT on the right, one bronchial artery on the right, and one common bronchial trunk origin to arteries on the right and on the left (1.4%)

The first six patterns described comprise approximately 90% of the anatomic patterns encountered in this series.

Aberrant Origins and Anatomic Variations of the Bronchial Arteries

The bronchial arteries may arise from the aortic arch or have an aberrant origin from other arteries in the greater circulation. They may be small but important when bleeding supervenes. Aberrant, replaced, and accessory bronchial arteries are supplied from other systemic arteries, including subclavian, innominate (brachiocephalic trunk), abdominal aorta, inferior phrenic arteries, thyrocervical trunk, pericardiophrenic, internal thoracic, and axillary arteries (Figs 7.24, 7.25).

Anastomotic Connections of the Thoracic Arteries

There are innumerable anastomotic channels in the chest (Fig. 7.26), related to the internal thoracic (mammary) arteries and systemic thoracic arteries (Fig. 7.27). Pathways are transverse anastomoses and vertical anastomoses (Fig. 7.27). Collaterals may develop in addition to the natural anastomoses, related to inflammatory and other pathologic problems (Fig. 7.29).

Radicular arteries originating from the ICBT may be present in 58.3% of the cases. The anterior spinal artery is supplied by a radiculomedullary branch which may originate from the right ICBT in 5% of the cases in one series, usually at the level of T_4-T_6.

Esophageal Arteries

There are four or five esophageal arteries, arising anteriorly from the descending thoracic aorta, forming a vascular network with anastomoses above with the esophageal branches of the inferior thyroid arteries and inferiorly with the phrenic arteries and branches of the left gastric artery. Esophageal arteries, may be branches of the bronchial arteries or may arise as a common trunk, together with bronchial arteries in a significant number of cases.

Mediastinal Branches

These branches are small arteries supplying mediastinal lymph nodes and areolar tissue of the posterior mediastinum.

Phrenic Branches

These branches arise from the lower thoracic aorta and vascularize the superior diaphragmatic surface and have anastomoses with the pericardiophrenic and musculophrenic arteries.

Posterior Intercostal Arteries

There are usually nine pairs of the posterior intercostal arteries, arising from the posterior aspect of the descending thoracic aorta and distributed to the intercostal spaces. The first two or three intercostal arteries usually arise from the superior intercostal artery (or trunk). The second and third right posterior intercostal arteries usually arise together with the right bronchial artery and it is called intercostobronchial trunk. The left posterior intercostal arteries are short-er and run backwards on the vertebral bodies and the right posterior intercostal arteries are longer, due to the aortic deviation to the left, and run in front of the vertebral body, turning posteriorly following the vertebral body curvature. Reaching the ribs, the posterior intercostal arteries run along the costal grooves. The posterior intercostal vein and nerve are parallel to the artery. The last paired branches of the thoracic aorta are called subcostal arteries and run a path below the 12th ribs (Figs. 7.28, 7.29).

Branches

Dorsal branch (anterior)
Spinal branch (posterior)
Collateral intercostal branch
Muscular branches
Unnamed branches
Anterior branch

The posterior intercostal artery runs dorsally between the necks of adjoining ribs. It has an anterior branch (intercostal) and a posterior branch (spinal branch) entering the vertebral canal, by the intervertebral foramen to supply the vertebrae, spinal cord and meninges.

Spinal Branch

The posterior branch of the intercostal artery originates muscular branches and the radiculomedullary arteries. The radiculomedullary artery after originating a ganglionic branch divides in anterior radiculomedullary artery and posterior radiculomedullary artery, which anastomoses with the anterior spinal artery and posterior spinal artery, respectively.

Collateral Intercostal Artery

This artery arises from the posterior intercostal artery near the costal angle and descends to the upper border of the subjacent rib. It runs along the upper border of the rib and anastomoses with branches from the anterior intercostal branch of the internal thoracic artery.

Muscular Branches

These branches supply the intercostal, pectoral muscles, and serratus muscles. The muscular branches give several lateral cutaneous branches and mammary branches.

Unnamed Branches

There are several unnamed branches of the posterior intercostal artery that supply all the other tissues of the chest wall, including bone, periosteum, and parietal pleura.

Anterior Intercostal Arteries

These arteries originate from the internal mammary artery (Fig. 7.30) and are usually smaller than the posterior intercostal arteries.

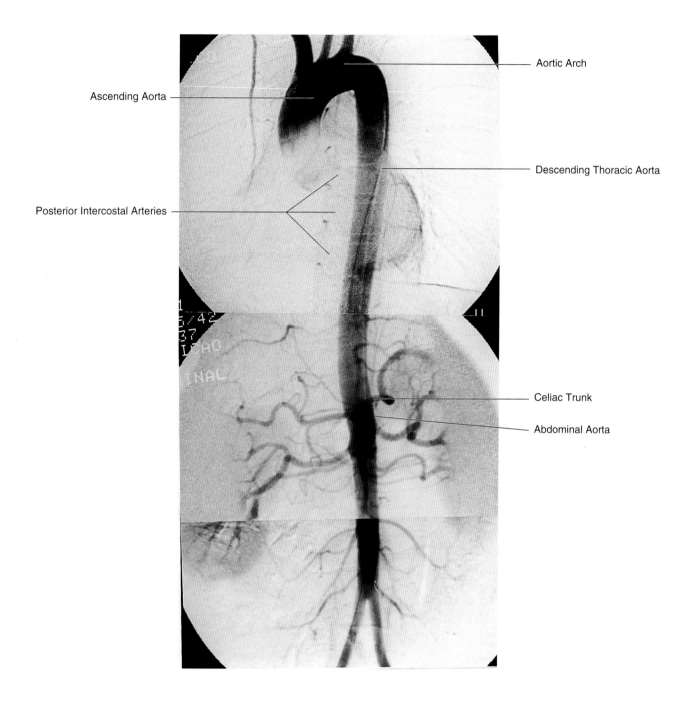

Figure 7.1. Aortic angiogram showing the ascending thoracic aorta, the aortic arch, the descending thoracic aorta, and the abdominal aorta. The posterior intercostal arteries, the right internal thoracic (mammary) artery are partially seen. The visceral arteries are well seen.

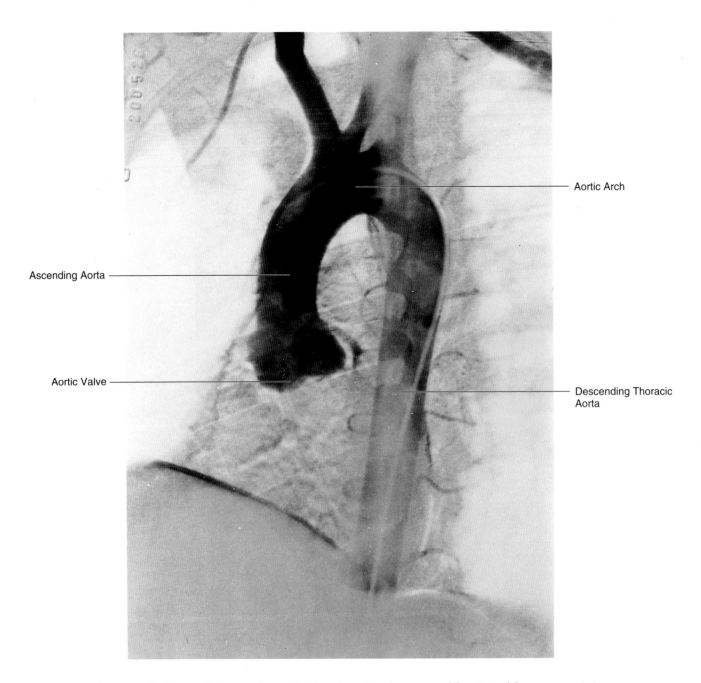

Figure 7.2. Angiogram of the ascending aorta. Note the aortic valve cusps and the origin of the coronary arteries. The aortic arch is partially filled.

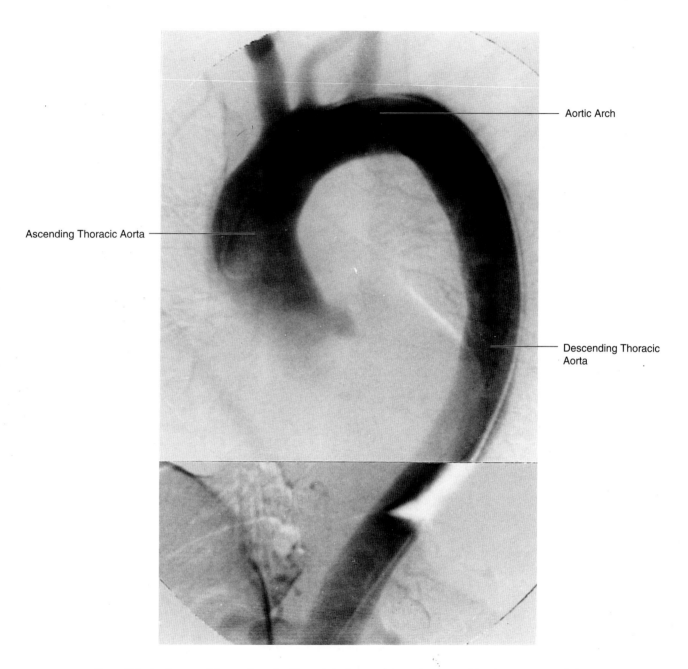

Aortic Arch

Ascending Thoracic Aorta

Descending Thoracic Aorta

Figure 7.3. Angiogram of the aortic arch. The arch is elongated. Note the origin of the three main vessels from the arch. The descending aorta is also visualized but is tortuous.

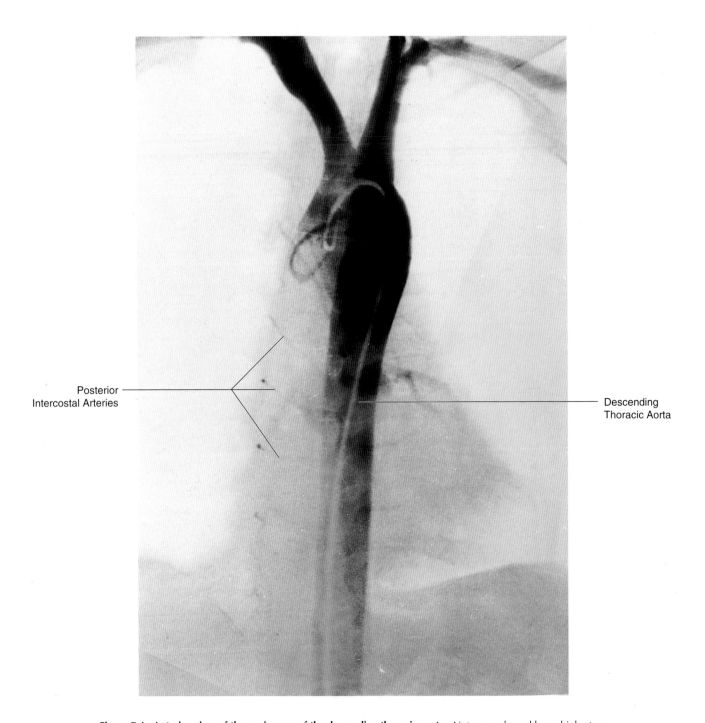

Posterior
Intercostal Arteries

Descending
Thoracic Aorta

Figure 7.4. Anterior view of the angiogram of the descending thoracic aorta. Note an enlarged bronchial artery appearing on the left. The intercostal arteries are partially observed.

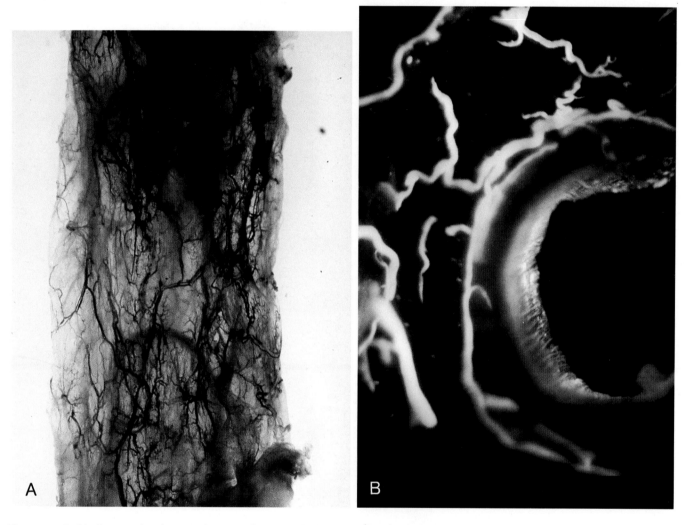

Figure 7.5. **A.** Diaphanography of a sagittal cut into the aorta of a dog, showing the arterial and venous vasa vasorum opacified by acrylic plastic. Note the reticulated pattern in a polygonal network, resulting from the bifurcation of the vasa vasorum and anastomoses with neighbor branches of vasa vasorum. The polygonal network is located mostly in the adventitia of the aorta. **B.** Axial cut into the aortal of a dog showing the vasa vasorum with origin in a Lumbar Artery. Note the multiple layers of vessels. (Provided by Dr. JM Pisco, Lisboa, Portugal).

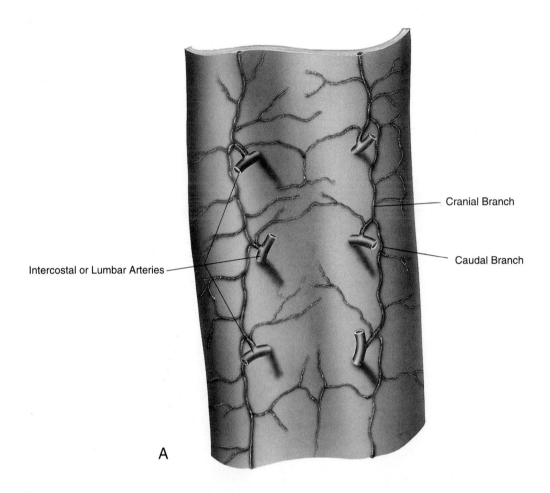

A

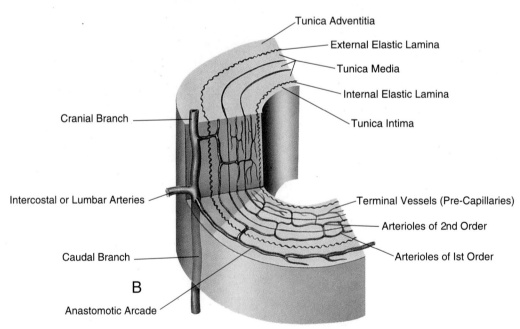

B

Figure 7.6. A. Sagittal cut of the aorta showing the polygonal network of vasa vasorum in the aortic wall. **B.** Axial cut of the aorta showing the multiple layers of vessels in the aortic wall.

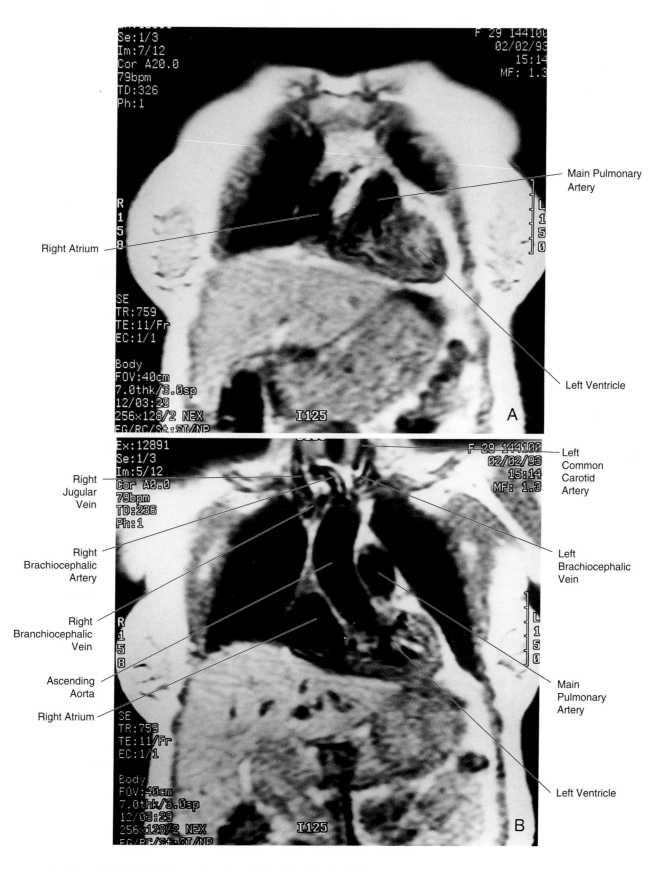

Figure 7.7. A-D. MRI coronal sections of the chest showing the heart and the great vessels, including the aorta.

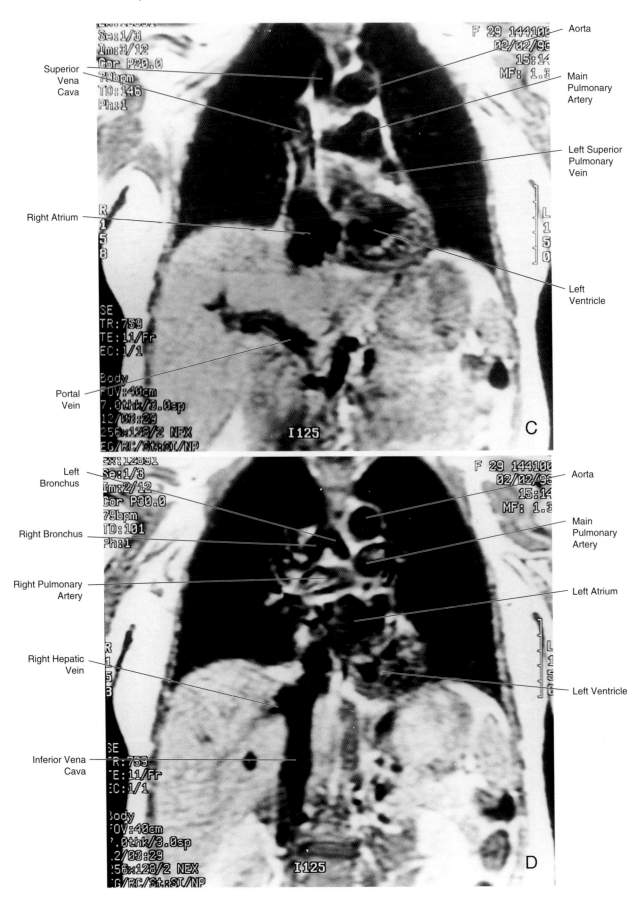

Figure 7.7. *Continued*

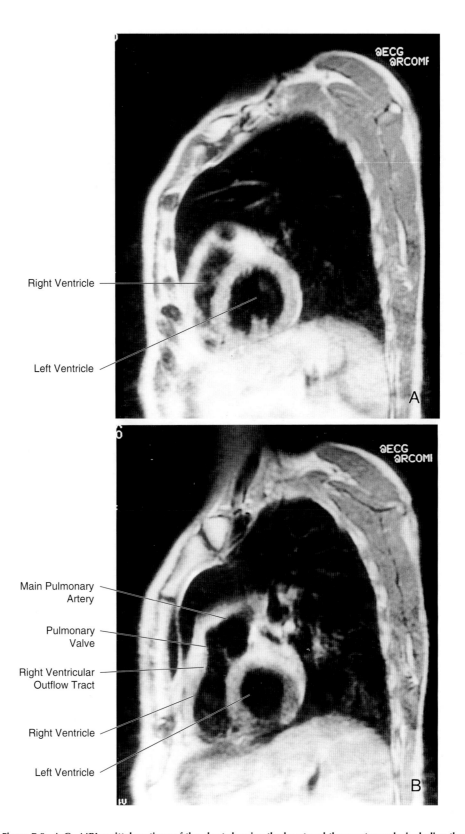

Figure 7.8. A-G. MRI sagittal sections of the chest showing the heart and the great vessels, including the aorta.

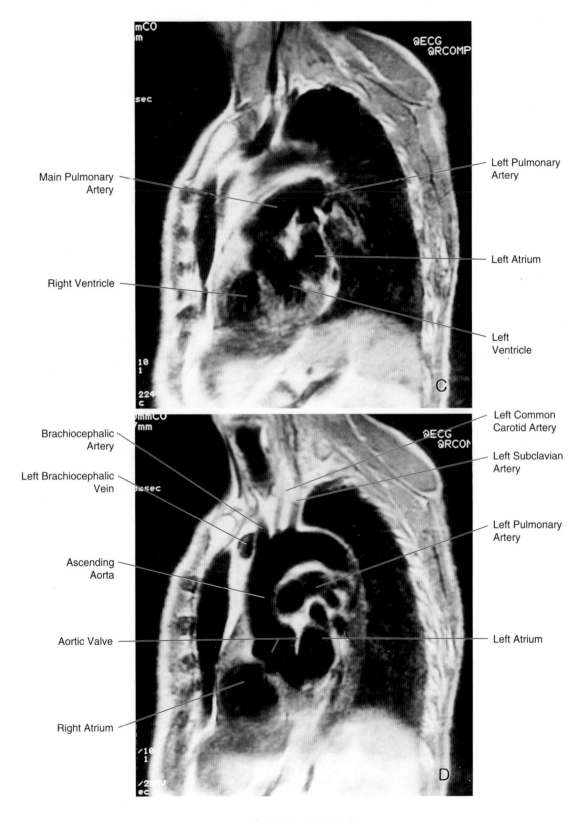

Figure 7.8. *Continued*

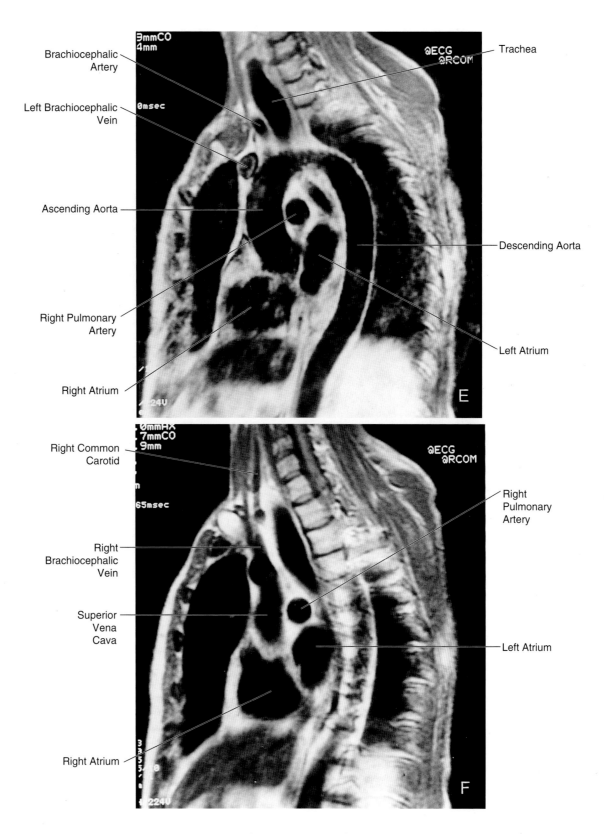

Figure 7.8. *Continued*

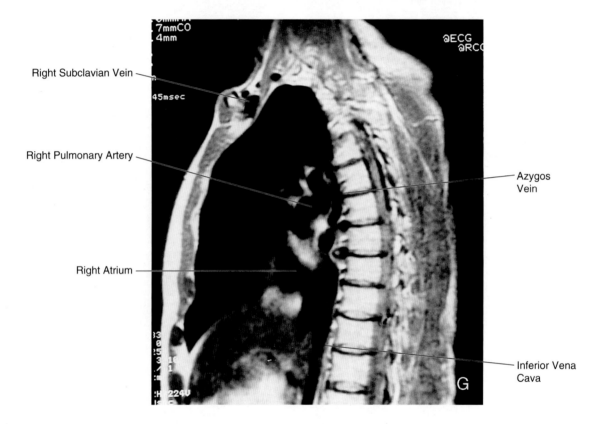

Figure 7.8. *Continued*

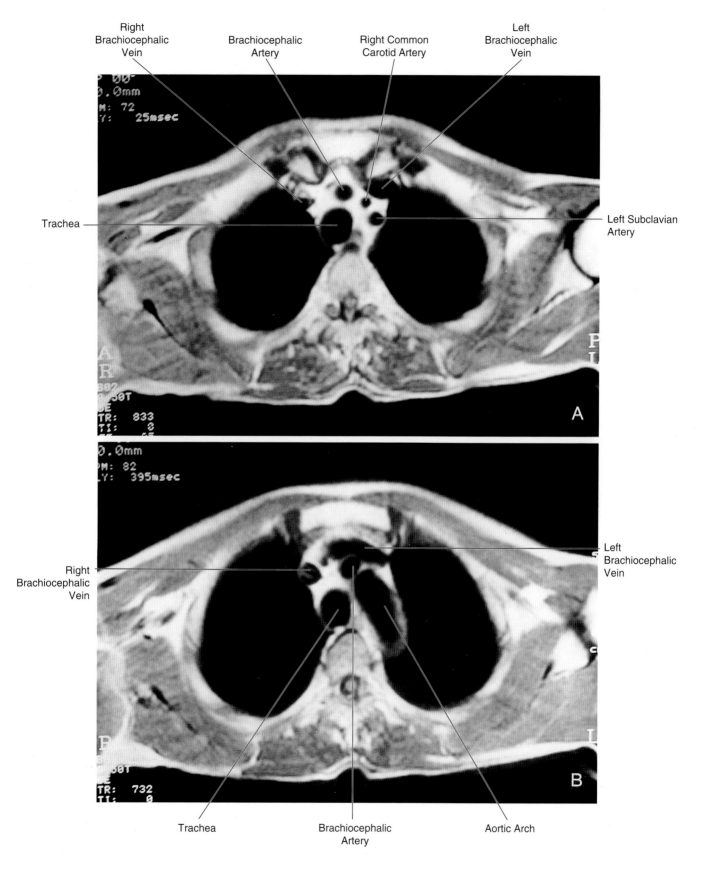

Figure 7.9. A-J. MRI axial sections of the chest showing the heart and the great vessels, including the aorta.

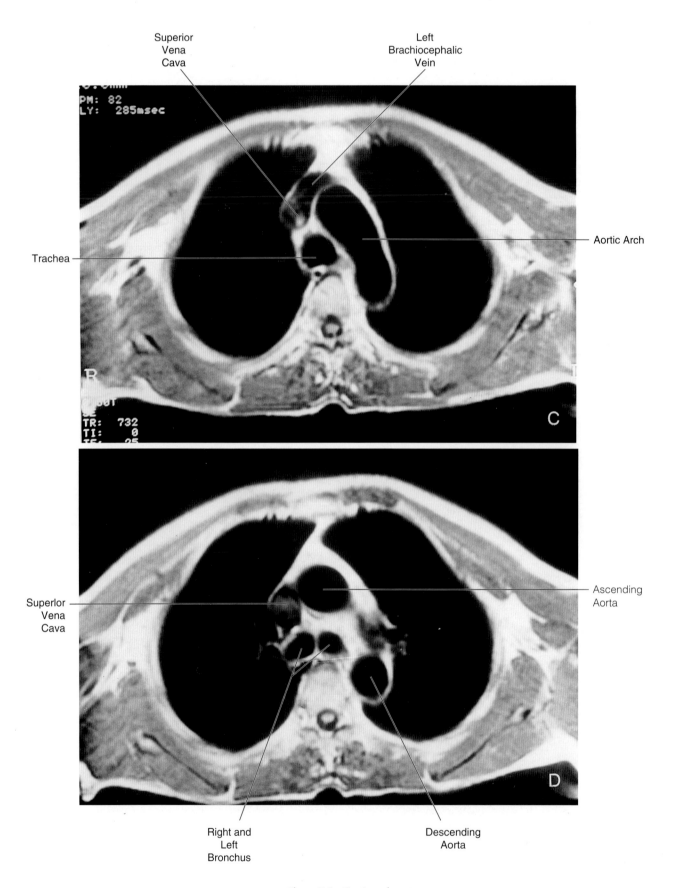

Figure 7.9. *Continued*

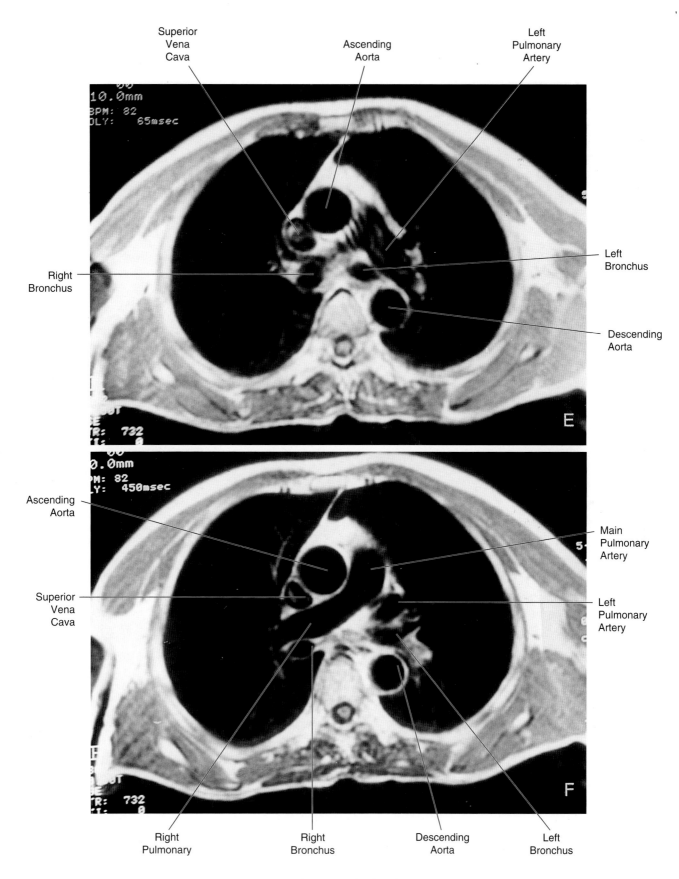

Figure 7.9. *Continued*

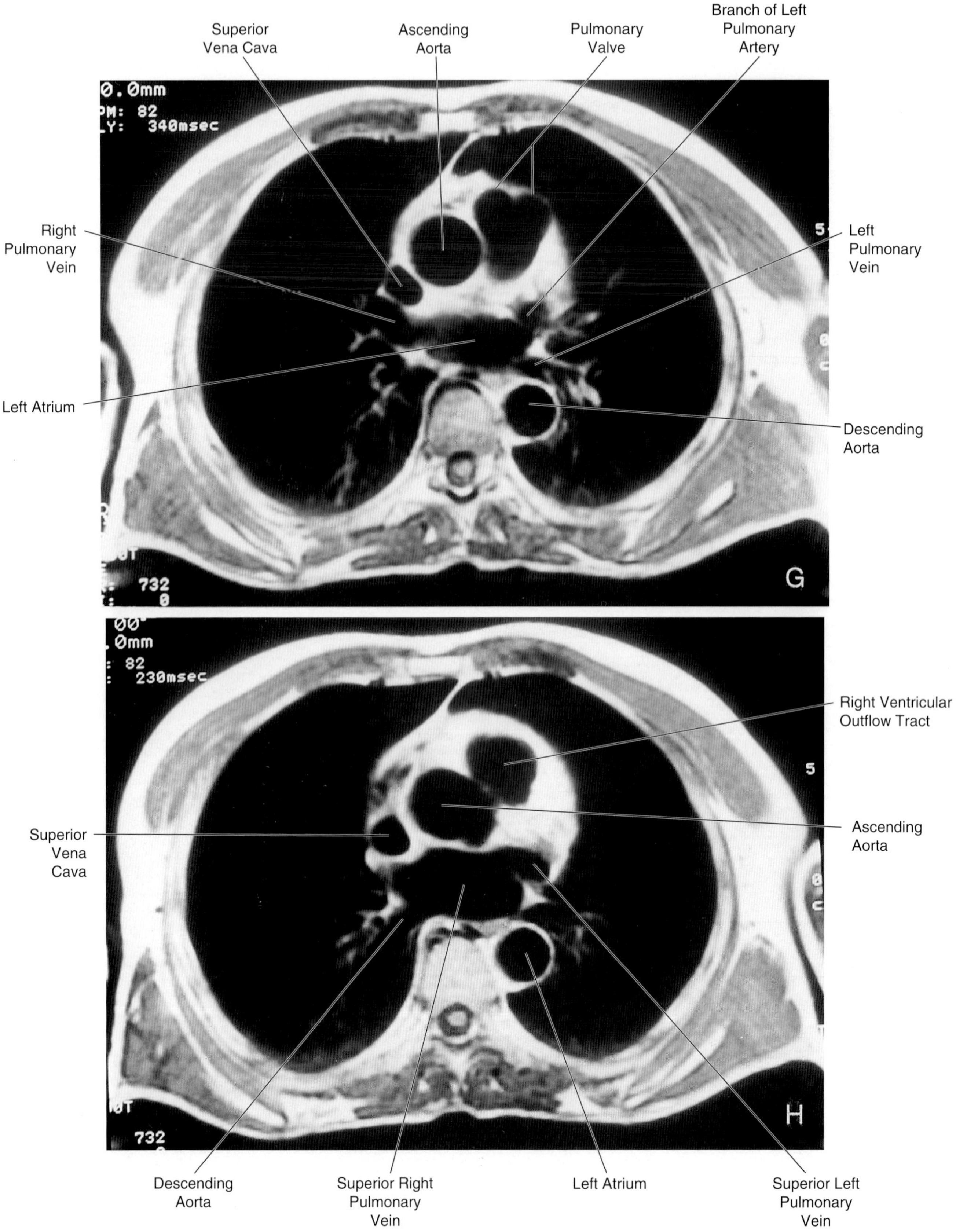

Figure 7.9. *Continued*

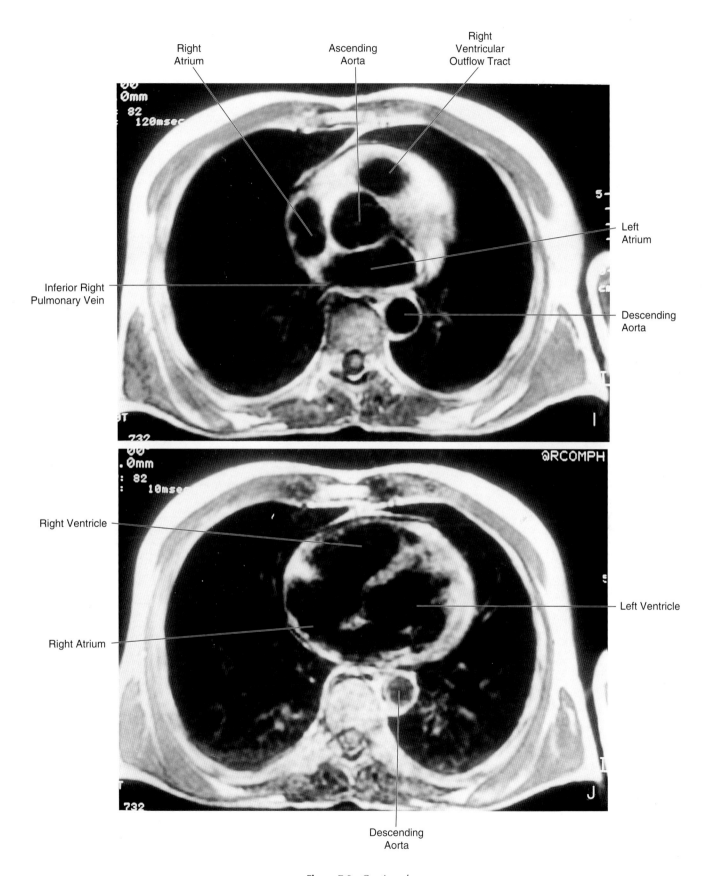

Figure 7.9. *Continued*

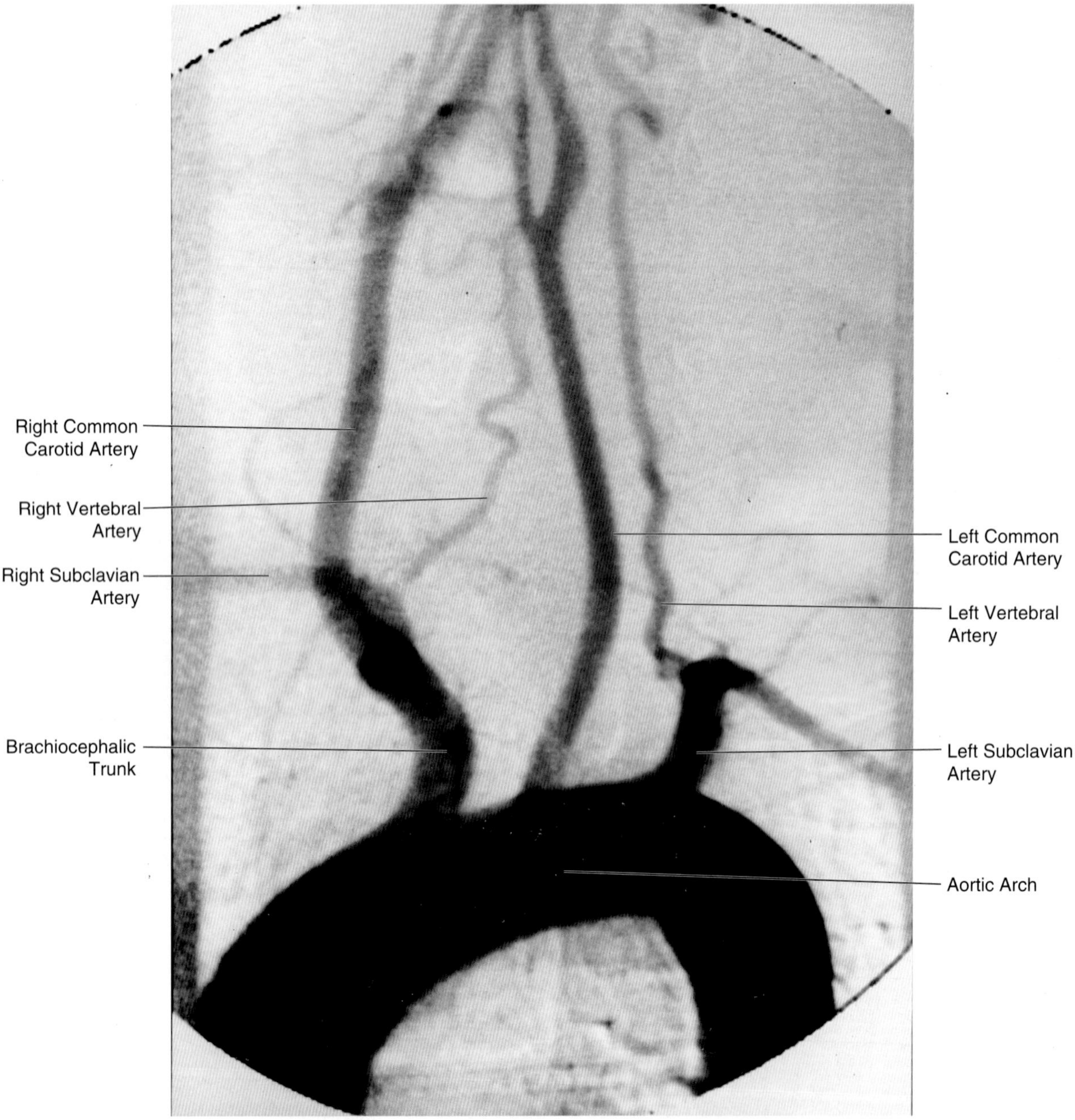

Right Common Carotid Artery

Right Vertebral Artery

Right Subclavian Artery

Brachiocephalic Trunk

Left Common Carotid Artery

Left Vertebral Artery

Left Subclavian Artery

Aortic Arch

Figure 7.10. Angiogram of the aortic arch showing the usual distribution of the origins of the main branches.

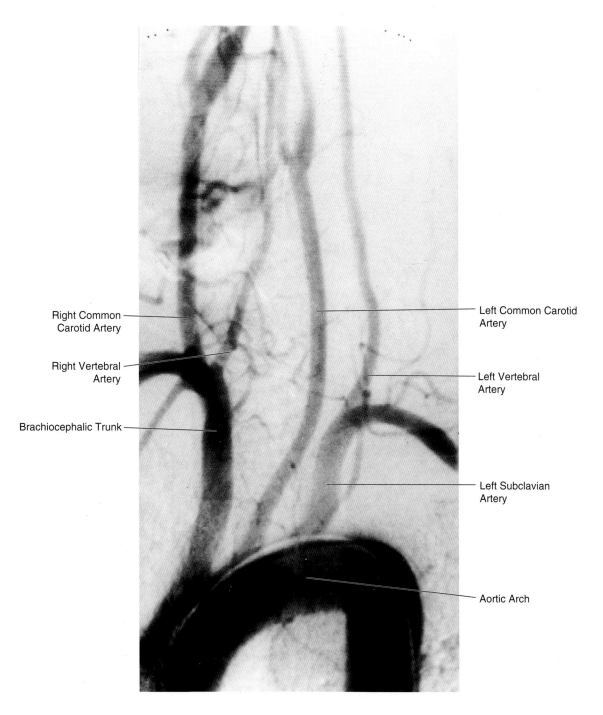

Right Common Carotid Artery

Right Vertebral Artery

Brachiocephalic Trunk

Left Common Carotid Artery

Left Vertebral Artery

Left Subclavian Artery

Aortic Arch

Figure 7.11. Angiogram of the aortic arch showing the origin of the main branches of the aortic arch.

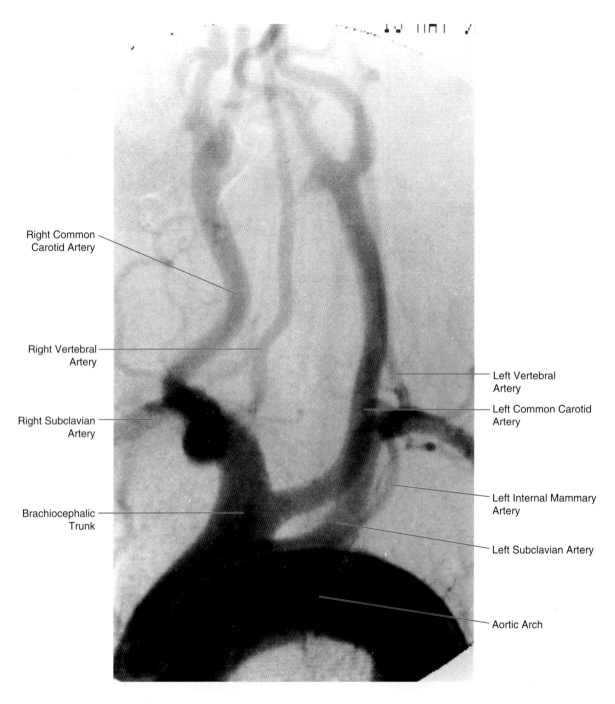

Right Common
Carotid Artery

Right Vertebral
Artery

Right Subclavian
Artery

Brachiocephalic
Trunk

Left Vertebral
Artery

Left Common Carotid
Artery

Left Internal Mammary
Artery

Left Subclavian Artery

Aortic Arch

Figure 7.12. Angiogram of the aortic arch showing the common origin of the left common carotid artery and the brachiocephalic trunk.

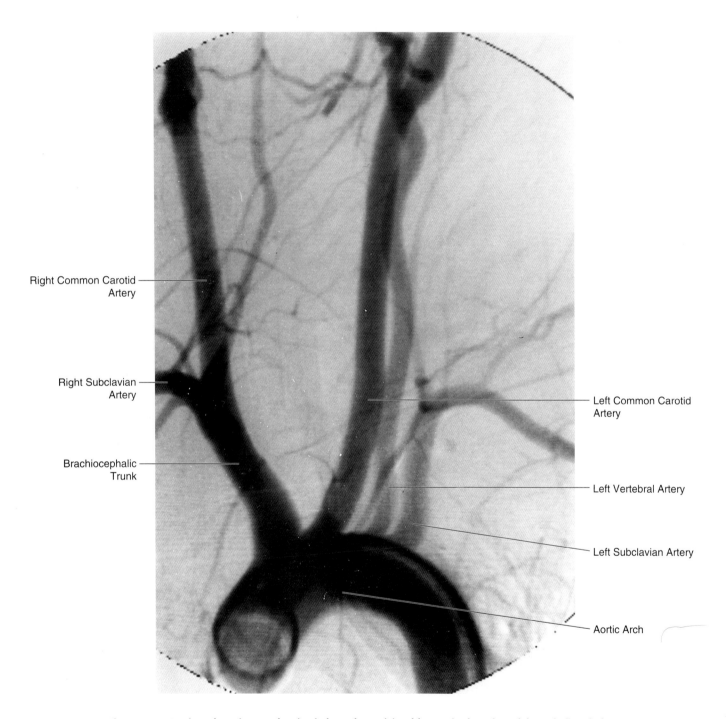

Right Common Carotid
Artery

Right Subclavian
Artery

Brachiocephalic
Trunk

Left Common Carotid
Artery

Left Vertebral Artery

Left Subclavian Artery

Aortic Arch

Figure 7.13. Aortic arch angiogram showing independent origin of four major branches of the arch directly from the arch. Note the dominant left vertebral artery directly from the aorta.

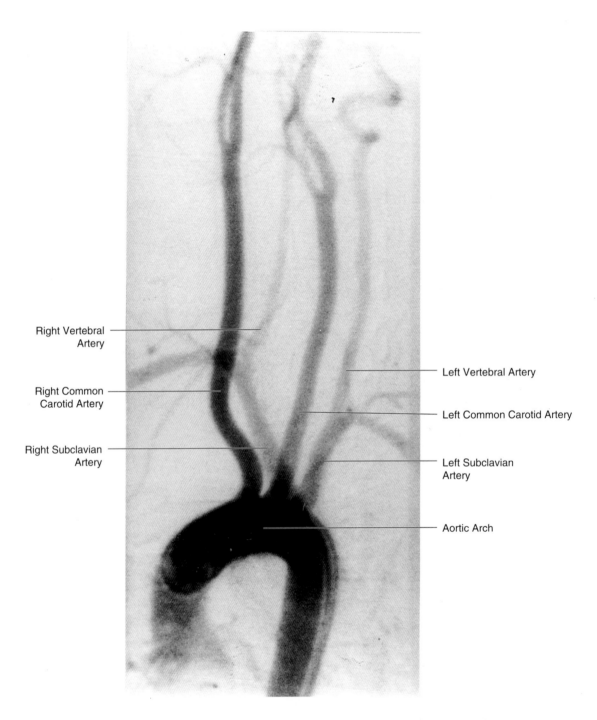

Right Vertebral Artery

Right Common Carotid Artery

Right Subclavian Artery

Left Vertebral Artery

Left Common Carotid Artery

Left Subclavian Artery

Aortic Arch

Figure 7.14. Aortic arch angiogram showing the origin of the right common carotid artery directly from the arch, as well as the left carotid artery and the left subclavian artery. The right subclavian artery arises directly from the distal aspect of the aortic arch.

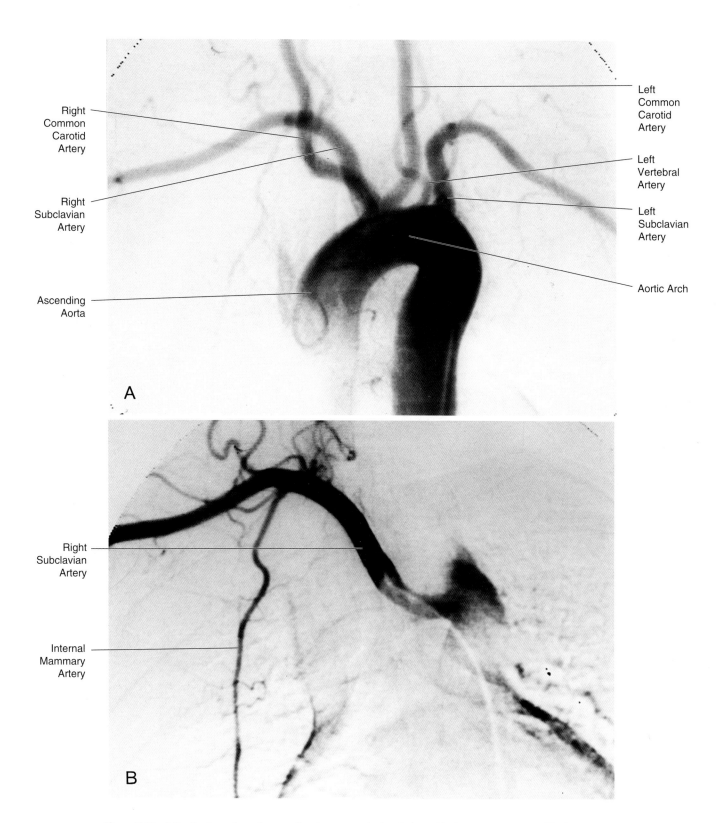

Right Common Carotid Artery

Right Subclavian Artery

Ascending Aorta

Left Common Carotid Artery

Left Vertebral Artery

Left Subclavian Artery

Aortic Arch

A

Right Subclavian Artery

Internal Mammary Artery

B

Figure 7.15. A-B. Aortic arch angiogram showing anatomical variation with the common origin of both common carotid arteries, direct origin of the left vertebral artery from the aorta, normal origin of the left subclavian artery, and independent posterolateral origin of the right subclavian artery from the arch. **C-D.** MRI of the chest showing the anatomical variation. The posterolateral origin of the right subclavian artery.

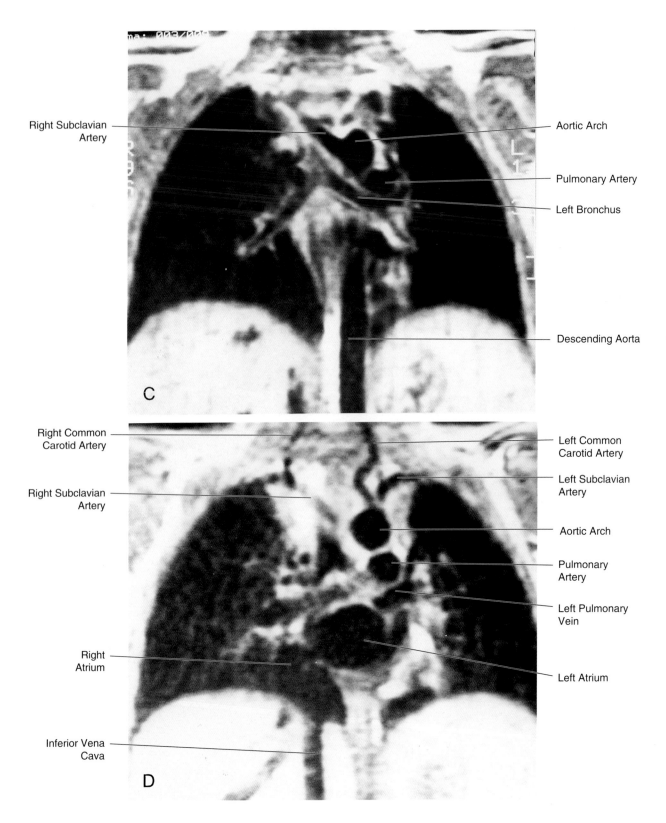

Right Subclavian Artery

Aortic Arch

Pulmonary Artery

Left Bronchus

Descending Aorta

C

Right Common Carotid Artery

Left Common Carotid Artery

Right Subclavian Artery

Left Subclavian Artery

Aortic Arch

Pulmonary Artery

Left Pulmonary Vein

Right Atrium

Left Atrium

Inferior Vena Cava

D

Figure 7.15. *Continued*

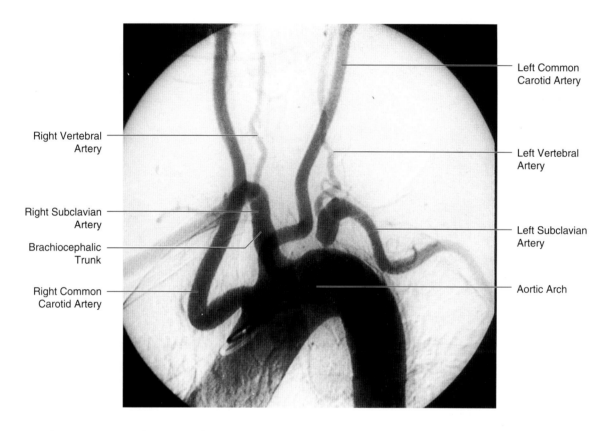

Figure 7.16. Aortic arch angiogram showing anatomical variation with the brachiocephalic trunk giving origin to the left common carotid artery, the right common carotid artery with independent origin directly from the aorta, as the first branch of the aortic arch.

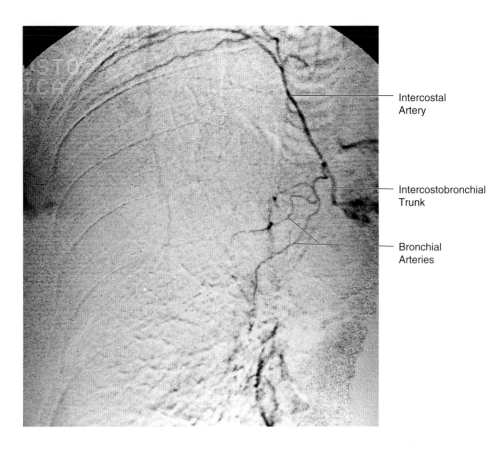

Figure 7.17. Selective angiogram of the intercostobronchial trunk showing filling of the two first intercostal arteries and simultaneous filling of the right superior and inferior bronchial arteries.

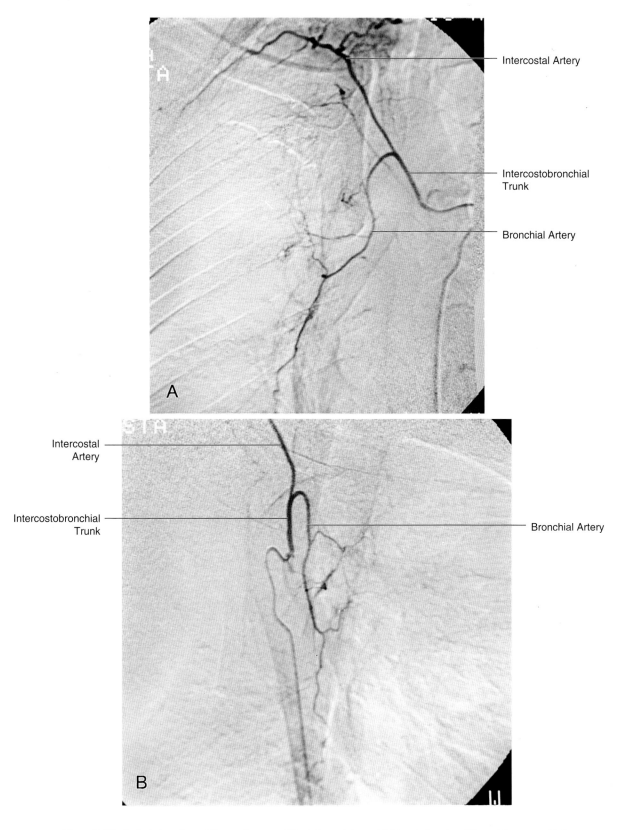

Figure 7.18. A. Anterior view of the angiogram of the intercostobronchial trunk showing filling of the second intercostal artery and right bronchial arteries. **B.** Lateral view of the angiogram of the same artery as in A, showing that the intercostal artery is posterior and the bronchial arteries follow a more central or anterior direction, along with the bronchus.

Bronchial
Arteries

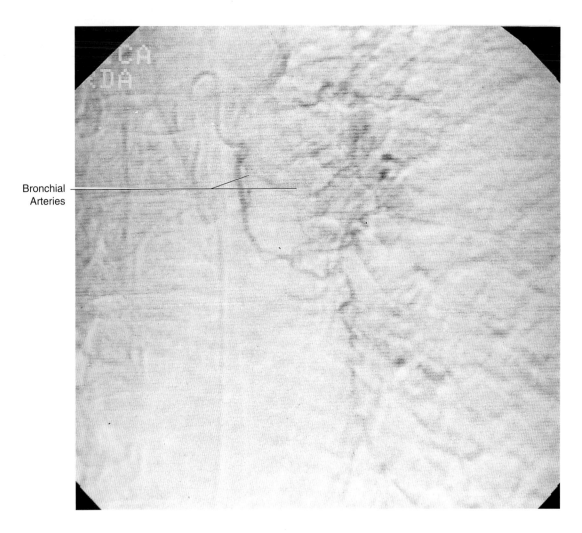

Figure 7.19. Left bronchial artery angiogram.

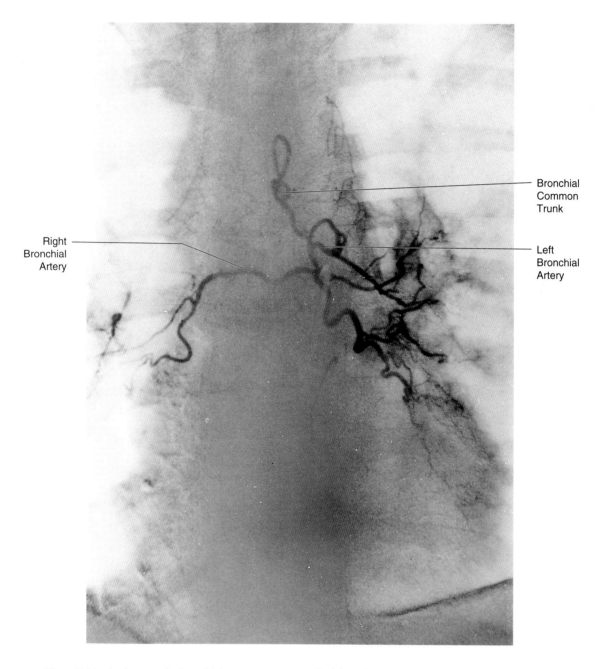

Figure 7.20. Angiogram of a bronchial artery common trunk giving origin to a right bronchial artery and a left bronchial artery. Note the right bronchial artery is inferior and on the left there are superior and inferior bronchial arteries.

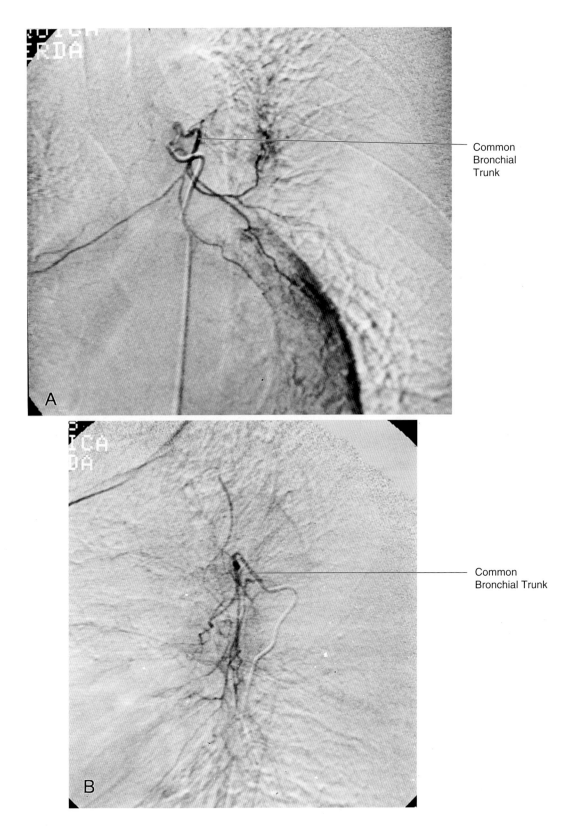

Common
Bronchial
Trunk

Common
Bronchial Trunk

Figure 7.21. A. Selective angiogram of a common bronchial trunk showing the branches to right and left.
B. Lateral view showing the right and left Bronchial Arteries following a central or anterior direction.
The origin of the Common Trunk is almost perpendicular to the aortic wall.

Common
Bronchial
Trunk

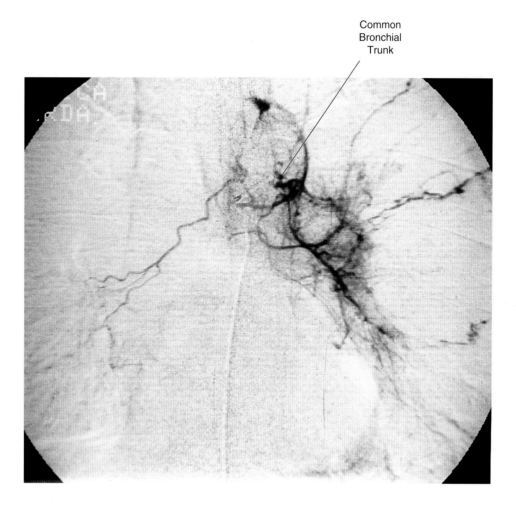

Figure 7.22. Selective angiogram of a common trunk showing the vascular components either in the bronchial wall and in peribronchial tissues. Due to the inflammatory changes the circulation is increased.

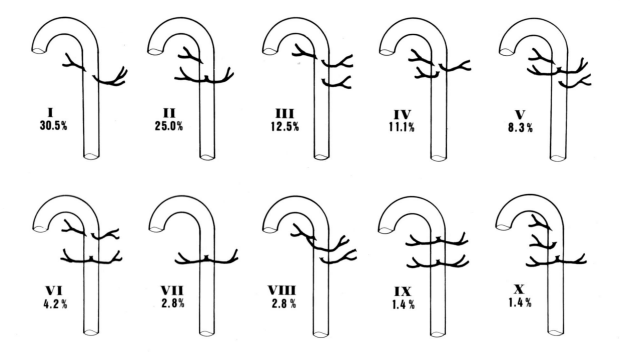

Figure 7.23. Ventral aspect of the types of bronchial arterial supply, based on the angiographic data of 72 patients. The right intercostobronchial trunk arises laterally or dorsally, the remaining single bronchial arteries and common bronchial trunk arise from the ventral aspect of the aorta. (From Uflacker et al. Radiology 1985;157:637-644).

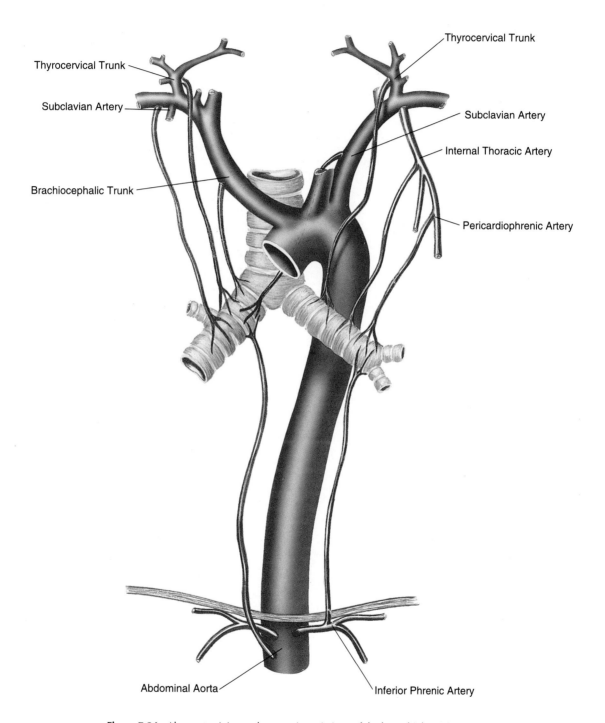

Figure 7.24. Aberrant origins and anatomic variations of the bronchial arteries.

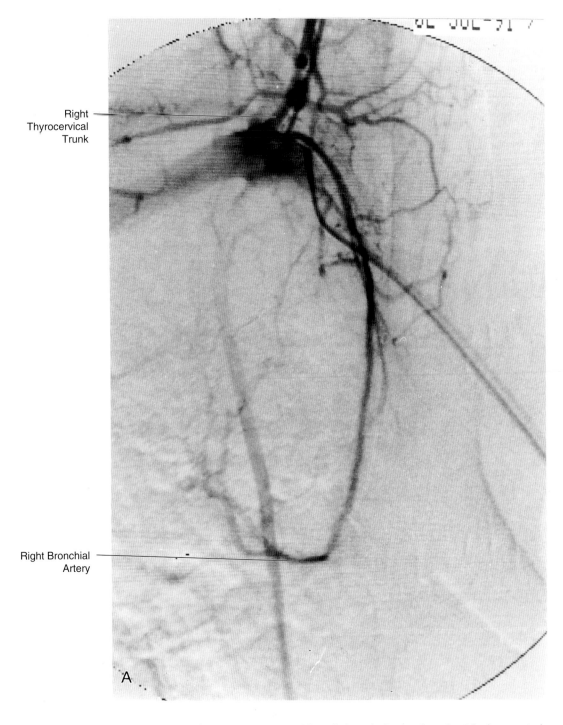

Right
Thyrocervical
Trunk

Right Bronchial
Artery

A

Figure 7.25. A. Angiogram showing aberrant origin of the right bronchial artery from the right thyrocervical trunk.
B. Angiogram showing aberrant origin of the Left Bronchial Artery from the Right Thyrocervical Trunk. **C.** Common
Bronchial Trunk with aberrant origin from the Left Thyrocervical Trunk. Note multiple Intercostal Arteries
originated from the same trunk.

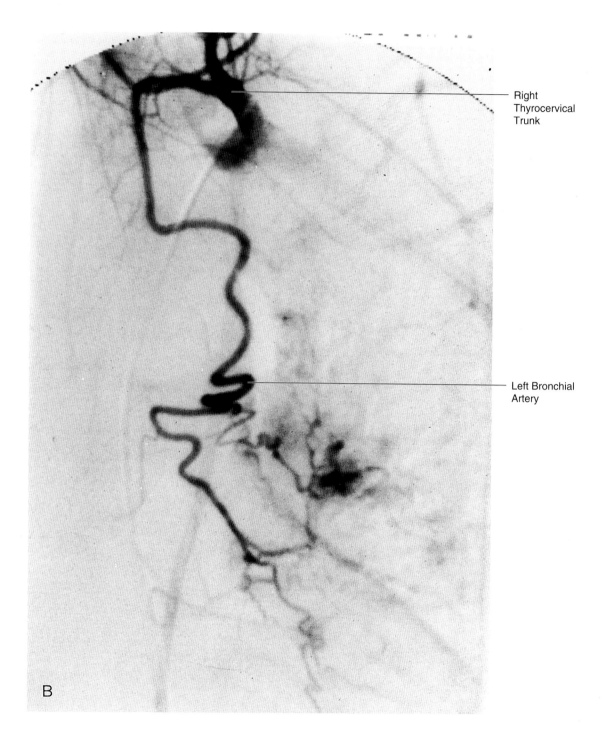

Right
Thyrocervical
Trunk

Left Bronchial
Artery

B

Figure 7.25. *Continued*

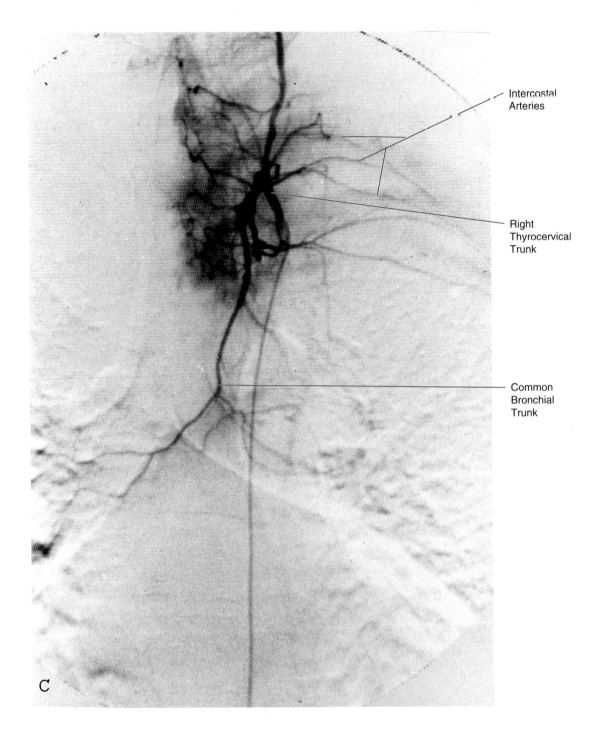

Intercostal
Arteries

Right
Thyrocervical
Trunk

Common
Bronchial
Trunk

C

Figure 7.25. *Continued*

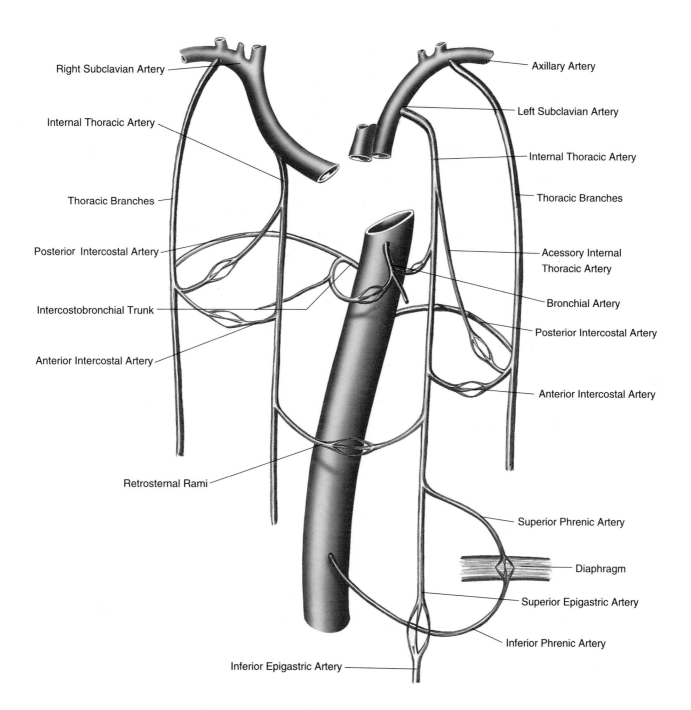

Figure 7.26. Anastomotic connections of the thoracic arteries.

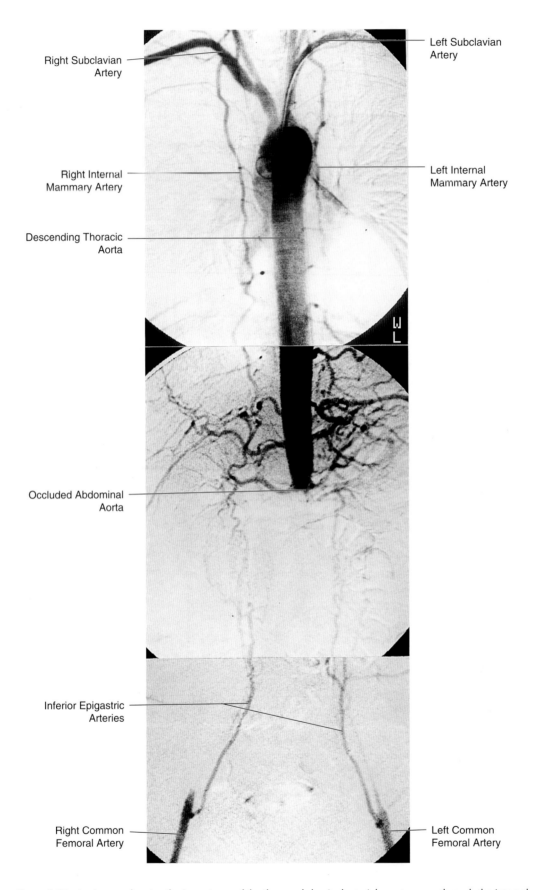

Right Subclavian Artery

Left Subclavian Artery

Right Internal Mammary Artery

Left Internal Mammary Artery

Descending Thoracic Aorta

Occluded Abdominal Aorta

Inferior Epigastric Arteries

Right Common Femoral Artery

Left Common Femoral Artery

Figure 7.27. Angiogram showing the importance of the thoracoabdominal arterial anastomoses through the internal mammary arteries, allowing reconstitution of the common femoral arteries, through the anastomoses with the inferior epigastric arteries.

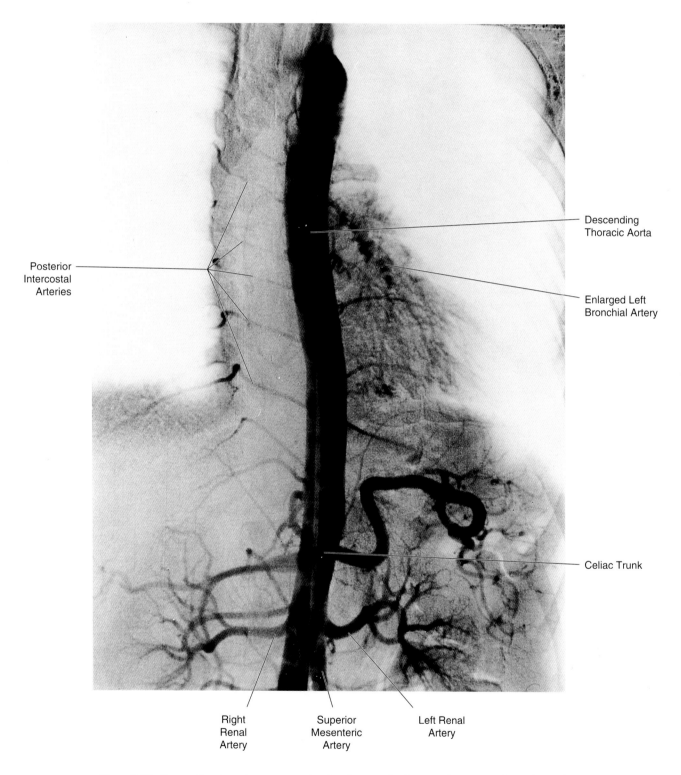

Posterior
Intercostal
Arteries

Descending
Thoracic Aorta

Enlarged Left
Bronchial Artery

Celiac Trunk

Right
Renal
Artery

Superior
Mesenteric
Artery

Left Renal
Artery

Figure 7.28. Descending thoracic aortogram showing the posterior intercostal arteries and an enlarged left bronchial artery. The visceral arteries are also seen.

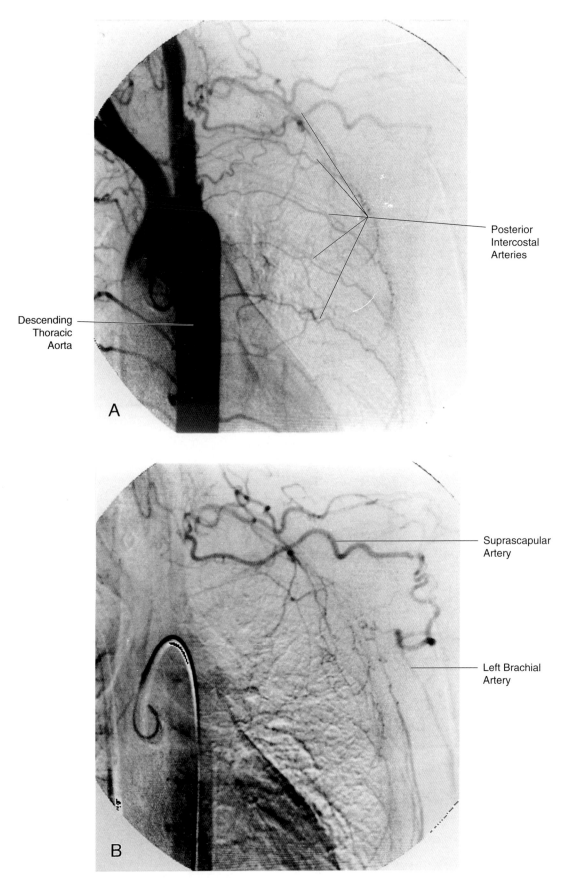

Figure 7.29. A. Thoracic aortogram showing the enlarged posterior intercostal arteries due to the occlusion of the left subclavian artery, in an attempt to reconstitute the left brachial artery. **B.** Later phase of the angiogram showing development of the suprascapular artery.

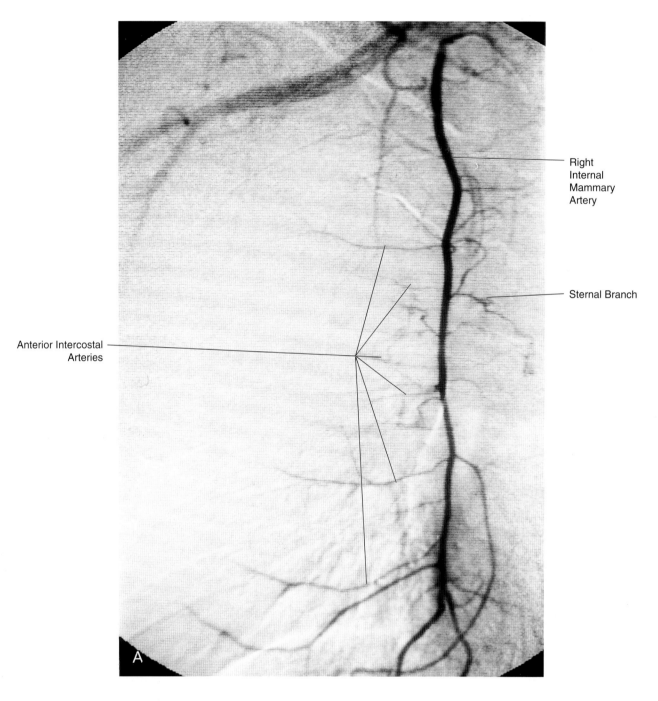

Figure 7.30. A. Selective angiogram of the right internal mammary artery, showing filling of the anterior intercostal arteries. The anterior intercostal arteries are much smaller than the posterior intercostal arteries. **B.** Selective angiogram of the left internal mammary artery.

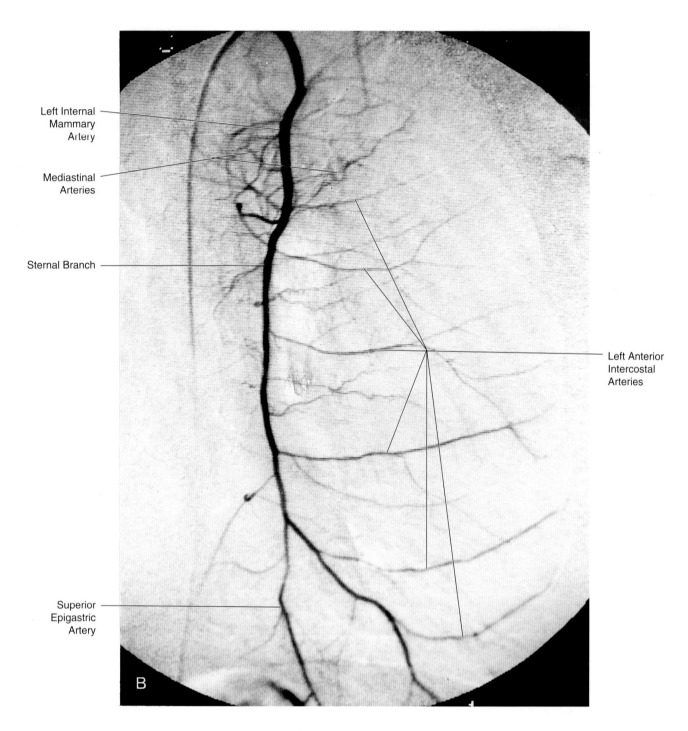

Left Internal
Mammary
Artery

Mediastinal
Arteries

Sternal Branch

Left Anterior
Intercostal
Arteries

Superior
Epigastric
Artery

B

Figure 7.30. *Continued*

8
VEINS OF THE THORAX

BRACHIOCEPHALIC VEINS

Branchiocephalic veins, also called innominate veins, are large veins at the upper thorax and represent united trunks of the internal jugular veins and subclavian veins. There are no valves in these veins (Figs. 8.1, 8.2, 8.3).

The right brachiocephalic vein is approximately 2.5 cm long, following an almost vertical direction, in front of the right brachiocephalic trunk, joining the left brachiocephalic vein, forming the superior vena cava. The tributaries are the right vertebral, internal thoracic, inferior thyroid, and occasionally the first right intercostal veins (Fig. 8.4).

The left brachiocephalic vein is 6 cm long, following an oblique path to the right direction to join the right brachiocephalic vein to form the superior vena cava. It is positioned anteriorly to the left subclavian and common carotid arteries. Tributaries are the left vertebral, internal thoracic, inferior thyroid, superior intercostal, thymic vein, and pericardiophrenic veins. Variations of the brachiocephalic veins include entering the right atrium separately and the configuration of a left vena cava.

INTERNAL THORACIC VEINS (MAMMARY) (FIG. 8.5)

The internal thoracic veins are venae comitans to the internal thoracic arteries, ending in the corresponding brachiocephalic veins. Tributaries are the intercostal veins and pericardiophrenic veins.

INFERIOR THYROID VEINS (FIG. 8.6)

The inferior thyroid veins originate in the glandular venous plexus, having connections with the middle and superior thyroid veins. There is a pretracheal venous plexus, from which the left inferior vein descends to enter the left brachiocephalic vein, and the right inferior thyroid vein crosses the neck to open in the right brachiocephalic vein.

LEFT SUPERIOR INTERCOSTAL VEIN (FIG. 8.1)

The left superior intercostal vein drains the second and third left posterior intercostal veins, directly to the left brachiocephalic vein.

SUPERIOR VENA CAVA (FIG. 8.7)

The superior vena cava is the main vein for venous drainage for the superior aspect of the body. It is around 7 cm in length and is formed by the confluence of the brachiocephalic veins. It has no valves. It ends in the right atrium. The superior vena cava is in contact with the right lung, pleura, trachea, right pulmonary hilum, and aorta. Tributaries are the azygos vein and small veins from the mediastinum.

PERICARDIOPHRENIC VEIN (FIG. 8.8)

The pericardiophrenic veins are the main venous drainage channel for the diaphragm and the pericardium. These veins are in contact with the pericardium and pleura.

THYMIC VEINS (FIGS. 8.9, 8.10, 8.11)

The thymic veins are small in adults, unless there is some enlargement of the gland thymus.

AZYGOS VEIN

The azygos vein is formed by the confluence of the ascending lumbar veins, subcostal veins, and lumbar azygos. It ascends in the posterior mediastinum up to the level of the 4th vertebra, where it arches anteriorly above the right pulmonary hilum, ending in the superior vena cava. Tributaries are the posterior intercostal veins, the hemiazygos, accessory hemiazygos veins, esophageal, mediastinal, and pericardial veins. The right bronchial veins also drain to the azygos vein, near the hilum. When present, the trunk formed by the subcostal and ascending lumbar veins are major tributaries. The azygos vein starts laterally to the vertebral bodies but turns anterior to the thoracic spine as it approaches the vena cava (Figs. 8.12, 8.13, 8.14, 8.15, 8.16, 8.17).

HEMIAZYGOS VEIN

The hemiazygos vein starts on the left side, ascending anteriorly to the spine, crossing the column and reaching the azygos vein. Tributaries are the lower three posterior intercostal veins, a common trunk formed by the left ascending lumbar vein and the subcostal vein (Figs. 8.12, 8.13, 8.14, 8.15, 8.17).

ACCESSORY HEMIAZYGOS VEIN

The accessory hemiazygos vein results from the confluence of several posterior intercostal veins, descending laterally to the thoracic spine, reaching the azygos vein. It may, however, join the hemiazygos vein (Figs. 8.12, 8.14).

POSTERIOR INTERCOSTAL VEINS

There are 11 pairs of posterior intercostal veins. They are companions of the posterior intercostal arteries, running along the subcostal groove. On the right, the 2nd, 3rd, and 4th posterior intercostal veins form the right superior intercostal vein (Figs. 8.12, 8.18).

There are anterior intercostal veins, tributaries of the internal thoracic and musculophrenic veins, but are small.

Bronchial veins are also found on each side, draining blood from larger hilar structures and the bronchial tree. The right bronchial vein joins the azygos, and the left joins the left superior intercostal or hemiazygos vein.

ESOPHAGEAL VEINS

The esophageal veins run along the esophagus and drain to the azygos vein and the more distal veins drain into the portal venous system through the left gastric vein (Fig. 8.19).

VEINS OF THE VERTEBRAL COLUMN (CHAPTER 6)

There is a large and complex venous plexus around the vertebral column. This is also called Batson's venous plexus. This plexus is internal and external to the spinal canal (Figs. 8.8, 20.33).

External Venous Plexuses
    Anterior external venous plexus
    Posterior external venous plexus
Internal vertebral venous plexus
    Anterior internal venous plexus
    Posterior internal venous plexus
Basivertebral veins
Intervertebral veins
Veins of the spinal cord

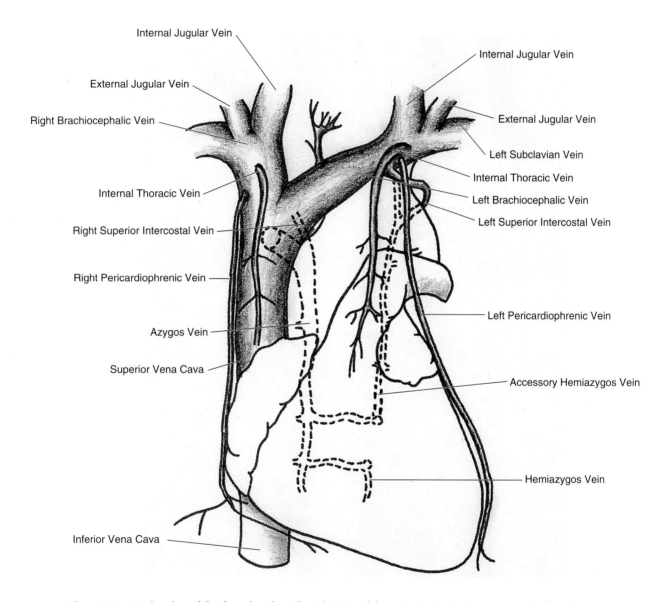

Internal Jugular Vein

External Jugular Vein

Right Brachiocephalic Vein

Internal Thoracic Vein

Right Superior Intercostal Vein

Right Pericardiophrenic Vein

Azygos Vein

Superior Vena Cava

Inferior Vena Cava

Internal Jugular Vein

External Jugular Vein

Left Subclavian Vein

Internal Thoracic Vein

Left Brachiocephalic Vein

Left Superior Intercostal Vein

Left Pericardiophrenic Vein

Accessory Hemiazygos Vein

Hemiazygos Vein

Figure 8.1. Anterior view of the thoracic veins. The right internal thoracic vein terminates more proximally on its brachiocephalic vein than does the left. The left pericardiophrenic vein terminates on the left brachiocephalic vein; it may also terminate on the internal thoracic vein or superior intercostal vein.

Right Internal
Jugular Vein

Right
Subclavian
Vein

Right
Brachiocephalic
Vein

Azygos
Vein

Superior
Vena Cava

Right
Atrium

Left Internal
Jugular Vein

Left Subclavian
Vein

Left Brachiocephalic
Vein

Pulmonary
Artery

Right Ventricle

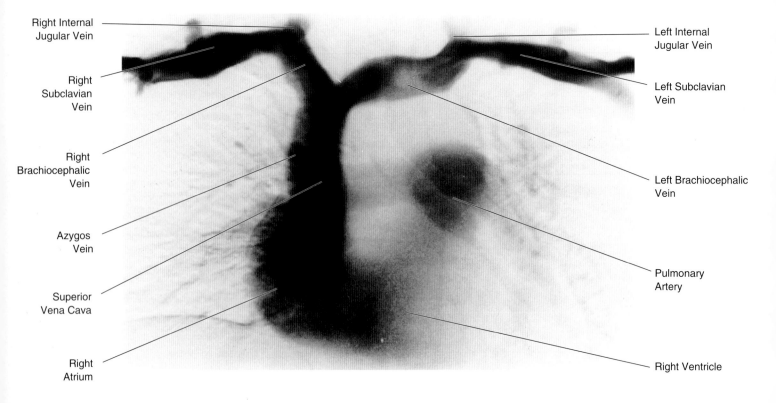

Figure 8.2. Anterior view of an angiogram of the main thoracic veins. Note the vertical course of the right
brachiocephalic vein and the horizontal course of the left brachiocephalic vein.

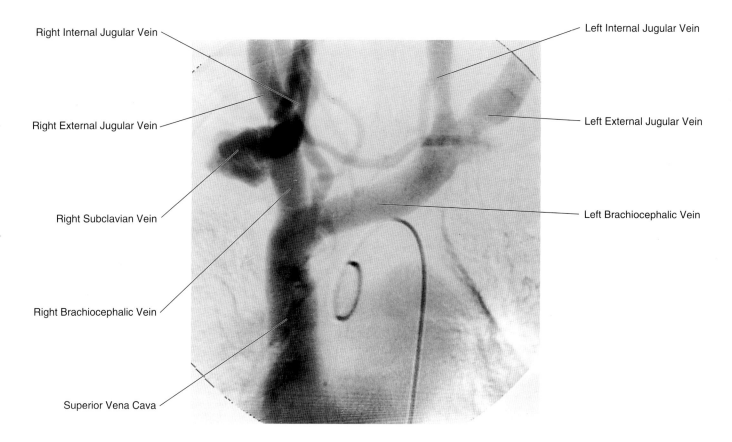

Right Internal Jugular Vein

Right External Jugular Vein

Right Subclavian Vein

Right Brachiocephalic Vein

Superior Vena Cava

Left Internal Jugular Vein

Left External Jugular Vein

Left Brachiocephalic Vein

Figure 8.3. Anterior view of an angiogram of the main thoracic veins showing the superior vena cava and some of the tributaries of the brachiocephalic veins.

Anterior Jugular Vein

Internal Jugular Vein

Subclavian Vein

Cephalic Vein

Right Brachiocephalic Vein

Superior Vena Cava

Right Atrium

External Jugular Vein

Intercostal Veins

Jugular Arch

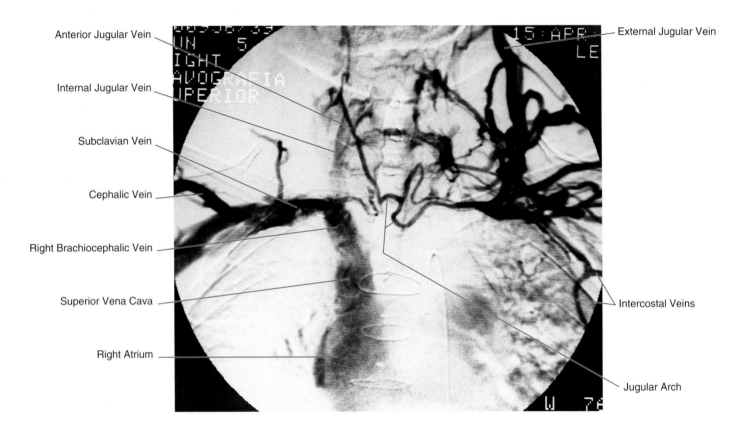

Figure 8.4. Anterior view of an angiogram of the main thoracic veins. Due to occlusion of the left brachiocephalic vein, there is marked development of collateral circulation around the neck and upper thorax.

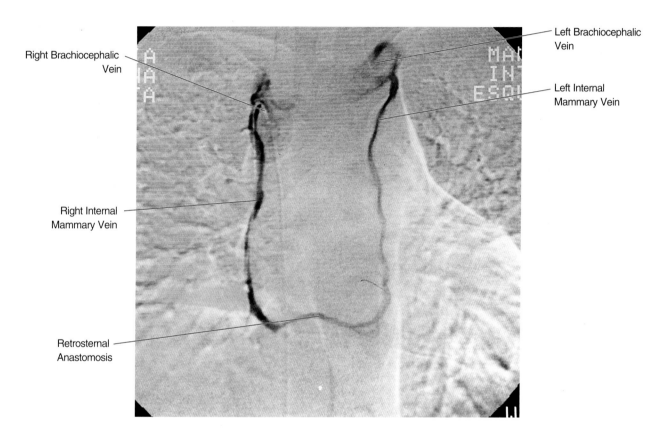

Right Brachiocephalic Vein

Left Brachiocephalic Vein

Left Internal Mammary Vein

Right Internal Mammary Vein

Retrosternal Anastomosis

Figure 8.5. Anterior view of an angiogram with selective injection at the right internal thoracic vein with contralateral filling of the left internal thoracic vein (internal mammary artery). Note the retrosternal anastomosis.

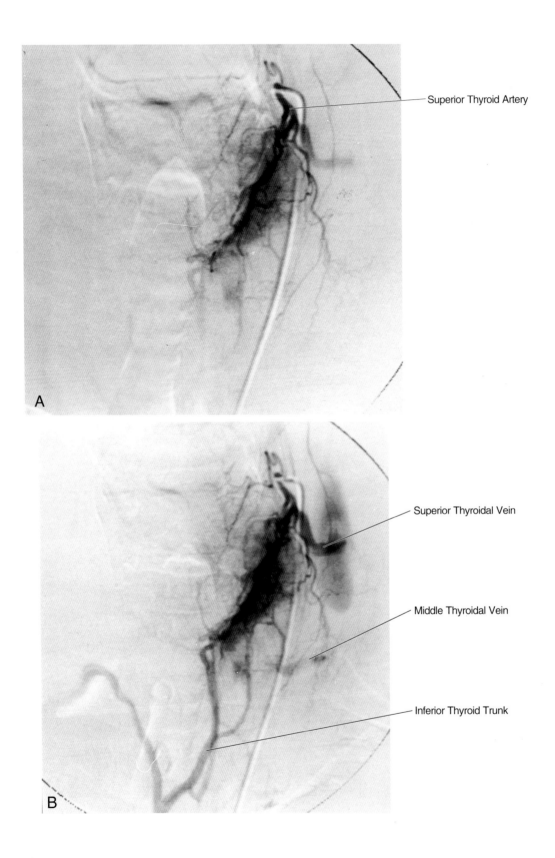

Figure 8.6. **A**, Left superior thyroid artery injection showing early filling of the upper and lower drainage veins. **B**, Late phase of the angiogram showing the thyroid venous drainage. **C**, Right side arterial injection showing the venous drainage. **D**, Selective venogram of the inferior thyroid vein showing the thyroid venous plexus.

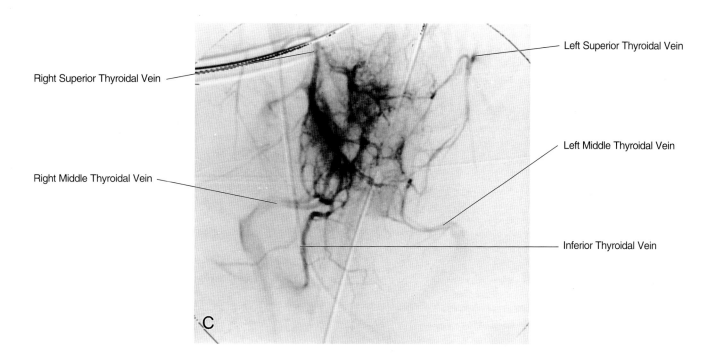

Figure 8.6. *Continued*

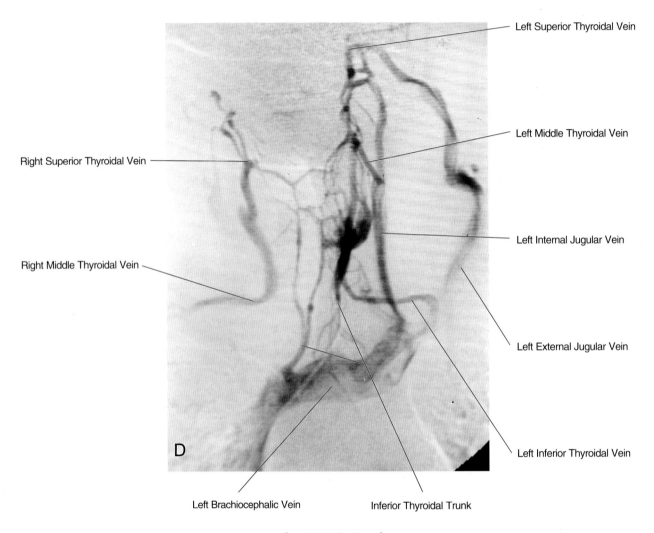

Left Superior Thyroidal Vein

Left Middle Thyroidal Vein

Right Superior Thyroidal Vein

Left Internal Jugular Vein

Right Middle Thyroidal Vein

Left External Jugular Vein

Left Inferior Thyroidal Vein

D

Left Brachiocephalic Vein

Inferior Thyroidal Trunk

Figure 8.6. *Continued*

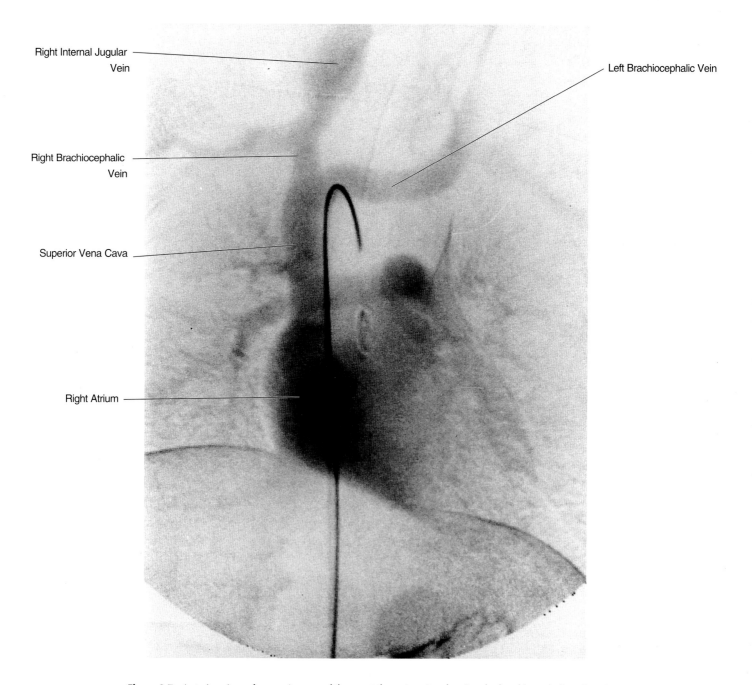

Right Internal Jugular Vein

Left Brachiocephalic Vein

Right Brachiocephalic Vein

Superior Vena Cava

Right Atrium

Figure 8.7. Anterior view of an angiogram of the great thoracic veins showing the brachiocephalic veins, the superior vena cava, and the right atrium and right ventricle.

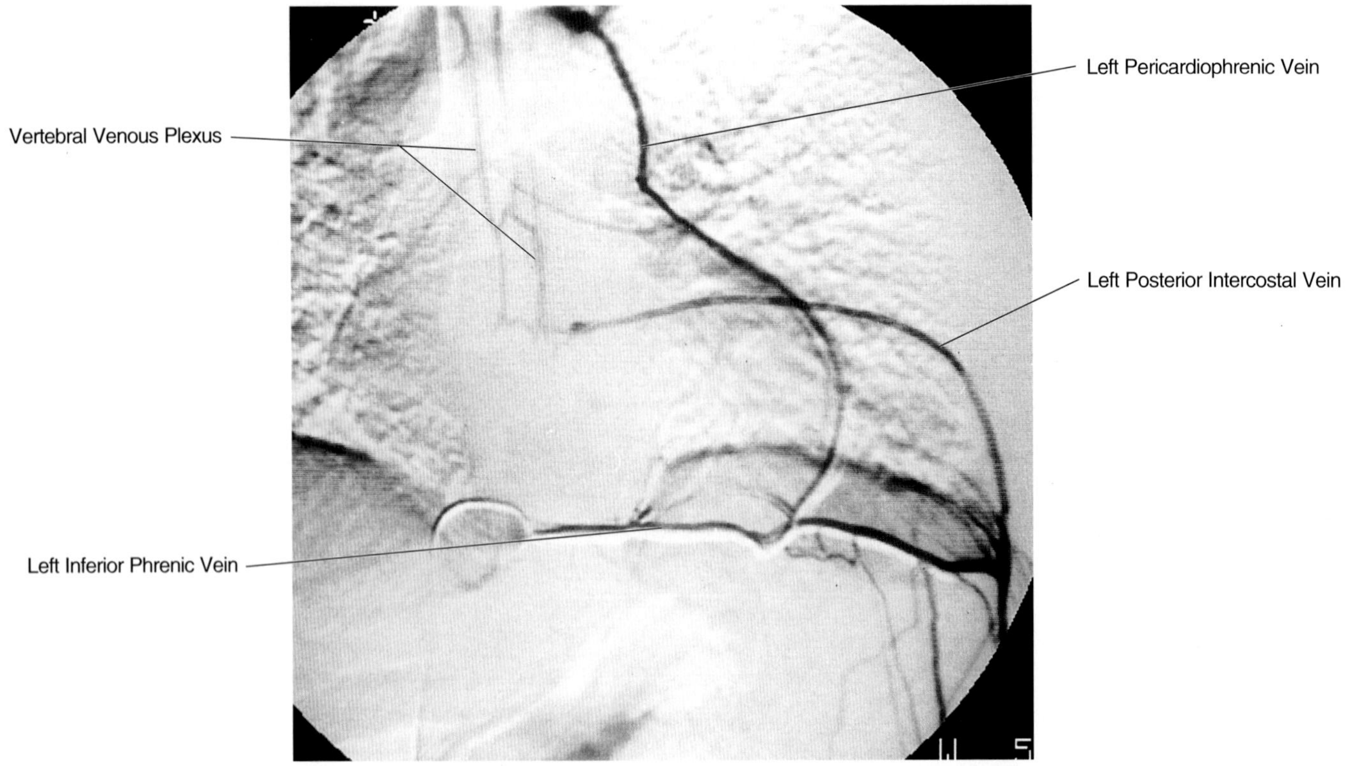

Figure 8.8. Anterior view of an angiogram showing the pericardiophrenic vein, one intercostal vein and the connections with the inferior phrenic vein catheterized from the inferior vena cava. Note the connections with the perivertebral venous plexus.

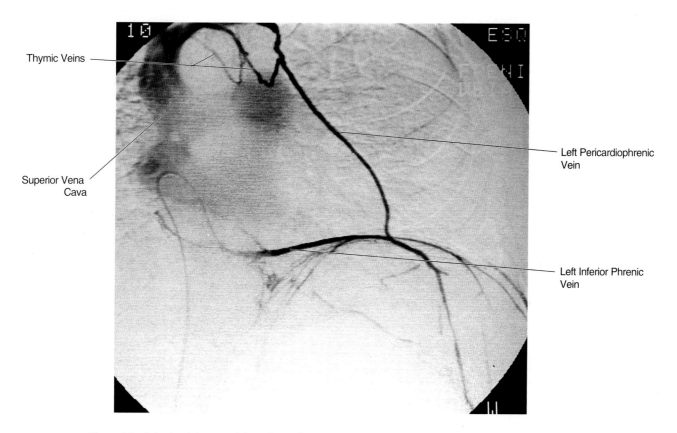

Figure 8.9. Selective injection of the inferior phrenic vein with opacification of the pericardiophrenic vein and the thymic veins in connection with the superior mediastinal venous drainage.

Right Internal Jugular Vein

Right Subclavian Veins

Right Brachiocephalic Vein

Vertebral Venous Plexus

Anterior Jugular Veins

Suprascapular Vein

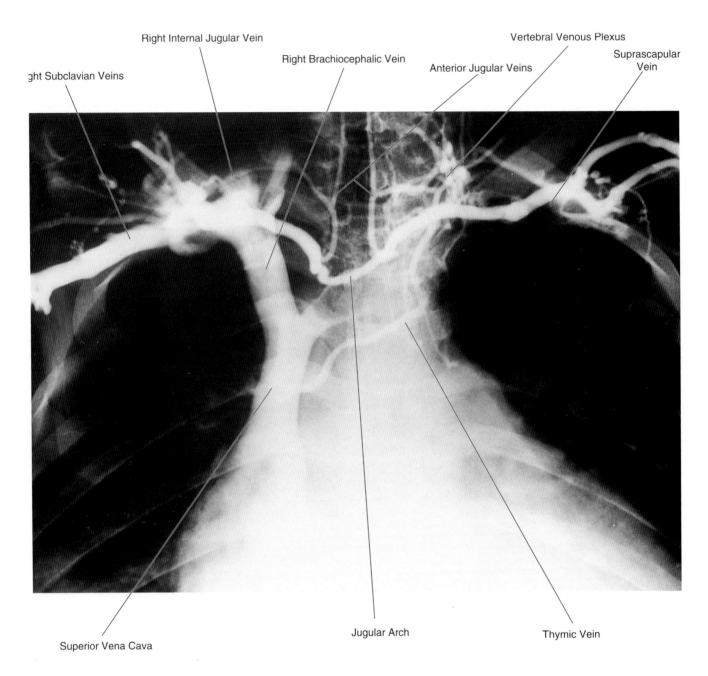

Superior Vena Cava

Jugular Arch

Thymic Vein

Figure 8.10. Angiogram of the great venous vessels of the thorax with occlusion of the left brachiocephalic vein and development of cervical and thoracic collaterals.

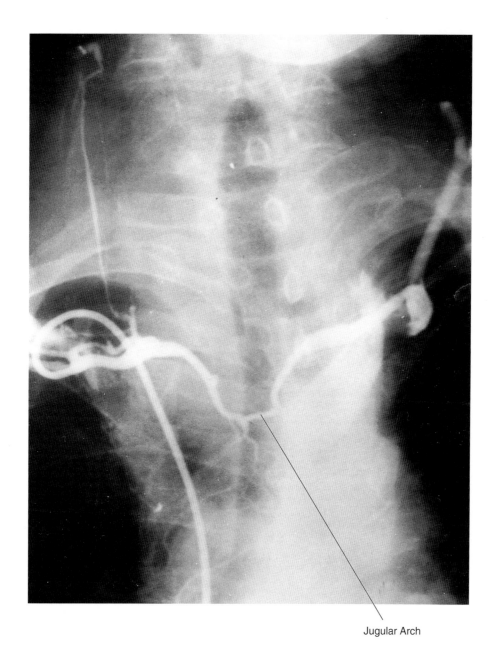

Jugular Arch

Figure 8.11. Selective angiogram of the jugular arch.

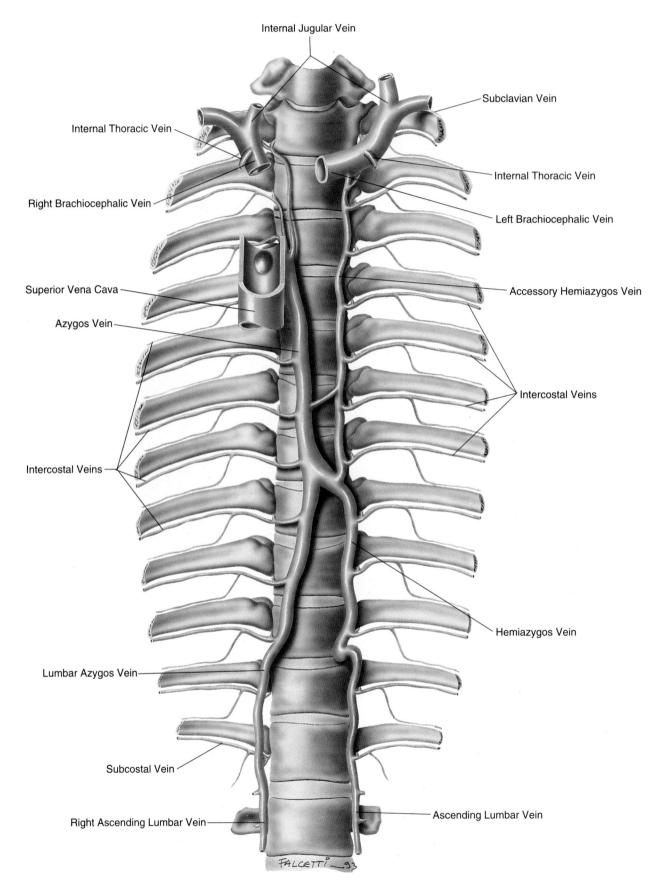

Internal Jugular Vein

Subclavian Vein

Internal Thoracic Vein

Internal Thoracic Vein

Right Brachiocephalic Vein

Left Brachiocephalic Vein

Superior Vena Cava

Accessory Hemiazygos Vein

Azygos Vein

Intercostal Veins

Intercostal Veins

Hemiazygos Vein

Lumbar Azygos Vein

Subcostal Vein

Ascending Lumbar Vein

Right Ascending Lumbar Vein

FALCETTI 93

Figure 8.12. Venous circulation of the thorax in an anterior view.

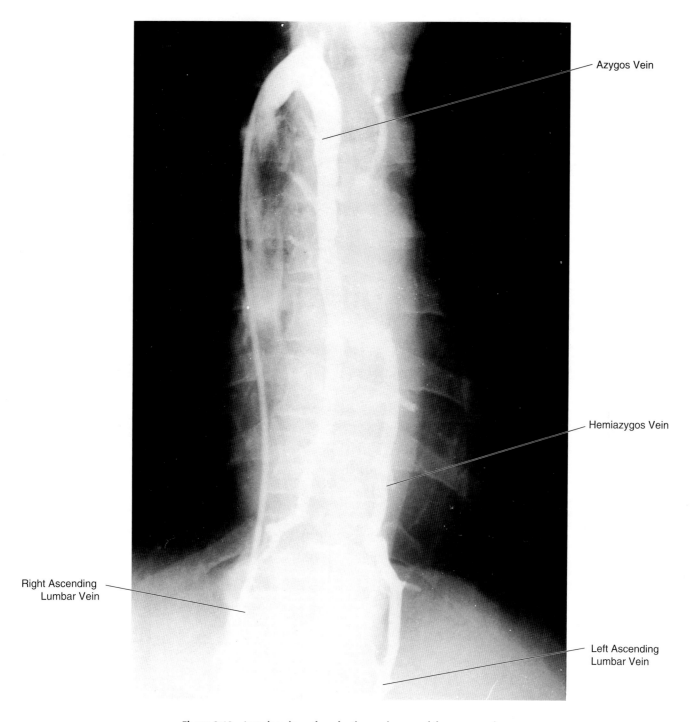

Azygos Vein

Hemiazygos Vein

Right Ascending Lumbar Vein

Left Ascending Lumbar Vein

Figure 8.13. Anterior view of a selective angiogram of the azygos vein.

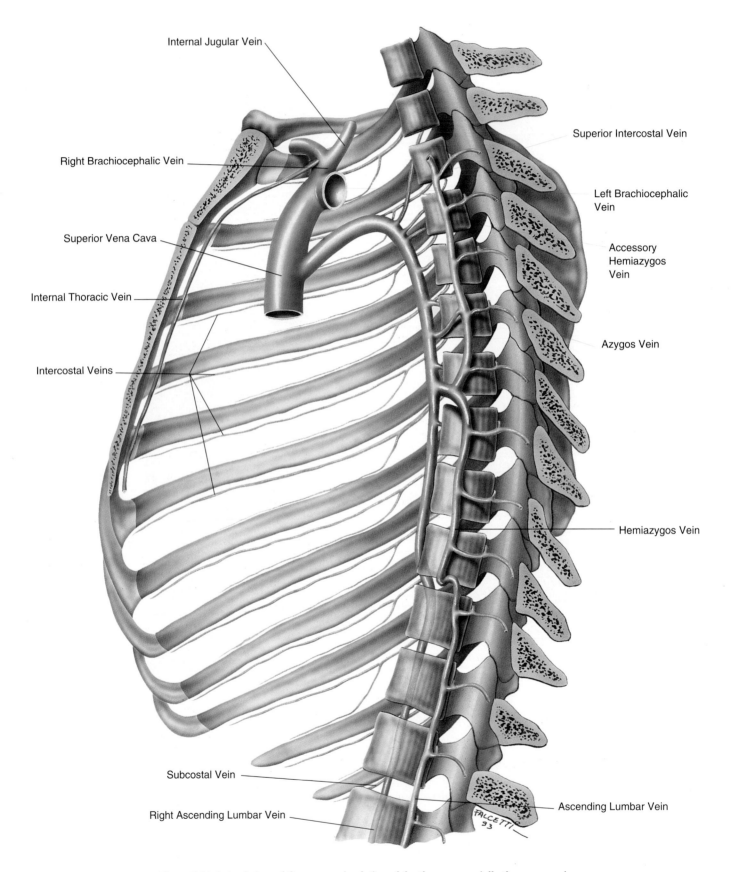

Internal Jugular Vein

Right Brachiocephalic Vein

Superior Vena Cava

Internal Thoracic Vein

Intercostal Veins

Subcostal Vein

Right Ascending Lumbar Vein

Superior Intercostal Vein

Left Brachiocephalic Vein

Accessory Hemiazygos Vein

Azygos Vein

Hemiazygos Vein

Ascending Lumbar Vein

FALCETTI 93

Figure 8.14. Lateral view of the venous circulation of the thorax, especially the azygos vein.

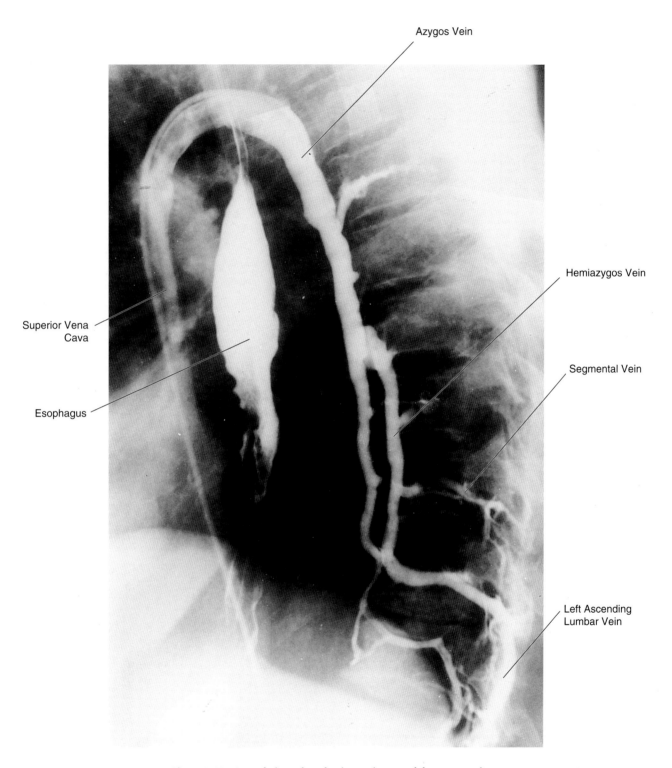

Figure 8.15. Lateral view of a selective angiogram of the azygos vein.

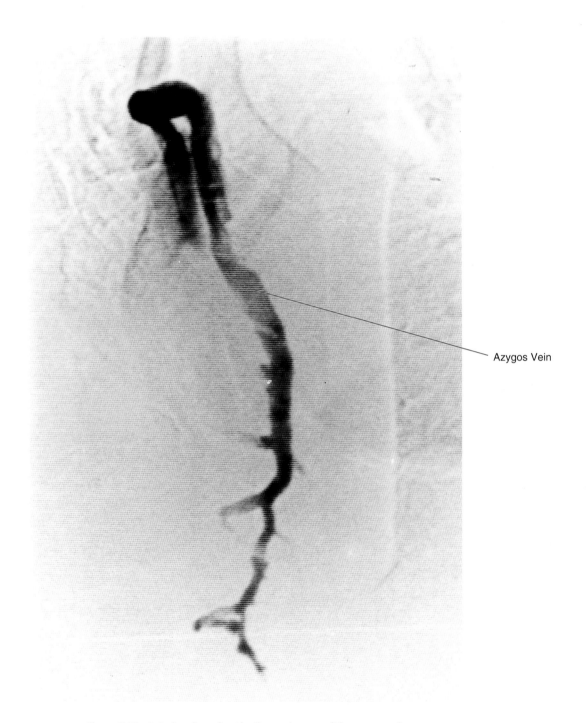

Azygos Vein

Figure 8.16. Anterior view of a selective angiogram of the azygos vein.

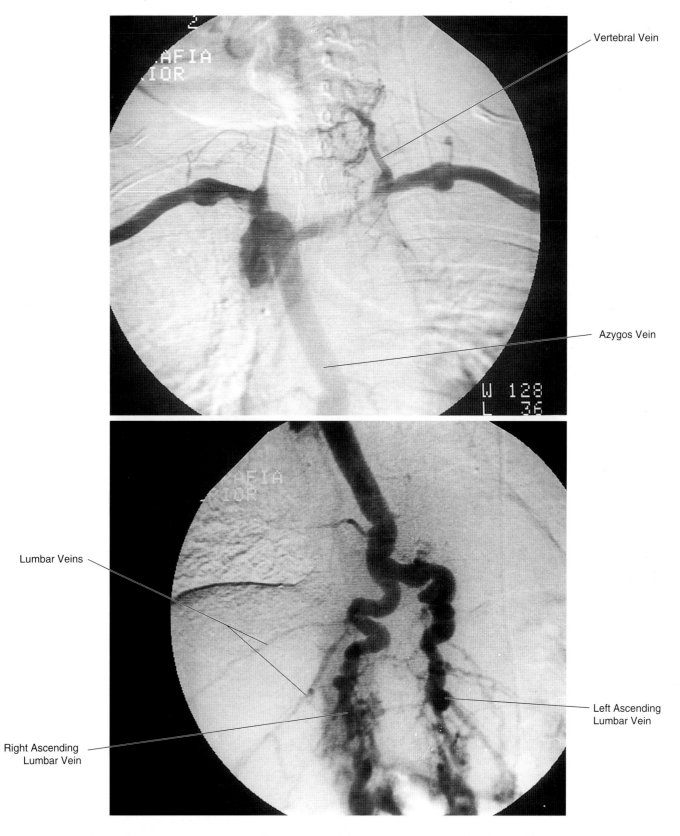

Figure 8.17. Anterior composite view of an angiogram of the azygos vein in a case of occlusion of the superior vena cava, with drainage of the thorax veins through the azygos system and inferior vena cava, not demonstrated in this angiogram.

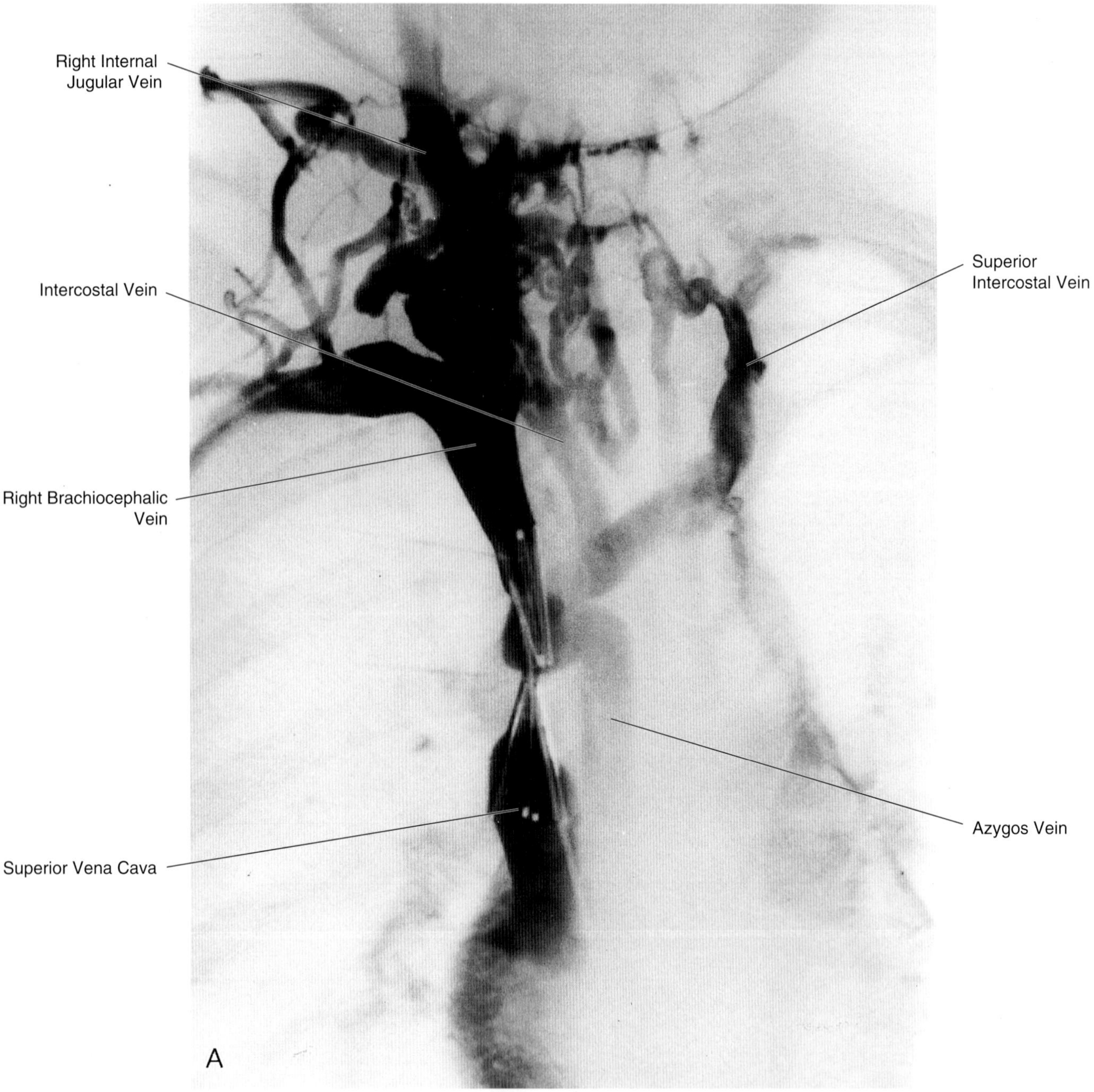

Figure 8.18. A, Venogram of the great veins of the thorax in a case with obstruction of the superior vena cava partially treated with a stent not fully opened. Note the development of collaterals and the azygos veins tribu-taries, including the posterior intercostal vein. **B**, Lateral view of the same patient before introduction of the stent showing the occlusion of the azy-gos vein, the superior vena cava, and the collateral circulation.

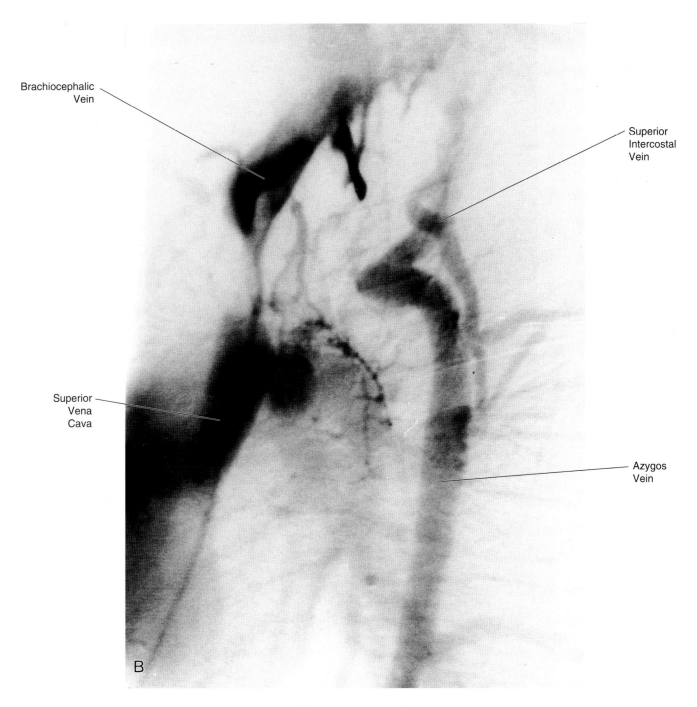

Brachiocephalic Vein

Superior Intercostal Vein

Superior Vena Cava

Azygos Vein

B

Figure 8.18. *Continued*

Azygos Vein

Esophageal Veins

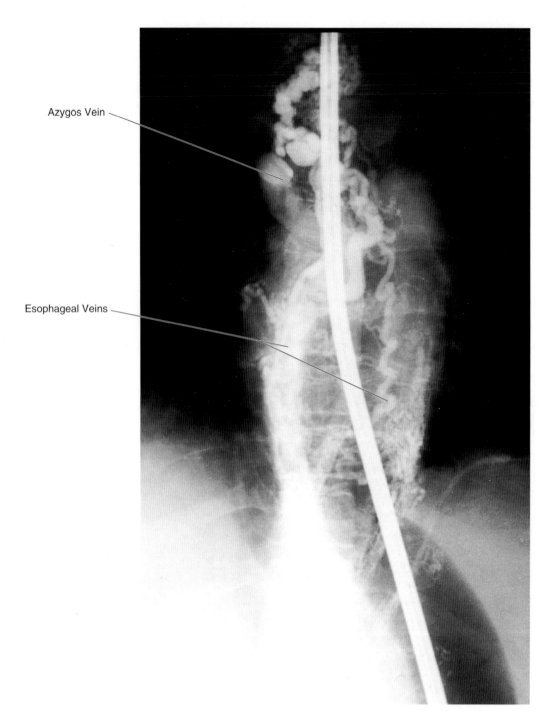

Figure 8.19. Selective venogram of the inferior esophageal veins draining into the azygos vein, in a patient with portal hypertension.

9

LYMPHATIC SYSTEM OF THE THORAX

THORACIC LYMPHATIC DRAINAGE

Peripheral lymph drainage is made to the venous circulation, via the right and left lymphovenous portals, which are located close to the junction of the large internal jugular and subclavian veins. On the right, there are three main lymphatic trunks; on the left, four main lymphatic trunks are identified, the three corresponding to the right and in addition the thoracic duct, which is the largest lymphatic trunk in the body (Figs. 9.1, 9.2, 9.3). The anatomy of the lymphovenous portals varies. In 80% of subjects, the right trunks open independently at the jugular-subclavian junction. In 1/5 of cases, a short right lymphatic trunk is formed.

Lymphovenous Portals

On the Right

There are three main lymphatic trunks converging to the junction of the right internal jugular vein with the right subclavian vein: 1) the right jugular trunk, which runs along the ventrolateral aspect of the internal jugular vein, carrying all the lymph from the right half of the head and neck; 2) the right subclavian trunk from the right apical axillary lymph nodes, running along the axillary and subclavian vein, and carrying lymph from the upper right limb and the superficial tissues of the right chest and abdominal wall; and 3) the right bronchomediastinal trunk, which runs along the trachea, carrying lymph from the right lung, diaphragm, bronchi, and trachea.

On the Left

The left portal receives the volume of lymph from all over the body, except the territories mentioned for the right lymphatic trunks. There are four main lymphatic trunks converging to the left lymphovenous portal: 1) the left jugular trunk, which runs along the ventrolateral aspect of the internal jugular vein, carrying lymph from the left half of the head and neck; 2) the left subclavian trunk draining lymph from the upper left limb and superficial tissues of the left chest and abdominal wall; 3) the left bronchomediastinal trunk, which drains more of the heart and esophagus,

besides the lung, bronchi, and trachea; and 4) the thoracic duct, which drains the remaining territories of the body. It is formed by the abdominal confluence of the lymphatic trunks to the cisterna chyli.

Thoracic Duct

The thoracic duct measures about 38-45 cm in length, in adults, extending from the abdomen to the neck, transgressing the diaphragm, ascending at the posterior mediastinum, right of the midline, between the descending thoracic aorta and the azygos vein and anterior of the vertebral column. The thoracic duct commences wide, forming in some cases a pouch called cisterna chyli, and diminishes in caliber up to the neck, where it arches laterally to the left and anteriorly and eventually descends in direction to the junction of the left internal jugular and left subclavian veins, opening into the venous system, through a bicuspid valve. At the termination, the thoracic duct may be multiple and the site or opening may be in any of the left great veins. The origin of the thoracic duct is the confluence of the four main abdominal lymph trunks (Figs. 9.1, 9.2).

Tributaries of the Thoracic Duct Proper

Confluence of the Abdominal Lymphatic Trunks

Lumbar lymph trunks
Intestinal lymph trunks
    Bilateral descending lymph trunks
    Bilateral ascending lymph trunks
Upper intercostal lymph trunks
Mediastinal lymph trunks
Left subclavian lymph trunk
Left jugular lymph trunk
Left bronchomediastinal lymph trunk

Lymphatic Drainage of the Thoracic Wall

Lymphatic Vessels

The superficial lymphatic vessels of the chest wall converge to the axillary nodes, subscapular nodes, pectoral nodes, and parasternal nodes (Fig. 9.4). The deeper lymphatic vessels of the chest walls drain mainly to the parasternal, intercostal, and diaphragmatic lymphatic nodes (Fig. 9.1).

Parasternal Lymph Nodes (Internal Thoracic)

There are four or five nodes on each side, at the anterior end of the intercostal spaces, following the path of the internal thoracic arteries and veins. They drain the internal, anterior thoracic wall, and the mammary glands. Their efferents form the bronchomediastinal trunk, together with the tracheobronchial and the brachiocephalic lymph nodes (Fig. 9.5).

Intercostal Lymph Nodes

The intercostal lymph nodes are located at the heads and necks of the ribs and receive lymphatic vessels from the posterolateral aspect of the chest and mammary gland. The lower four to seven intercostal spaces unite, forming the descending trunk, which joins the thoracic duct or the abdominal confluence of the lymphatic trunks (Figs. 9.1, 9.4).

Diaphragmatic Lymph Nodes

There are anterior, right and left lateral, and posterior groups of diaphragmatic lymph nodes on the thoracic surface of the diaphragm.

Lymphatic Drainage of the Thoracic Contents

The lymph from the thoracic organs is drained through one of the three groups of lymph nodes in the chest before entering the thoracic duct or the right lymphatic duct: the brachiocephalic, the posterior mediastinal, or tracheobronchial lymph nodes.

Brachiocephalic Lymph Nodes

The brachiocephalic lymph nodes are located in the superior mediastinum, anteriorly to the brachiocephalic veins and the large arterial trunks. They receive lymph from the thymus, thyroid gland, pericardium, heart, and lateral diaphragmatic nodes. They drain to the right and left bronchomediastinal trunks after joining the efferent lymphatics from the tracheobronchial nodes.

Posterior Mediastinal Lymph Nodes

The posterior mediastinal lymph nodes are located behind the pericardium, close to the esophagus and the descending thoracic aorta. They receive afferent lymphatic vessels from the esophagus, posterior pericardium, diaphragm, and sometimes from the left lobe of the liver. They are mostly connected to the thoracic duct.

Tracheobronchial Lymph Nodes (Chapter 12, see Fig. 12.2)

There are five foremost groups of tracheobronchial lymph nodes.
1. Paratracheal
2. Superior Tracheobronchial
3. Inferior Tracheobronchial (Carinate Nodes)
4. Bronchopulmonary (Hilar Nodes)
5. Pulmonary

These groups are continuous and without clear differentiation. The afferent vessels drain the lungs parenchyma, the pleura, the bronchi, thoracic trachea, and heart and connect with some posterior mediastinal nodes. The efferent vessels ascend to the trachea to join the efferent vessels of the parasternal and brachiocephalic nodes forming the right and left bronchomediastinal trunks. On the right side, this trunk may join a right lymphatic duct or another lymphatic trunk. On the left side, the trunk may connect to the thoracic duct, but more often open independently at the jugulosubclavian junction.

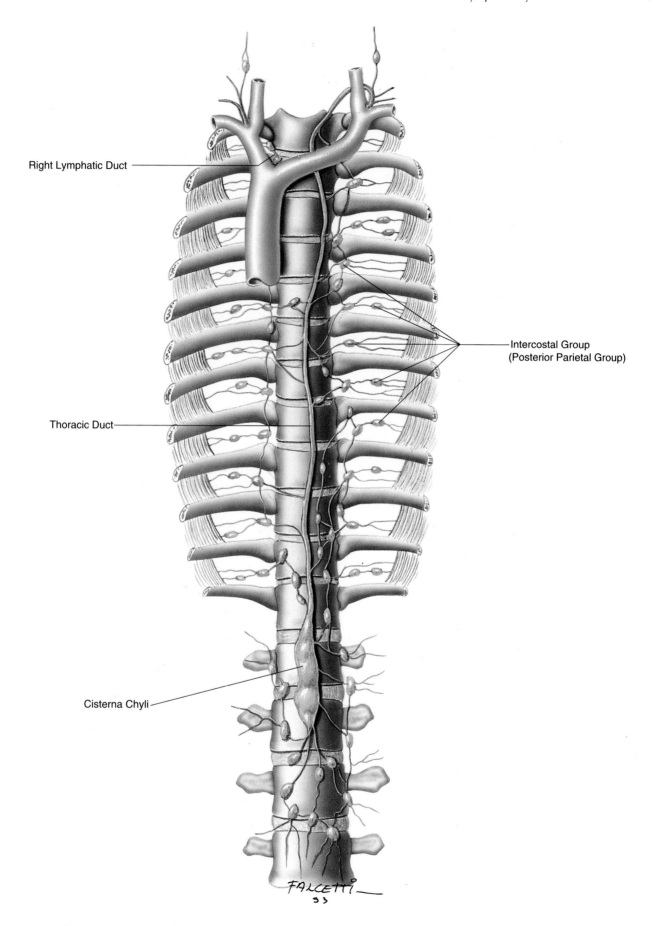

Right Lymphatic Duct

Intercostal Group
(Posterior Parietal Group)

Thoracic Duct

Cisterna Chyli

Figure 9.1. Posterior mediastinal lymphatic system with the thoracic duct, intercostal lymphatic nodes group, and the cisternal chyli. Note the right lymphatic duct entering the right subclavian vein.

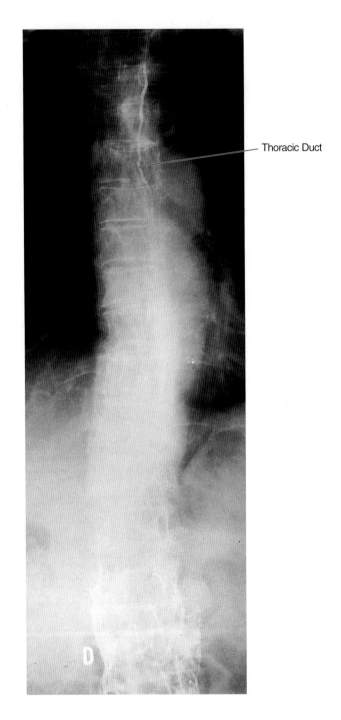

Thoracic Duct

Figure 9.2. Lymphangiogram showing the thoracic duct.

Confluence of the Thoracic Duct with the Vein

Supraclavicular Lymph Nodes

Thoracic Duct

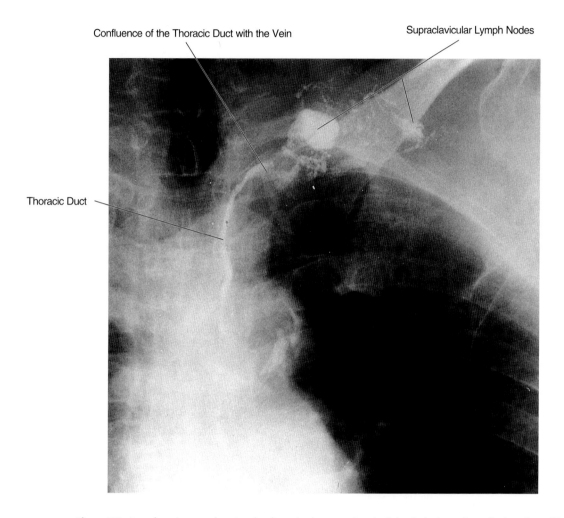

Figure 9.3. Lymphangiogram showing the thoracic duct entering the left subclavian vein at the junction with the right internal jugular vein. Note the lymph nodes opacified by the contrast.

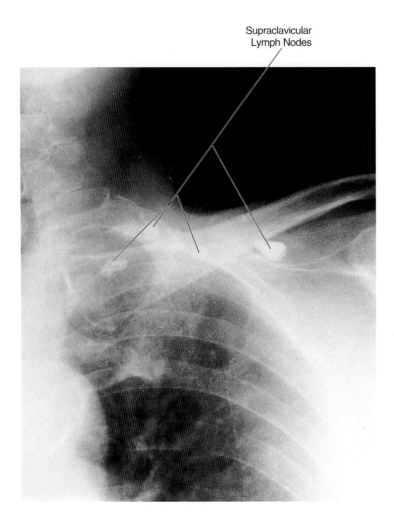

Figure 9.4. Supraclavicular lymph nodes opacified 24 hours after the lymphangiogram.

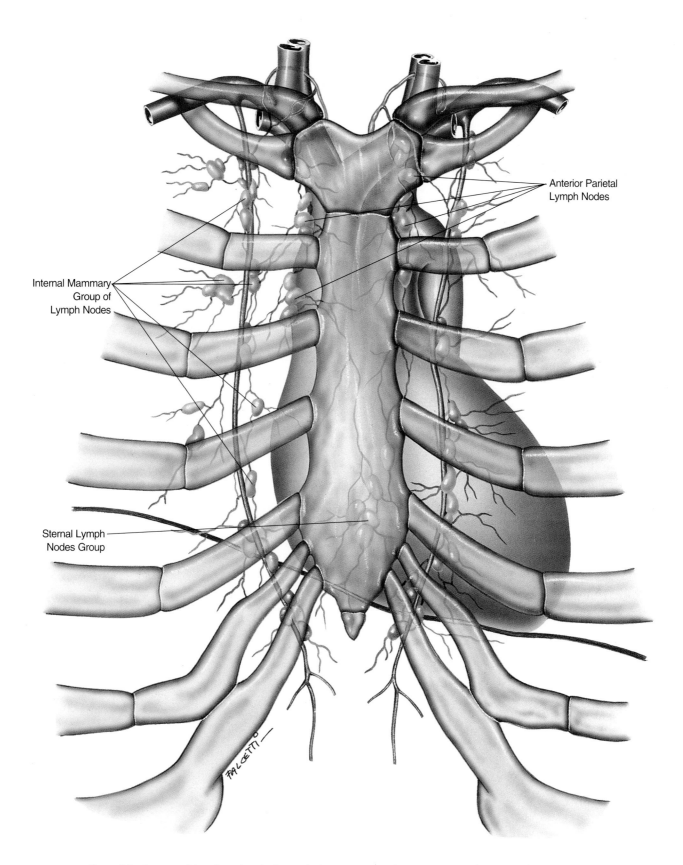

Anterior Parietal
Lymph Nodes

Internal Mammary
Group of
Lymph Nodes

Sternal Lymph
Nodes Group

Figure 9.5. Parasternal lymph nodes, the internal mammary group, the anterior parietal group, and retrosternal lymph nodes group.

10

PULMONARY ARTERIAL CIRCULATION

Anatomically, the pulmonary arteries are elastic, with little mural musculature down to their 5th or 6th divisions. Peripherally, the amount of smooth muscle in the walls of intrapulmonary arteries increases. The branches with 1.0 mm to 0.1 mm in diameter are mainly muscular. Branches less than 0.1 mm in diameter are nonmuscular and are chiefly poorly supported endothelial tubes, with profuse anastomotic, alveolar capillary networks — the principal structural elements in the walls of the respiratory membranes. The pulmonary circulation is a low-resistance, low-pressure system with high distensibility and little vasomotor control. The pulmonary resistance is about a sixth of the systemic, with a pressure averaging 22/8 mm Hg (mean, 13 mm Hg). The pulmonary blood flow can triple without significant increase in pulmonary artery pressure due to the high degree of distensibility of the normal pulmonary vasculature. The large and small pulmonary arteries carry about 30% of the blood in the lungs, while the capillaries carry around 20% of the blood in the lungs.

PULMONARY TRUNK

The pulmonary trunk carries deoxygenated blood from the right ventricle of the heart to the lung circulation. It has about 5 cm in length and 3 cm in diameter, arising from the right ventricle base above and left to the supraventricular crest. It is a short vessel arising from the pulmonary conus of the right ventricle at the pulmonary semilunar valves. It has an ascending and posterior orientation, in front of the ascending aorta towards its left aspect (Fig. 10.1). The pulmonary trunk lies totally within the pericardium. It divides in the left and right pulmonary arteries, with about the same sizes. The bifurcation of the main pulmonary artery varies in appearance, its angle ranging between 100 and 180 degrees (Fig. 10.2). The diameter of the right pulmonary artery ranges between 17 and 30 mm (mean, 23.4 mm). The caliber of the main pulmonary artery is between 20 and 30 mm (mean, 26.4 mm). The sum of the diameter of the left and right main branches is greater than the diameter of the main pulmonary artery.

RIGHT PULMONARY ARTERY

The right pulmonary artery is only slightly smaller in caliber than the main artery, as seen in angiograms. It runs a horizontal, sometimes slightly downward, course across the heart image on the frontal view, to the hilum of the right lung, where it divides into superior and inferior branches. Anatomically, it lies behind the ascending aorta and the superior vena cava and in front of the tracheal bifurcation and esophagus (Fig. 10.3).

The right pulmonary artery divides at the right hilum into two main branches: the ascending branch, to the right upper lobe, and the descending branch, to the right middle lobe and the right lower lobe (Figs. 10.4, 10.5, 10.6).

The ascending branch of the right pulmonary artery supplies the right upper lobe, coursing upward for a short distance and divides into three branches: the apical segmental artery, the posterior segmental artery, and the anterior segmental artery.

The apical segmental artery divides into two major rami: the apical and the posterior rami, supplying the apical bronchopulmonary segment of the right upper lobe.

The posterior segmental artery often arises as a trifurcation, with the apical and posterior segmental arteries supplying the posterior bronchopulmonary segment of the right upper lobe. There are two main rami: a posterior ramus and a lateral ramus.

The anterior segmental artery of the right upper lobe supplies the bronchopulmonary segment of the same name and is the most inferior artery of the trifurcation of the ascending branch of the right pulmonary artery. There are two main rami: an anterior ramus and a lateral ramus.

The descending branch of the right pulmonary artery supplies the right middle and lower lobes. It originates at the bifurcation of the right pulmonary artery and is caudally oriented. The first branch is the middle lobe artery and the superior segmental artery of the right lower lobe. The next branches are the basal segmental artery and the anterior basal segmental artery. The parent vessel splits to form the posterior basal segmental artery and the lateral basal segmental artery. Each branch supplies the corresponding named bronchopulmonary segment of the right lower lobe.

The middle lobe artery arises from the descending branch of the right pulmonary artery, at the opposite aspect of the origin of the superior segmental artery. It has an anterior and inferiorly oriented direction, bifurcating into a lateral and a medial segmental artery, which supply the respective bronchopulmonary segments of the right middle lobe (Fig. 10.5).

The superior segmental artery of the right lower lobe courses posteriorly upward and laterally, supplying the upper part of the right lower lobe. The medial basal segmental artery of the right lower lobe arises as the third major branch of the right pulmonary artery, and arises just distally to the point of origin of the superior segmental artery. The anterior basal segmental artery of the right lower lobe arises from the anterolateral aspect of the descending branch of the right pulmonary artery, slightly distal to the point of origin of the medial basal segmental artery. The posterior basal segmental artery of the right lower lobe arises together with the lateral basal segment, as a bifurcation of the descending branch of the right pulmonary artery, reaching the most posterior and dependent portion of the right lower lobe. The lateral basal segmental artery of the right lower lobe arises together with the posterior basal segmental artery as a bifurcation of the descending branch of the right pulmonary artery and supplies the lateral basal bronchopulmonary segment (Fig. 10.7).

LEFT PULMONARY ARTERY

The left pulmonary artery is a short continuation of the main pulmonary artery. It runs upward, to the back and to the left, when it turns sharply to the left and caudally to the hilum of the left lung. It lies in front of the descending aorta, beneath the curve of the aortic arch, being connected to the arch by the ligamentum arteriosum.

The left pulmonary artery is short and bifurcates in the left hilum into ascending and descending branches supplying the left upper and lower lobes, respectively (Figs. 10.8, 10.9, 10.10).

The ascending branch of the left pulmonary artery arises about 2 to 4 cm from the origin of the main artery. It runs cranially and bifurcates into two segmental arteries: the posterior apical segmental artery and the anterior segmental artery to the left upper lobe (Figs. 10.11, 10.12). The apical posterior segmental artery of the left upper lobe, the larger to the upper lobe, is short and bifurcates into two major rami: apical and posterior, supplying the corresponding named apical posterior bronchopulmonary segment of the left upper lobe. The apical ramus is medial and the posterior ramus is lateral. The anterior segmental artery of the left upper lobe arises as an inferior branch of the ascending branch of the left pulmonary artery and courses anteriorly. It bifurcates into the anterior and lateral rami, supplying the named portions of the anterior bronchopulmonary segment of the left upper lobe.

The descending branch of the left pulmonary artery courses downward into the lung as a smooth continuation of the main left pulmonary artery, giving origin to the lingular artery, the superior segmental artery, and to the arteries to the basal bronchopulmonary segments of the left lower lobe (Figs. 10.12, 10.13, 10.14).

The lingular artery arises about 2 cm distal from the origin of the ascending branch of the left pulmonary artery, laterally and immediately bifurcates in two segmental components, the superior and inferior lingular segmental arteries.

The segmental arteries to the left lower lobe are similar to those of the contralateral lower lobe, but there are usually three instead of four bronchopulmonary segments in the left. The superior segmental artery is posterior and arises distal to the lingular artery. The anterior and medial segmental arteries are combined and called anteromedial basal segment, being larger than the anterior or medial basal segmental artery of the right lower lobe. The posterior basal segmental artery arises with the lateral basal segmental artery as a bifurcation of the descending branch of the left pulmonary artery and proceeds inferiorly and posteriorly to the posterior bronchopulmonary segment. The lateral basal segmental artery proceeds inferiorly and laterally to supply the lateral bronchopulmonary segment.

PULMONARY MICROCIRCULATION

The pulmonary circulation plays a role of a universal blood filter among the venous and arterial territories. Particles larger than 75 µm are usually retained at the level of the pulmonary arterioles. The pulmonary arterioles reduce their caliber rapidly from 100 to 50 µm. The sizes of the capillaries are about 8 to 9 µm in diameter and 6 to 18 µm in length. The size of the capillaries varies markedly accordingly to the gravity and position of the individual. Experimentally, it was established that particles up to 400 µm in size could be recovered in the venous side of the pulmonary circulation, indicating precapillaries shunts between pulmonary arteries and veins (Fig. 10.15).

The peripheral pulmonary artery and alveolar capillary network are large vascular beds of about 70 to 90 m², in the adult, allowing very intimal contact of the blood circulation with the oxygen from the air in the alveoli. The process of O_2-CO_2 exchange is performed by diffusion of the gases through the alveolar and capillary membranes due to a concentration gradient. The pulmonary capillaries develop a dense network enclosed in the alveolar wall. The basic elements of this network, the capillary segments are short cylindric tubes joined at both ends by two adjacent segments, making a network of hexagonal aspect.

The pulmonary artery, despite high volume and flow, has no capability of lung nutrition. The blood supply to the bronchial connective tissue of the lung is part of the systemic circulation. There is free communication between the capillaries of the pulmonary and bronchial systems, and these capillary beds may drain into either the systemic venous system through the azygos vein or through the pulmonary veins into the left atrium. The interrelation of the two circulations at the capillary level provides a potential shunt, which can serve to prevent elevation of capillary hydrostatic pressure should increase in either right or left atrial pressure occur unilaterally. The bronchial vessels can provide collateral circulation to the lungs when the pulmonary arterial supply is interrupted (Fig. 10.15).

From the lung hilum, the bronchial arteries go into two different directions. They follow the bronchial tree and the visceral pleura. The bronchial arteries are significant in size up to the terminal bronchiole, where the pulmonary artery circulation takes over the nutrition. The small arteriolar branches of the bronchial artery may, however, extend to the alveolar ducts and occasionally even into the lung parenchyma around the alveolar sacs.

The bronchial arteries vascularize the bronchial walls, muscles, glands, and cartilage. The bronchial arteries supply the vasa vasorum to the walls of the pulmonary arteries and the vasa nervorum to the nerves.

The bronchial arteries are unique in that they have a dual venous drainage. The blood from the bronchial arteries drains into the systemic veins, bronchial veins, tributaries of the azygos vein or superior vena cava. From the secondary or tertiary bronchi, the blood of the bronchial arteries drains into the alveolar capillary network at precapillary, capillary, and postcapillary sites, and subsequently into the pulmonary veins. Dense vascular networks around the bronchi are arteriolar networks terminating in bronchial capillaries and numerous bronchial venous plexus with a characteristic irregular shape and course. There are connections of bronchial capillaries with the bronchial venous plexuses, and these vascular components exist either in the bronchial wall or in the peribronchial connective tissue. These microvascular structures are observed along the entire length of the bronchial tree as far distally as the terminal bronchioles, but with decreased number in proportion to the reduction of the caliber of the bronchi and bronchioles. The connective tissue around the pulmonary arteries contains a similar vascular network, but with less numerous vessels. The majority of the juxtapleural bronchial artery's blood drains into the pulmonary capillary network. A fine vascular network exists in the mediastinal pleura, and the bronchial venous plexus in the pleura communicates with branches of the pulmonary vein. There are precapillary and postcapillary anastomoses between the bronchial artery circulation and the pulmonary arterial circulation. There are communications of bronchial venous plexus with small branches of the pulmonary vein. Bronchial vessels around the pulmonary vein also communicate with small branches of the pulmonary vein. Thus all bronchial venous systems around the airway and blood vessels are connected with the pulmonary vein through small branches. There are direct communications of bronchial venous plexuses with the surrounding alveolar capillaries through small venules, and observed in both bronchi and bronchioles.

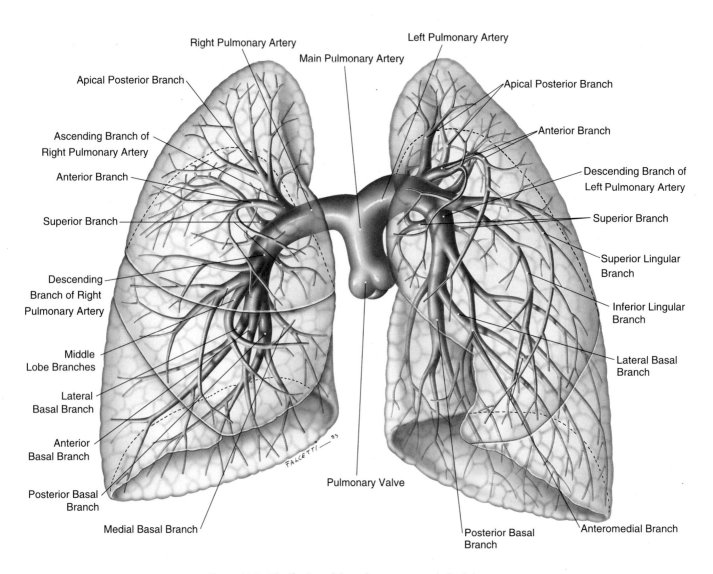

Figure 10.1. Distribution of the pulmonary artery in both lungs.

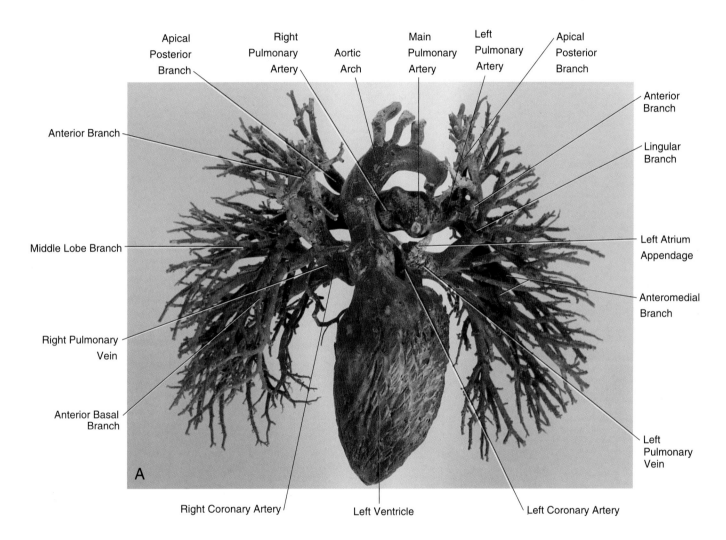

Apical Posterior Branch

Right Pulmonary Artery

Aortic Arch

Main Pulmonary Artery

Left Pulmonary Artery

Apical Posterior Branch

Anterior Branch

Anterior Branch

Lingular Branch

Middle Lobe Branch

Left Atrium Appendage

Anteromedial Branch

Right Pulmonary Vein

Anterior Basal Branch

Left Pulmonary Vein

A

Right Coronary Artery

Left Ventricle

Left Coronary Artery

Figure 10.2. A, Anterior view of an injection cast of the pulmonary arteries, pulmonary veins, left ventricle, and aortic arch. **B**, Posterior view of the cast.

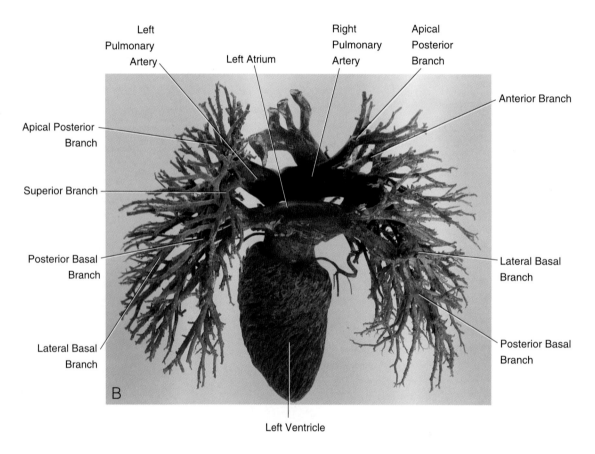

Figure 10.2. *Continued*

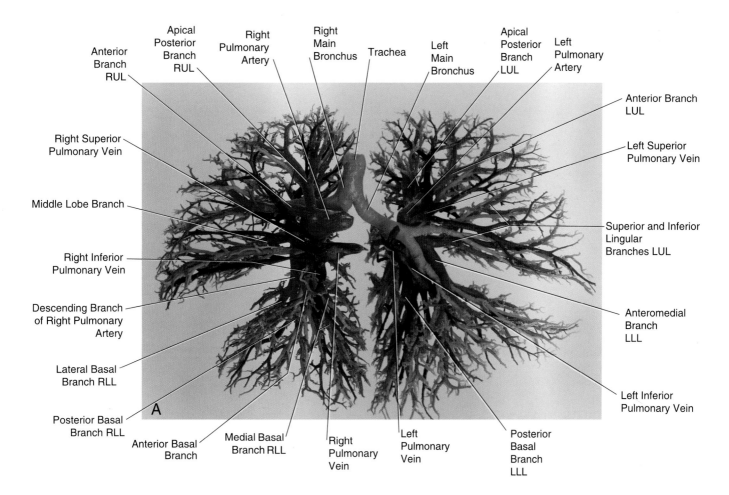

Figure 10.3. A, Anterior view of an injection cast of the pulmonary arteries, pulmonary veins, and tracheo-bronchial tree. **B**, Posterior view of the cast. Some degree of deformation of the structures is seen due to technique artifacts.

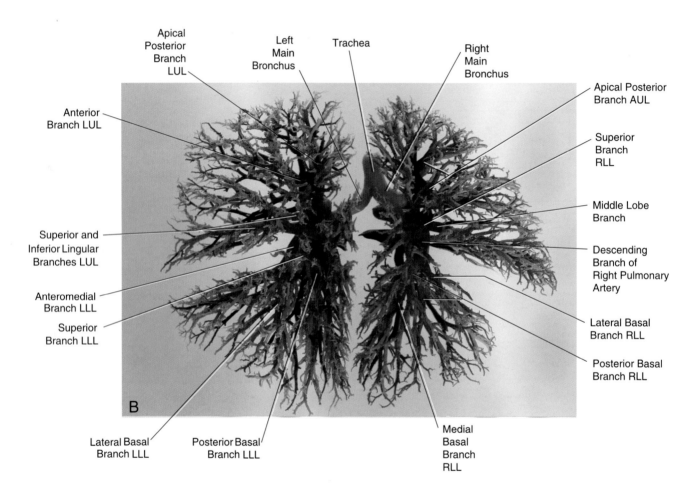

Figure 10.3. *Continued*

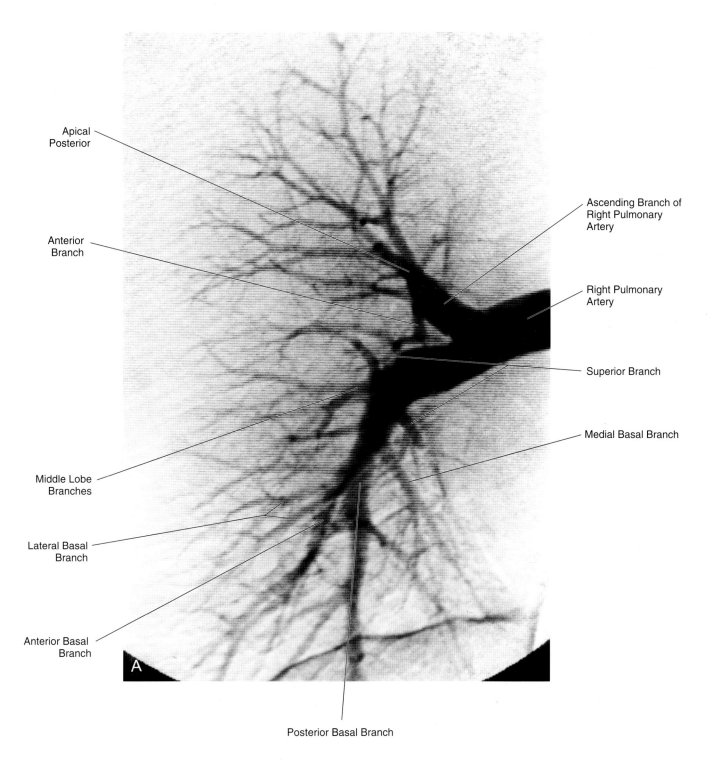

Apical
Posterior

Anterior
Branch

Ascending Branch of
Right Pulmonary
Artery

Right Pulmonary
Artery

Superior Branch

Medial Basal Branch

Middle Lobe
Branches

Lateral Basal
Branch

Anterior Basal
Branch

Posterior Basal Branch

Figure 10.4. **A**, Anterior view of an angiogram of the right pulmonary artery. **B**, Late-phase angiography shows the
right pulmonary veins.

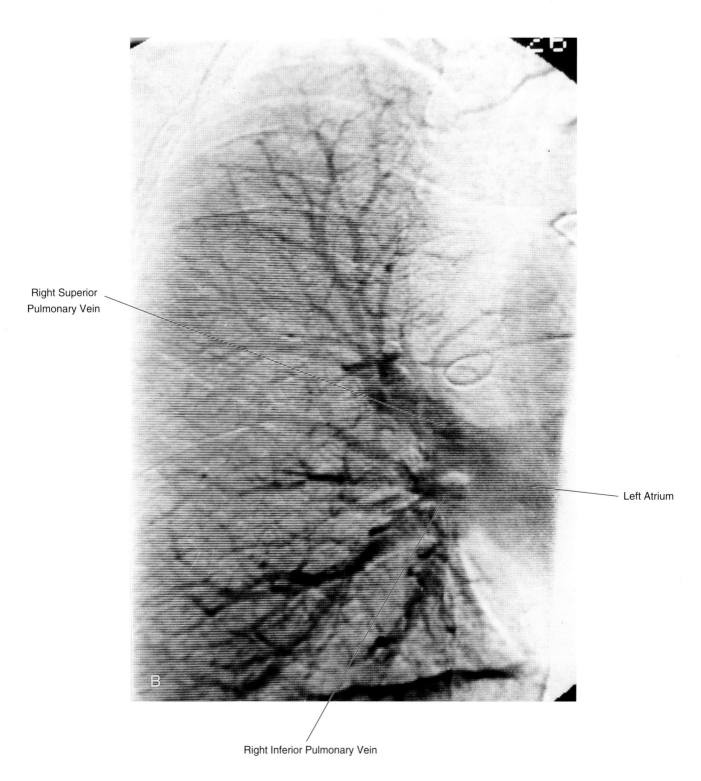

Right Superior
Pulmonary Vein

Left Atrium

Right Inferior Pulmonary Vein

Figure 10.4. *Continued*

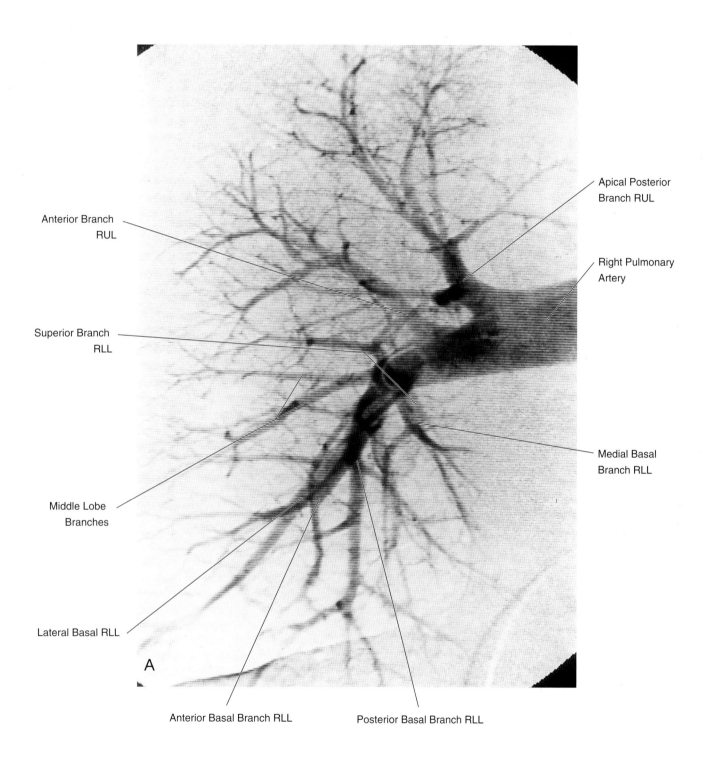

Figure 10.5. **A**, Anterior view of an angiogram of the right pulmonary artery. **B**, Late-phase angiography shows the right pulmonary veins. **C**, Right oblique view of the angiogram of the right pulmonary artery. **D**, Right oblique view of the late phase of the angiography shows the pulmonary veins.

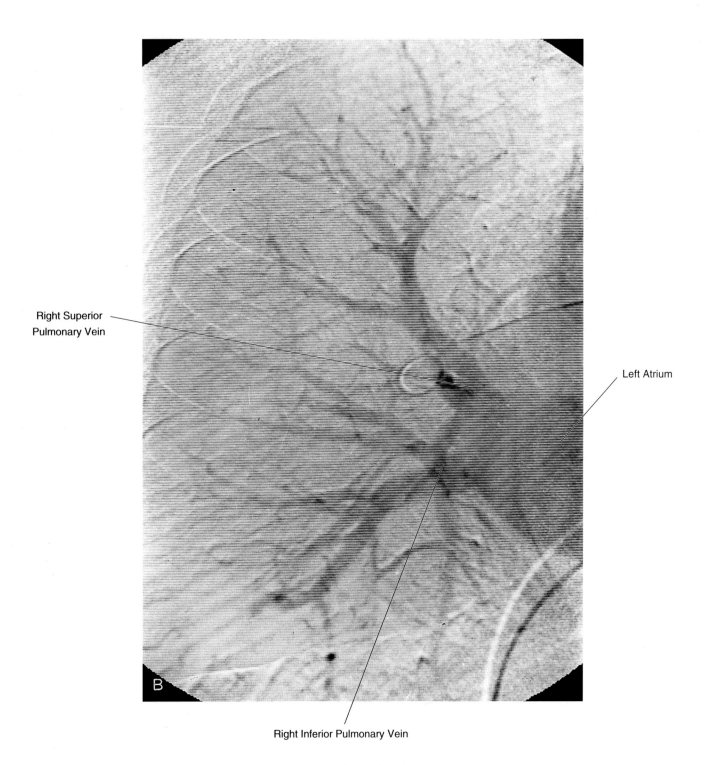

Right Superior
Pulmonary Vein

Left Atrium

Right Inferior Pulmonary Vein

Figure 10.5. *Continued*

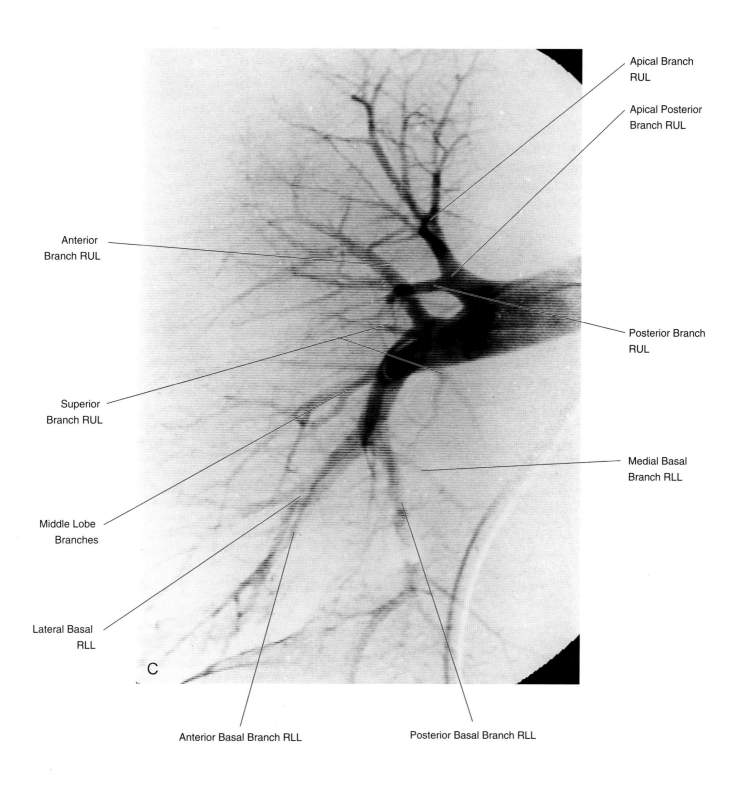

Apical Branch
RUL

Apical Posterior
Branch RUL

Anterior
Branch RUL

Posterior Branch
RUL

Superior
Branch RUL

Middle Lobe
Branches

Medial Basal
Branch RLL

Lateral Basal
RLL

C

Anterior Basal Branch RLL

Posterior Basal Branch RLL

Figure 10.5. *Continued*

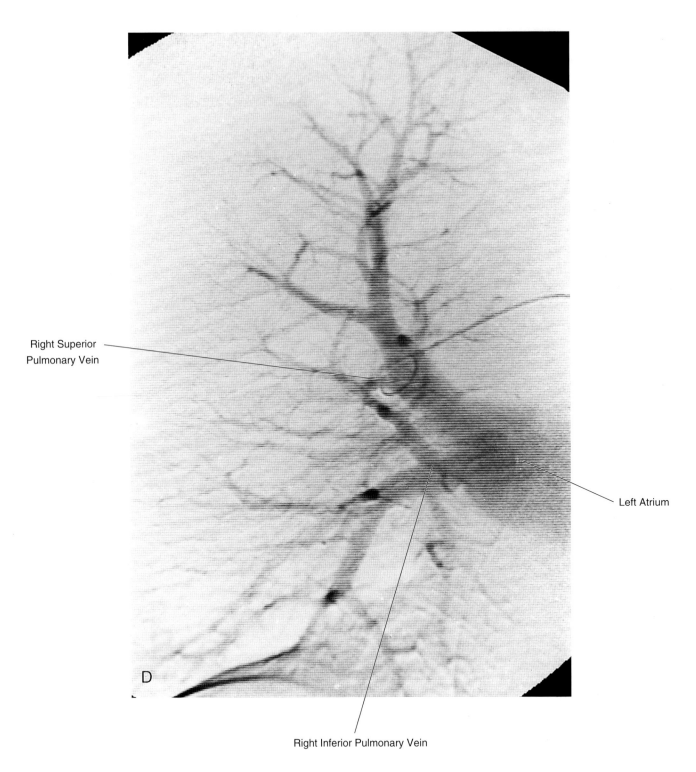

Right Superior
Pulmonary Vein

Left Atrium

D

Right Inferior Pulmonary Vein

Figure 10.5. *Continued*

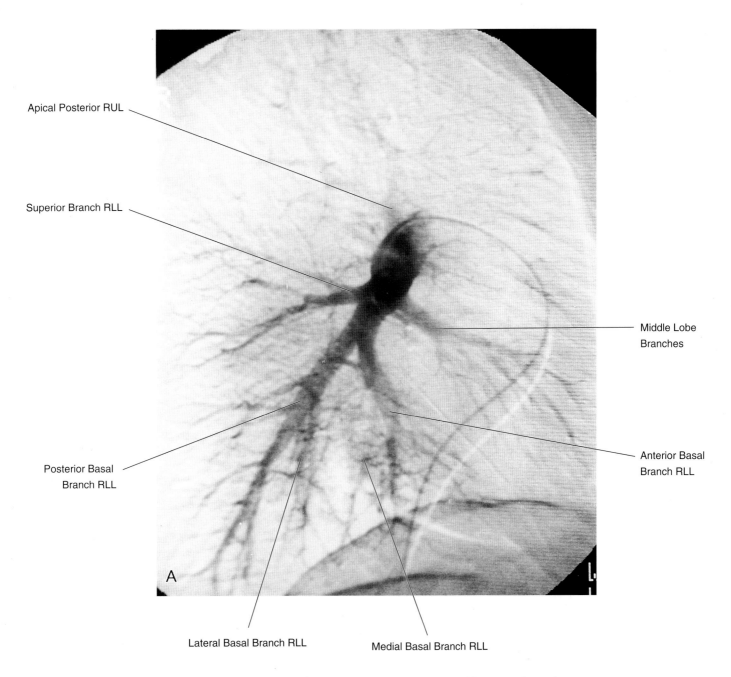

Apical Posterior RUL

Superior Branch RLL

Middle Lobe
Branches

Posterior Basal
Branch RLL

Anterior Basal
Branch RLL

A

Lateral Basal Branch RLL

Medial Basal Branch RLL

Figure 10.6. A, Lateral view of an angiogram of the right pulmonary artery (in the same subject of Figure 10.5).
B, Late-phase angiography shows the right pulmonary artery.

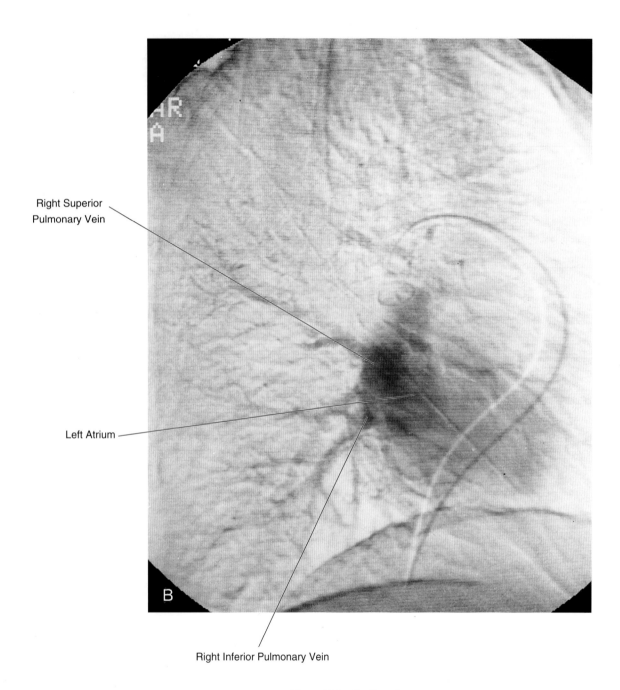

Right Superior
Pulmonary Vein

Left Atrium

Right Inferior Pulmonary Vein

Figure 10.6. *Continued*

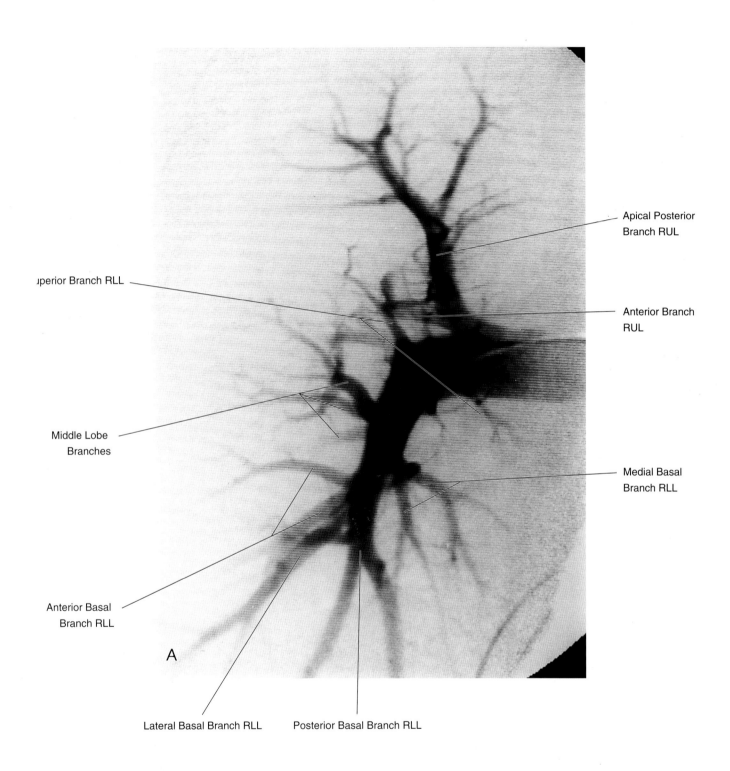

Figure 10.7. A, Early phase of the anterior view of an angiogram of the right pulmonary artery. **B**, Later phase of the right pulmonary angiography. **C**, Late phase of the right pulmonary angiography showing the pulmonary veins.

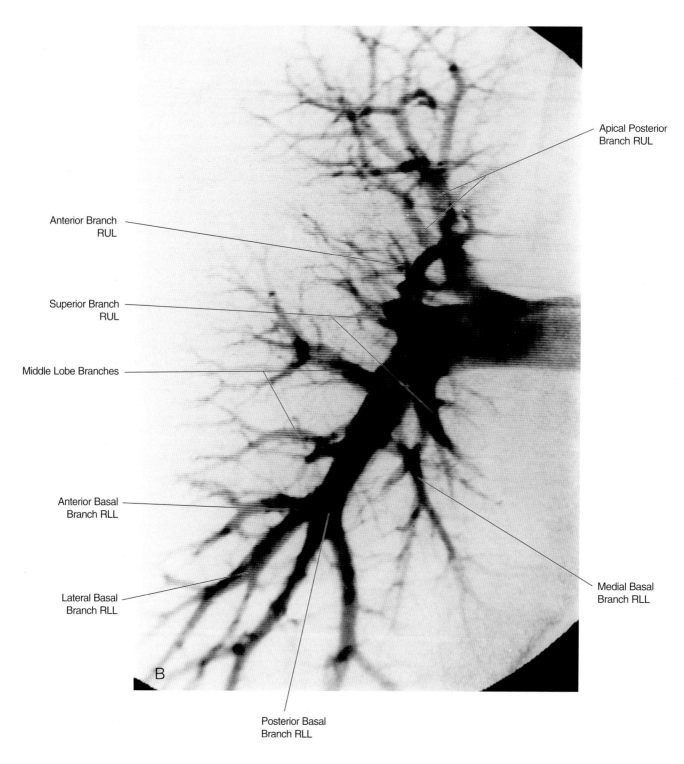

Apical Posterior
Branch RUL

Anterior Branch
RUL

Superior Branch
RUL

Middle Lobe Branches

Anterior Basal
Branch RLL

Lateral Basal
Branch RLL

Medial Basal
Branch RLL

B

Posterior Basal
Branch RLL

Figure 10.7. *Continued*

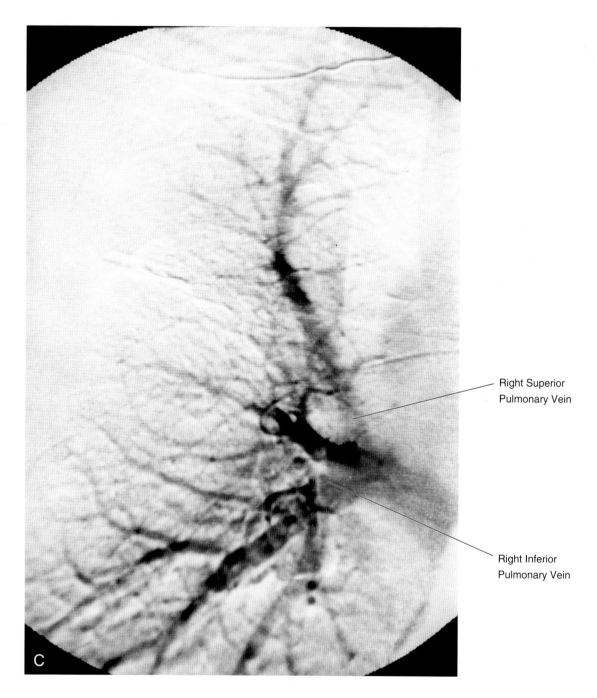

Right Superior
Pulmonary Vein

Right Inferior
Pulmonary Vein

Figure 10.7. *Continued*

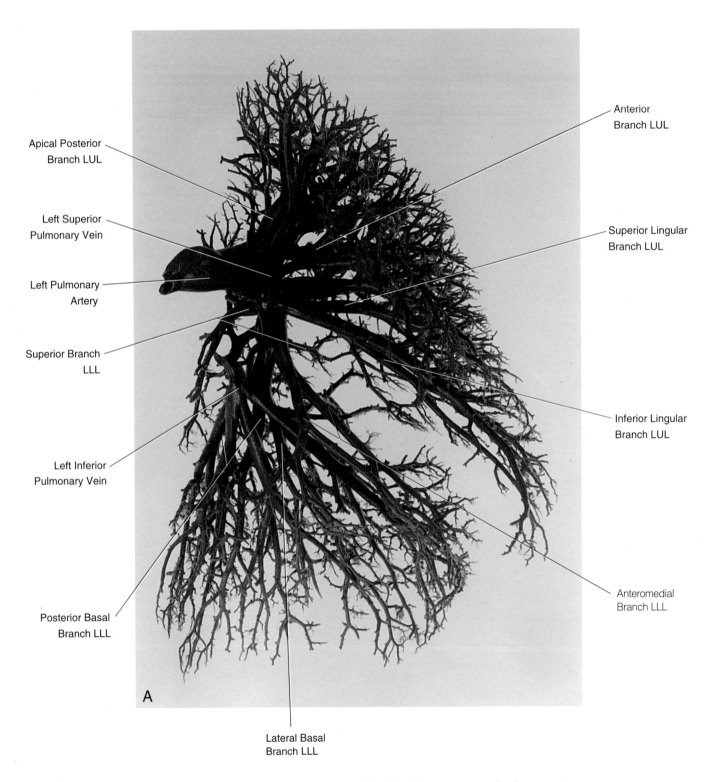

Apical Posterior
Branch LUL

Left Superior
Pulmonary Vein

Left Pulmonary
Artery

Superior Branch
LLL

Left Inferior
Pulmonary Vein

Posterior Basal
Branch LLL

Anterior
Branch LUL

Superior Lingular
Branch LUL

Inferior Lingular
Branch LUL

Anteromedial
Branch LLL

Lateral Basal
Branch LLL

A

Figure 10.8. A, Anterior view of an injection cast of the left pulmonary artery and pulmonary veins.
B, Posterolateral view of the cast.

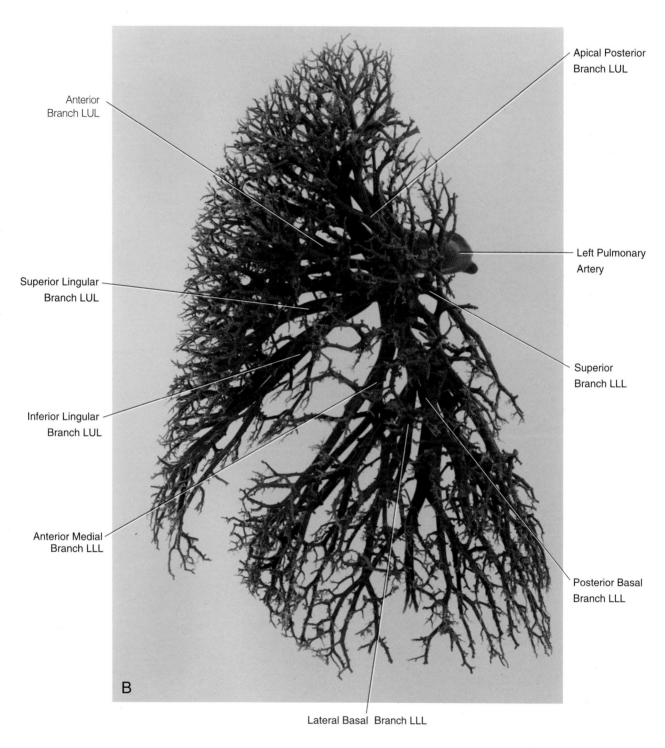

Apical Posterior
Branch LUL

Anterior
Branch LUL

Left Pulmonary
Artery

Superior Lingular
Branch LUL

Superior
Branch LLL

Inferior Lingular
Branch LUL

Anterior Medial
Branch LLL

Posterior Basal
Branch LLL

B

Lateral Basal Branch LLL

Figure 10.8. *Continued*

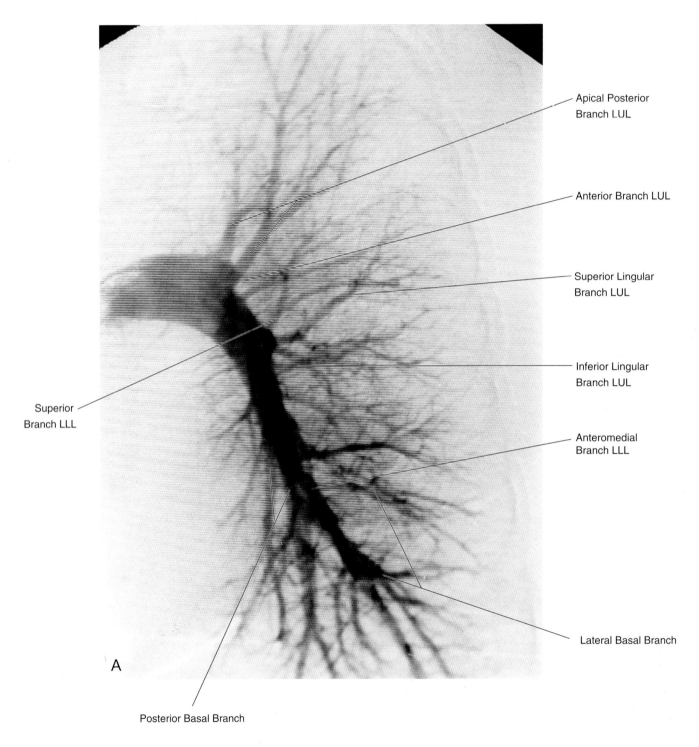

Apical Posterior
Branch LUL

Anterior Branch LUL

Superior Lingular
Branch LUL

Inferior Lingular
Branch LUL

Anteromedial
Branch LLL

Superior
Branch LLL

Lateral Basal Branch

A

Posterior Basal Branch

Figure 10.9. A, Anterior view of the early phase of the angiogram of the left pulmonary artery. **B**, Late phase of the
left pulmonary angiogram shows the pulmonary veins.

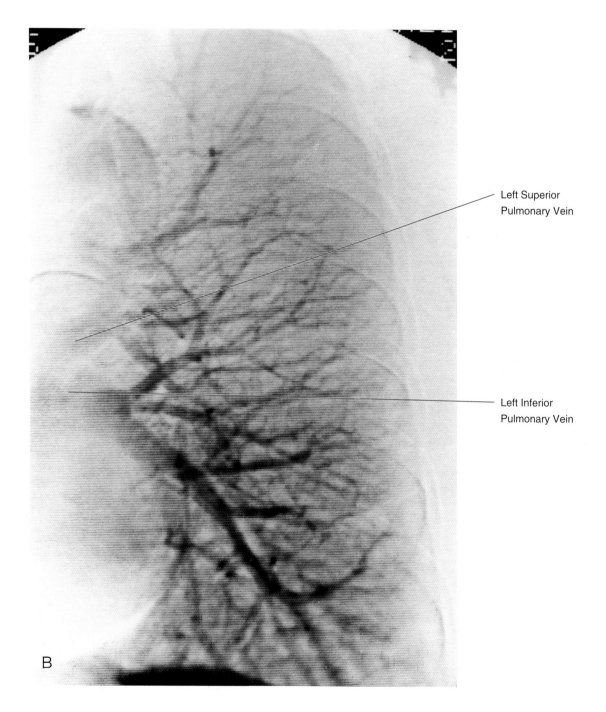

Left Superior
Pulmonary Vein

Left Inferior
Pulmonary Vein

B

Figure 10.9. *Continued*

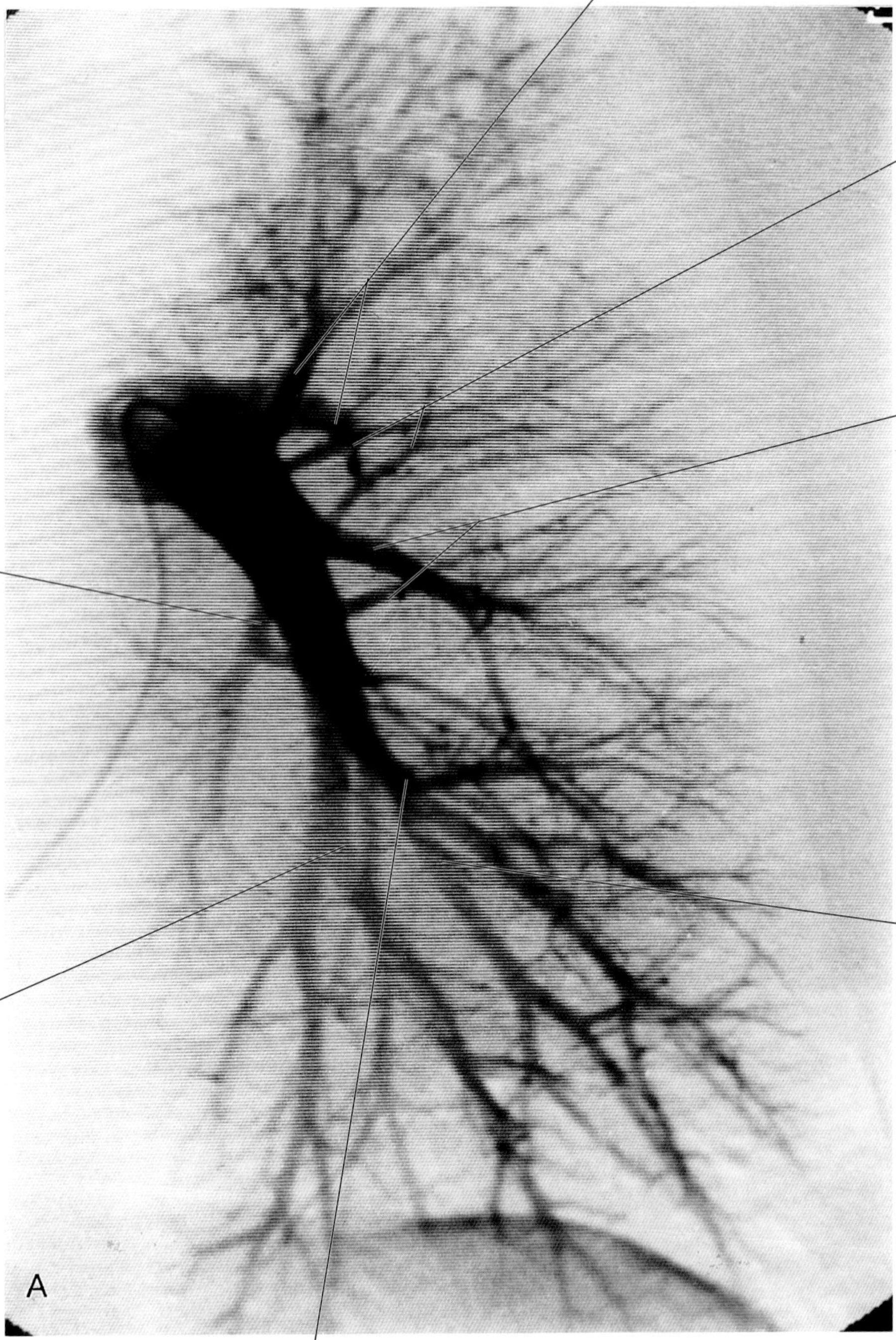

Apical Posterior Branch LUL

Anterior Branch LUL

Lingular Branch LUL

Superior Branch
LLL

Lateral Basal LLL

Posterior
Basal LLL

A

Anteromedial Branch LLL

Figure 10.10. **A**, Left oblique angiography of the left pulmonary artery. **B**, Late phase of the left angiography
showing the pulmonary veins.

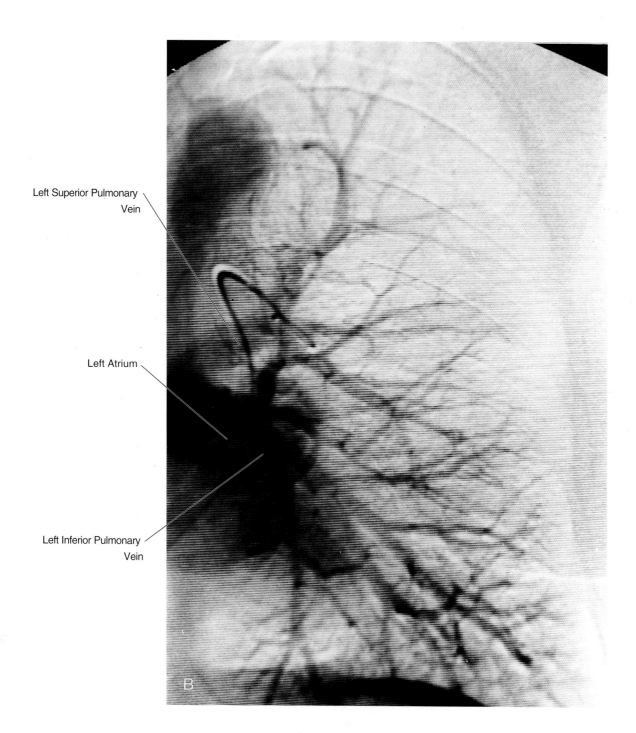

Left Superior Pulmonary Vein

Left Atrium

Left Inferior Pulmonary Vein

Figure 10.10. *Continued*

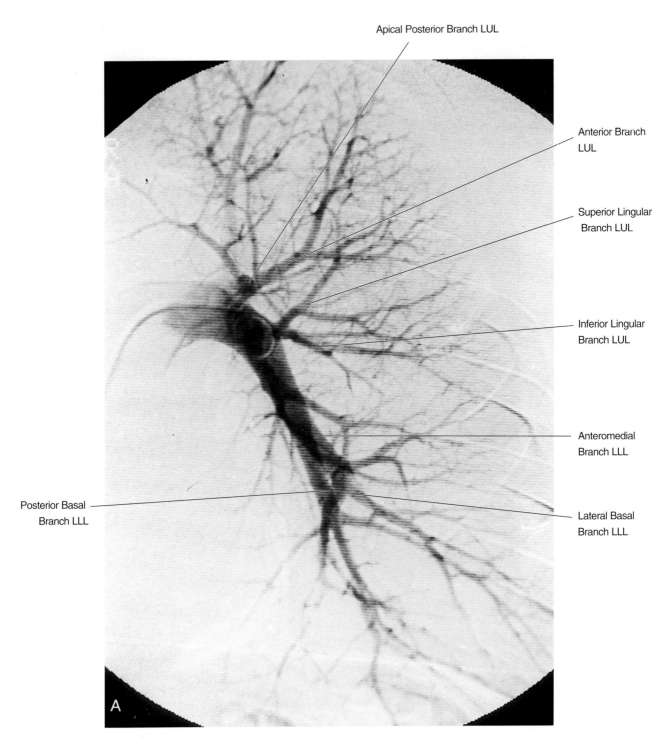

Apical Posterior Branch LUL

Anterior Branch
LUL

Superior Lingular
Branch LUL

Inferior Lingular
Branch LUL

Anteromedial
Branch LLL

Posterior Basal
Branch LLL

Lateral Basal
Branch LLL

A

Figure 10.11. A, Left oblique angiography of the left pulmonary artery. **B**, Late phase of the left angiography showing the pulmonary veins.

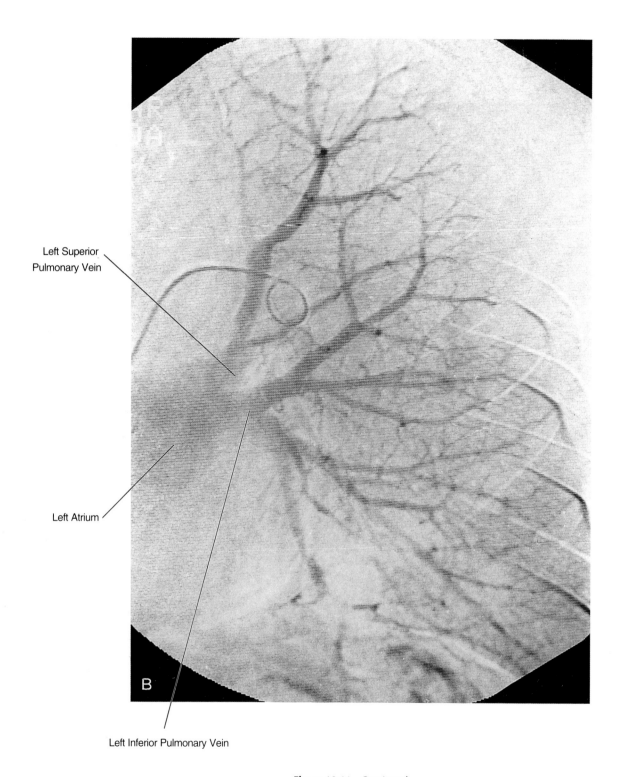

Left Superior
Pulmonary Vein

Left Atrium

Left Inferior Pulmonary Vein

Figure 10.11. *Continued*

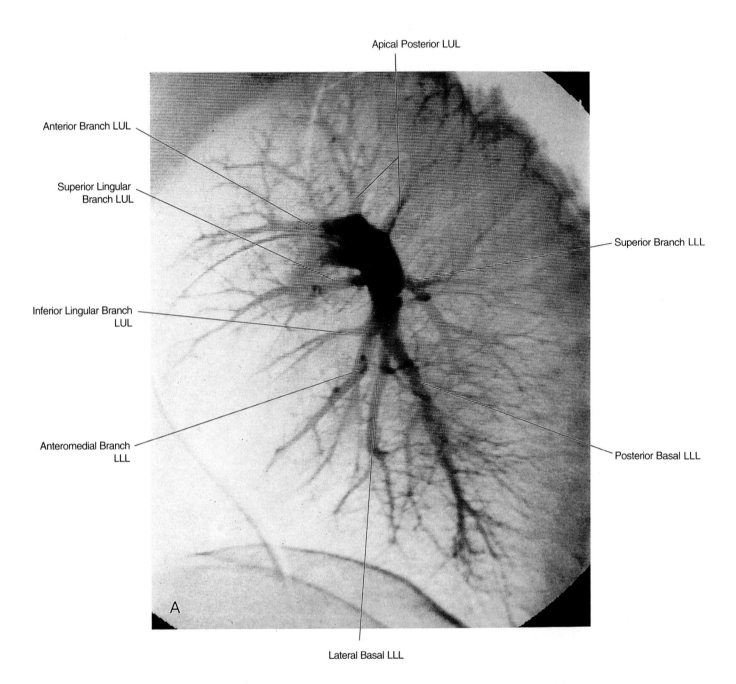

Apical Posterior LUL

Anterior Branch LUL

Superior Lingular
Branch LUL

Superior Branch LLL

Inferior Lingular Branch
LUL

Anteromedial Branch
LLL

Posterior Basal LLL

A

Lateral Basal LLL

Figure 10.12. A, Lateral angiogram of the left pulmonary artery. **B**, Late phase of the left angiography showing the lateral view of the pulmonary veins.

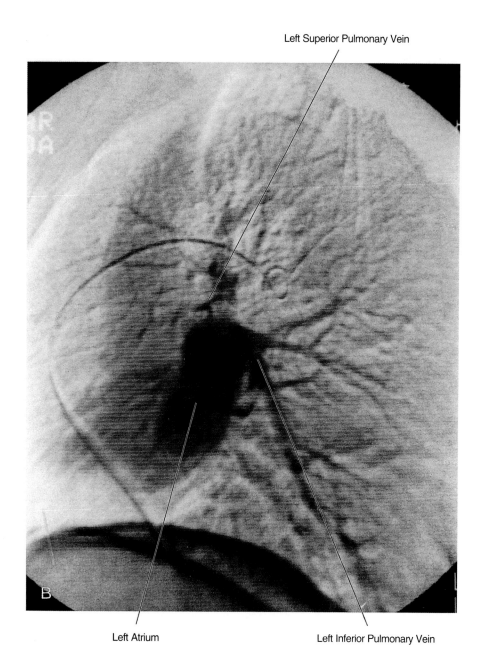

Left Superior Pulmonary Vein

Left Atrium

Left Inferior Pulmonary Vein

Figure 10.12. *Continued*

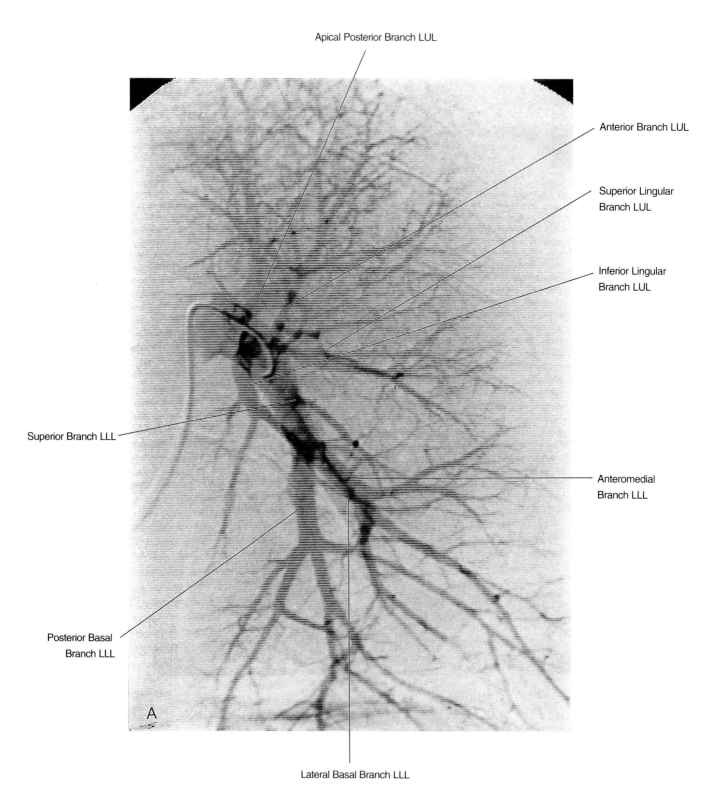

Apical Posterior Branch LUL

Anterior Branch LUL

Superior Lingular
Branch LUL

Inferior Lingular
Branch LUL

Superior Branch LLL

Anteromedial
Branch LLL

Posterior Basal
Branch LLL

A

Lateral Basal Branch LLL

Figure 10.13. **A**, Anterior view of the left pulmonary artery angiography. **B**, Late phase of the left angiogram
showing the pulmonary veins.

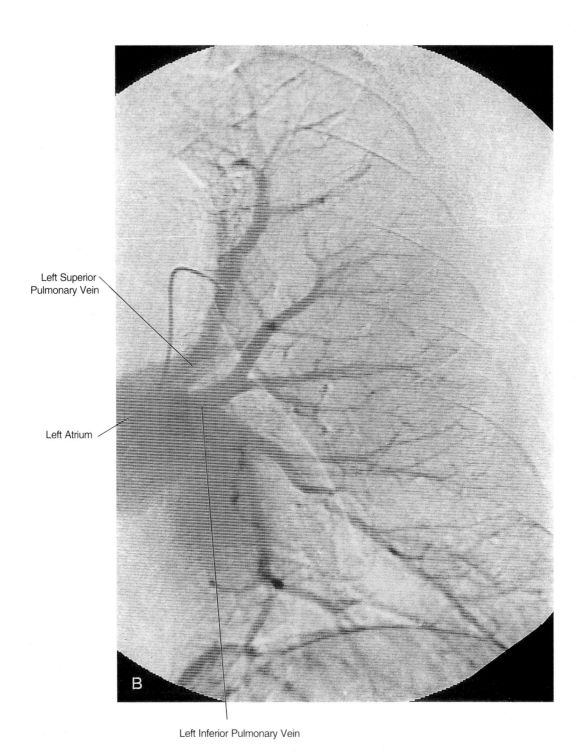

Left Superior
Pulmonary Vein

Left Atrium

Left Inferior Pulmonary Vein

Figure 10.13. *Continued*

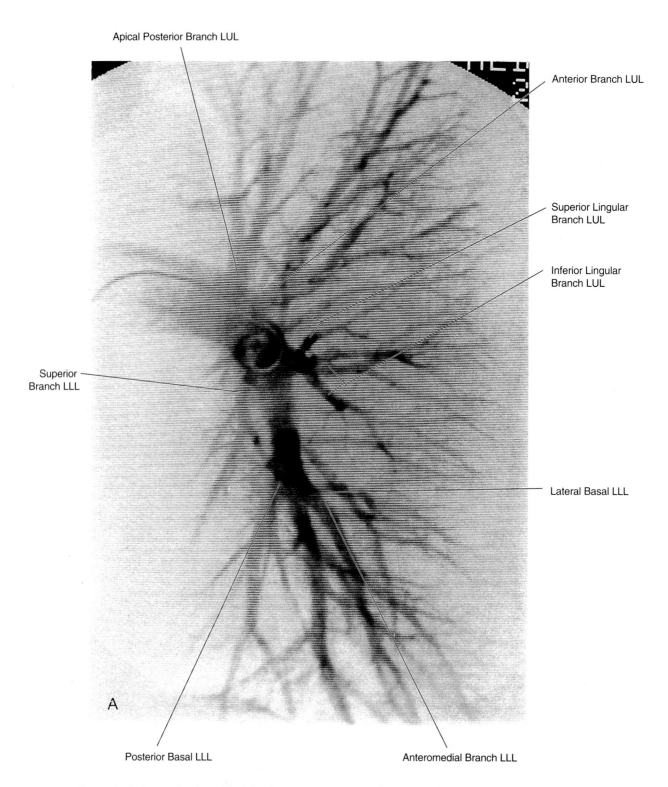

Apical Posterior Branch LUL

Anterior Branch LUL

Superior Lingular Branch LUL

Inferior Lingular Branch LUL

Superior Branch LLL

Lateral Basal LLL

A

Posterior Basal LLL

Anteromedial Branch LLL

Figure 10.14. A, Anterior view of the left pulmonary artery angiography. **B,** Late phase of the left angiogram showing the pulmonary veins. **C,** Oblique view of the left pulmonary artery angiography.

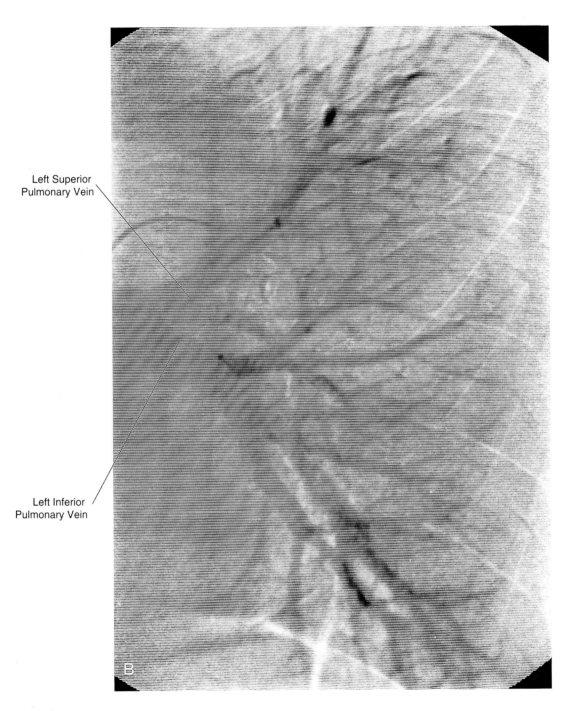

Left Superior
Pulmonary Vein

Left Inferior
Pulmonary Vein

Figure 10.14. *Continued*

Apical Posterior Branch LUL

Anterior Branch LUL

Superior Lingular
Branch LUL

Inferior Lingular
Branch LUL

Superior Branch LLL

Lateral Basal LLL

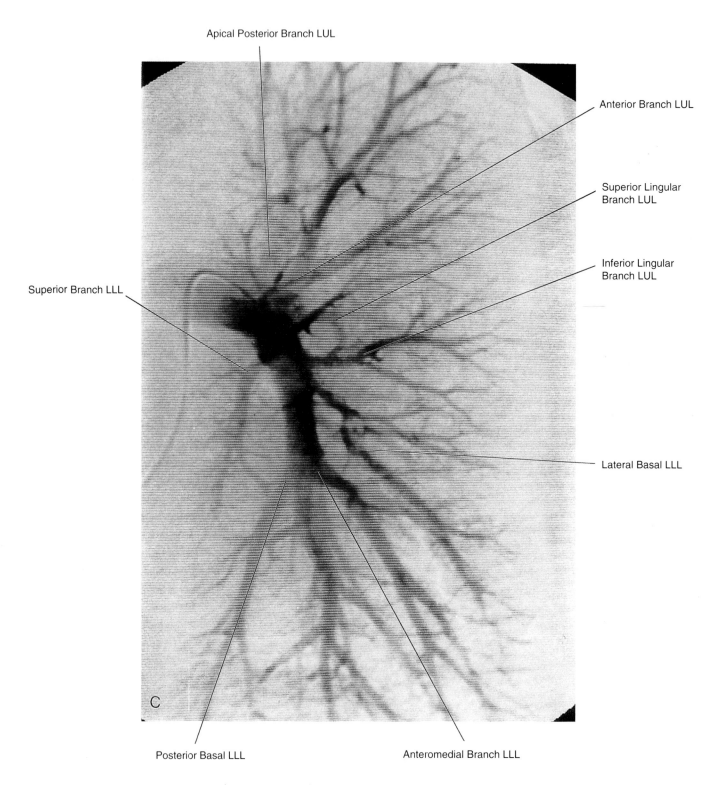

C

Posterior Basal LLL

Anteromedial Branch LLL

Figure 10.14. *Continued*

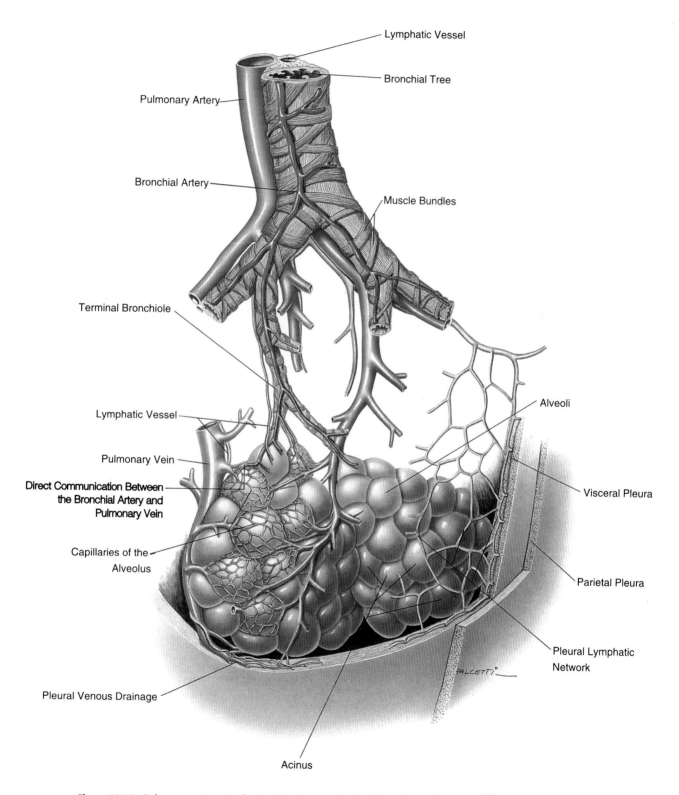

Figure 10.15. Pulmonary microcirculation, showing the relationships of the pulmonary artery, bronchial artery, capillaries of the alveolus, pulmonary vein, and lymphatic network.

11

PULMONARY VENOUS CIRCULATION

PULMONARY VEINS

The pulmonary veins arise from the capillaries of the alveolar meshwork and from the capillary network of the pleura. The larger branches run within the interlobular septa and are, therefore, separate from the pulmonary bronchoarterial pathways. Histologically, the smaller pulmonary veins are identical to the arterioles. As the diameter of the veins increases, smooth muscle cells and elastica lamina are identifiable, and at a diameter of 60 and 100 μm, they become evident as veins and enter the interlobular septa (see Fig. 10.15).

There is a dense vascular network around the bronchi, which is an arteriolar network terminating in bronchial capillaries and numerous bronchial venous plexuses with a characteristic irregular shape and course. There are also connections between the bronchial capillaries with the bronchial venous plexuses. The bronchial venous plexus communicates with the smaller branches of the pulmonary vein.

There are usually two superior and two inferior main pulmonary veins, the former draining the middle and upper lobes on the right side and the upper lobe on the left. The inferior pulmonary veins drain the inferior lobes (Fig. 11.1). The pulmonary veins drain the oxygenated pulmonary blood to the left atrium. There is, however, occasional variations with anomalous pulmonary venous drainage directly to the superior vena cava or to the right atrium.

The right veins reach the hilum beneath the main pulmonary artery and posteriorly to the superior vena cava. The veins usually reach the left atrium independently as two separate veins. The left veins cross in front of the descending aorta and may enter the left atrium separately as on the right side or may join each other already within the pericardial cavity to enter the atrium as a common vein (Figs. 11.2, 11.3, 11.4, 11.5).

The pulmonary venous system carries approximately 50% of the blood in the lungs at any given time.

ANOMALOUS PULMONARY VENOUS DRAINAGE

When partial anomalous pulmonary venous drainage exists, it usually involves part or all of one lung. In most cases, there is an associated reduction in size of the pulmonary arteries supplying the anomalous drained lung segment (Fig. 11.6). Other anomalies of the pulmonary venous drainage are related to pulmonary sequestration, Halasz' syndrome, or can be the sole anomaly. Halasz' syndrome refers to dextrocardia, hypoplasia of the right pulmonary artery, and scimitar-like pulmonary venous drainage. The venous drainage in the scimitar vein may be through the inferior vena cava and less frequently through the azygos vein, whereas the anomalous pulmonary venous drainage may be to the superior vena cava or the brachiocephalic vein.

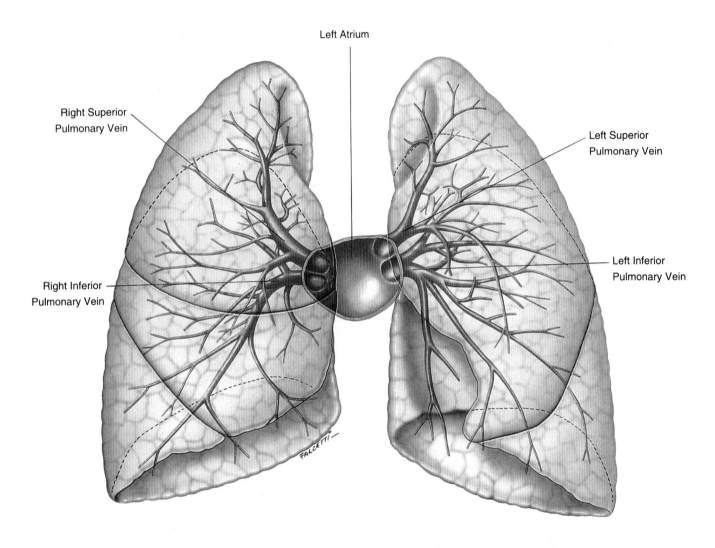

Left Atrium

Right Superior
Pulmonary Vein

Left Superior
Pulmonary Vein

Left Inferior
Pulmonary Vein

Right Inferior
Pulmonary Vein

Figure 11.1. Schematic drawing of the pulmonary veins and left atrium. Note the two superior pulmonary veins
and the two inferior pulmonary veins.

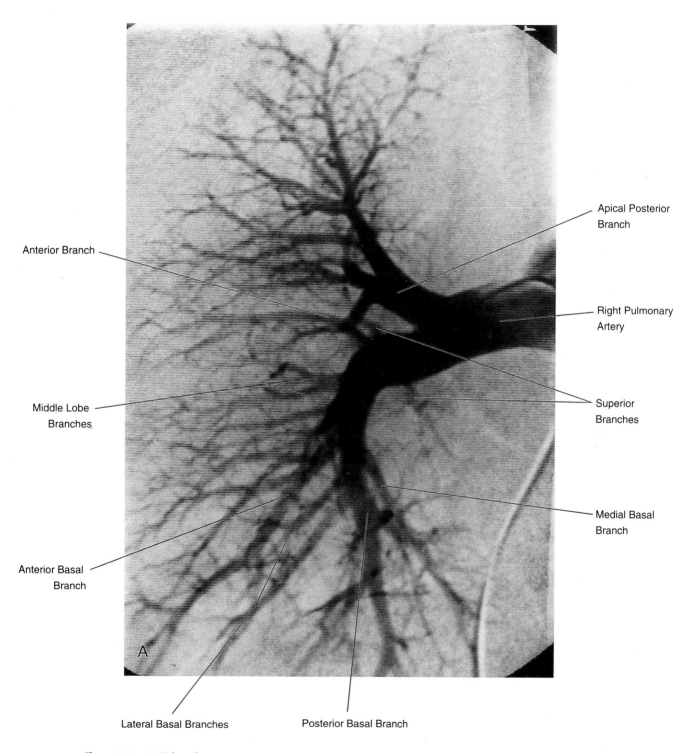

Apical Posterior
Branch

Anterior Branch

Right Pulmonary
Artery

Middle Lobe
Branches

Superior
Branches

Medial Basal
Branch

Anterior Basal
Branch

Lateral Basal Branches

Posterior Basal Branch

Figure 11.2. **A,** Right pulmonary artery angiogram showing the pulmonary artery to the superior, middle, and inferior pulmonary lobes. **B,** Late-phase angiogram showing the drainage of the right lung by the superior and inferior pulmonary veins. The left atrium and the ascending aortic arch are also visualized.

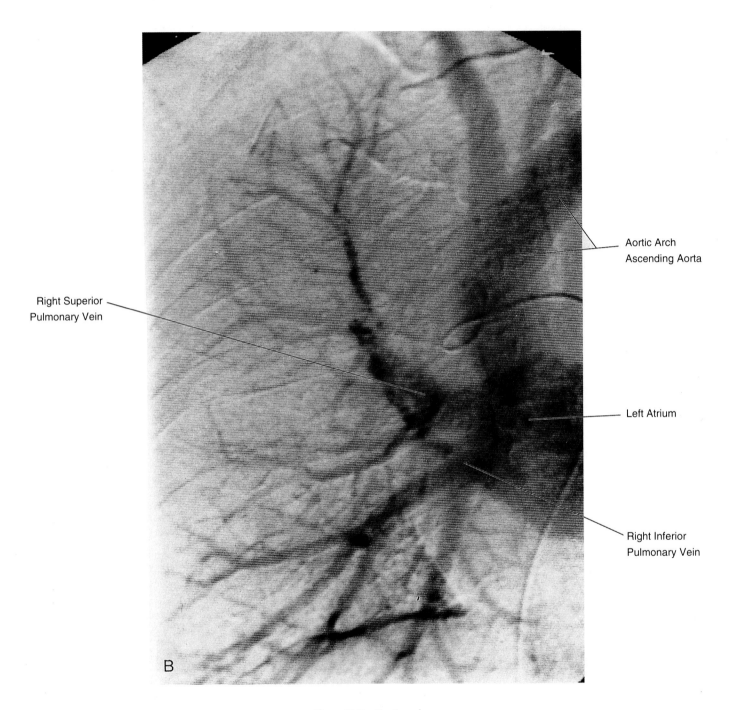

Right Superior
Pulmonary Vein

Aortic Arch
Ascending Aorta

Left Atrium

Right Inferior
Pulmonary Vein

B

Figure 11.2. *Continued*

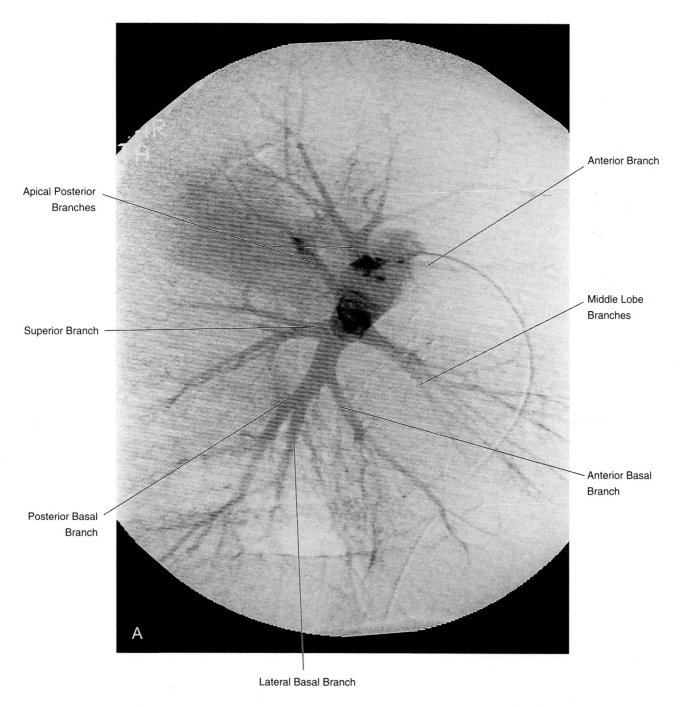

Apical Posterior
Branches

Superior Branch

Posterior Basal
Branch

Anterior Branch

Middle Lobe
Branches

Anterior Basal
Branch

A

Lateral Basal Branch

Figure 11.3. A, Lateral view of the right pulmonary artery angiogram showing the segments to the superior, middle, and inferior lobes. **B,** Late-phase angiogram showing the venous drainage from the superior and inferior pulmonary veins. The left atrium is also visualized.

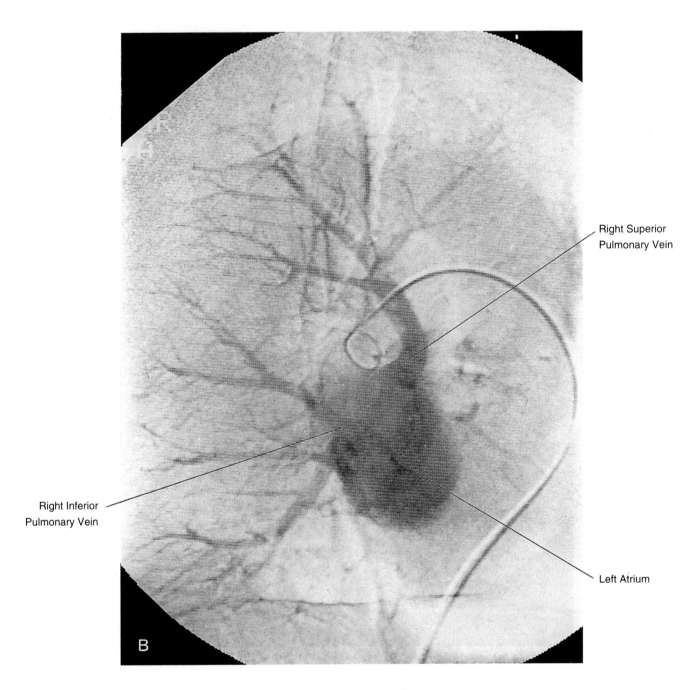

Figure 11.3. *Continued*

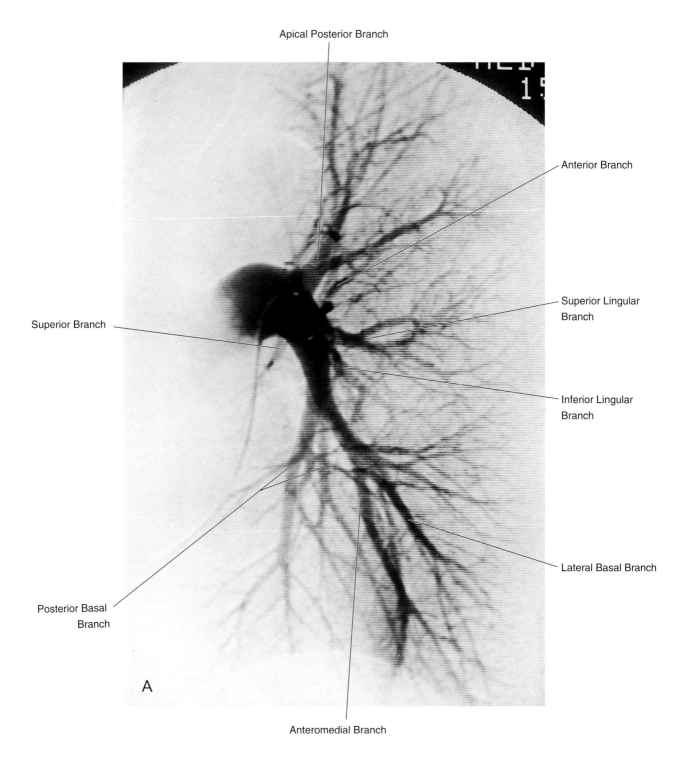

Figure 11.4. A, Anterior view of the left pulmonary artery angiogram showing the segments to the superior and inferior lobes. **B,** Late-phase angiogram showing the venous drainage from the superior and inferior pulmonary veins. The left atrium is partially visible.

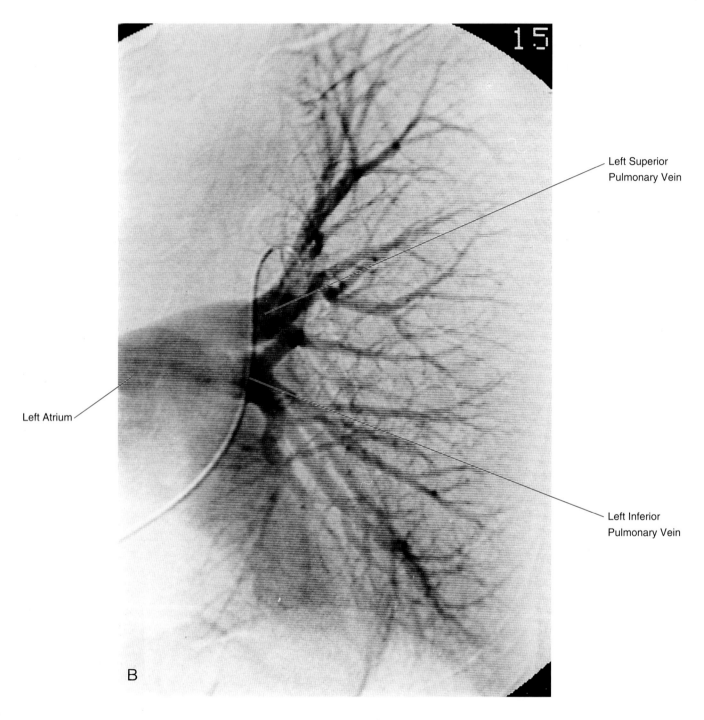

Left Superior
Pulmonary Vein

Left Atrium

Left Inferior
Pulmonary Vein

B

Figure 11.4. *Continued*

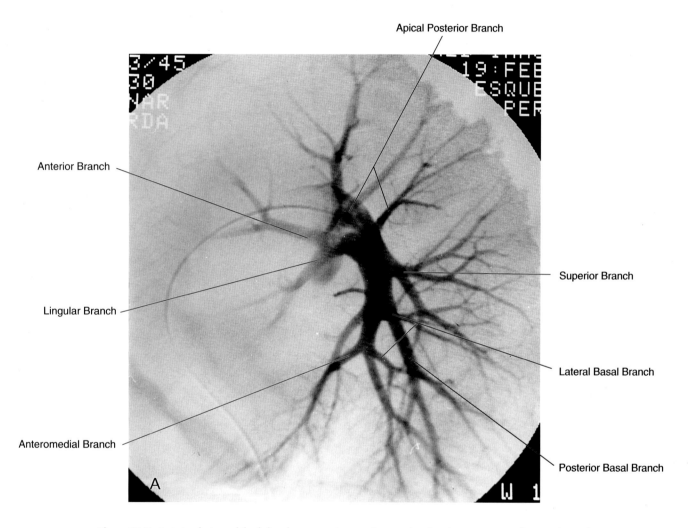

Figure 11.5. A, Lateral view of the left pulmonary artery angiogram showing the segments to the superior and inferior lobes. **B,** Late-phase angiogram showing the venous drainage. The upper pulmonary vein is not seen well. The left atrium is visualized as well as the left ventricle.

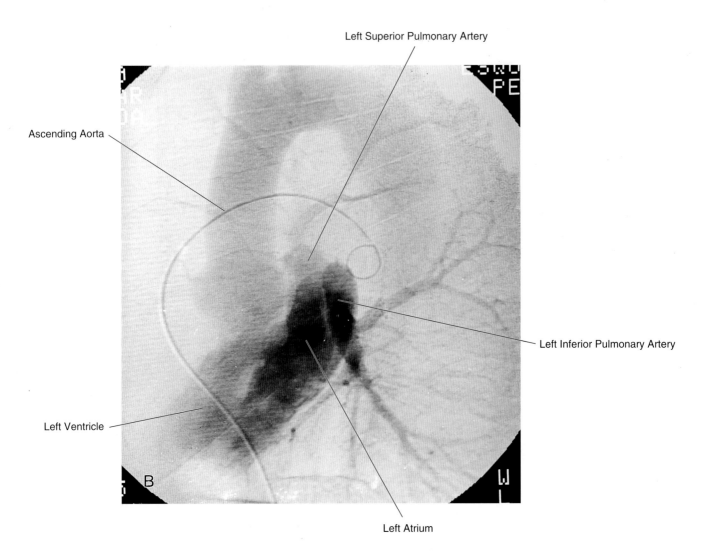

Figure 11.5. *Continued*

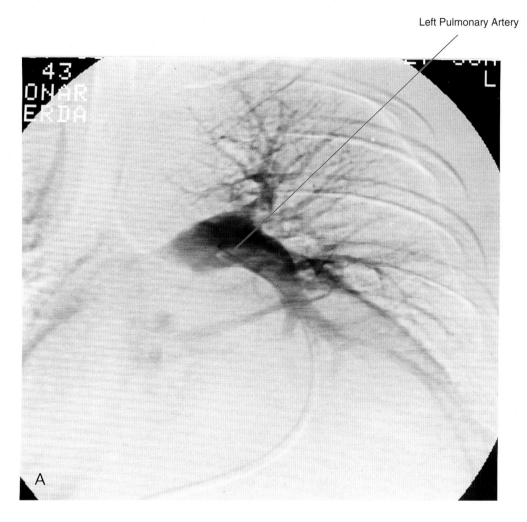

Figure 11.6. Pulmonary anomalous venous drainage. A, Anterior view of the arterial injection. **B,** Late phase of the pulmonary angiography showing the anomalous pulmonary drainage directly to the left brachiocephalic vein with opacification of the superior vena cava. **C,** Lateral view of the pulmonary angiography showing posterior displacement of the lung and artery. **D,** Late phase of the angiography showing the anomalous venous drainage to the left brachiocephalic vein and opacification of the superior vena cava.

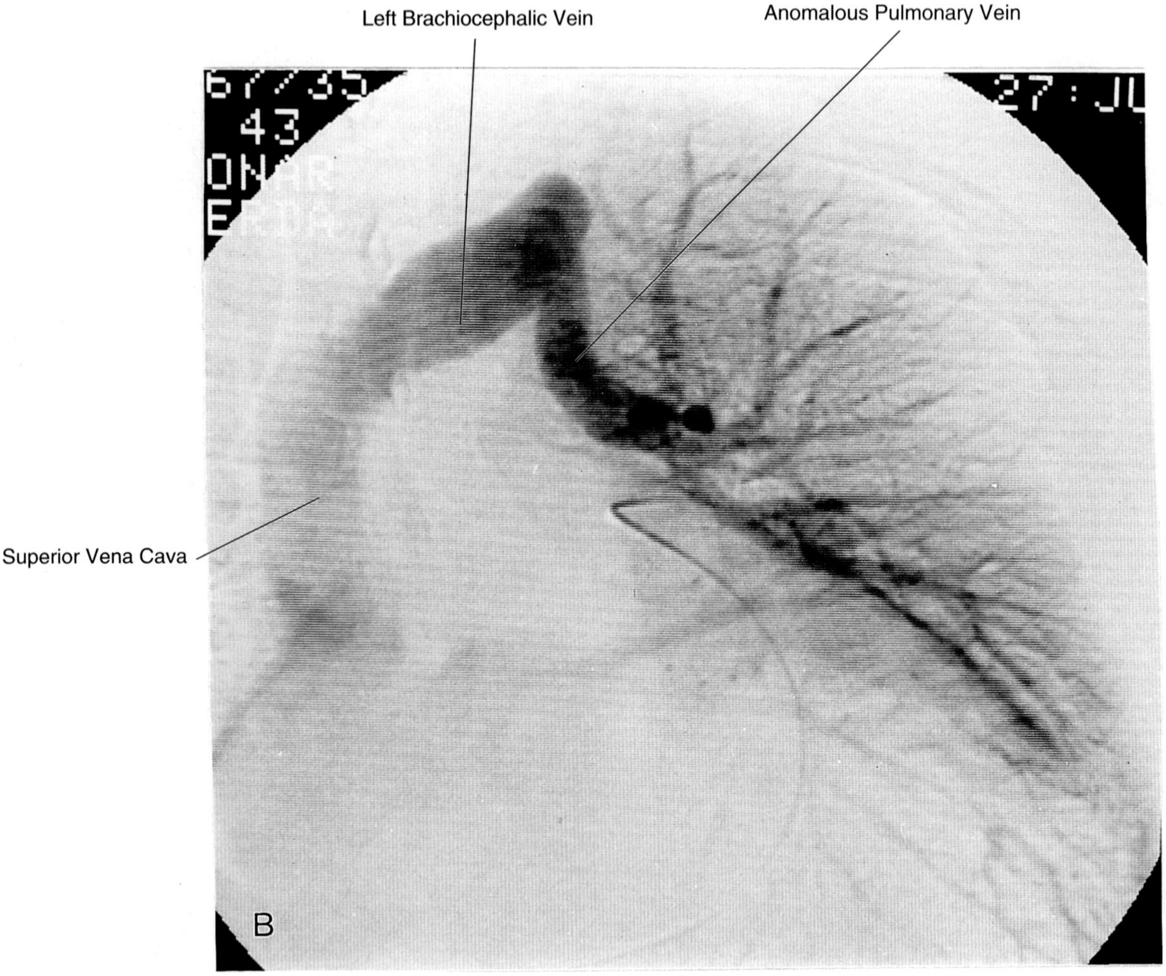

Figure 11.6. *Continued*

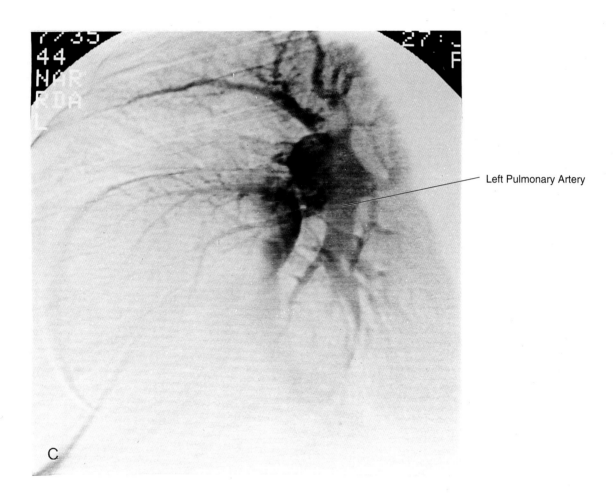

Left Pulmonary Artery

Figure 11.6. *Continued*

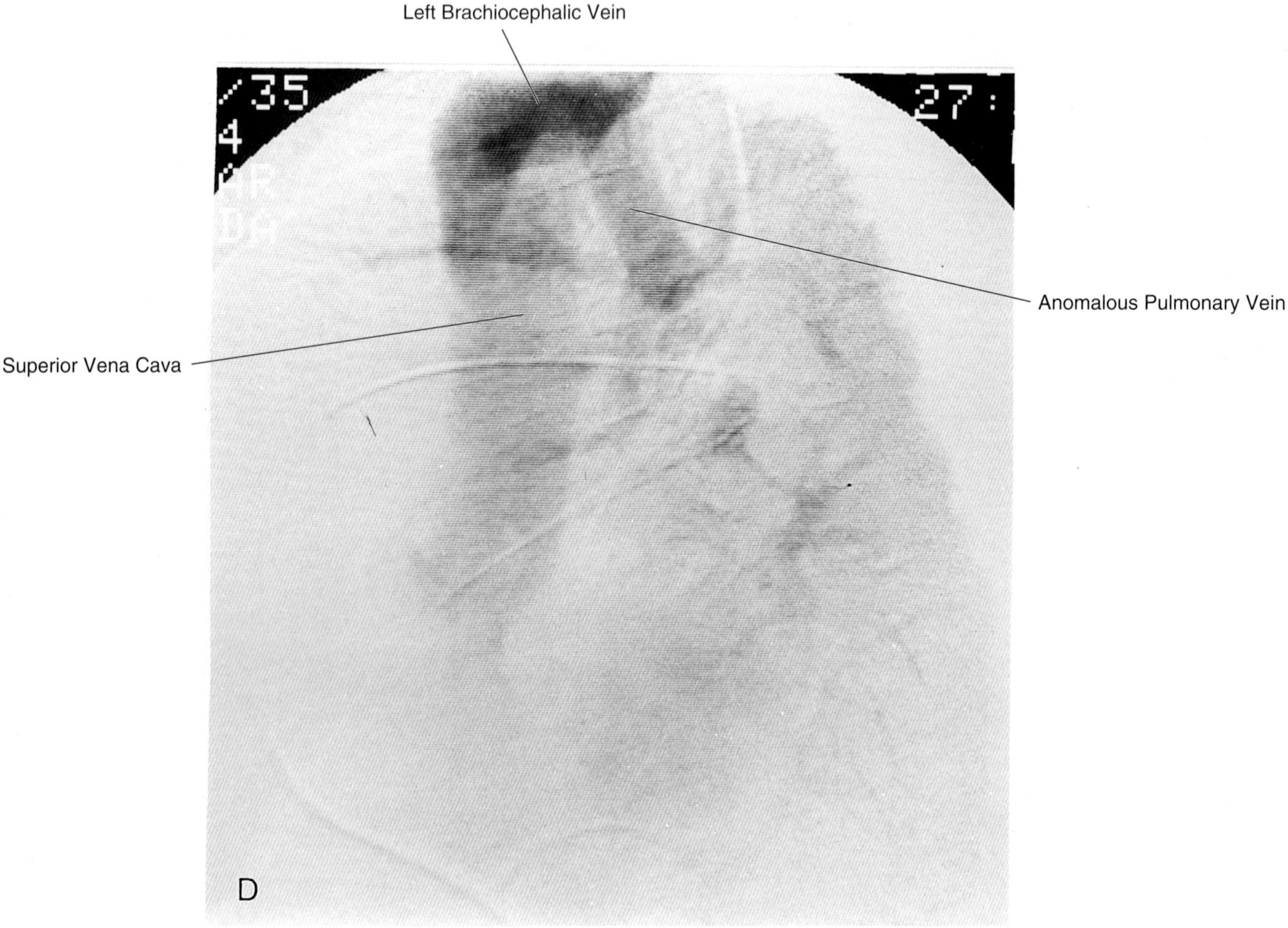

Figure 11.6. *Continued*

12

PULMONARY AND THORACIC LYMPHATIC SYSTEM

LYMPHATICS OF THE LUNGS AND PLEURA

The pleural Lymphatics are variable in size, number, and distribution. They distribute in a plexus with broad channels. There are abundant anastomoses with the pulmonary lymphatics. The lymphatic network is more prominent over the lower than the upper pulmonary lobes. The pleural lymphatics drain to the medial aspect of the lung near the hilum, where there are anastomoses with the lymphatics of the parenchymal plexus (Fig. 12.1, Fig. 12.2).

In the lungs, the lymphatic channels form two major paths: the first in the bronchoarterial and the other in the interlobular septal connective tissue. In both systems, the lymph flows toward the hilum, reaching the bronchial and mediastinal lymph nodes. Multiple anastomoses connect the interlobular perivenous lymphatics with those in the bronchoarterial sheathing. Anastomoses also exist among the bronchoarterial and pleural plexuses. The bronchoarterial lymphatics begin in the region of the distal respiratory bronchioles (Fig. 12.1).

The lungs are subdivided into three main lymphatic drainage areas: superior, middle, and inferior, without correspondence to the pulmonary lobes. On the right lung, the superior area drains directly into the paratracheal and upper bronchopulmonary nodes. The middle zone drains into the paratracheal bifurcation, and the central group of bronchopulmonary lymph nodes. The inferior zone drains into the inferior bronchopulmonary and bifurcation nodes and the posterior mediastinal chain. The right lymphatic duct is, therefore, the main drainage system of the right lung. On the left lung, the left superior area drains in the prevascular group of anterior mediastinal nodes and the left paratracheal nodes. The middle zone drains through the bifurcation and central group of bronchopulmonary nodes and also directly through the paratracheal group. The inferior zone drains into the bifurcation and inferior bronchopulmonary nodes and into the posterior mediastinal group. The left lung, therefore drains lymph from the superior and part of the middle zone to the left paratracheal nodes and into the thoracic duct. The remainder lymph drainage of the left lung ends up in the right lymphatic duct (Fig. 12.3).

THORACIC DUCT AND RIGHT LYMPHATIC DUCT

The right lymphatic duct drains the great majority of lymph from both lungs, while the thoracic duct drains the apical portion of the left lung (Fig. 12.3).

The thoracic duct originates at the cisterna chyli on the anterior aspect of the vertebral column at the lever T12 to L2, resulting from the junction of the lumbar lymphatic trunks. The thoracic duct enters the posterior mediastinum through the aortic hiatus of the diaphragm. The thoracic duct ascends cephalad at the right side of the aorta, approximately at the midline or slightly towards the right side. High up in the thorax the thoracic duct crosses to the left and leaves the thorax between the esophagus and left subclavian artery, joining the left subclavian vein from the posterior aspect. The diameter of the thoracic duct ranges from 1 to 7 mm, and valves are found in the majority of the cases.

The right lymphatic duct is poorly documented, but the duct is an inconstant channel and it may consist of multiple fine vessels or a network of small ducts instead of a single channel.

LYMPH NODES OF THE MEDIASTINUM

The intrathoracic lymph nodes are composed of parietal and visceral components. The parietal lymph nodes lie outside the parietal pleura in the extramediastinal tissue, where they drain the thoracic wall and other extrathoracic structures. The visceral lymph nodes are located within the mediastinum between the pleural membranes and are related to the drainage of the intrathoracic content (Chapter 9, Figs. 9.1 and 9.5).

Parietal Lymph Nodes

Anterior Parietal Nodes (Internal Mammary Nodes)

The anterior parietal nodes are located bilateral, either medial or lateral to the internal mammary vessels. They drain the afferent lymph vessels from the upper anterior abdominal wall, anterior thoracic wall, anterior portion of the diaphragm, and medial portion of the breasts. They communicate with the anterior mediastinal nodes and the cervical nodes. The main efferent vessel is the right lymphatic duct or thoracic duct (see Fig. 9.5).

Posterior Parietal Nodes (Intercostal nodes and Juxtavertebral nodes)

The posterior parietal nodes drain the intercostal spaces, parietal pleura, and vertebral column. There are communications with other posterior mediastinal lymph nodes. The efferent channels drain superiorly to the thoracic duct and to the cisterna chyli inferiorly (see Fig. 9.1).

Diaphragmatic Lymph Nodes (Anterior-prepericardiac-group, Middle-juxtaphrenic-group, Posterior-retrocrural-nodes)

The diaphragmatic lymph nodes drain the diaphragm and the anterosuperior portion of the liver.

Visceral Lymph Nodes

Anterosuperior Mediastinal Nodes (Prevascular)

The anterosuperior mediastinal nodes are located along the anterior aspect of the superior vena cava, right and left innominate veins, and ascending aorta. They drain most of the structures in the anterior mediastinum, including the pericardium, thymus, thyroid, diaphragmatic and mediastinal pleura, part of the heart, and the anterior portion of the hilum. Efferents drain into the right lymphatic duct or thoracic duct.

Posterior Mediastinal Nodes

Periesophageal Nodes

These nodes are located around the esophagus.

Periaortic Nodes

The periaortic nodes are located anterior and lateral to the descending aorta. They communicate with the tracheobronchial group, particularly with the subcarinal group and drain mainly to the thoracic duct.

Tracheobronchial Lymph Nodes Group

Paratracheal Lymph Nodes

The paratracheal lymph nodes are located in front and to the right and left of the trachea. Posterior nodes are occasionally found. The azygos node is one of the large lower paratracheal nodes, medial to the azygos vein arch. The paratracheal nodes receive afferents from the bronchopulmonary and tracheal bifurcation nodes. They also receive afferents from the trachea, esophagus, and right and left lungs. Efferents are the right lymphatic duct and thoracic duct.

Tracheal Bifurcation Nodes (Carinal)

These nodes are located in the precarinal and subcarinal fat, as well as around the right and left main bronchi. On the left, the aortopulmonary window nodes are found between the left pulmonary artery and aortic arch. They receive afferents from the bronchopulmonary nodes, anterior and posterior mediastinal nodes, heart, esophagus, pericardium, and lungs. Efferents drain to the paratracheal group.

Bronchopulmonary Nodes (Hilar)

The bronchopulmonary nodes are located around the bronchi and vessels, especially at the bifurcation. They receive lymph vessels from the pulmonary lobes. Efferent vessels drain to the carinal and paratracheal nodes (Fig. 12.3).

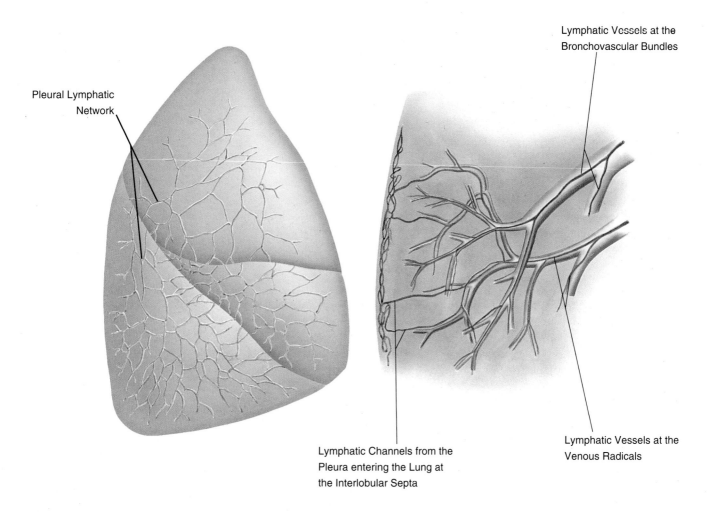

Pleural Lymphatic
Network

Lymphatic Vessels at the
Bronchovascular Bundles

Lymphatic Channels from the
Pleura entering the Lung at
the Interlobular Septa

Lymphatic Vessels at the
Venous Radicals

Figure 12.1. Pleural lymphatic drainage. The lateral view of the right lung shows the pleural lymphatic network. The lymphatic network is more prominent over the lower than the upper pulmonary lobes. On close up, the lymphatic channels, in the lungs, form two major paths, the first in the bronchoarterial bundles and the other in the interlobular septal connective tissue. In both systems, the lymph flows toward the hilum, reaching the bronchopulmonary nodes and mediastinal lymph nodes.

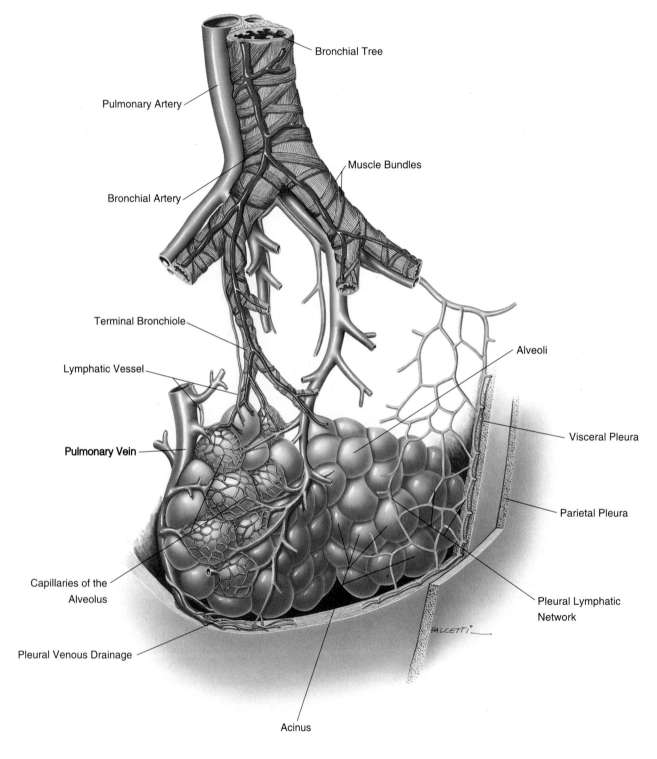

Figure 12.2. Pulmonary microcirculation, showing the relationships of the pulmonary artery, bronchial artery, capillaries of the alveolus, pulmonary vein, and lymphatic network.

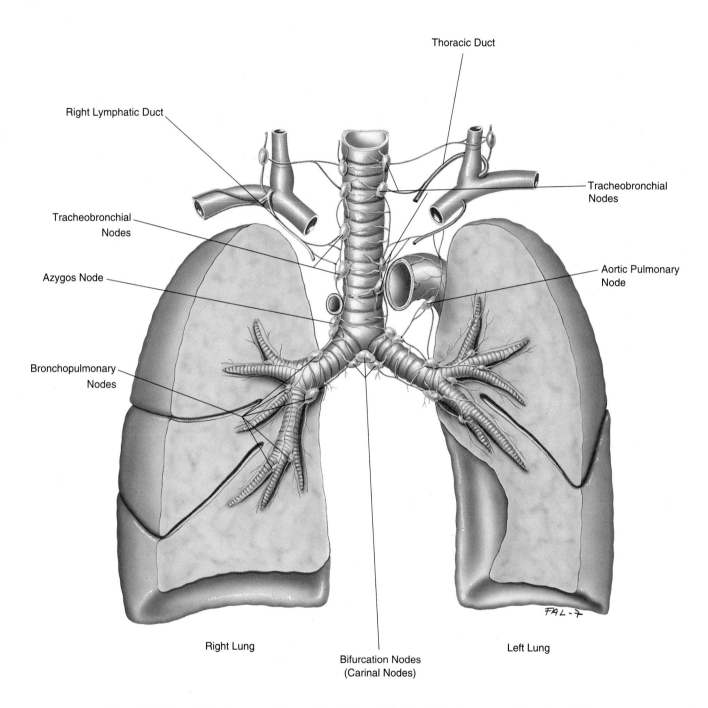

Right Lymphatic Duct

Thoracic Duct

Tracheobronchial Nodes

Tracheobronchial Nodes

Aortic Pulmonary Node

Azygos Node

Bronchopulmonary Nodes

Right Lung

Left Lung

Bifurcation Nodes
(Carinal Nodes)

FAL-7

Figure 12.3. Lymphatic pulmonary drainage. The right lymphatic duct drains the great majority of lymph from both lungs while the apical portion of the left lung drains preferentially to the left system or the thoracic duct.

13

HEART AND CORONARY ARTERIES

The heart is an organ asymmetrically situated in the mediastinum. It is protected by a mesodermal derived structure, the pericardial sac, consisting of two sheets: the external or parietal, which is fibrous, and the internal or visceral, which is a thin serous membrane attached to the heart muscle surface.

The heart is located in the middle portion of the inferior mediastinum bordered laterally by the medial face of the lungs, anteriorly by the chest wall and posteriorly by the dorsal spine. In the majority of the individuals a large part of the heart lies in the left hemithorax and is partially covered by the lingula of the left lung (Figs. 13.1, 13.2).

In humans, the heart is a double valvulae pump that works physiologically in serial sequence. The superior and the inferior vena cava drain the systemic venous blood into the right atrium, which is connected with the right ventricle through the tricuspid valve. The right ventricle pumps the blood to the pulmonary artery across the pulmonary valve. The arterial blood returning from the lungs drains into the left atrium through two left and two right pulmonary veins. The atrioventricular ring where the mitral valve is attached separates the left atrium from the left ventricle, which ejects the blood into the aorta across the aortic valve (Fig. 13.3).

The longitudinal axis of the heart is most frequently oriented anteriorly, inferiorly, and toward the left. If oriented toward the right, it characterizes the so-called dextrocardia and if the longitudinal axis is in the sagittal plane and the heart occupies the middle mediastinum, it is called mesocardia (Fig. 13.4).

When the heart is faced in frontal view, the right border is formed by the lateral wall of the right atrium. The left margin is cranially outlined by the left atrium appendage and caudally by the lateral wall of the left ventricle (Figs. 13.1, 13.5A). The right atrium and the right ventricle are ventral to the left atrium and the left ventricle is dorsal (Figs. 13.1, 13.5B).

The heart has roughly the form of an inverted pyramid, with the base, formed by right and left atria and the root of the great vessels, located at the upper mediastinum. The apex of the pyramid corresponds to the apex of the left ventricle and is situated in the left

hemithorax toward the diaphragm. The anterior face of the heart or sternocostal face is related to the anterior wall of the chest. The inferior face lies on the diaphragm and the lateral or pulmonary face is covered by the lingula of the left lung (Figs. 13.4, 13.6). The junction of the sternocostal face with the inferior or diaphragmatic face defines a sharp border called the acute margin. On the left side, the junction of the left face with the diaphragmatic face is the obtuse margin with a rounded and ill-defined border (Fig. 13.7). The divisions of the four cardiac chambers are seen externally as sulks or grooves. Between the atria and ventricles, there is the atrioventricular sulcus divided in right and left. The ventricle's separation is marked externally by the interventricular sulcus, which is divided into anterior and inferior. The point where the atrioventricular sulcus meets the inferior interventricular sulcus is termed the crux of the heart.

CARDIAC CHAMBERS

In angiography, the axial projections for identification of the cardiac structures are used. These projections permit the visualization of the septum and the surrounding structures of the heart in more detail than the classical frontal and lateral views.

The routine of the angiographic study of the heart consists of three projections:

Long axial view — 30º cranio-caudal image intensifier inclination and 60° left anterior oblique patient inclination

Elongated right anterior oblique view — 30º cranio-caudal inclination of the image intensifier and 30º right anterior oblique patient inclination

Four chambers view — 30º cranio-caudal image intensifier inclination and 30º left anterior oblique patient inclination

Additional views may be necessary in special situations. Frontal and lateral views may be the elected projections for adequate visualization of the interventricular septum in same complex cardiac defects. The pulmonary trunk and its bifurcation are better visualized in the sitting up projection with the patient lying supine and the image intensifier rotating 30º cranially.

Right Atrium

Anatomic Aspects

The right atrium is a somewhat quadrangular chamber that forms the right surface of the heart. It presents two main portions: the posterior smooth wall called sinus venarum and the anterior with a trabeculated wall called atrium proper and auricle. The crista terminalis is a smooth muscular ridge in the lateral wall of the right atrium separating the sinus venarum from the proper atrium. The anterior trabeculated wall of the right atrium extends anteriorly with the auricle or right atrium appendage, which is a conical pouch expanding in front of the root of the ascending aorta. The left wall of the right atrium corresponds to the interatrial septum, which separates this chamber from the left atrium. The right face of the interatrial septum presents a central depression called fossa ovalis which is encircled by a prominent margin: the limbus of the fossa ovalis. The most inferior part of the interatrial septum, near the atrioventricular anulus, is formed by the atrioventricular septum (Fig. 13.8).

Angiographic Aspects

Long Axial View

In this view, the left border of the right atrium corresponds to the anterior portion of the interatrial septum, and the superior border is formed by the free superior wall of the right atrium. The lateral border is represented by a continuous line between the superior and inferior caval veins. The inferior border of the right atrium is the tricuspid valve and it overlaps the junction of the inferior vena cava. The anterior wall and the right auricle are not seen in this projection (Fig. 13.9).

Elongated Right Anterior Oblique View

The superior and inferior vena cava are separated by a straight line that is the right posterior wall of the right atrium. The tricuspid valve seen in profile is in the inferior and left aspect of the atrial chamber. There is an inferior contour between the inferior vena cava and the tricuspid anulus, where is located the entrance of the coronary sinus and is formed partially by the atrioventricular septum. The left and superior aspect of the right atrium corresponds to the right atrial appendage or right auricle (Fig. 13.10).

Four Chambers View

In this projection, the right atrium has a globular form, very similar to that seen in the long axial view. The left border corresponds to the more posterior portion of the atrial septum and the right border is related with the anterolateral atrial wall. The atrial appendage and the vena cava are overlapped by the right atrium contour. The tricuspid valve is not well defined in this projection although it forms the left inferior contour (Fig. 13.11).

Right Ventricle

Anatomic Aspects

The right ventricle is a triangular-shaped chamber and is located at the ventral portion of the heart. The base of the right ventricle is more cranial and to the right and the apex is caudal and projected toward the left. The base is formed at the right by the atrioventricular anulus and the leaflets of the tricuspid valve. At the left and more cranially is located the pulmonary valve. These two valves are separated by a smooth and prominent muscular invagination of the right ventricular wall called ventriculo-infundibular fold. The rest of the right ventricle, including the apex, has a coarse trabeculation (Figs. 13.12, 13.13). The right ventricular chamber is divided in three portions: the inlet, the outlet, and the trabecular zones (Fig. 13.14). The inlet zone includes the tricuspid valve and extends until the implantation line of the papillary muscles. The outlet zone or infundibulum is a tubular muscular formation with the pulmonary valve on its top. The trabeculated zone extends from the papillary muscle's insertion until the apex. The right ventricle is limited by three walls: the anterior or free wall, the inferior, and the septal wall, which corresponds to the interventricular septum. The interventricular septum is formed by two components: the membranous septum and the muscular septum. The membranous septum is a small fibrous structure divided in two portions by the septal tricuspid leaflet attachment: the superior is the atrioventricular portion and the inferior is the interventricular portion. The atrioventricular portion is above the tricuspid anulus and separates the left ventricle from the right atrium. The interventricular portion is related to both ventricles. The muscular component, the largest part of the interventricular septum, is divided in three portions: the inlet portion, which divides the inlet of the ventricles; the infundibular portion, which separates the outlet of the ventricles; and the trabeculated portion, situated more apical. The outlet or infundibulum of the right ventricle is limited anteriorly by the free anterior ventricular wall. The posterior wall is the ventriculo-infundibular fold, the muscular formation which separates the tricuspid from the pulmonary valve. The third wall of the infundibulum is the infundibular or outlet portion of the interventricular septum. In normal hearts, the muscular structure, which separates the tricuspid from the pulmonary valve, is called supraventricular crest and is formed in its greater part by the ventriculo-infundibular fold and a small portion of the outlet septum. On the right side of the muscular interventricular septum, there is a

well-marked muscular band called septomarginal trabecula, which has two limbs embracing the body of
the supraventricular crest. These three structures,
the ventriculo-infundibular fold, the outlet septum,
and the septomarginal trabecula, characterize the
normal right ventricle (Fig. 13.15).

The tricuspid valve consists of an atrioventricular
orifice surrounded by a fibrous ring, three somewhat
triangular cusps or leaflets, various types of chordae
tendineae and papillary muscles. The cusps are
named anterior, septal and posterior. The anterior
cusp is the largest and is interposed between the atrioventricular ring and the infundibulum. The septal
cusp is attached to the membranous portion of the
interventricular septum. The posterior cusp is
attached in the inferior portion of the tricuspid annulus. The papillary muscles in the right ventricle are:
the anterior with the base arising from the anterolateral ventricular wall and related with the septomarginal trabecula and the posterior, smaller than the
anterior, arising from the inferior portion of the septum. There are small, papillary muscles arising from
the infundibular septal wall.

The pulmonary valve is situated at the summit of the
infundibulum. It consists of three semilunar segments
or cusps attached to a fibrous annulus. Two of the cusps
are anterior (right and left) and the third is posterior.

Angiographic Aspects

Long Axial View

In this view, the right ventricle has a triangular
shape with the base at the top. The tricuspid valve is
at the right and the pulmonary valve is at the left and
in an upper level. The right contour corresponds to the
free anterior wall. The upper left border is formed by
the anterior portion of the interventricular septum and
the posterior portion is a straight line toward the apex.
The right ventricular outflow tract is limited by the
supraventricular crest on the right side and by part of
the septomarginal trabecula on the left. It looks like as
a wide channel with the pulmonary valve on the top.
The negative shadow of the tricuspid valve lies in the
right and upper contour of the right ventricle. The
anterior leaflet can be visualized superiorly and to the
right on the tricuspid anulus. The septal leaflet is seen
near and parallel to the interventricular septum. The
posterior or mural leaflet is not visualized (Fig. 13.16).

Elongated Right Anterior Oblique View

The tricuspid valve seen in the lateral view is in the
posterior border and to the right. The outflow tract is
superior and to the left and is limited posteriorly by
the supraventricular crest and anteriorly by the free
wall of the right ventricle (Fig. 13.17).

Four Chambers View

The morphologic aspect of the right ventricle in
this projection is similar to that of the long axial view

but the outflow tract is not visualized, and the tricuspid valve is localized more medial.

Left Atrium

Anatomic Aspects

The arterial blood returns from the lungs to the left
heart through two pulmonary veins in each side of the
left atrium. This is the most dorsal chamber and is
localized in front of the lumbar spine and esophagus.
It communicates with the left ventricle through the
mitral valve. The left atrium has a quadrangular
shape and a smooth posterior wall where the four pulmonary veins converge to. To the right, there is the
interatrial septum and to the left there is an elongated pouch with a trabeculated wall that encircles the
left aspect of the pulmonary artery; that is the left
auricle or left atrium appendage. The left appendage
is a finger-like formation that communicates with the
left atrium through a narrow orifice. It is different
from the right appendage, where the communication
with the right atrium is wide and has a triangular
form. The inferior wall of the left atrium corresponds
to the mitral valve (Fig. 13.18).

Angiographic Aspects

Long Axial View

The right contour of the left atrium is formed by the
anterior portion of the atrial septum. In the right
upper corner, there is the entrance of the right superi-
or right pulmonary vein. The left pulmonary veins and
the left atrial appendage are not seen. At the floor of
the left atrium, there is the mitral valve (Fig. 13.19).

Elongated Right Anterior Oblique View

In this view, the most prominent structure is the
left atrial appendage which forms the anterior and
lateral border of the left atrium. This is an irregular
and elongated finger-shaped structure that protrudes
towards the left between the superior wall and the
mitral valve. The entrance of the right superior pulmonary vein is localized on the right in continuation
with the roof of the left atrium (Figs. 13.20, 13.21).

Four Chambers View

This view shows a similar appearance described in
the long axial view but the atrial septum is visualized
in its posterior portion (Fig. 13.22).

Left Ventricle

Anatomic Aspects

The left ventricle has the thickest chamber wall of
the heart and is located at the left and posteriorly to
the right ventricle (Fig. 13.23). It has an elongated
and triangular shape with the base upwards where
the mitral and aortic valves are located. The apex is

oriented inferiorly toward the left. The left ventricle is divided in three portions: the inlet tract with the mitral valve complex, the trabeculated zone with less coarse trabeculation than in the right ventricle and the outlet tract which supports the aortic valve. Unlike the right ventricle, in the left ventricle the inlet and the outlet tracts are not separated by a well developed infundibulum and the aortic and mitral annuli are in continuity. The left ventricle has a lateral free wall, an inferior or diaphragmatic wall and a septal wall. This one is a nontrabeculated wall that extends from the aortic annulus to the apex (Figs. 13.19, 13.24—13.26).

The mitral valve is formed by two leaflets or cusps attached to a fibrous anulus, a number of chordae tendineae and two papillary muscles: the anterolateral and the posterior. The cusps or leaflets are the anterior or septal and the posterior or parietal, separated, one of the other, by two indentations: the anterolateral and the posteromedial commissures. The anterior cusp is longer and narrower than the posterior, but both have about the same area.

At the top of the left ventricular outlet tract is located the aortic valve that consists of three cusps attached to the aortic anulus. Two cusps are posterior, right and left and one is anterior. The anterior cusp is related to the right coronary artery above and to the membranous portion of the ventricular septum below and is called right coronary or septal cusp. The left posterior cusp is related to the left main coronary artery and is called left coronary cusp. The right posterior cusp is the noncoronary cusp.

Angiographic Aspects

Long Axial View

In this projection, the right contour of the left ventricle corresponds to the trabecular portion of the interventricular septum. A small cranial portion of the septum is formed by the outlet septum located just below the aortic valve. The outlet of the left ventricle is limited anteriorly and at the right by the outlet portion of the ventricular septum and posteriorly by the anterior leaflet of the mitral valve. The free wall of the left ventricle corresponds to the posterolateral contour and extends from the mitral valve to the apex. The mitral valve is seen as negative shadow in the superior and lateral contour of the left ventricle. The papillary muscles are seen as a negative shadow in the middle portion of the left ventricle (Fig. 13.27).

Elongated Right Anterior View

In this view the outflow tract is limited anteriorly, and to the left, by the infundibular septum as a straight vertical line below the right coronary cusp and posteriorly, to the right, by a smooth contour extending from the noncoronary cusp to the crux cordis. It represents the atrioventricular portion of the interventricular septum. The anterior free wall of the left ventricle extends from the infundibular septum toward the apex and the inferior wall corresponds to the contour from the crux cordis to the apex. The mitral valve is not well seen in this view. The aortic valve is localized in the uppermost aspect of the outlet tract and the coronary cusps cover one each other at the left. The noncoronary cusp is at the right (Fig. 13.28).

Four Chambers View

The left ventricle in this view has a semioval shape with a left rounded contour and a right straight line. The apex is localized inferiorly towards the right. The left contour corresponds to the free anterolateral wall and the right limit is formed in the superior half by the atrioventricular portion of the interventricular septum which separates the left ventricle from the right atrium. The mural leaflet of the mitral valve is localized laterally near this portion of the septum (the crux cordis). The inferior half of the right contour is formed by the posterior portion of the muscular septum. The aortic valve is visualized above the septal wall. The right coronary and the non coronary cusps are overlying one each other on the right side. The left coronary cusp is on the left side. The mitral orifice is fully exposed and the mural leaflet implantation is seen in all its length. The septal leaflet is not visualized and the papillary muscles appear as two filling defects: anterolateral and posteromedial. They are oriented toward the commissures of the mitral valve (Fig. 13.29). As a rule the left ventricle shows a smooth trabeculated contour at the angiography and it differs from the coarse trabeculation of the right ventricle (Figs. 13.12, 13.24).

CORONARY ARTERIES

The coronary arteries, the vascular network of the heart, are the arteries that provide arterial blood to the myocardium. They are the left and right coronaries that originate from the left (posterior) and right (anterior) coronary sinus of the aortic root (Figs. 13.30–13.34).

The left main coronary artery has a variable length and a diameter ranging from 5 to 10 mm. In about 1% of the hearts studied, in a series, there was no left main coronary artery and two orifices were found in the left coronary sinus with the left anterior descending and circumflex arteries originating separately from each one. The left main coronary artery bifurcates into two vessels: the left anterior descending artery (LAD), running over the anterior interventricular sulcus and the circumflex artery related to the left atrioventricular sulcus. The left main coronary artery in a few cases may give rise to a third vessel: the intermediary artery, also called diagonalis artery, which is located between the anterior descending and circumflex artery and supplies the free lateral wall of the left ventricle (Fig. 13.45).

The left anterior descending artery extends down ending proximal, at or distal to the apex. In this last situation, the LAD goes up in the posterior interventricular sulcus. The length of the LAD is thus extremely variable. The main branches of the LAD are the diagonal and septal branches. The diagonals vary in number and size. These vessels arise in acute angle from the LAD and supply the anterolateral wall of the left ventricle. Most frequently, there is a major artery, which is identified as the first diagonal branch. The septal branches in number of four to six, or more, originate from the LAD in right angle, coursing close to the endocardium on the right side of the interventricular septum. They anastomose with the septal branches coming from the posterior descending artery. In the majority of the hearts, it is possible to identify a bigger septal branch called first septal artery, originating from the proximal portion of the LAD. In some hearts, the LAD has an unusual configuration: it is short and divided in two parallel vessels called "dual" LAD (Fig. 13.48). One running over the interventricular sulcus gives off the septal branches and the other, lying in the anterior left ventricular wall, originates the diagonal branches (Figs. 13.35–13.39).

The circumflex artery is the other principal vessel originating from the left main coronary artery. It emerges in a right or acute angle and is covered by the left atrial appendage in its proximal portion, and then takes position in the left atrioventricular sulcus. The circumflex artery may terminate proximal to the obtuse margin of the left ventricle, before, at or beyond the crux cordis. The principal branches of the circumflex artery are the marginal arteries and the left atrial branch. In 40% of hearts, the sinus node artery arises from the circumflex artery. The marginal arteries are variable in number, but are usually three. The most prominent marginal artery runs on the obtuse margin of the heart and extends distally close to the apex. When the circumflex artery reaches the crux cordis, it gives origin to the posterior descending and to the atrioventricular node arteries (Figs. 13.33–13.39, 13.49).

The right coronary artery has its origin at the right coronary aortic sinus. Often a small branch may arise directly from the aortic sinus in an isolated ostium and supply the right ventricle infundibulum. This branch is called the conus artery, which anastomoses with a left conus branch coming from the left coronary artery to form the arterial anulus of Vieussens. Close to its origin, the right coronary artery gives rise to the sinus node artery in 60% of the hearts. The right coronary artery goes into the right atrioventricular sulcus and has a variable form of termination. If it is a short artery, it terminates between the acute margin of the right ventricle and the crux cordis as a small branch (left dominance). When there is a dominant right coronary artery, it extends further from the crux supplying the posterolateral wall of the left ventricle with a variable number of posterolateral branches. Near the acute margin of the heart, the right coronary artery gives origin to the right marginal or acute marginal artery that supplies the free anterior wall of the right ventricle. The shorter the left circumflex artery, the longer will be the terminal posterolateral branches of the right coronary artery. At the crux cordis, the right coronary gives origin to the posterior descending artery, which runs into the posterior interventricular sulcus and supplies the inferior portion of the interventricular septum through a variable number of septal branches. Several of these small septal branches anastomose with the septal branches coming from the anterior descending artery. Just distal to the crux, the right coronary artery makes an inverted "U" turn, giving origin to the atrioventricular node artery (Fig. 13.40). The coronary arterial anatomy at this region of the heart has a variable configuration. It is possible to find two parallel posterior descending arteries and the diaphragmatic surface of the heart may be irrigated by vessels coming from the right coronary artery, from the circumflex or from both (Figs. 13.39–13.45).

Angiographic Aspects

It is important to visualize all the segments of the main coronary arteries, their branches, anatomic variations, and anastomosis that occasionally occur. All the details of the lesions as well as their locations should be properly defined. To reach these goals, several angiographic projections are used.

Since the anatomic aspects of the coronary arteries are so variable, a number of appropriated projections with special angles of the x-ray bean are used for each different individual. All the principal vessels must be visualized in at least two orthogonal projections.

The elongated or cranial left oblique view shows the left main coronary artery, the LAD and the diagonal branches (Fig. 13.37). The caudal left oblique projection (spider view) shows the left main coronary artery, its bifurcation, and the proximal circumflex artery (Fig. 13.46). To visualize the LAD, the septal and the diagonal branches either the cranial and the caudal right oblique views are indicated. The circumflex artery and its marginal branches are well defined in the elongated left oblique and in the caudal right anterior oblique projections (Figs. 13.46–13.49).

The anteroposterior view is a good projection to study the left main coronary artery and its bifurcation. In some cases, the caudal anteroposterior or the true lateral views may help visualize the proximal portion of the LAD and of the circumflex artery.

The right coronary artery is well visualized in the majority of the cases in the conventional right and left oblique projections (Figs. 13.50, 13.51). The origin of the posterior descending and the posterolateral branches are defined in the caudal left anterior oblique view.

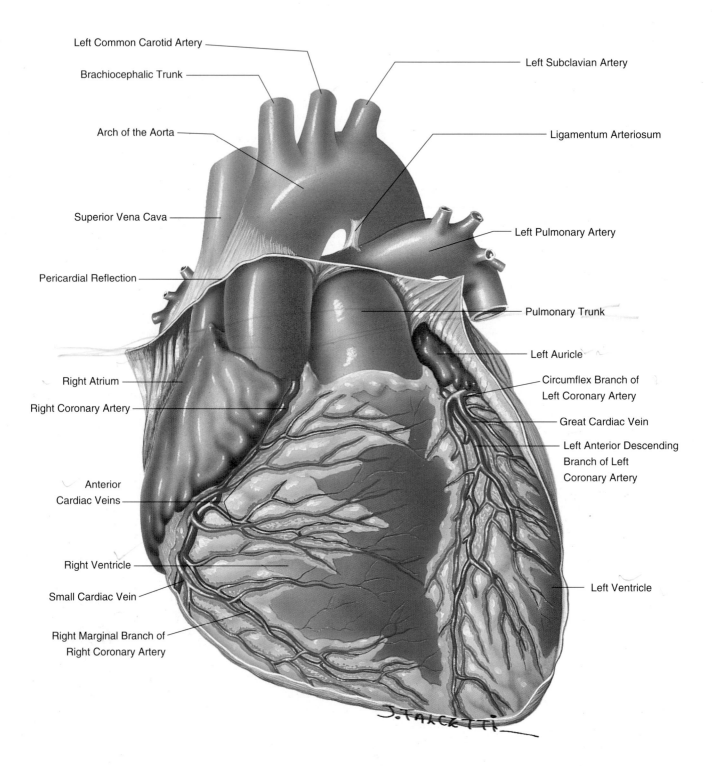

Left Common Carotid Artery

Brachiocephalic Trunk

Arch of the Aorta

Superior Vena Cava

Pericardial Reflection

Right Atrium

Right Coronary Artery

Anterior
Cardiac Veins

Right Ventricle

Small Cardiac Vein

Right Marginal Branch of
Right Coronary Artery

Left Subclavian Artery

Ligamentum Arteriosum

Left Pulmonary Artery

Pulmonary Trunk

Left Auricle

Circumflex Branch of
Left Coronary Artery

Great Cardiac Vein

Left Anterior Descending
Branch of Left
Coronary Artery

Left Ventricle

Figure 13.1. A. External aspect of the heart in the frontal view. Note the relationship of the great vessels and the ventricular cavities. **B.** External aspect of the heart in a posterior view. Note the relationship of the left atrium, pulmonary veins, and the large size of the coronary sinus.

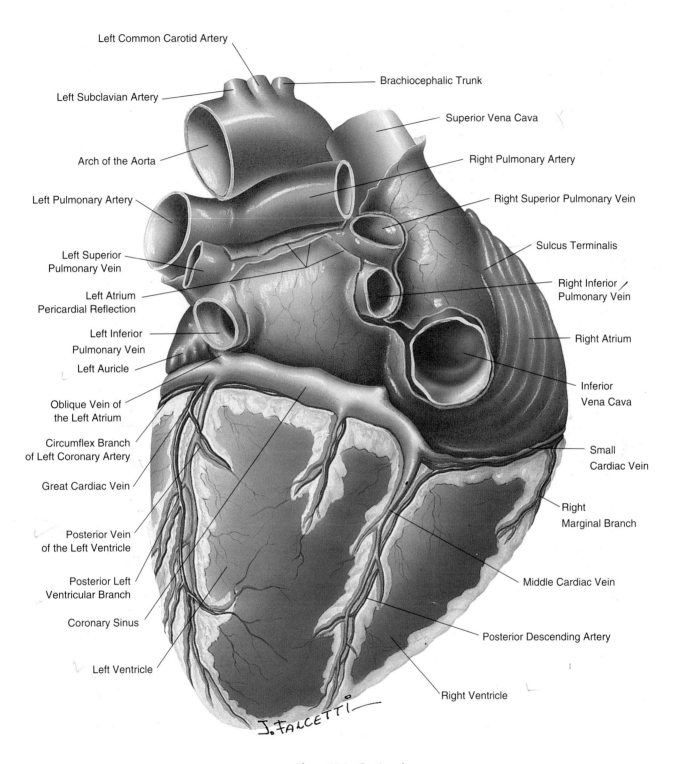

Left Common Carotid Artery

Brachiocephalic Trunk

Left Subclavian Artery

Superior Vena Cava

Arch of the Aorta

Right Pulmonary Artery

Left Pulmonary Artery

Right Superior Pulmonary Vein

Sulcus Terminalis

Left Superior
Pulmonary Vein

Right Inferior
Pulmonary Vein

Left Atrium
Pericardial Reflection

Left Inferior
Pulmonary Vein

Right Atrium

Left Auricle

Inferior
Vena Cava

Oblique Vein of
the Left Atrium

Small
Cardiac Vein

Circumflex Branch
of Left Coronary Artery

Great Cardiac Vein

Right
Marginal Branch

Posterior Vein
of the Left Ventricle

Posterior Left
Ventricular Branch

Middle Cardiac Vein

Coronary Sinus

Posterior Descending Artery

Left Ventricle

Right Ventricle

J. FALCETTI

Figure 13.1. *Continued*

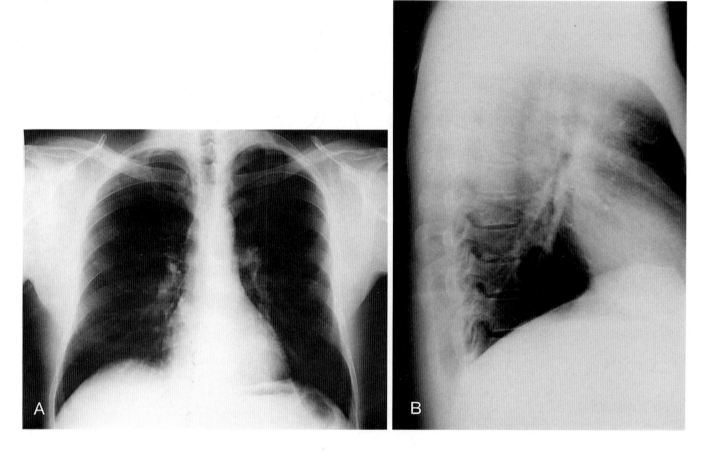

Figure 13.2. **A.** Thoracic roentgenogram in posteroanterior projection. The heart is located in the middle portion of the inferior mediastinum. The apex of the heart lies in the left hemithorax. **B.** Thoracic roentgenogram in lateral projection. Anteriorly the heart is bordered by the anterior chest wall and posteriorly by the dorsal spine.

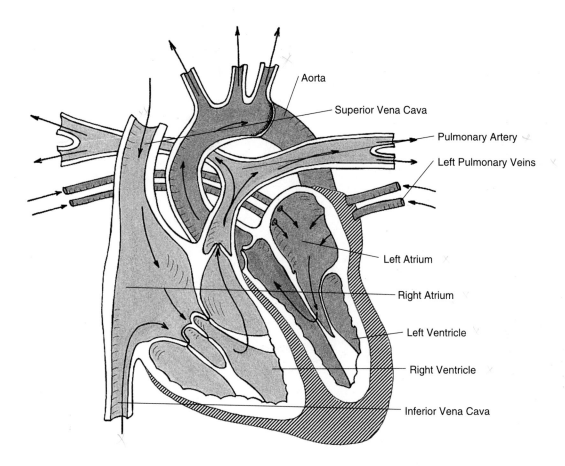

Figure 13.3. Pathways of the blood circulation inside the heart. In blue color is the venous blood and in red is the arterial blood. The pathways are marked by the arrows.

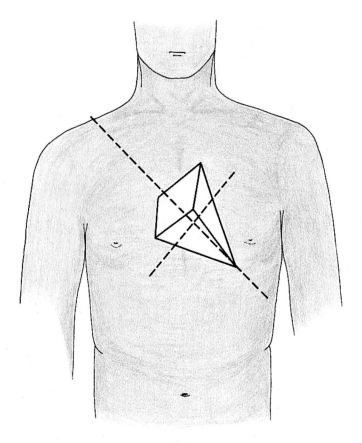

Figure 13.4. The heart looks like an inverted pyramid, with the longitudinal axis oriented anteriorly, inferiorly and toward the left. The dashed lines show the orientation.

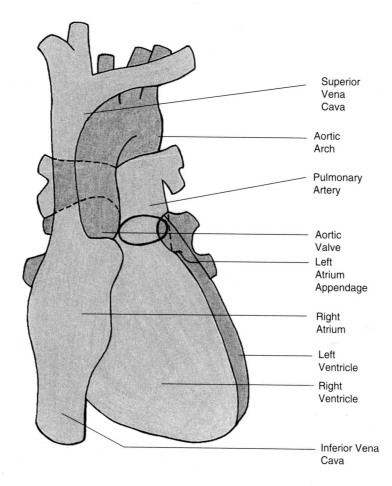

Superior
Vena
Cava

Aortic
Arch

Pulmonary
Artery

Aortic
Valve

Left
Atrium
Appendage

Right
Atrium

Left
Ventricle

Right
Ventricle

Inferior Vena
Cava

Figure 13.5. A. Frontal view of the heart. The right and left borders are outlined. Right heart is in blue and left heart and aorta in red. **B.** Lateral view of the heart. The anterior border corresponds to the anterior wall of the right ventricle and the posterior or dorsal border to the posterior wall of the left atrium and the inferior vena cava.

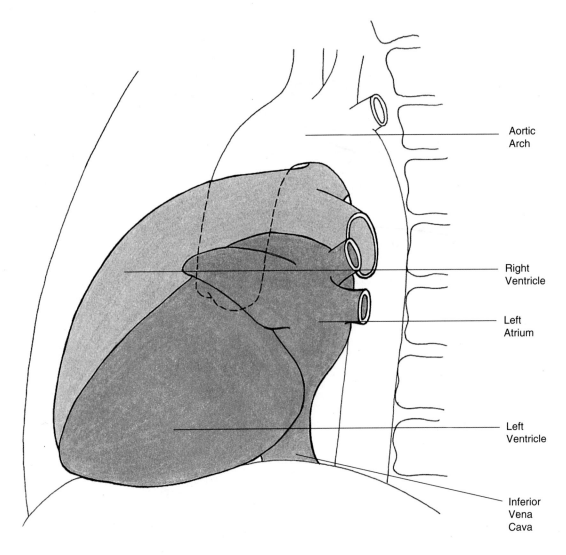

Figure 13.5. *Continued*

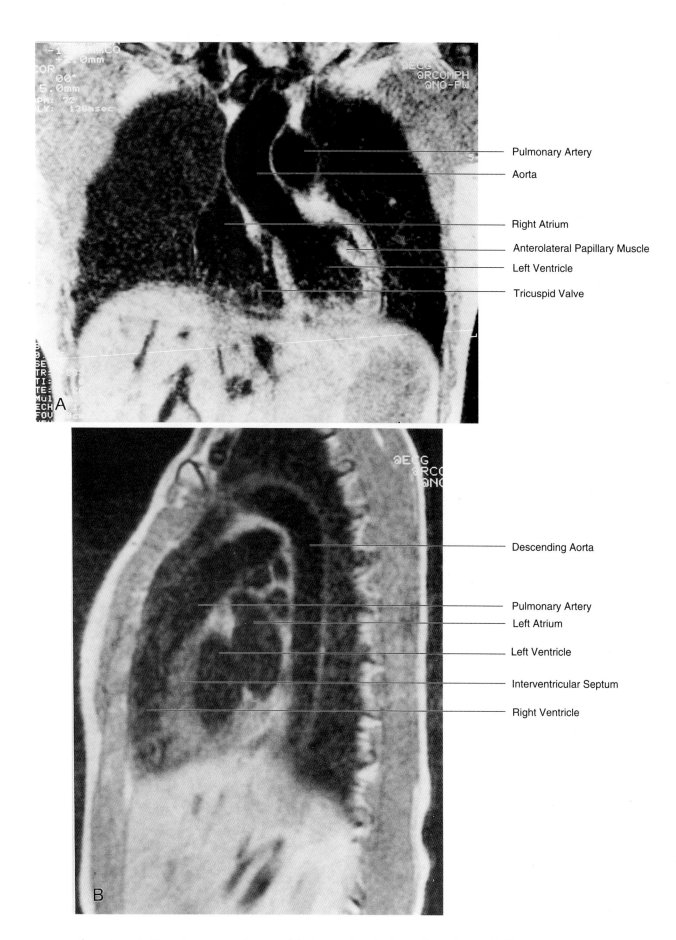

—— Pulmonary Artery

—— Aorta

—— Right Atrium

—— Anterolateral Papillary Muscle

—— Left Ventricle

—— Tricuspid Valve

A

—— Descending Aorta

—— Pulmonary Artery

—— Left Atrium

—— Left Ventricle

—— Interventricular Septum

—— Right Ventricle

B

Figure 13.6. A. Magnetic resonance imaging of the heart and mediastinum. Coronal plane. **B.** Magnetic resonance imaging of the heart and mediastinum. Sagittal plane. **C.** Magnetic resonance imaging of the heart and mediastinum. Axial plane.

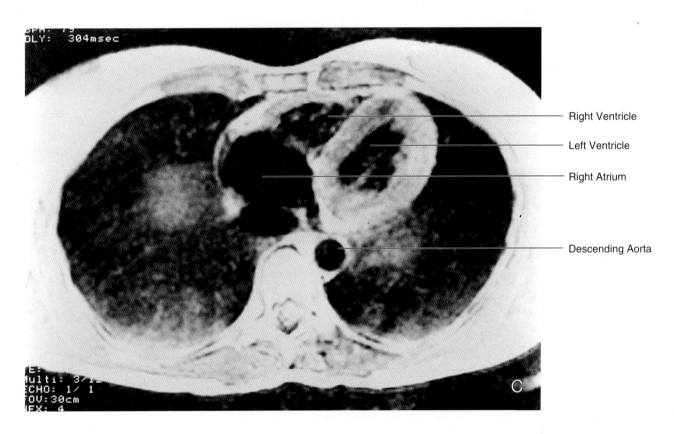

Figure 13.6. *Continued*

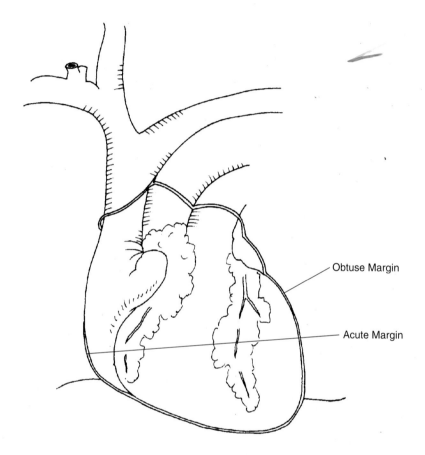

Figure 13.7.   The acute margin of the heart is sharp and is formed mainly by the right ventricle. The obtuse margin
is round and corresponds mainly to the left ventricle.

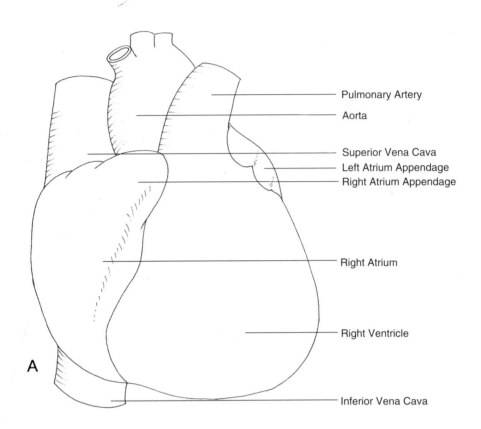

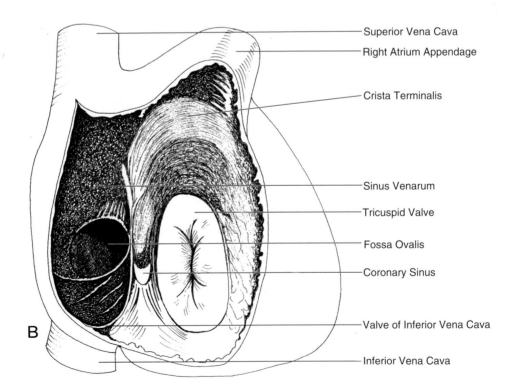

Figure 13.8. A. External features of the right atrium. The lateral wall of the right atrium forms most of the right cardiac border. **B.** Internal features of the right atrium. The atrial septum has a central circular depression: the fossa ovalis.

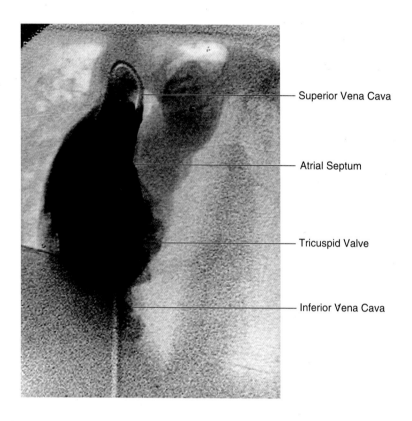

Superior Vena Cava

Atrial Septum

Tricuspid Valve

Inferior Vena Cava

Figure 13.9. Right atrial angiography. The left superior border corresponds to the most anterior portion of the atrial septum. The atrial appendage is not seen in this view. The tricuspid valve is located inferior and to the left. This is a long axial view.

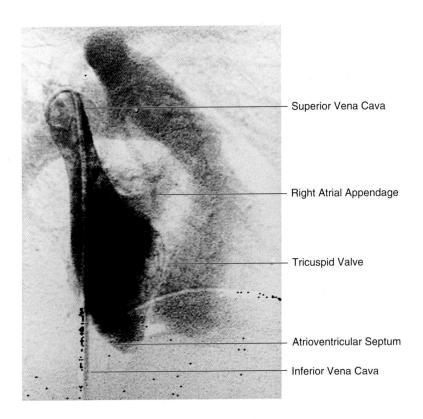

— Superior Vena Cava

— Right Atrial Appendage

— Tricuspid Valve

— Atrioventricular Septum

— Inferior Vena Cava

Figure 13.10. Right atrium in elongated right anterior oblique view. The posterior wall is seen as a continuity of the superior and inferior caval veins in the right border. The right atrial appendage is located superiorly and to the left. Between the inferior vena cava and the tricuspid anulus is the atrioventricular septum.

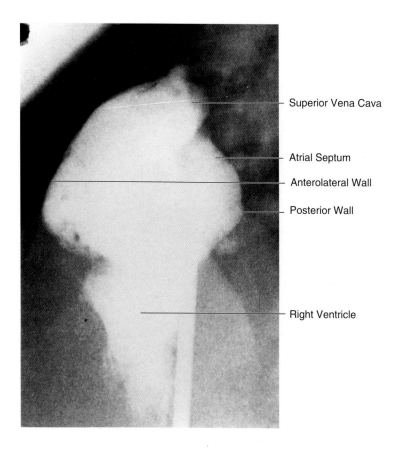

Superior Vena Cava

Atrial Septum

Anterolateral Wall

Posterior Wall

Right Ventricle

Figure 13.11. Right atrial angiogram in the so-called four chamber view. The atrial appendage is overlapped.

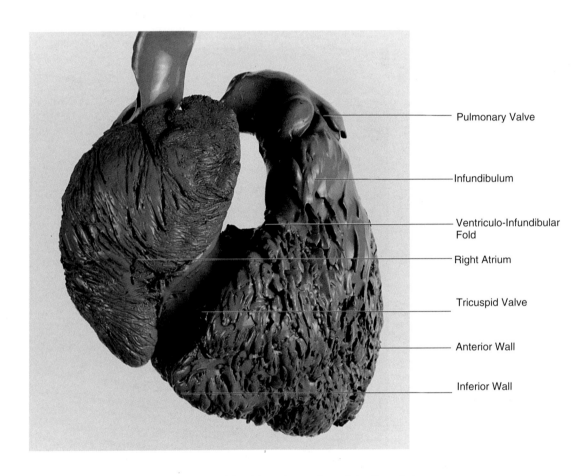

Pulmonary Valve

Infundibulum

Ventriculo-Infundibular
Fold

Right Atrium

Tricuspid Valve

Anterior Wall

Inferior Wall

Figure 13.12. Luminal cast of the right atrium and ventricle. Frontal view.

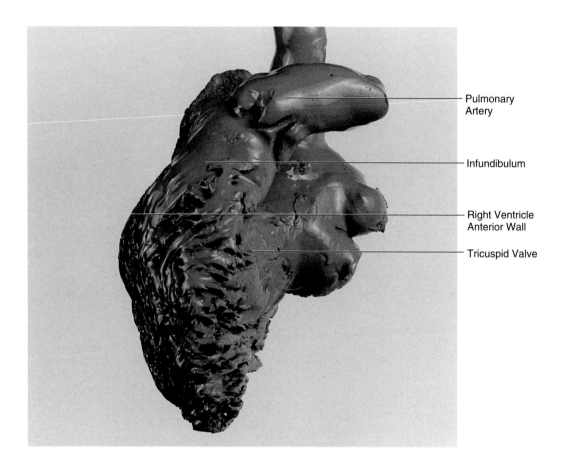

Figure 13.13. Luminal cast of the right ventricle. Lateral view.

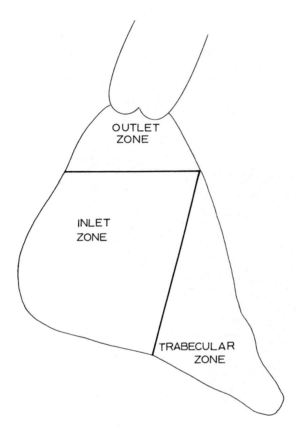

Figure 13.14. The three portions of the right ventricular chamber.

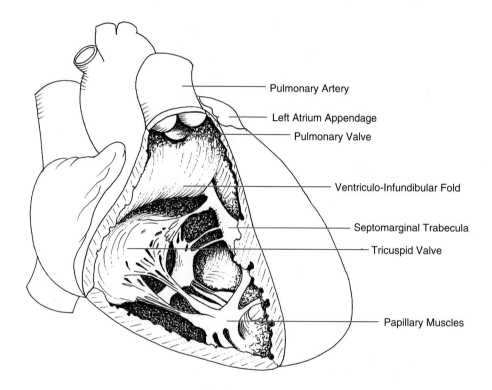

Figure 13.15. Internal features of the right ventricle.

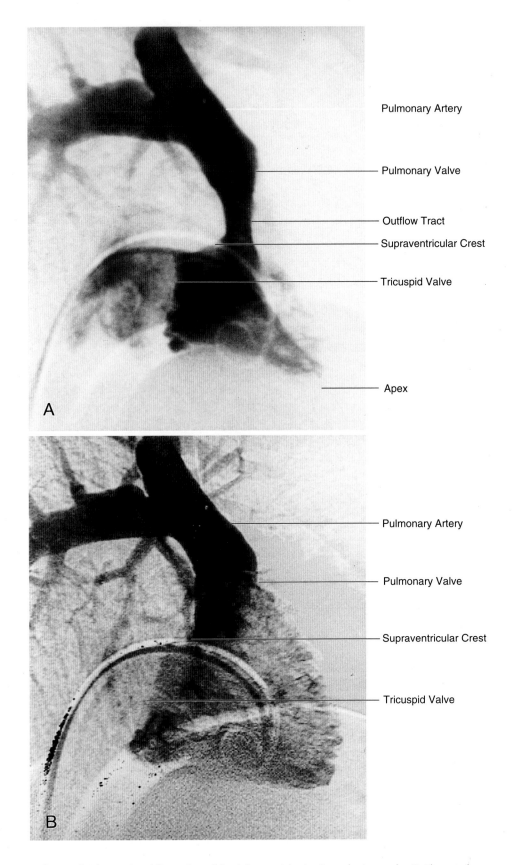

Figure 13.16. **A.** Elongated right anterior oblique view of the right ventricle. Angiography in systole. **B.** Elongated right anterior oblique view of the right ventricle. Angiography in diastole.

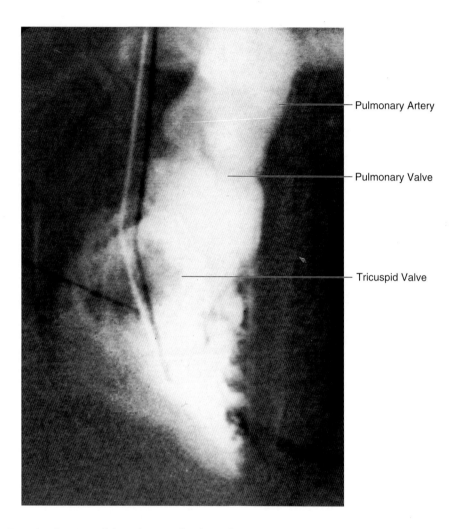

— Pulmonary Artery

— Pulmonary Valve

— Tricuspid Valve

Figure 13.17. Four chamber view of the right ventricle. The outflow tract is not well defined as it is in the long axial view.

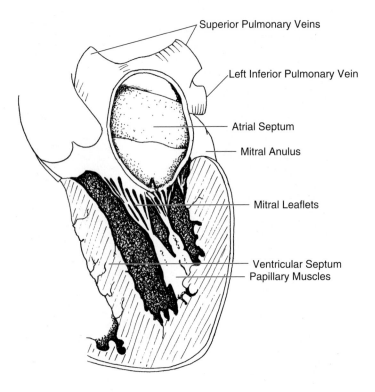

Figure 13.18. Internal features of the left atrium and ventricle.

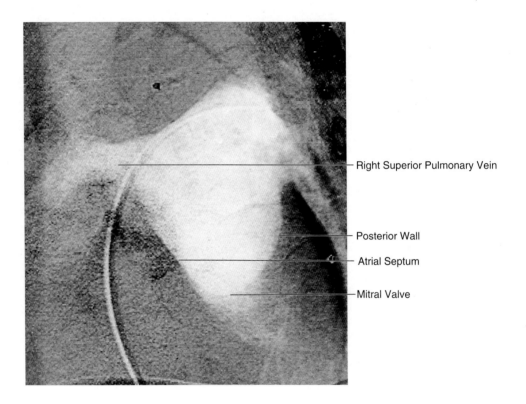

Right Superior Pulmonary Vein

Posterior Wall

Atrial Septum

Mitral Valve

Figure 13.19. Left atrial angiogram in long axial view. The left pulmonary veins and the left atrium appendage are not seen in this view.

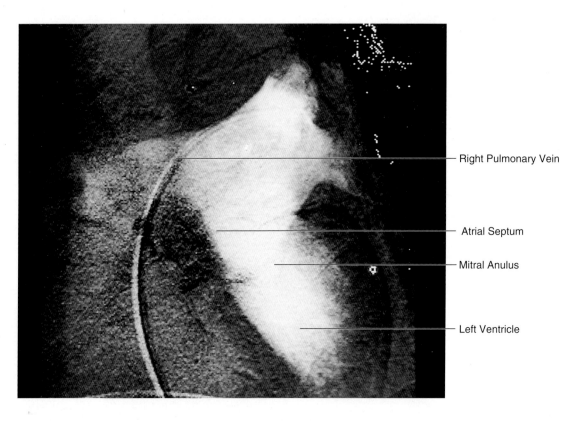

— Right Pulmonary Vein

— Atrial Septum

— Mitral Anulus

— Left Ventricle

Figure 13.20. Long axial view of the left atrium. The anterior portion of the left atrial septum is the right wall of the left atrium. The left atrial appendage is not seen in this projection.

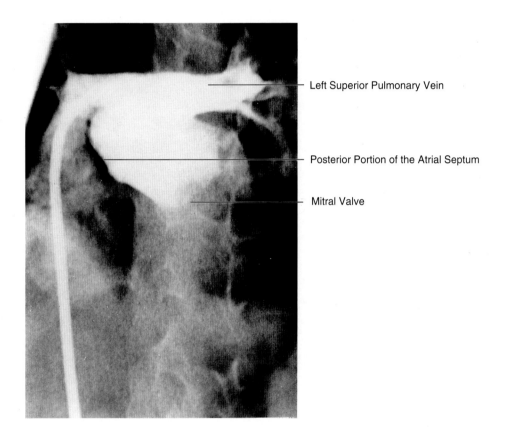

Left Superior Pulmonary Vein

Posterior Portion of the Atrial Septum

Mitral Valve

Figure 13.21. Four chamber view of the left atrium. The posterior portion of the atrial septum is seen as the right border of the left atrium. (Courtesy of Dr. Benigno Soto from University of Alabama, Birmingham.)

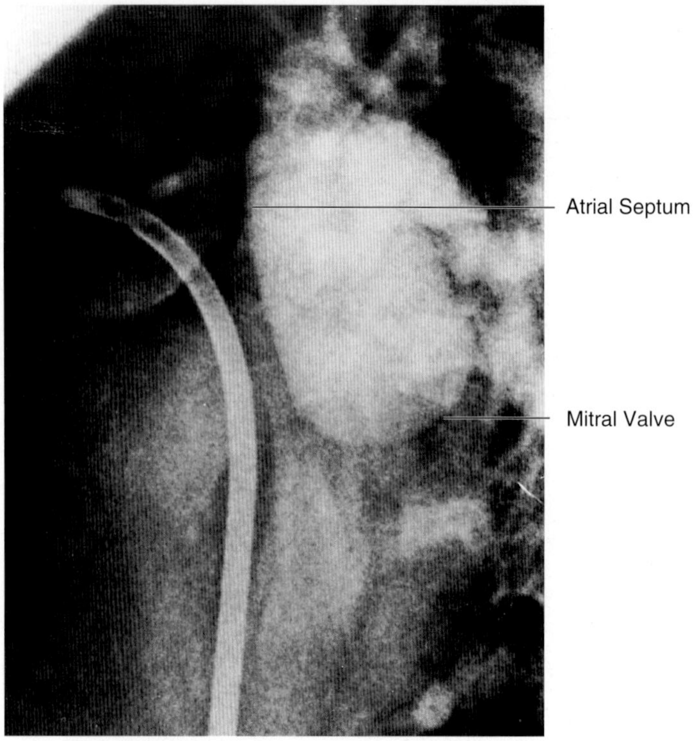

Figure 13.22. Left atrial angiogram in the so-called four chamber view.

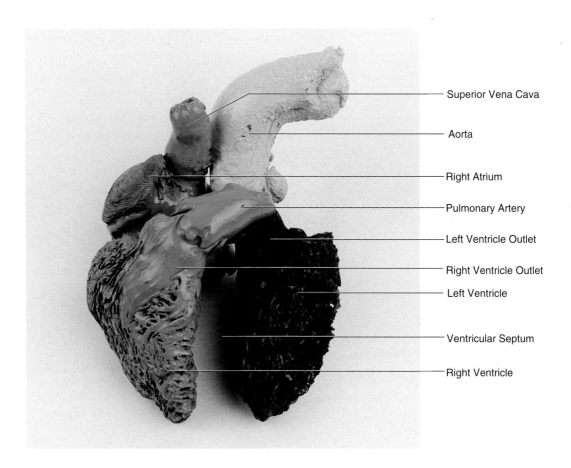

Superior Vena Cava

Aorta

Right Atrium

Pulmonary Artery

Left Ventricle Outlet

Right Ventricle Outlet

Left Ventricle

Ventricular Septum

Right Ventricle

Figure 13.23. Cast of the heart showing the spatial relationships of the ventricular chambers. Note that the left ventricle is red, the aortal is yellow, the right ventricle, right atrium, superior vena cava, and pulmonary artery are blue.

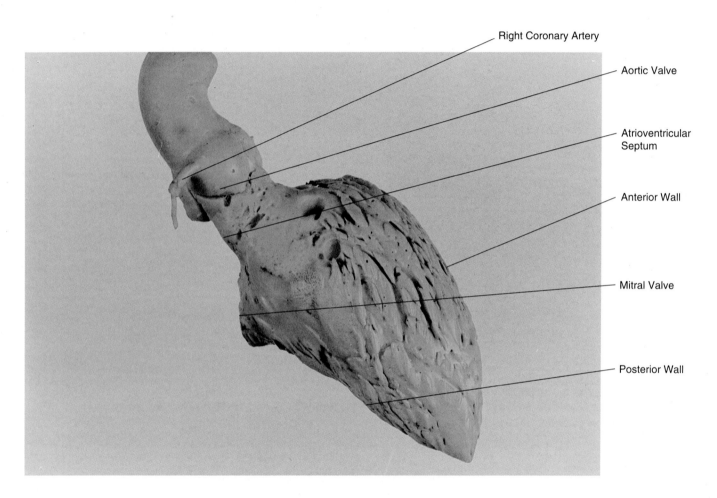

Right Coronary Artery

Aortic Valve

Atrioventricular
Septum

Anterior Wall

Mitral Valve

Posterior Wall

Figure 13.24. Luminal cast of the left ventricle and aorta in a frontal view.

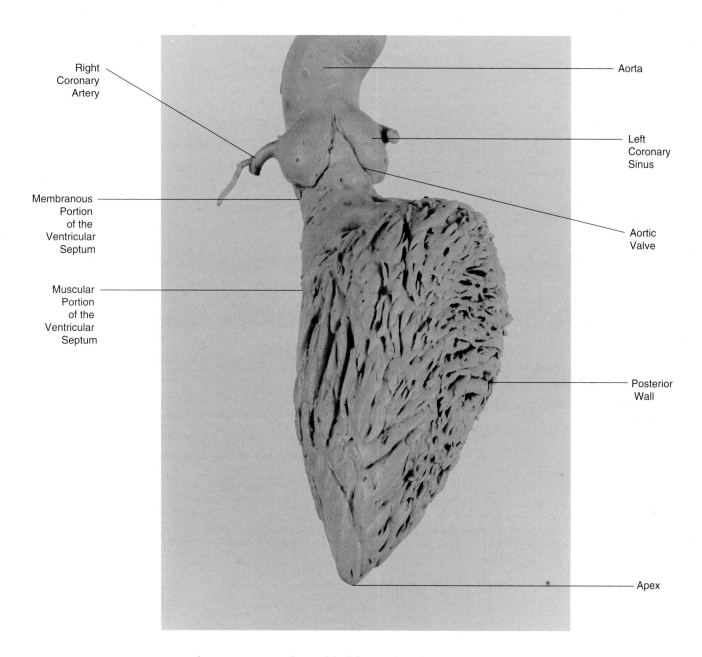

Right Coronary Artery

Membranous Portion of the Ventricular Septum

Muscular Portion of the Ventricular Septum

Aorta

Left Coronary Sinus

Aortic Valve

Posterior Wall

Apex

Figure 13.25. Luminal cast of the left ventricle and aorta in lateral view.

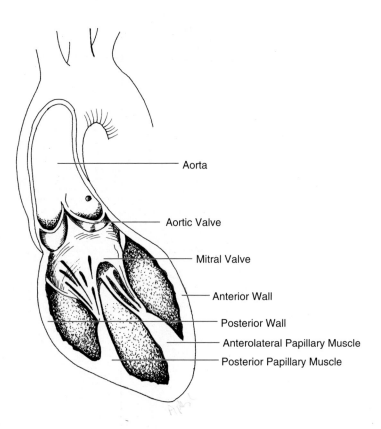

Figure 13.26. Internal features of the left ventricle.

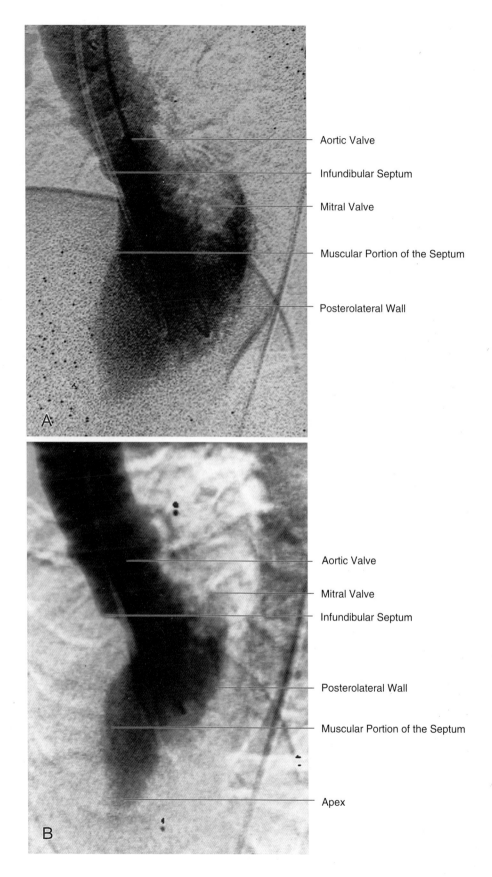

Aortic Valve

Infundibular Septum

Mitral Valve

Muscular Portion of the Septum

Posterolateral Wall

Aortic Valve

Mitral Valve

Infundibular Septum

Posterolateral Wall

Muscular Portion of the Septum

Apex

Figure 13.27. **A.** Left ventricle angiogram in long axial view. Diastolic phase. **B.** Left ventricle angiogram in long axial view. Systolic phase. The superior portion of the interventricular septum is formed by the infundibular septum just below the Aortic Valve.

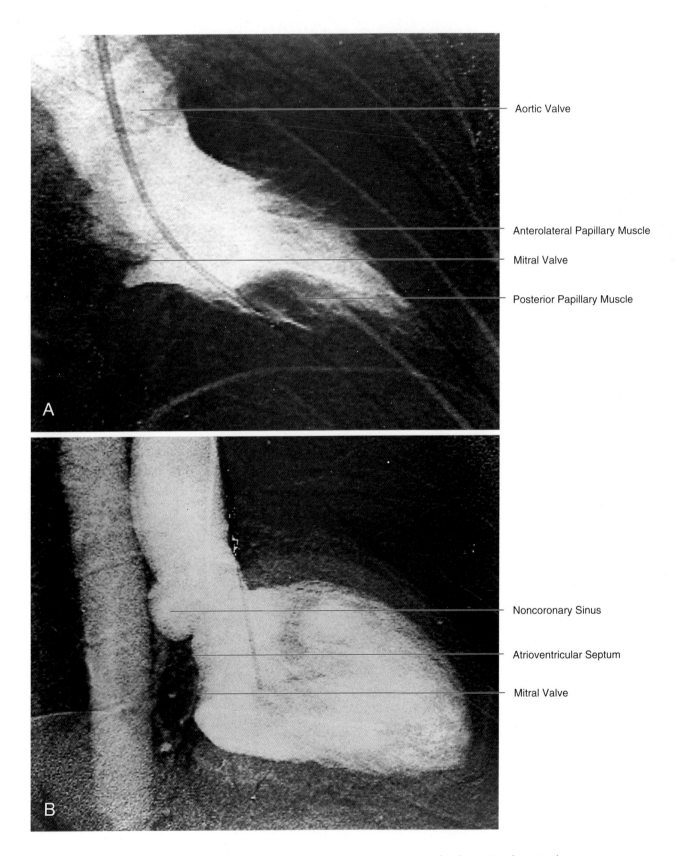

Figure 13.28. A. Left ventricular angiogram in elongated right anterior view. Systolic phase. **B.** Left ventricular angiogram in elongated right anterior view. Diastolic phase.

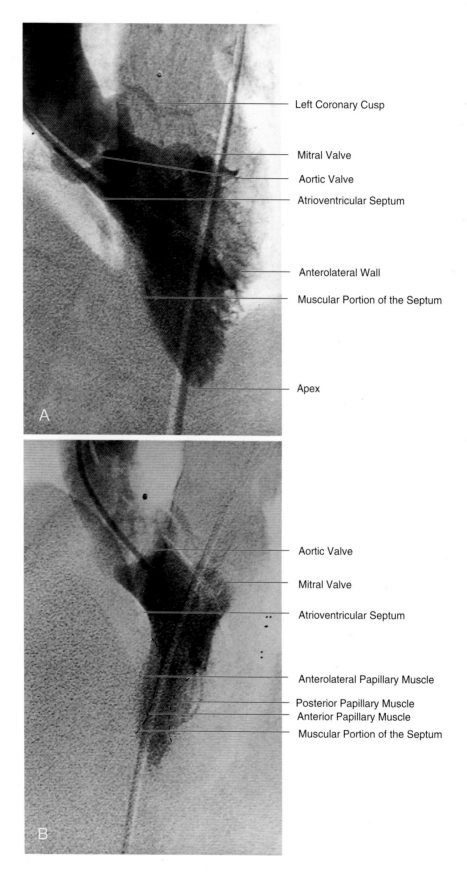

Left Coronary Cusp

Mitral Valve

Aortic Valve

Atrioventricular Septum

Anterolateral Wall

Muscular Portion of the Septum

Apex

A

Aortic Valve

Mitral Valve

Atrioventricular Septum

Anterolateral Papillary Muscle

Posterior Papillary Muscle
Anterior Papillary Muscle
Muscular Portion of the Septum

B

Figure 13.29. A. Left ventricle angiogram in four chamber view. Diastolic phase. The atrioventricular portion of the interventricular septum separates the left ventricle from the Right Atrium. **B.** Left ventricle angiogram in four chamber view. Systolic phase. The two papillary muscles appear as two filling defects in the body of the left ventricle.

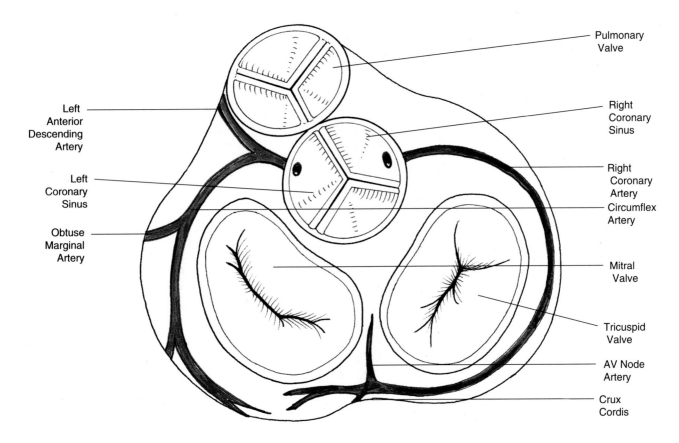

Figure 13.30. A. Relationships of the coronary arteries around the heart. The left coronary artery is in red color and the right coronary artery is in blue. **B.** The right coronary and the circumflex arteries form a circle around the atrioventricular sulci. The left anterior descending and the posterior descending arteries form a semicircle around the interventricular sulci.

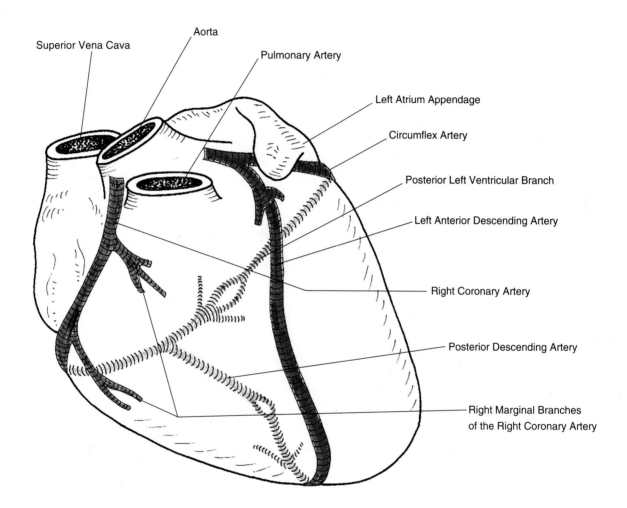

Superior Vena Cava

Aorta

Pulmonary Artery

Left Atrium Appendage

Circumflex Artery

Posterior Left Ventricular Branch

Left Anterior Descending Artery

Right Coronary Artery

Posterior Descending Artery

Right Marginal Branches
of the Right Coronary Artery

Figure 13.30. *Continued*

Left Coronary Artery   Aorta

Branch to Sinoatrial (SA) Node

Right Coronary Artery

Acute Marginal Artery

Posterior Descending Artery

Posterolateral Branches

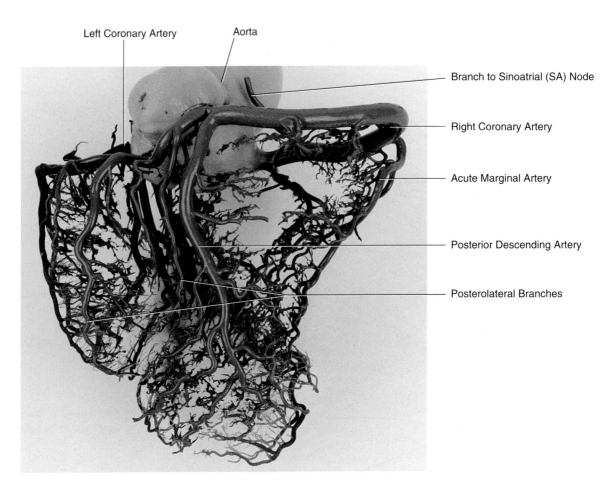

Figure 13.31. Cast of the coronary arteries viewed from the inferior face of the heart. The right coronary artery is blue. It is dominant and supplies all the inferior wall and part of the left lateral wall of the heart. The aorta is in yellow. The left coronary artery is in red.

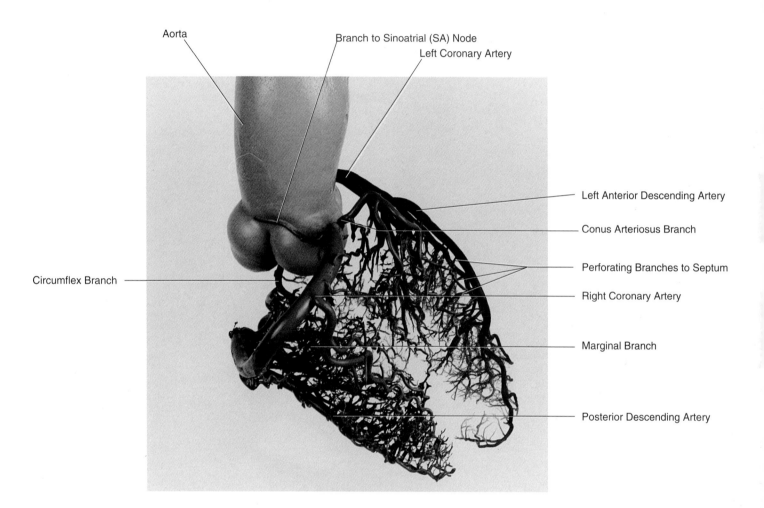

Aorta

Branch to Sinoatrial (SA) Node

Left Coronary Artery

Left Anterior Descending Artery

Conus Arteriosus Branch

Perforating Branches to Septum

Right Coronary Artery

Marginal Branch

Circumflex Branch

Posterior Descending Artery

Figure 13.32. Cast of the coronary arteries in lateral view. The right coronary artery is in blue. The left coronary branches are in red and supply the anterior part of the left lateral wall of the heart.

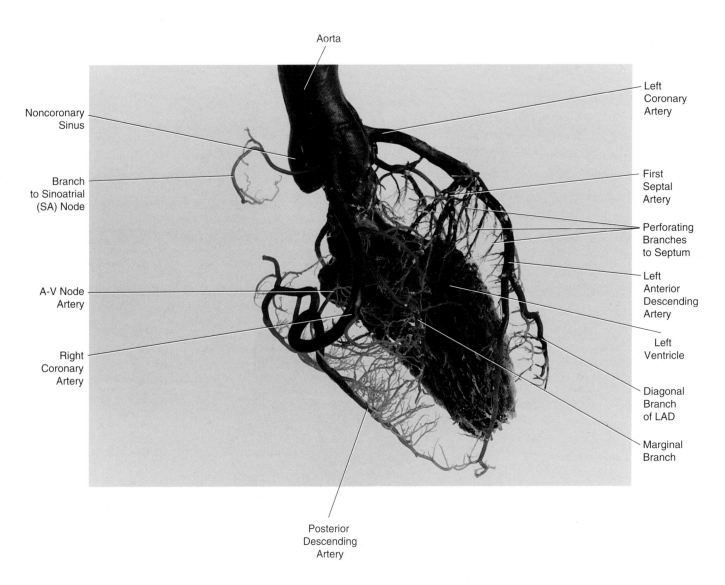

Figure 13.33. Cast of the coronary arteries in right oblique view and their relationships with the left ventricle.
The right coronary artery is in blue and gives rise to the posterior descending artery which goes towards the
apex of the heart close to the distal portion of the left anterior descending artery in red.

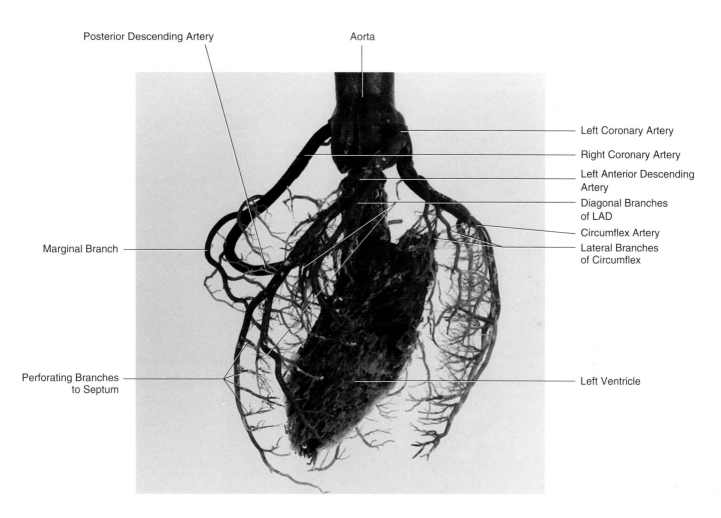

Posterior Descending Artery

Aorta

Left Coronary Artery

Right Coronary Artery

Left Anterior Descending Artery

Diagonal Branches of LAD

Circumflex Artery

Lateral Branches of Circumflex

Marginal Branch

Perforating Branches to Septum

Left Ventricle

Figure 13.34. Cast of the coronary arteries in a left oblique view and their relations with the left ventricle. The left coronary artery and its branches are in red. The right coronary artery is in blue.

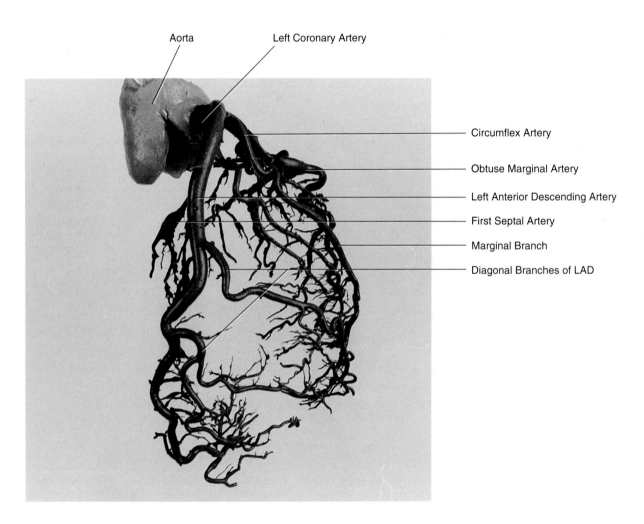

Aorta   Left Coronary Artery

Circumflex Artery

Obtuse Marginal Artery

Left Anterior Descending Artery

First Septal Artery

Marginal Branch

Diagonal Branches of LAD

Figure 13.35. Cast of the left coronary artery in a left oblique view. The coronary artery is in blue and the aorta
is in yellow.

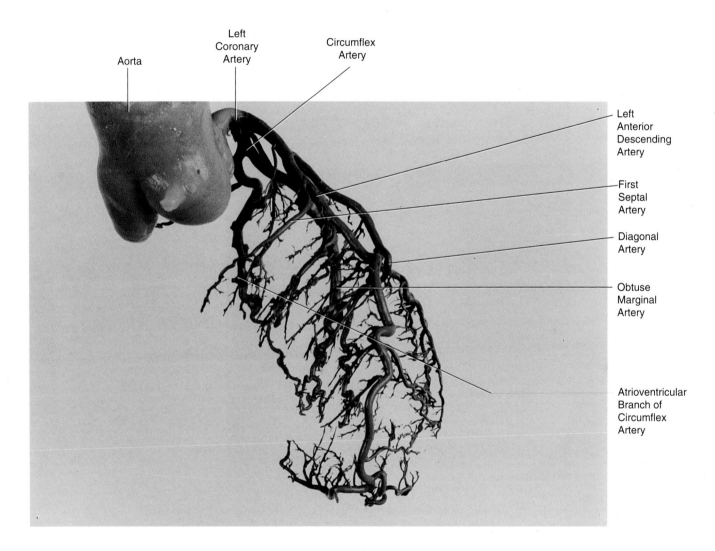

Figure 13.36. Cast of the left coronary artery in a right oblique view. The coronary artery is in blue and the aortal is in yellow.

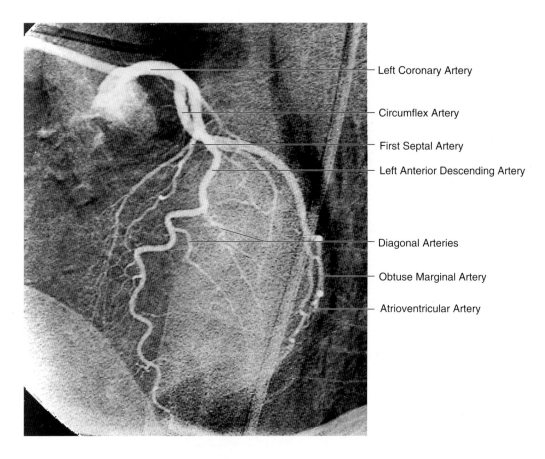

Left Coronary Artery

Circumflex Artery

First Septal Artery

Left Anterior Descending Artery

Diagonal Arteries

Obtuse Marginal Artery

Atrioventricular Artery

Figure 13.37. Angiogram of the left coronary artery in the cranial left anterior oblique projection.

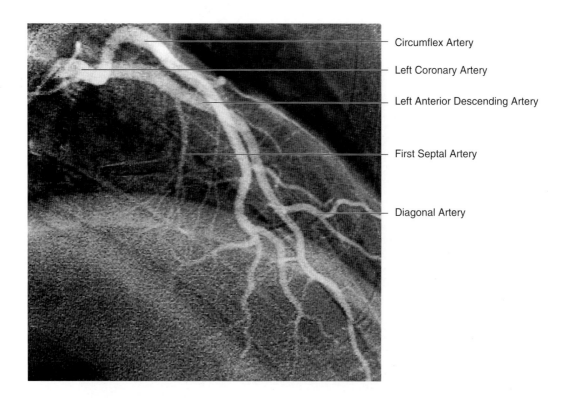

Circumflex Artery

Left Coronary Artery

Left Anterior Descending Artery

First Septal Artery

Diagonal Artery

Figure 13.38. Angiogram of the left coronary artery in the cranial right anterior oblique view. The origin of the septal and diagonal arteries are well demonstrated in this projection.

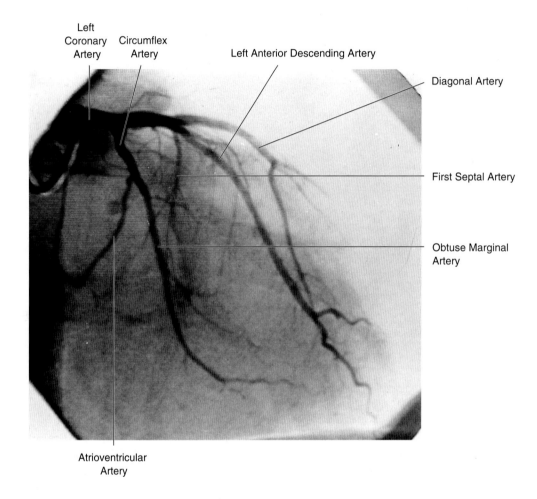

Figure 13.39. Angiogram of the left coronary artery in the right anterior oblique view.

Right
Coronary
Artery

Aorta

Acute
Marginal
Artery

Branches
to the
Back
of Left
Ventricle
(Posterolateral
Arteries)

Posterior
Descending
Artery

Marginal
Branches

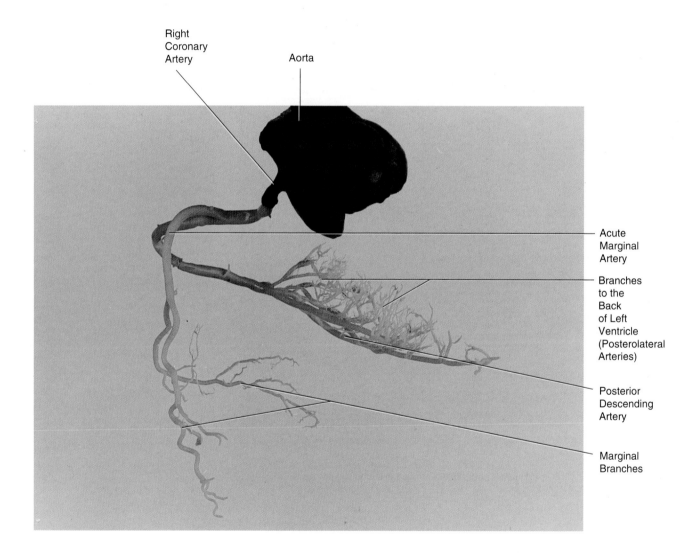

Figure 13.40. Cast of the right coronary artery in a left oblique view.

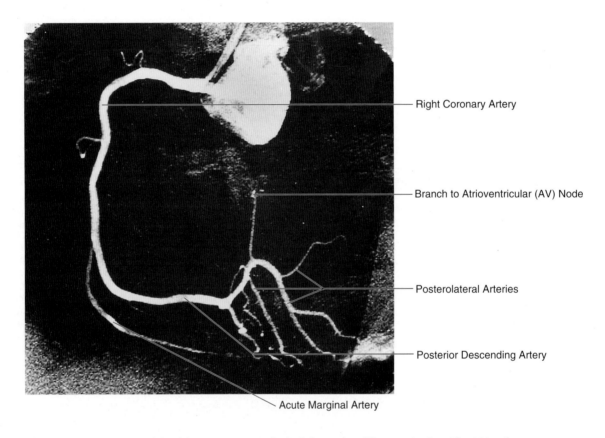

Right Coronary Artery

Branch to Atrioventricular (AV) Node

Posterolateral Arteries

Posterior Descending Artery

Acute Marginal Artery

Figure 13.41. Angiogram of the right coronary artery in the left anterior oblique projection. The A-V node artery arises from an inverted U turn.

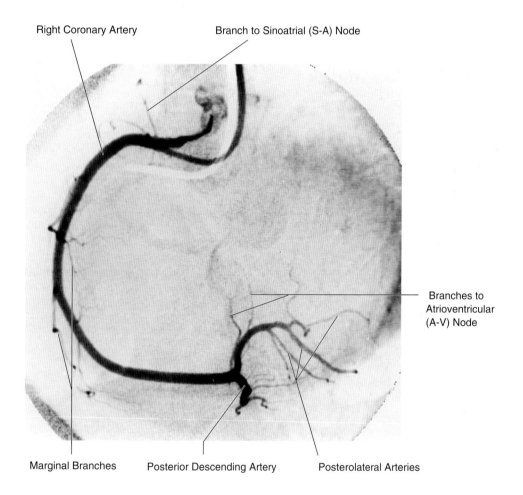

Right Coronary Artery

Branch to Sinoatrial (S-A) Node

Branches to Atrioventricular (A-V) Node

Marginal Branches

Posterior Descending Artery

Posterolateral Arteries

Figure 13.42. Angiogram of the right coronary artery in the left anterior oblique projection. The branches to the A-V node are multiple.

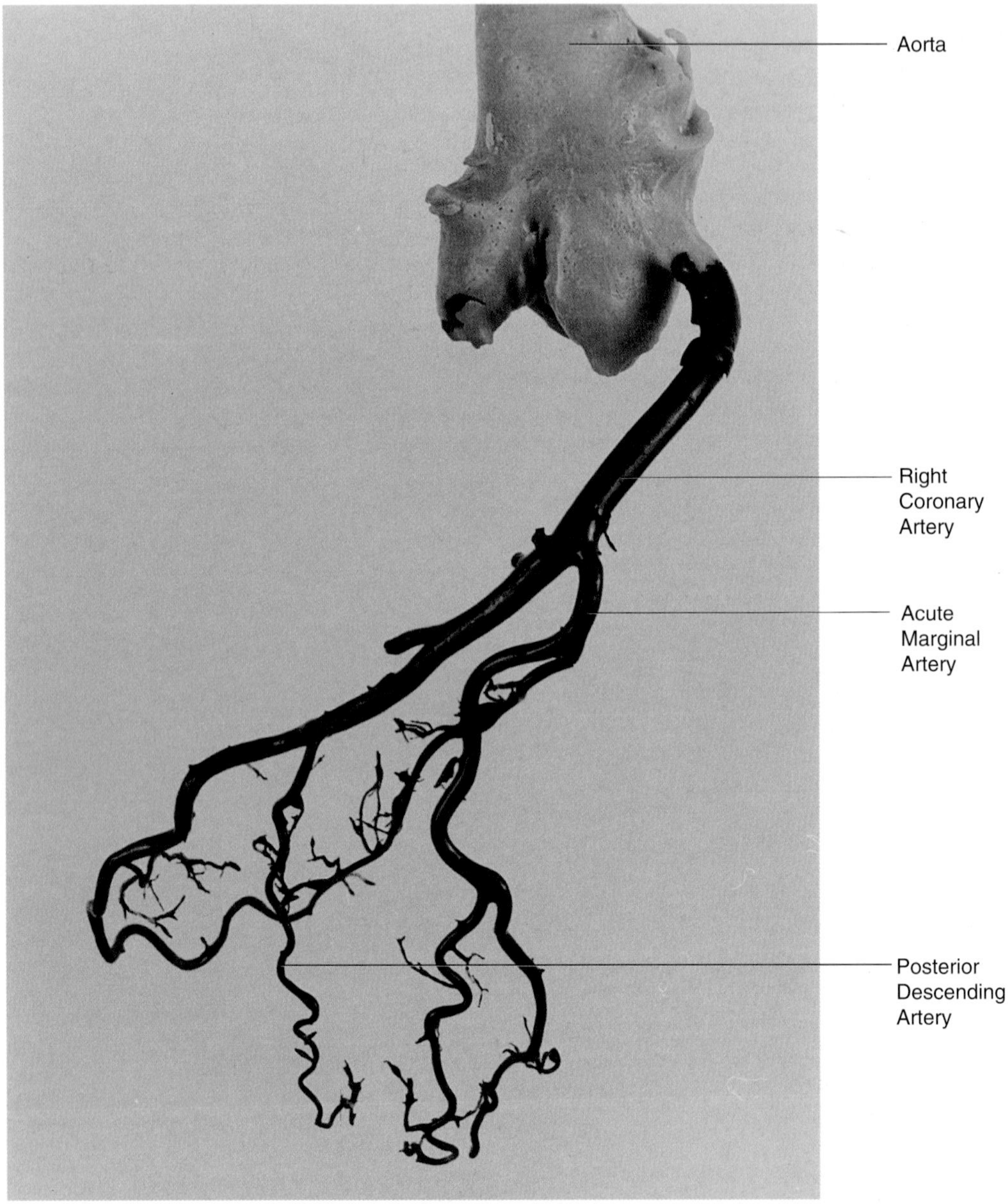

— Aorta

— Right
Coronary
Artery

— Acute
Marginal
Artery

— Posterior
Descending
Artery

Figure 13.43. Cast of the right coronary.artery in a right oblique view. The posterior descending artery is the
terminal branch. There are no posterolateral arteries.

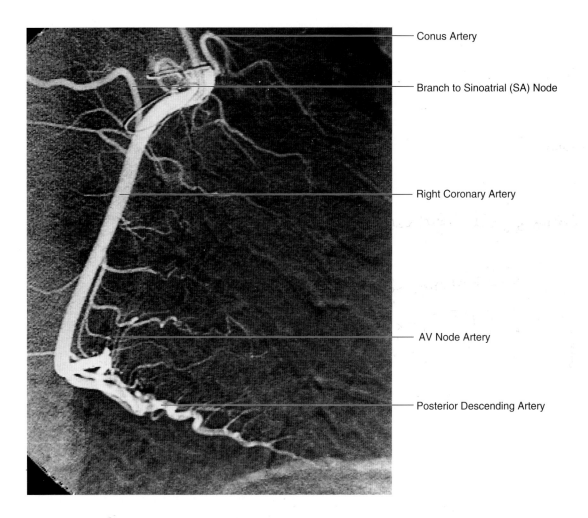

Conus Artery

Branch to Sinoatrial (SA) Node

Right Coronary Artery

AV Node Artery

Posterior Descending Artery

Figure 13.44. Angiogram of the right coronary artery in the right anterior oblique projection.

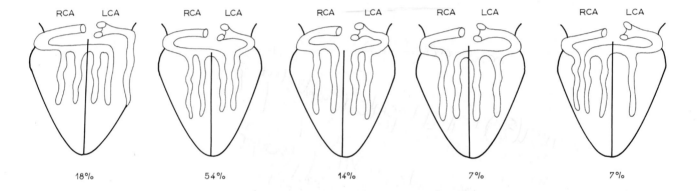

Figure 13.45. Distribution of the coronary branches to the posterior surface of the heart. (According to Campbell 1929).

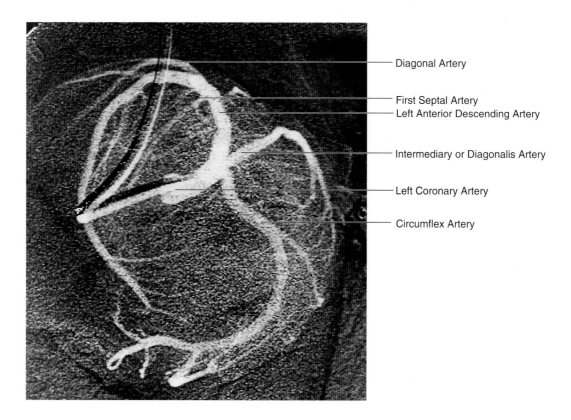

Diagonal Artery

First Septal Artery
Left Anterior Descending Artery

Intermediary or Diagonalis Artery

Left Coronary Artery

Circumflex Artery

Figure 13.46. Left coronary artery angiogram obtained in the caudal left anterior oblique or spider projection showing the origin of the left anterior descending artery, the circumflex artery and the diagonalis branch.

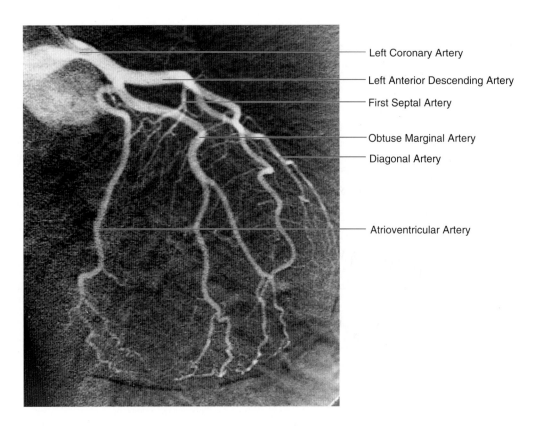

Left Coronary Artery

Left Anterior Descending Artery

First Septal Artery

Obtuse Marginal Artery

Diagonal Artery

Atrioventricular Artery

Figure 13.47. Left coronary artery angiogram in the caudal right anterior oblique projection. The circumflex artery is very short and divides into a well developed obtuse marginal artery and an atrioventricular artery.

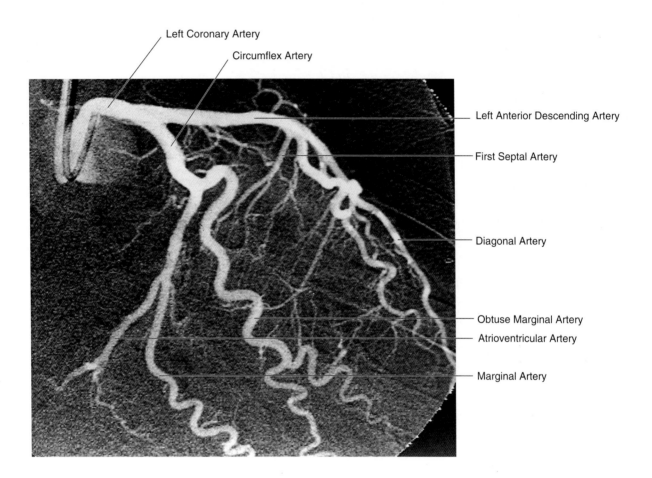

Left Coronary Artery

Circumflex Artery

Left Anterior Descending Artery

First Septal Artery

Diagonal Artery

Obtuse Marginal Artery

Atrioventricular Artery

Marginal Artery

Figure 13.48. Left coronary artery in the caudal right anterior oblique projection. The left anterior descending artery is short and divides in two parallel arteries: one running over the interventricular sulcus supplying the interventricular septum. The other runs in the anterior wall of the left ventricle and originates the diagonal arteries. It is called dual left anterior descending artery.

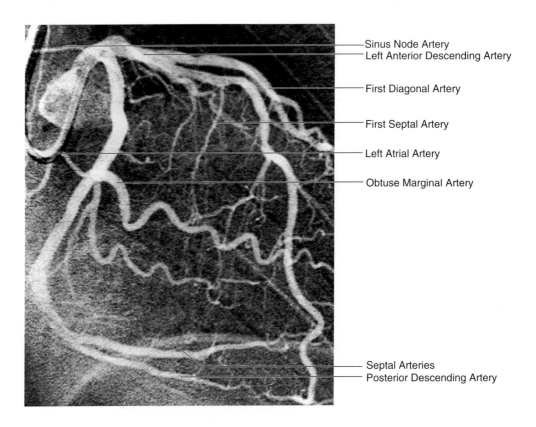

— Sinus Node Artery
— Left Anterior Descending Artery

— First Diagonal Artery

— First Septal Artery

— Left Atrial Artery

— Obtuse Marginal Artery

— Septal Arteries
— Posterior Descending Artery

Figure 13.49. Dominant left coronary artery: the posterior descending artery arises distally from the circumflex artery. The sinus node artery is originated from the proximal circumflex artery. This is an angiogram in the cranial right anterior oblique projection.

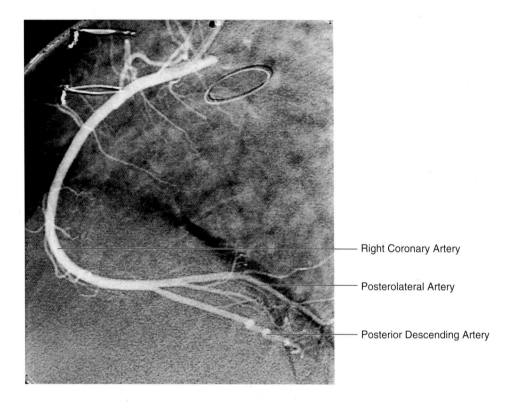

Right Coronary Artery

Posterolateral Artery

Posterior Descending Artery

Figure 13.50. Dominant right coronary artery in the left anterior oblique view. The posterior descending artery arises from the right coronary artery at the crux cordis.

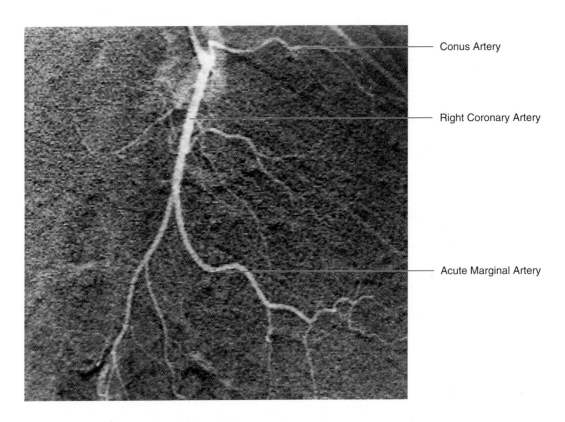

Conus Artery

Right Coronary Artery

Acute Marginal Artery

Figure 13.51. Angiogram showing a nondominant right coronary artery in the right anterior oblique projection.

14

CARDIAC VEINS

The human heart has three systems of veins: the left ventricular, the right ventricular, and the thebesian veins. They are separate but intercommunicating systems.

The left ventricular system drains most of the left ventricular venous blood and is formed by the anterior interventricular vein, the posterior ventricular vein, the left marginal vein, the middle cardiac vein, and the right marginal vein. The anterior interventricular vein ascends parallel to the LAD artery and enters into the left atrioventricular sulcus where it becomes the great cardiac vein that follows in continuity with the coronary sinus that ends in the right atrium (see Fig. 13.1). The posterior ventricular vein or middle cardiac vein running in the posterior interventricular sulcus may drain into the right atrium or in the coronary sinus. The left marginal vein drains into the great cardiac vein. The right marginal vein ends in the coronary sinus or in the right atrium (Fig. 14.1).

The right ventricle veins are known as the anterior cardiac veins and are two to four long veins crossing the anterior surface of the right ventricle and draining directly into the right atrium.

The small thebesian veins drain directly into the right atrium and right ventricle.

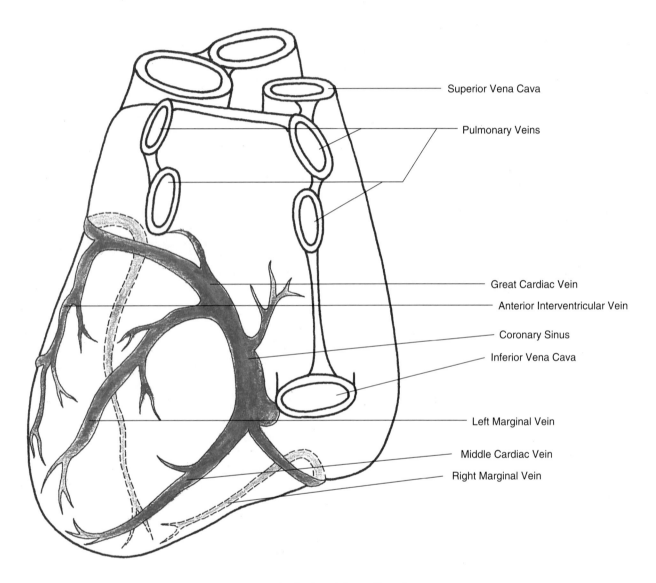

Figure 14.1. Distribution of the cardiac veins.

Superior Vena Cava

Pulmonary Veins

Great Cardiac Vein

Anterior Interventricular Vein

Coronary Sinus

Inferior Vena Cava

Left Marginal Vein

Middle Cardiac Vein

Right Marginal Vein

15

ARTERIES OF THE UPPER EXTREMITY

SUBCLAVIAN ARTERY

This artery arises from the brachiocephalic trunk at the right side, from the division of the brachiocephalic trunk (Part I), behind the right sternoclavicular joint passing upward behind the scalenus anterior muscle (Part II) and coursing horizontally slightly downwards to the outer border of the first rib (Part III), about the origin of the superior thoracic artery (Figs. 15.1, 15.2).

The left subclavian artery arises from the aortic arch, after the origin of the left common carotid artery at the level of the third and fourth thoracic vertebra, ascending in direction of the neck and bending laterally crossing behind the left scalenus anterior muscle (Part I), following the same pattern of the right subclavian artery on parts II and III.

Branches

Vertebral artery
Internal thoracic artery (internal mammary artery)
Thyrocervical trunk
Costocervical trunk
Dorsal scapular artery

Vertebral Artery

This artery is described in the head and neck section (Chapter 2).

Internal Thoracic Artery (Internal Mammary Artery)

This artery arises within 2 cm from the origin of the subclavian artery. It courses forward and downward behind the cartilages of the upper ribs and divides into the musculophrenic and superior epigastric arteries at the level of the sixth intercostal space (Figs. 15.3, 15.4, 15.5).

Branches

Pericardiophrenic artery
Mediastinal artery
Pericardial branches
Intercostal branches
Perforating branches
Musculophrenic artery
Superior epigastric artery

Thyrocervical Trunk

The thyrocervical trunk arises from the first part of the subclavian artery and gives three branches (Fig. 15.2).

Inferior Thyroid Artery (Figs. 15.6, 15.7)

Branches

Muscular branches
    Ascending cervical artery
    Inferior laryngeal artery
Pharyngeal branches
Tracheal branches
Esophageal branches
Large glandular branches
    Ascending (parathyroid)
    Descending (thyroid)

Variation: A bronchial artery may originate from the thyrocervical trunk (Fig. 15.8).

Suprascapular Artery (May be a branch of the Subclavian or Internal Thoracic Artery (Figs. 15.9, 15.10, 15.11)

Branches

Suprasternal branch
Acromial branch
Articular branches
    Clavicle nutrients
    Scapula nutrients

Superficial Cervical Artery (Fig. 15.12)

This artery anastomoses with the superficial branch of the descending branch of the occipital artery.

Costocervical Trunk

The costocervical trunk arises from the back of the second part of the subclavian artery on the right side, but on the first part on the left side (Fig. 15.13).

Superior Intercostal Artery

The superior intercostal artery anastomoses with third posterior intercostal artery. It may be supplied by a branch from the aorta.

Deep Cervical Artery

The deep cervical artery arises in most cases from the costocervical trunk, but may be a branch of the subclavian artery.

Dorsal Scapular Artery (Figs. 15.14, 15.15)

This artery arises from the 3rd or 2nd part of the subclavian artery.

AXILLARY ARTERY
(FIGS. 15.1, 15.2, 15.3, 15.16)

The axillary artery is a continuation of the subclavian artery.

Proximal Limit—Outer border of the first rib.

Distal Limit—Lower border of the teres major muscle tendon.

Branches

Superior thoracic artery (highest)
Thoracoacromial (acromiothoracic) artery
    Pectoral branch
    Acromial branch
    Clavicular branch
    Deltoid branch
Lateral thoracic (lateral mammary branches)
Subscapular artery
Anterior circumflex humeral artery
Posterior circumflex humeral artery

Superior Thoracic Artery (Highest Thoracic Artery or Arteria Thoracica Suprema)

The superior thoracic artery is a small vessel and arises from the first part of the axillary artery. It may branch from the thoracoacromial artery.

Thoracoacromial Artery (Acromiothoracic Artery) (Figs. 15.17, 15.18)

Branches

Pectoral branch
Acromial branch
Clavicular branch
Deltoid branch (may arise from the acromial branch)

Lateral Thoracic Artery (External Mammary or Inferior Thoracic Artery)

This artery anastomoses with the internal thoracic, subscapular, and intercostal arteries and pectoral branches of the thoracoacromial artery. In females, it is larger and gives off lateral mammary branches reaching the breast.

Subscapular Artery (Inferior Scapular Artery)

This artery is the largest branch of the axillary artery. It anastomoses with the lateral thoracic, inter-costal arteries and deep branch of the transverse cervical artery, and supplies muscles of the chest wall.

Branches

Circumflex scapular artery
Infrascapular artery
Lateral border of the scapula (dorsal thoracic artery)
Muscular branches

Anterior Circumflex Humeral Artery

This artery is a small branch, located in front of the surgical neck of the humerus. It supplies the head of the humerus and shoulder joint and may have common origin with the posterior circumflex humeral artery.

Posterior Circumflex Humeral Artery (Figs. 15.2, 15.3, 15.16)

This artery is larger than the anterior circumflex humeral artery. It arises from the 3rd part of the axillary artery and winds around the surgical neck of the humerus and distributes branches to the shoulder joint, deltoid, teres major and minor, long and lateral heads of triceps. The descending branch anastomoses with the deltoid branch of the arteria profunda brachii and with the anterior circumflex humeral artery, with the acromial branches of the suprascapular and thoracoacromial arteries.

Alar Thoracic Artery (Variation) (Fig. 15.21)

The subscapular, circumflex humeral, and profunda brachii arteries may arise as a common trunk (Fig. 15.20). The axillary artery may divide into radial and ulnar arteries or give off the anterior interosseous artery of the forearm. The radial artery may arise from the distal axillary artery (Fig. 15.19). The arteria profunda brachii may originate from the axillary artery (Fig. 15.21A). The subscapular, the lateral thoracic, and pectoral arteries may be part of a common trunk (Fig. 15.21B).

BRACHIAL ARTERY

The brachial artery is the continuation of the axillary artery. It begins at the lower border of the tendon of the teres major, ending a centimeter below the elbow dividing into radial and ulnar arteries. It runs down the arm, medially to the humerus and gradually moving to the front of the bone (Figs. 15.21, 15.22, 15.23, 15.24, 15.25, 15.26).

Branches

Arteria profunda brachii (profunda brachial) (Figs. 15.21, 15.22)

Nutrient of the humerus (Fig. 15.24)
Muscular (Fig. 15.24)
Superior ulnar collateral (Fig. 15.25)
Inferior ulnar collateral (Fig. 15.26)
Radial artery (Fig. 15.26)
Ulnar artery (Fig. 15.26)

Arteria Profunda Brachii (Brachial Profunda)

Branches

Nutrient artery of the humerus
Deltoid artery (ascending anastomoses with posterior humeral artery)
Middle collateral artery (posterior descending)
Anastomoses with interosseous recurrent artery
Radial collateral artery
Continuation of arteria profunda brachii
Muscular branches

Main Nutrient Artery

Main nutrient canal—downwards

Muscular Branches

Three or four in number—coracobrachialis, biceps, and brachialis

Superior Ulnar Collateral Artery

This small artery descends between medial epicondyle and the olecranon. It anastomoses with the posterior ulnar recurrent and inferior ulnar collateral.

Inferior Ulnar Collateral Artery (Supratrochlear)

This anastomotic branch forms an arch above the olecranon fossa by junction with the middle collateral branch. It anastomoses with the anterior ulnar recurrent artery.

Radial Artery (Figs. 15.19, 15.26, 15.27)

The radial artery is the more direct continuation of the brachial artery, arising about 1 cm below the bend of the elbow coursing along the radius bone, reaching the hand. There are three main parts of the radial artery: one in the forearm, one at the wrist, and one in the hand.

Variation

The radial artery may originate at the axillary or upper part of the brachial artery (Fig. 15.19).

Branches at the Forearm and Wrist (Fig. 15.27)

Radial recurrent artery (anastomoses with the radial collateral branch)
Muscular branches
Palmar carpal branch (anastomoses with the palmar carpal branch of the ulnar artery)

Ulnar Artery (Fig. 15.27)

The ulnar artery is the larger of the two distal branches of the brachial artery. It begins at the level of the neck of the radius, passing downwards and medially, reaching the ulnar side of the forearm. When it reaches the wrist, it crosses lateral to the pisiform bone and gives off a deep branch continuing across the palm as the superficial palmar arch.

Branches at the Forearm and Wrist (Figs. 15.22, 15.28)

Anterior ulnar recurrent artery
Posterior ulnar recurrent artery
Common interosseous artery
Anterior interosseous artery
Posterior interosseous artery
Muscular branches
Palmar carpal branch

ARTERIES OF THE HAND

The arteries of the hand are distal branches of the radial and ulnar arteries, with anastomosis with the posterior and anterior interosseous arteries (Figs. 15.29, 15.30).

Radial Branches in the Hand

Superficial Palmar Branch

The superficial palmar branch is located at the thenar eminence; it anastomoses with the terminal part of the ulnar artery to complete the superficial palmar arch (arcus volaris superficialis).

Dorsal Carpal Branch

The dorsal carpal branch of the radial artery anastomoses with the dorsal carpal branch of the ulnar artery and anterior and posterior interosseous arteries, forming the dorsal carpal arch (dorsal carpal rete). The dorsal metacarpal arteries descend on the 2nd, 3rd, and 4th dorsal interosseous muscles and bifurcate into dorsal digital branches for the fingers. They anastomose with the palmar digital branches of the superficial palmar arch. The dorsal metacarpal arteries anastomose with the deep palmar arch by the proximal perforating arteries and near their points of bifurcation with the palmar digital vessels of the superficial palmar digital arteries, branches of the superficial palmar arch by the distal perforating arteries.

Arteria Princeps Pollicis (Figs. 15.31, 15.32, 15.33)

The arteria princeps pollicis is the main artery of the thumb. It arises from the radial artery as it turns medially into the palm of the hand. It divides into two branches running along the sides of the thumb.

Arteria Radialis Indicis

The arteria radialis indicis arises from the deep palmar arch and frequently from the arteria princeps pollicis. It runs along the lateral borders of the 2nd finger.

Deep Palmar Arch (Arcus Volaris Profundus) (Figs. 15.29, 15.31, 15.32, 15.33)

The deep palmar arch is formed by the anastomosis of the terminal part of the radial artery with the deep palmar branch of the ulnar artery.

Branches

Three palmar metacarpal arteries
  From the convexity of the deep palmar arch
    (anastomoses with the common digital
    branches of the superficial palmar arch)
Three perforating branches
  Anastomoses with the dorsal metacarpal arteries
Recurrent branches
  Anastomoses with the palmar carpal arch

Ulnar Branches in the Hand

Palmar Carpal Branch

The palmar carpal branch anastomoses with the palmar carpal branch of the radial artery, receiving branches from the anterior interosseous artery, forming the palmar carpal arch at the wrist and carpus.

Dorsal Carpal Branch

The dorsal carpal branch arises above the pisiform bone and anastomoses with the dorsal carpal branch of radial artery.

Deep Palmar Branch

The deep palmar branch is often double and anastomoses with the radial artery to complete the deep palmar arch.

Superficial Palmar Arch (Arcus Volaris Superficialis) (Figs. 15.29, 15.30)

The superficial palmar arch is the main anastomosis of the ulnar artery. One third of the superficial palmar arch is formed by the ulnar artery alone. One third is completed by the superficial palmar branch of radial artery. An additional third is completed by either the arteria radialis indicis, branch of arteria princeps pollicis, or by the median artery.

Three Common Palmar Digital Arteries

These arteries arise from the convexity of the superficial palmar arch and are joined distally by the corresponding palmar metacarpal arteries (from deep palmar arch) and divides into a pair of proper palmar digital arteries, which run along the contiguous sides of the fingers. They are free to anastomose with the dorsal digital arteries by small branches at the level of the joints and at the finger tip vascular tufts (Fig. 15.34).

Variations

The persistent median artery may be the largest artery feeding the hand (Fig. 15.35). The arch is complete in 78.5% of the cases (Figs. 15.30, 15.33) and incomplete in 21.5% of the cases (Figs. 15.36, 15.37).

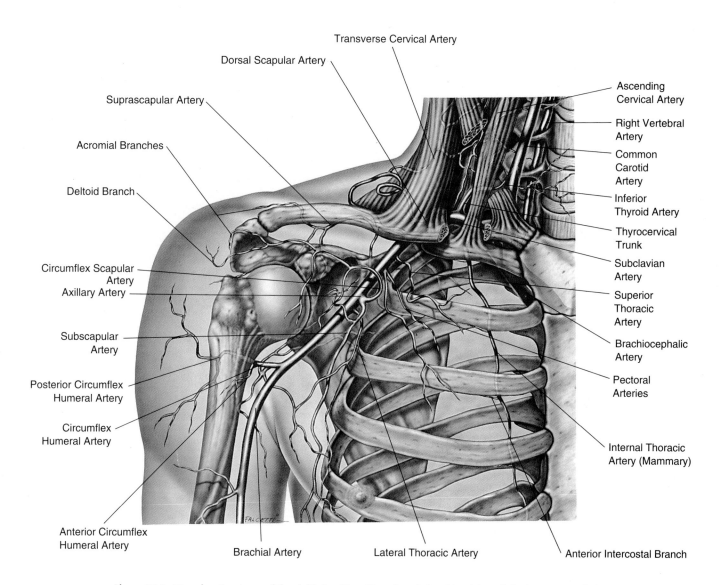

Figure 15.1. Vascular structures of the right shoulder. Note the relationship of the subclavian artery with the clavicle, first rib, and scalenus anterior muscle. The clavicle has been partially removed. Art based on an actual angiogram.

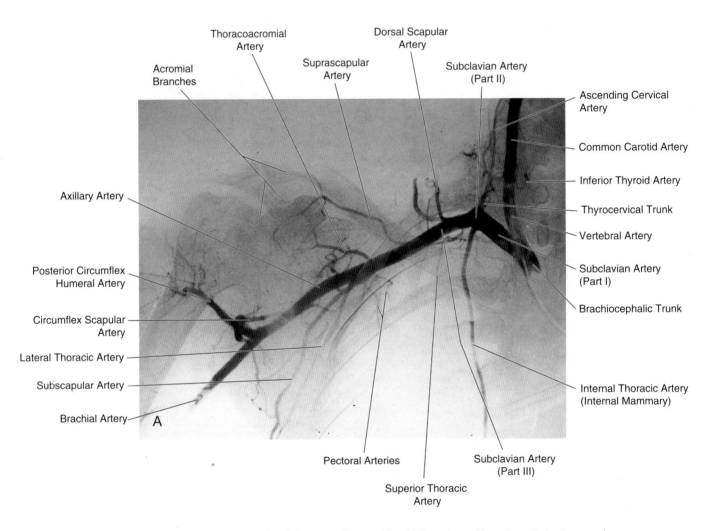

Thoracoacromial
Artery

Dorsal Scapular
Artery

Acromial
Branches

Suprascapular
Artery

Subclavian Artery
(Part II)

Ascending Cervical
Artery

Common Carotid Artery

Inferior Thyroid Artery

Axillary Artery

Thyrocervical Trunk

Vertebral Artery

Posterior Circumflex
Humeral Artery

Subclavian Artery
(Part I)

Circumflex Scapular
Artery

Brachiocephalic Trunk

Lateral Thoracic Artery

Subscapular Artery

Internal Thoracic Artery
(Internal Mammary)

Brachial Artery

A

Pectoral Arteries

Subclavian Artery
(Part III)

Superior Thoracic
Artery

Figure 15.2. **A.** Angiogram of the right subclavian, axillary, and brachial arteries and branches. **B.** Angiogram of the left subclavian artery. Note the origin of the vertebral artery arising in the second portion of the subclavian artery.

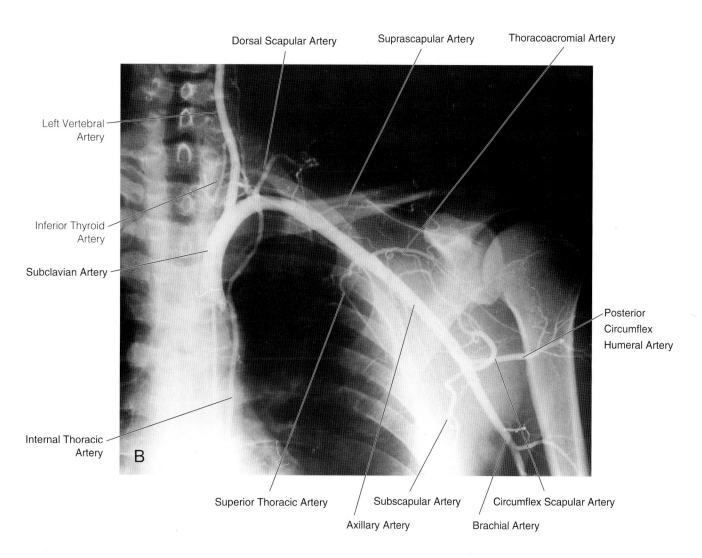

Figure 15.2. *Continued*

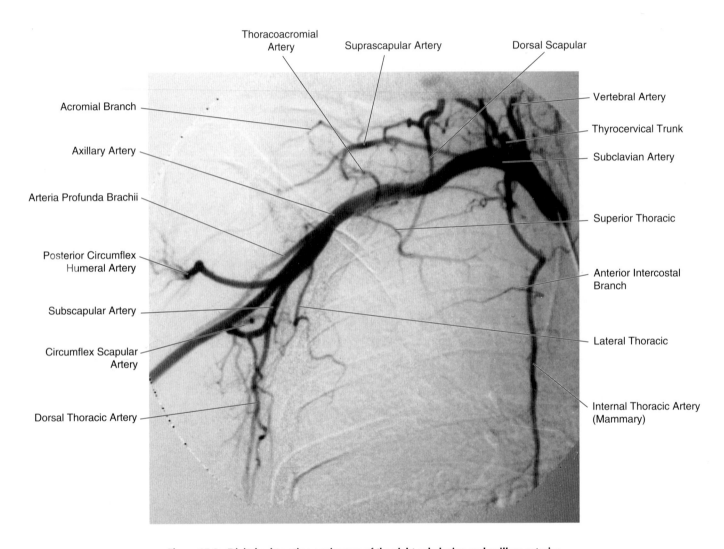

Figure 15.3. Digital subtraction angiogram of the right subclavian and axillary arteries.

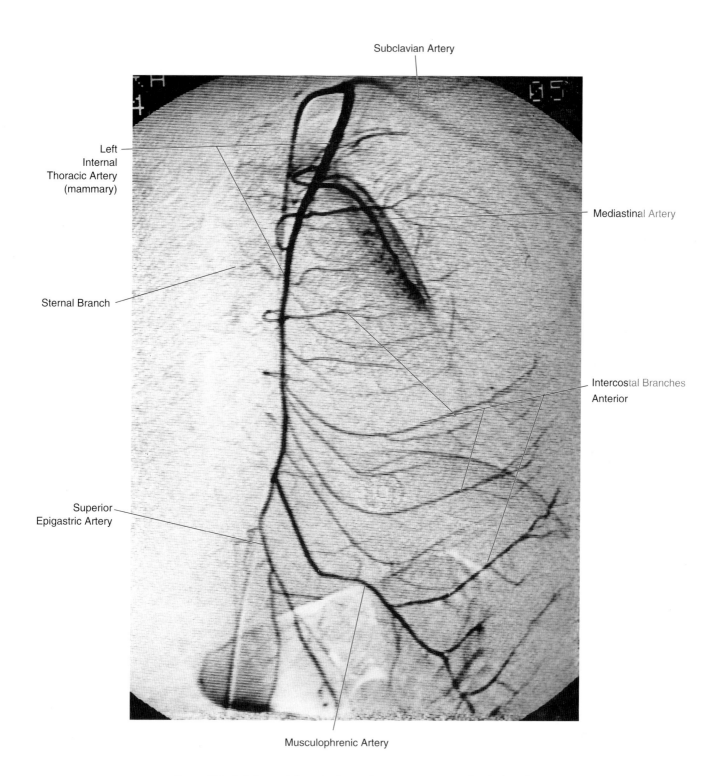

Subclavian Artery

Left
Internal
Thoracic Artery
(mammary)

Mediastinal Artery

Sternal Branch

Intercostal Branches
Anterior

Superior
Epigastric Artery

Musculophrenic Artery

Figure 15.4. Left internal thoracic (internal mammary) artery and main branches.

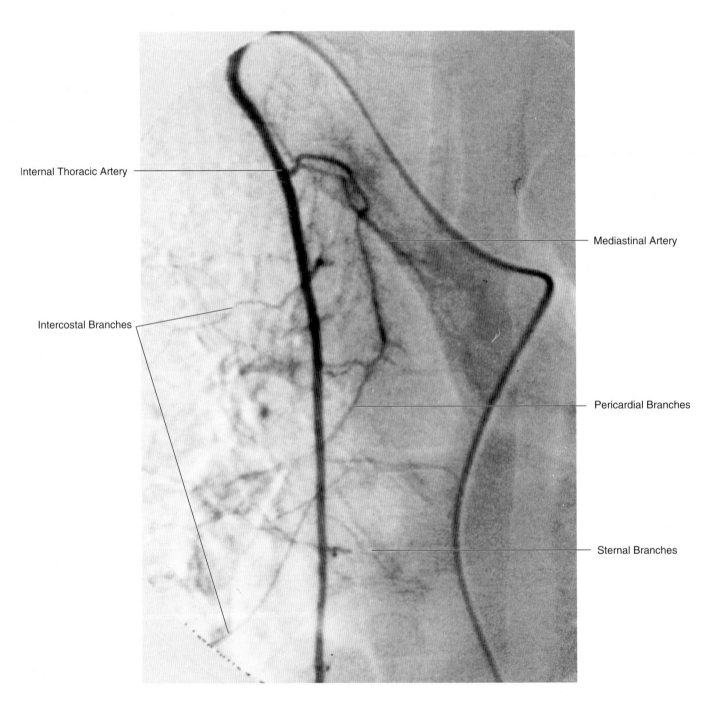

Internal Thoracic Artery

Intercostal Branches

Mediastinal Artery

Pericardial Branches

Sternal Branches

Figure 15.5. Right internal thoracic artery and the mediastinal and pericardial branches.

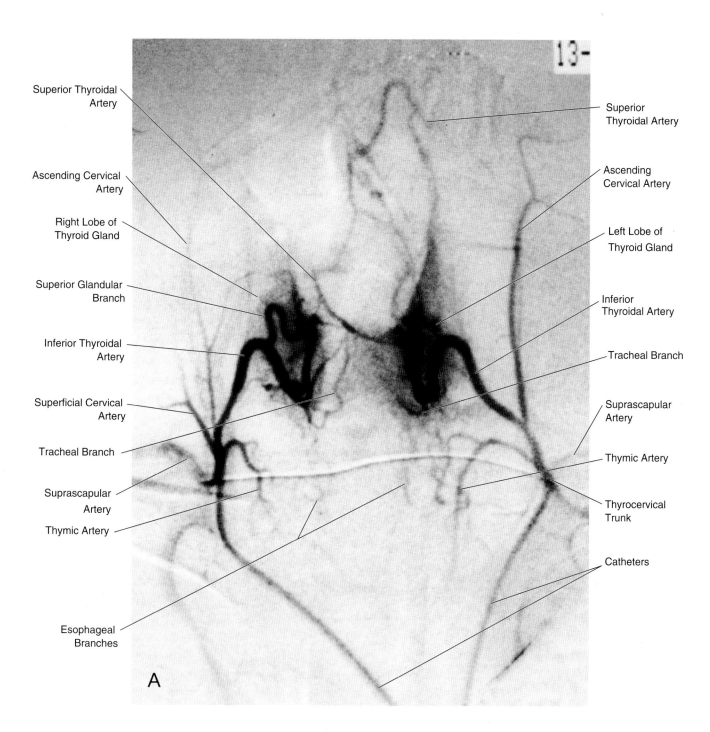

Figure 15.6. Simultaneous angiogram of the right and left thyrocervical trunks. Note the thyroid gland blush and named vessels, as well as the veins in (B).

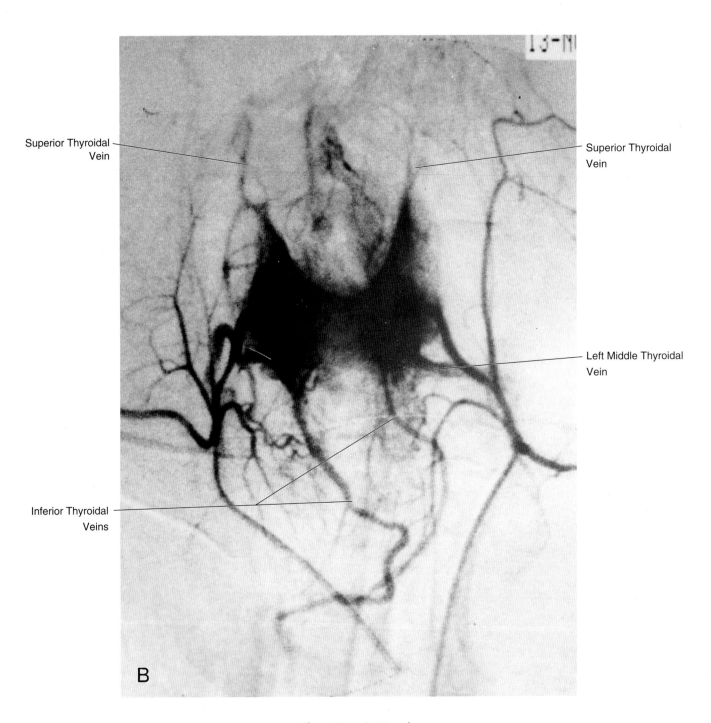

Superior Thyroidal
Vein

Superior Thyroidal
Vein

Left Middle Thyroidal
Vein

Inferior Thyroidal
Veins

B

Figure 15.6. *Continued*

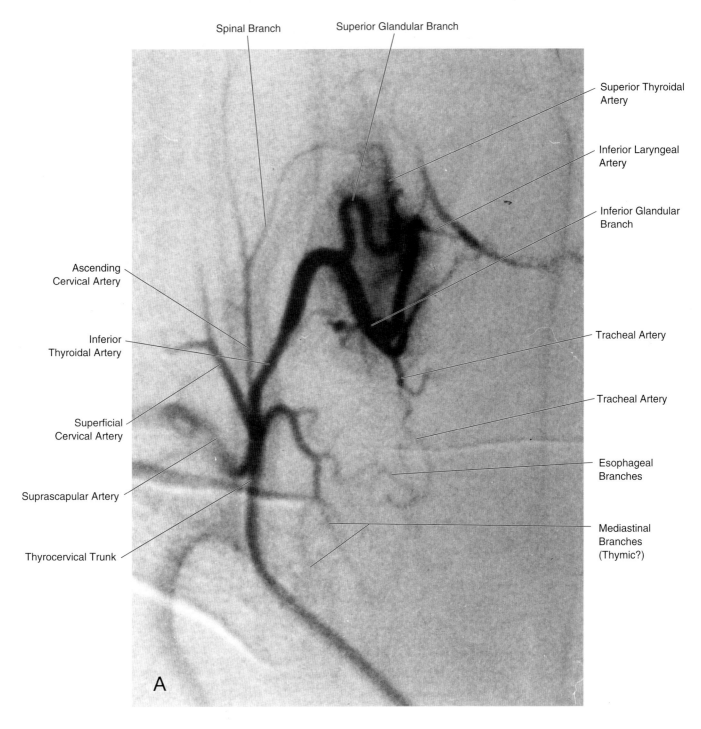

Figure 15.7. **A.** Close up view of the right thyroid vessels. **B.** Close up view of the left thyroid vessels. **C.** Selective injection into the right thyrocervical trunk. **D.** Selective injection into the left thyrocervical trunk.

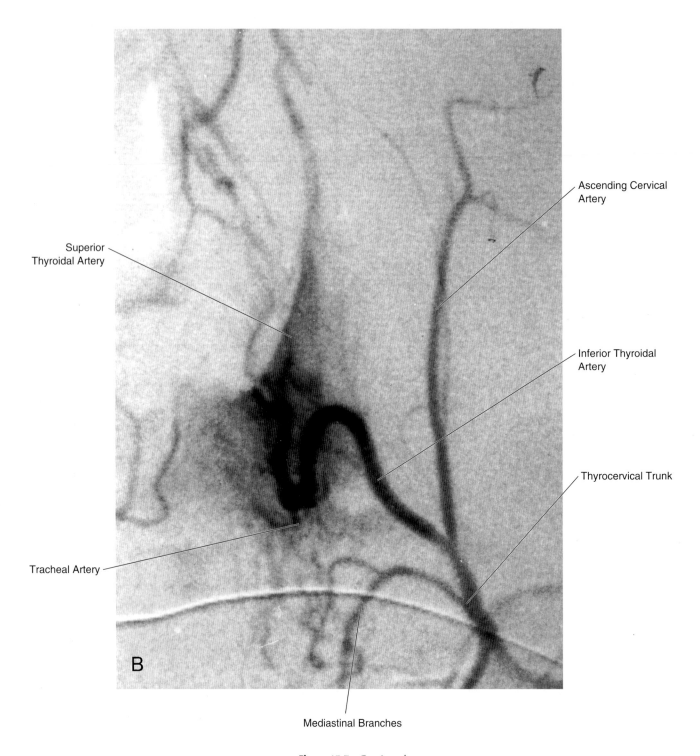

Ascending Cervical Artery

Superior Thyroidal Artery

Inferior Thyroidal Artery

Thyrocervical Trunk

Tracheal Artery

B

Mediastinal Branches

Figure 15.7. *Continued*

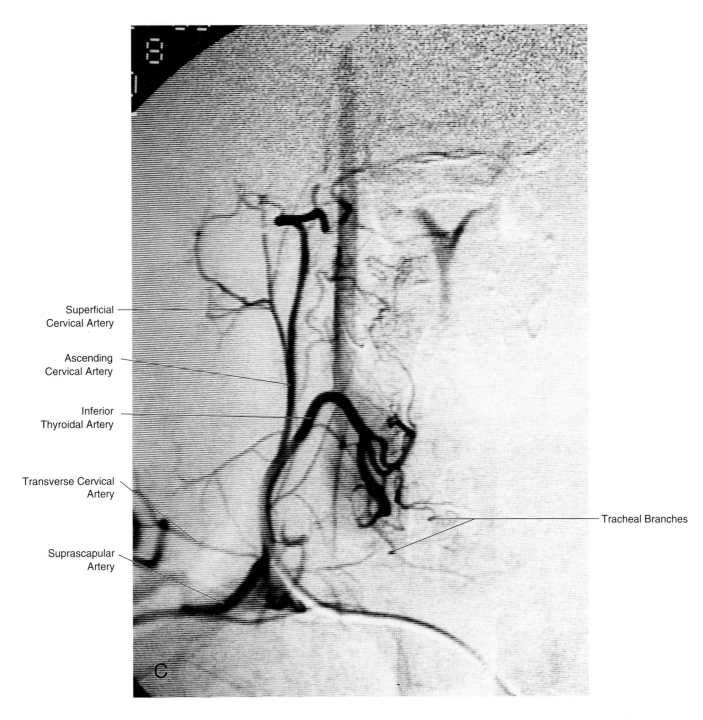

Superficial
Cervical Artery

Ascending
Cervical Artery

Inferior
Thyroidal Artery

Transverse Cervical
Artery

Suprascapular
Artery

Tracheal Branches

Figure 15.7. *Continued*

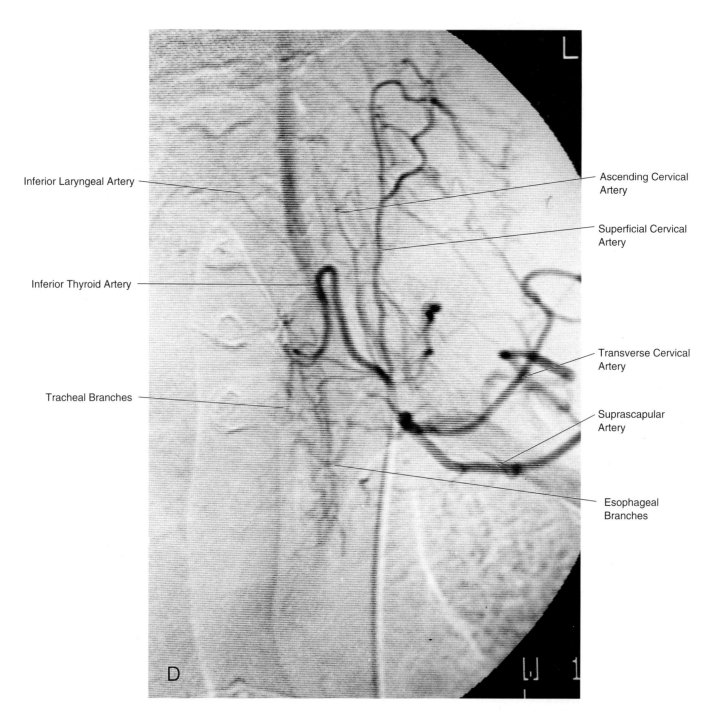

Inferior Laryngeal Artery

Inferior Thyroid Artery

Tracheal Branches

Ascending Cervical Artery

Superficial Cervical Artery

Transverse Cervical Artery

Suprascapular Artery

Esophageal Branches

Figure 15.7. *Continued*

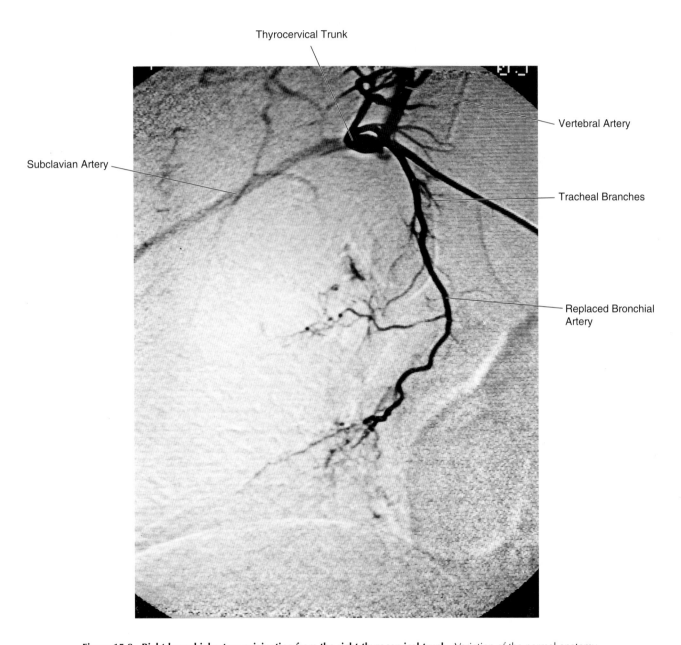

Figure 15.8. Right bronchial artery originating from the right thyrocervical trunk. Variation of the normal anatomy. (See bronchial artery anatomy).

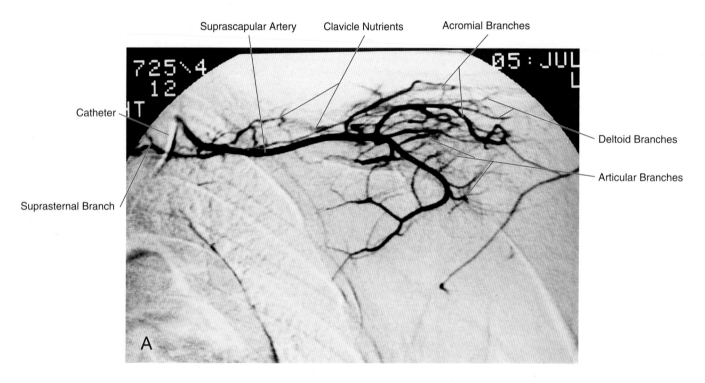

Figure 15.9. **A.** Selective angiogram of the left suprascapular artery and branches. **B.** Selective angiogram of the right subclavian artery showing the main branches.

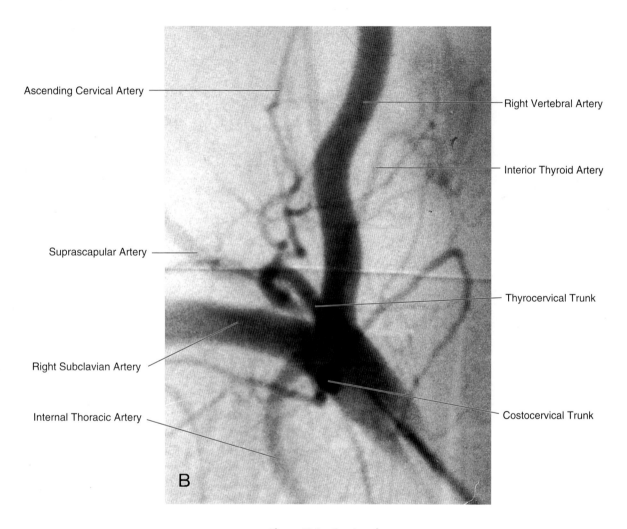

Ascending Cervical Artery

Right Vertebral Artery

Interior Thyroid Artery

Suprascapular Artery

Thyrocervical Trunk

Right Subclavian Artery

Internal Thoracic Artery

Costocervical Trunk

B

Figure 15.9. *Continued*

Acromial Branches

Deltoid Branches

Suprascapular Artery

Internal Mammary Artery

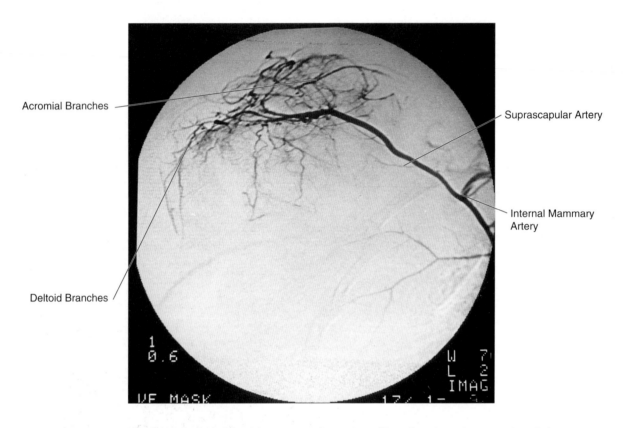

Figure 15.10. Selective angiogram of the right suprascapular artery and branches. Note the anatomic variation. The suprascapular artery originates from the right internal thoracic (internal mammary) artery. The peripheral arteries are displaced by a glenoid aneurysmatic bone cyst.

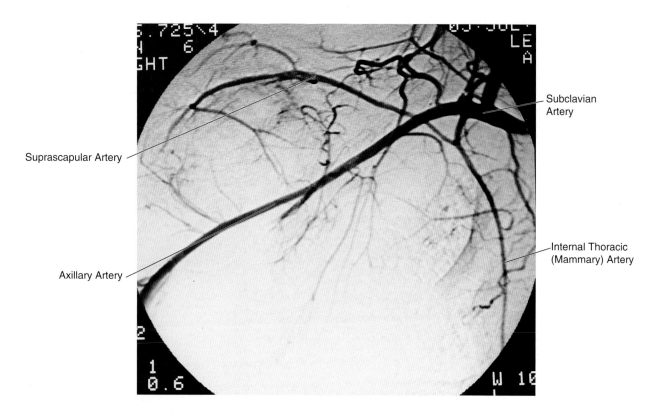

Figure 15.11. Suprascapular artery arising from the internal thoracic artery. Note the relationship with the subclavian artery.

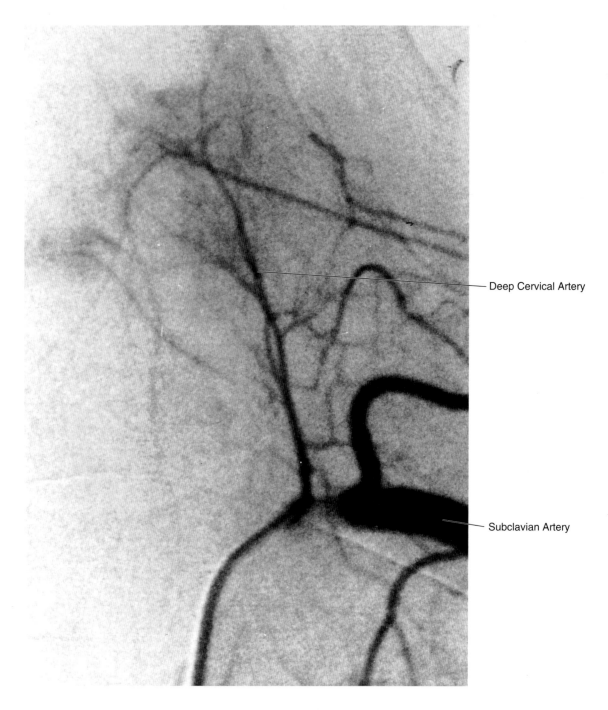

Figure 15.12. Deep cervical artery arising from the internal thoracic artery. Note the relationship with the subclavian artery.

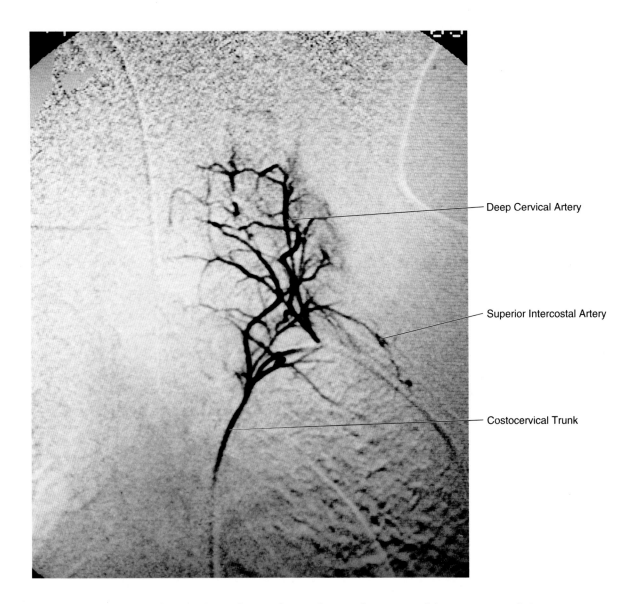

Deep Cervical Artery

Superior Intercostal Artery

Costocervical Trunk

Figure 15.13. Deep cervical artery, shorter than usual. Note the muscular arteries and the anastomosis with the intercostal artery. Origin from the costocervical trunk.

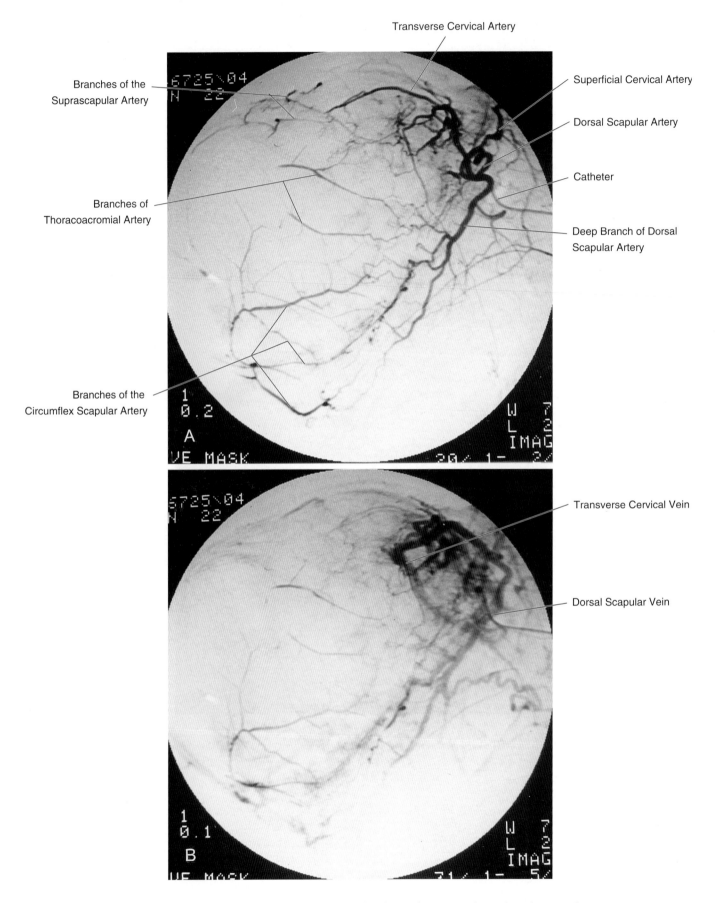

Transverse Cervical Artery

Branches of the
Suprascapular Artery

Superficial Cervical Artery

Dorsal Scapular Artery

Catheter

Branches of
Thoracoacromial Artery

Deep Branch of Dorsal
Scapular Artery

Branches of the
Circumflex Scapular Artery

Transverse Cervical Vein

Dorsal Scapular Vein

Figure 15.14. A. Scapular anastomosis. Angiogram of the dorsal scapular artery and main branches. Distal anastomoses are visible because of embolization of other arteries. **B.** Late phase of the angiogram showing the veins.

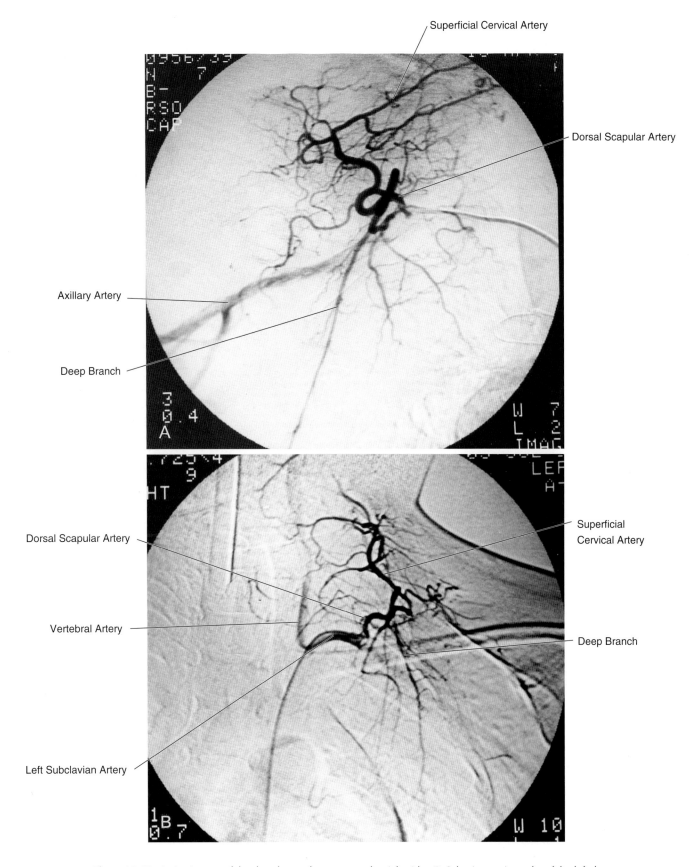

Figure 15.15. **A.** Angiogram of the dorsal scapular artery on the right side. **B.** Selective angiography of the left dorsal scapular artery, showing the superficial cervical artery and the deep branch.

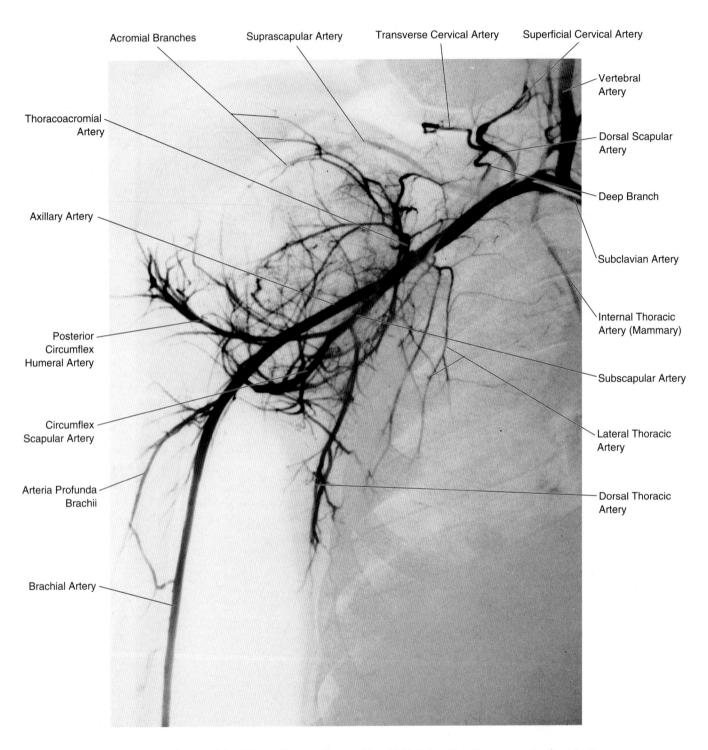

Figure 15.16. Angiogram of the right subclavian, axillary, and brachial arteries. Note the common trunk originating the subscapular, the circumflex scapular, and posterior circumflex scapular arteries.

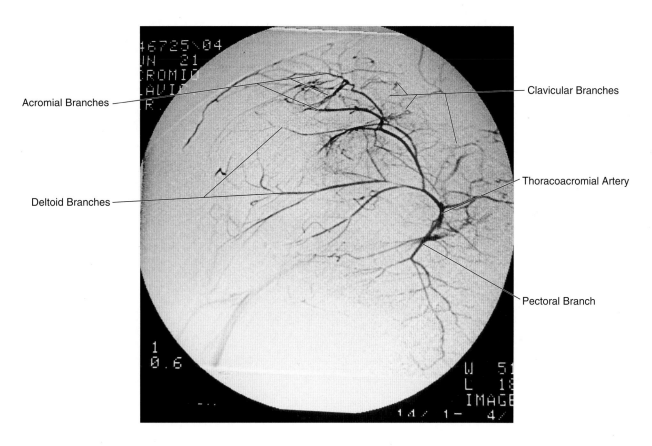

Acromial Branches

Clavicular Branches

Thoracoacromial Artery

Deltoid Branches

Pectoral Branch

Figure 15.17. Right thoracoacromial artery and main branches.

Catheter —

Thoracoacromial
Artery —

Pectoral Branches —

Acromial and
Clavicular
Branches

Deltoid Branches

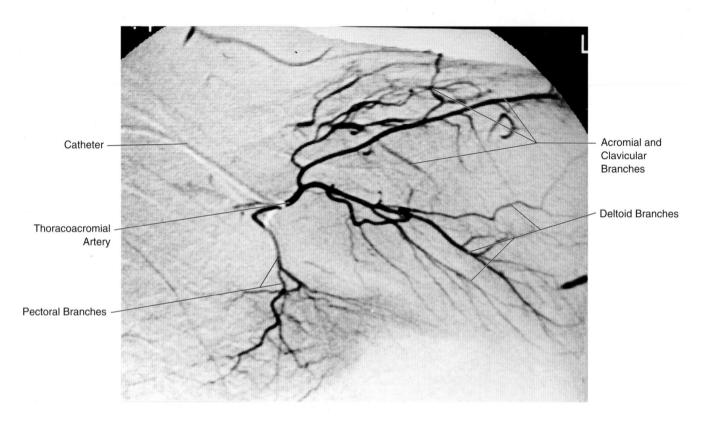

Figure 15.18. Left thoracoacromial artery and main branches.

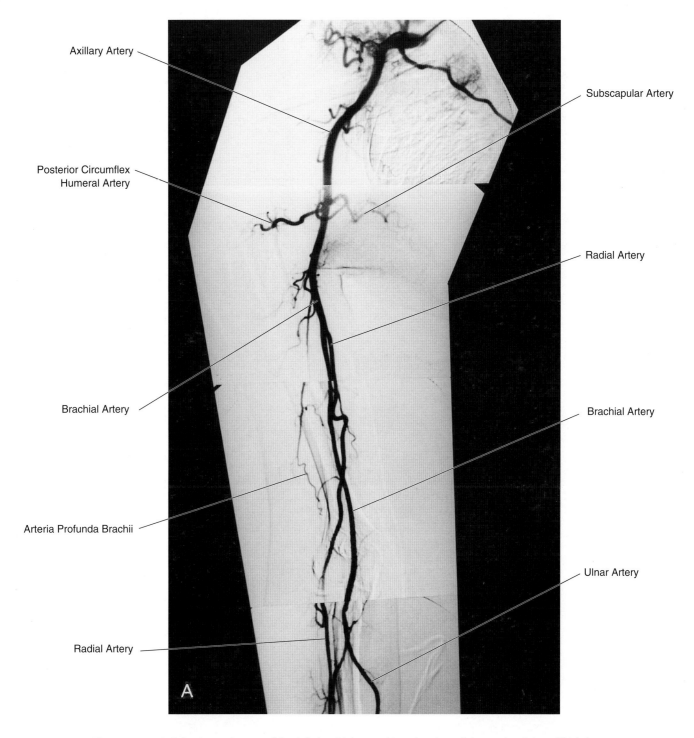

Figure 15.19. A. Selective angiogram of the right brachial artery. Note that the radial artery is originated high from the brachial artery. **B.** Distal angiogram showing the radial artery reaching the wrist.

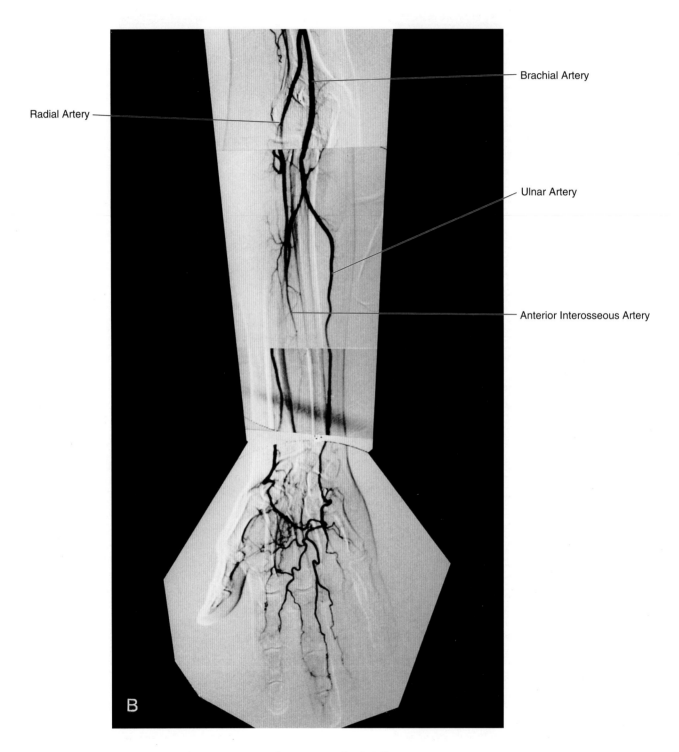

Brachial Artery

Radial Artery

Ulnar Artery

Anterior Interosseous Artery

B

Figure 15.19. *Continued*

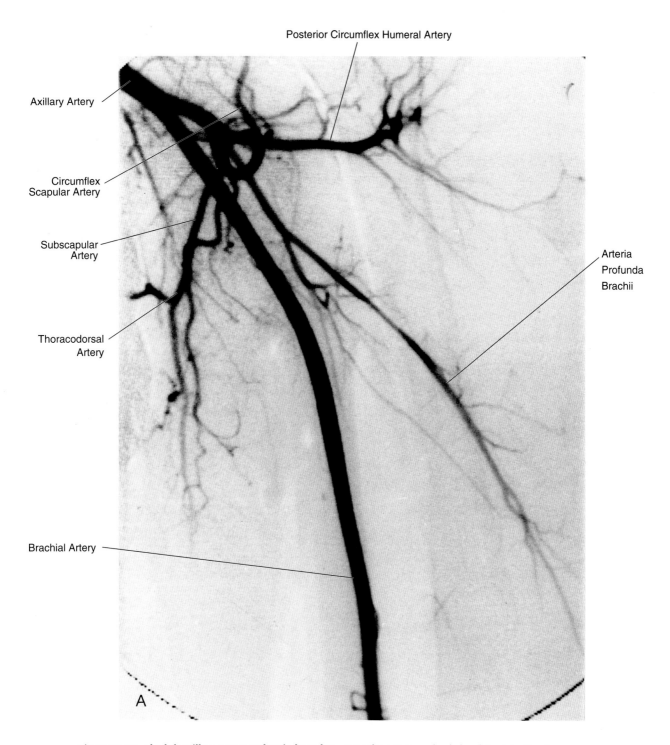

Posterior Circumflex Humeral Artery

Axillary Artery

Circumflex
Scapular Artery

Subscapular
Artery

Thoracodorsal
Artery

Arteria
Profunda
Brachii

Brachial Artery

A

Figure 15.20. The left axillary artery and main branches. Note the arteria profunda brachii originating from a common trunk together with the subscapular, posterior circumflex humeral, and circumflex scapular arteries

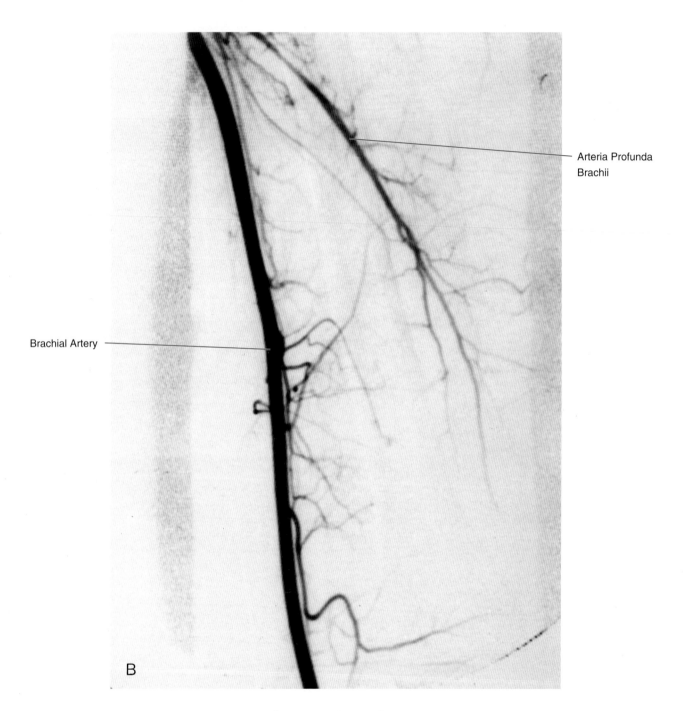

Arteria Profunda
Brachii

Brachial Artery

B

Figure 15.20. *Continued*

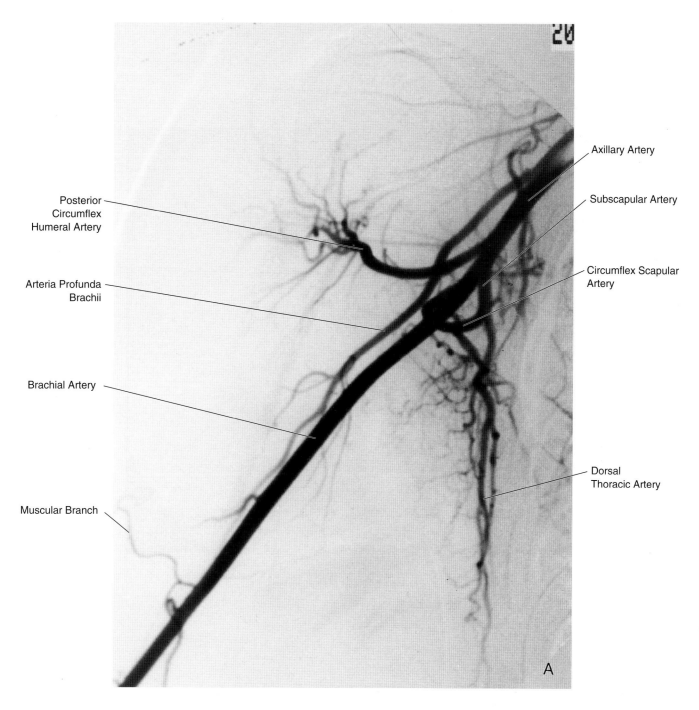

Axillary Artery

Subscapular Artery

Circumflex Scapular
Artery

Posterior
Circumflex
Humeral Artery

Arteria Profunda
Brachii

Brachial Artery

Dorsal
Thoracic Artery

Muscular Branch

A

Figure 15.21. A. High origin of the arteria profunda brachii from the axillary artery. **B.** Common trunk giving
origin to the pectoral, lateral thoracic, and subscapular arteries.

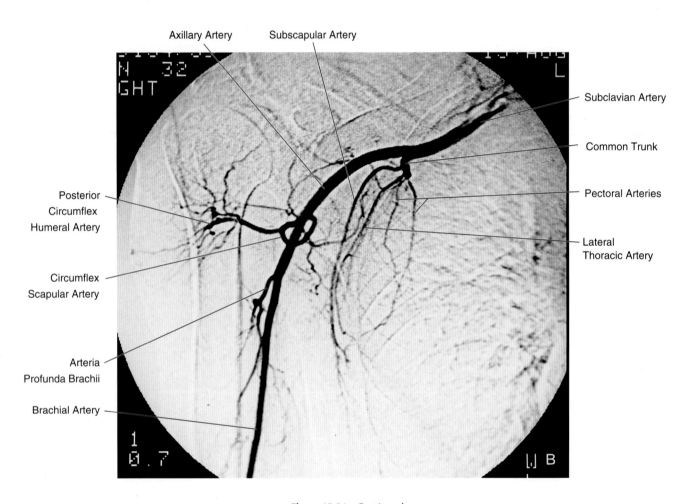

Figure 15.21. *Continued*

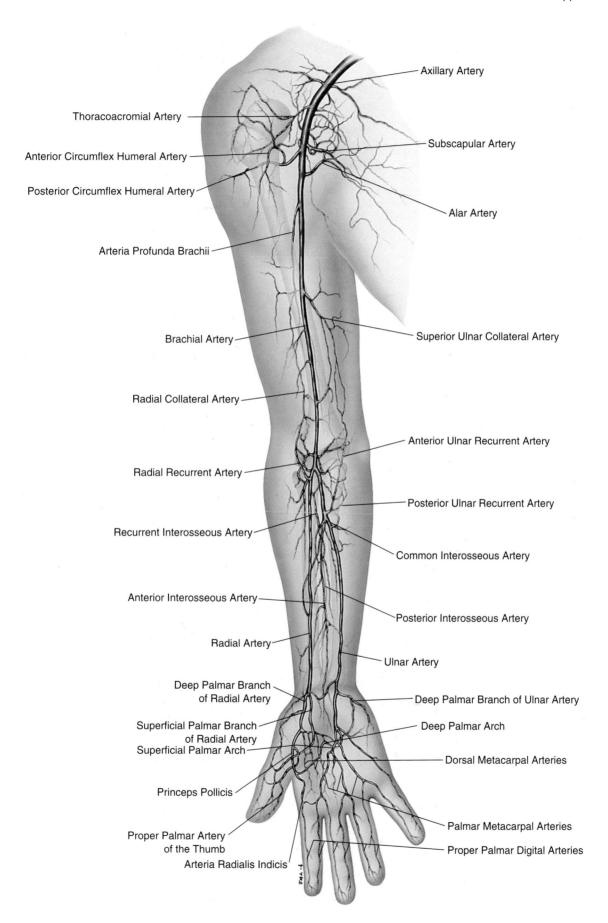

Axillary Artery

Thoracoacromial Artery

Anterior Circumflex Humeral Artery

Posterior Circumflex Humeral Artery

Subscapular Artery

Alar Artery

Arteria Profunda Brachii

Brachial Artery

Superior Ulnar Collateral Artery

Radial Collateral Artery

Anterior Ulnar Recurrent Artery

Radial Recurrent Artery

Posterior Ulnar Recurrent Artery

Recurrent Interosseous Artery

Common Interosseous Artery

Anterior Interosseous Artery

Posterior Interosseous Artery

Radial Artery

Ulnar Artery

Deep Palmar Branch
of Radial Artery

Deep Palmar Branch of Ulnar Artery

Superficial Palmar Branch
of Radial Artery
Superficial Palmar Arch

Deep Palmar Arch

Dorsal Metacarpal Arteries

Princeps Pollicis

Palmar Metacarpal Arteries

Proper Palmar Artery
of the Thumb
Arteria Radialis Indicis

Proper Palmar Digital Arteries

Figure 15.22. The right brachial artery and its branches. Art based on an actual angiogram.

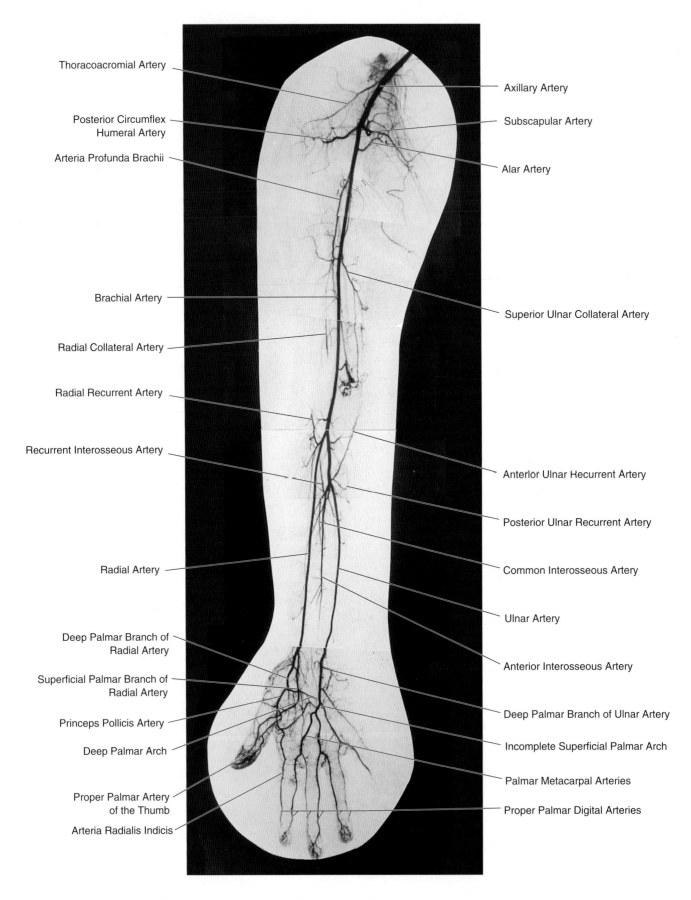

Thoracoacromial Artery

Posterior Circumflex Humeral Artery

Arteria Profunda Brachii

Brachial Artery

Radial Collateral Artery

Radial Recurrent Artery

Recurrent Interosseous Artery

Radial Artery

Deep Palmar Branch of Radial Artery

Superficial Palmar Branch of Radial Artery

Princeps Pollicis Artery

Deep Palmar Arch

Proper Palmar Artery of the Thumb

Arteria Radialis Indicis

Axillary Artery

Subscapular Artery

Alar Artery

Superior Ulnar Collateral Artery

Anterlor Ulnar Hecurrent Artery

Posterior Ulnar Recurrent Artery

Common Interosseous Artery

Ulnar Artery

Anterior Interosseous Artery

Deep Palmar Branch of Ulnar Artery

Incomplete Superficial Palmar Arch

Palmar Metacarpal Arteries

Proper Palmar Digital Arteries

Figure 15.23. Digital subtraction angiogram of the right arm. Brachial artery and main branches.

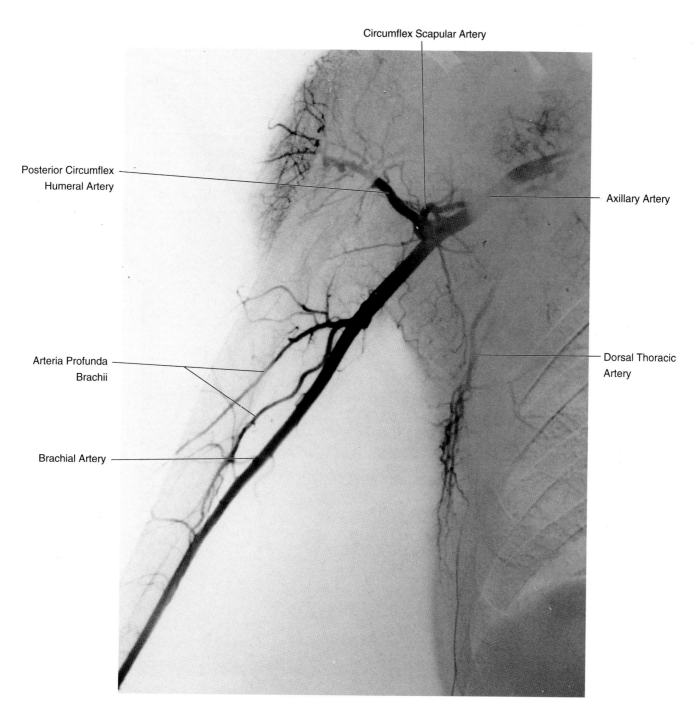

Figure 15.24. **Subtraction angiogram of the axillary and brachial artery and main branches.**

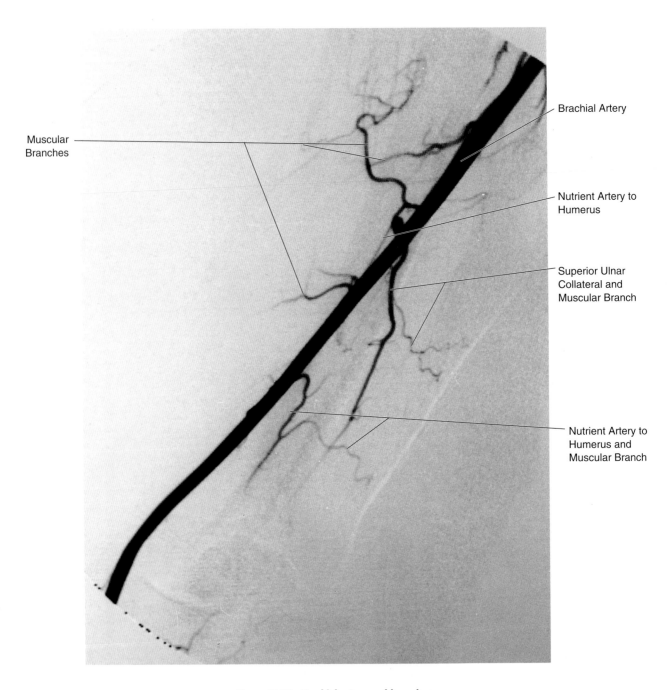

Muscular
Branches

Brachial Artery

Nutrient Artery to
Humerus

Superior Ulnar
Collateral and
Muscular Branch

Nutrient Artery to
Humerus and
Muscular Branch

Figure 15.25. Brachial artery and branches.

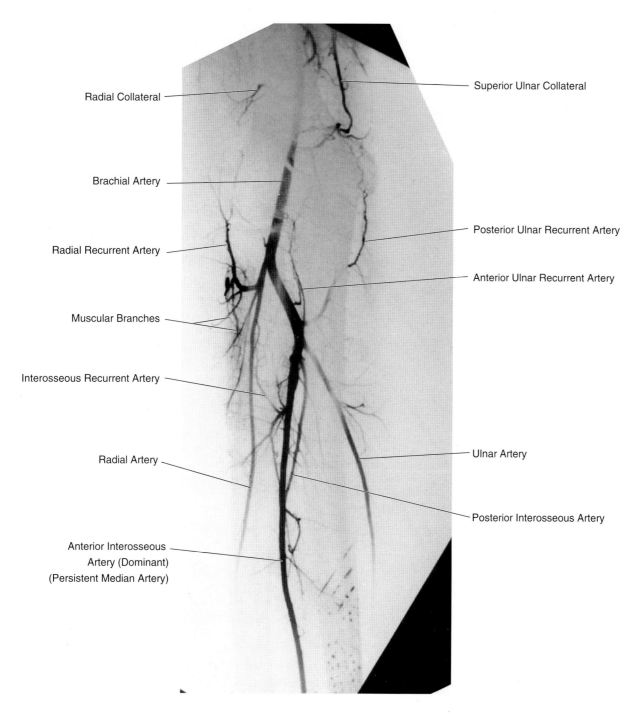

Figure 15.26. Bifurcation of the brachial artery. Note the dominant persistent median artery.

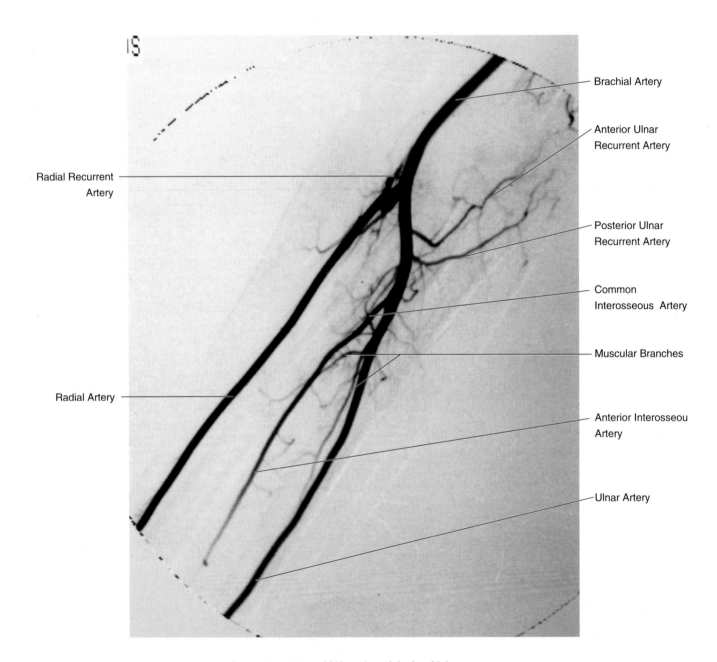

Figure 15.27. Normal bifurcation of the brachial artery.

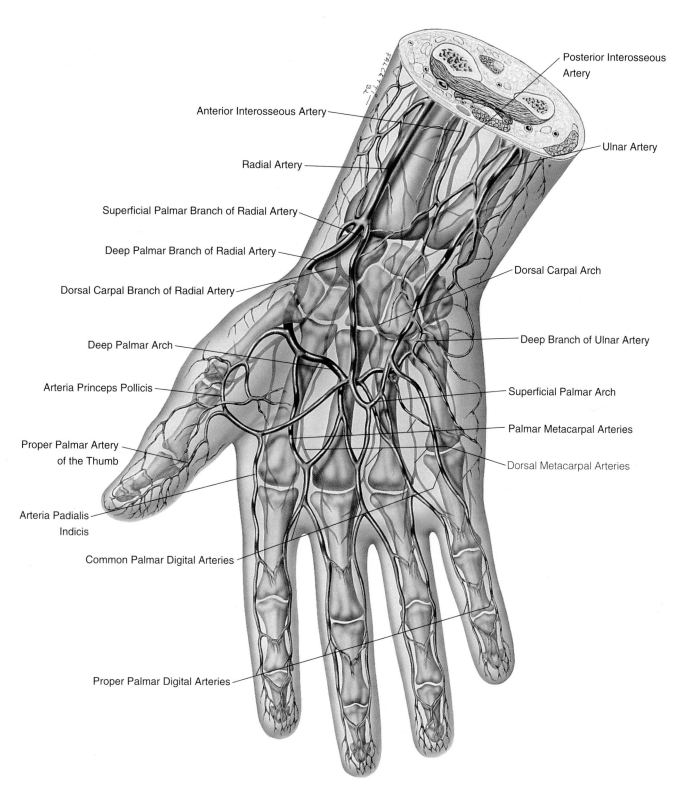

Posterior Interosseous Artery

Anterior Interosseous Artery

Radial Artery

Superficial Palmar Branch of Radial Artery

Deep Palmar Branch of Radial Artery

Dorsal Carpal Branch of Radial Artery

Deep Palmar Arch

Arteria Princeps Pollicis

Proper Palmar Artery of the Thumb

Arteria Padialis Indicis

Common Palmar Digital Arteries

Proper Palmar Digital Arteries

Ulnar Artery

Dorsal Carpal Arch

Deep Branch of Ulnar Artery

Superficial Palmar Arch

Palmar Metacarpal Arteries

Dorsal Metacarpal Arteries

Figure 15.28. Right hand. Radial and ulnar branches. The hand is in anatomic position with the palmar aspect showed ventrally. The art is based on an actual angiogram.

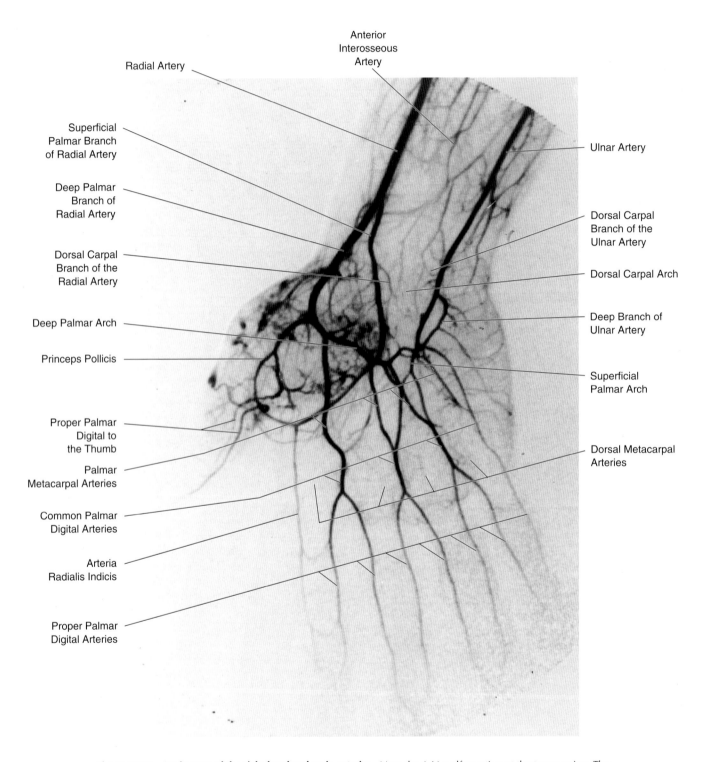

Radial Artery

Anterior
Interosseous
Artery

Superficial
Palmar Branch
of Radial Artery

Deep Palmar
Branch of
Radial Artery

Dorsal Carpal
Branch of the
Radial Artery

Deep Palmar Arch

Princeps Pollicis

Proper Palmar
Digital to
the Thumb

Palmar
Metacarpal Arteries

Common Palmar
Digital Arteries

Arteria
Radialis Indicis

Proper Palmar
Digital Arteries

Ulnar Artery

Dorsal Carpal
Branch of the
Ulnar Artery

Dorsal Carpal Arch

Deep Branch of
Ulnar Artery

Superficial
Palmar Arch

Dorsal Metacarpal
Arteries

Figure 15.29. Angiogram of the right hand and main arteries. Note the A-V malformation at the tenar region. The deep and superficial palmar arches are complete.

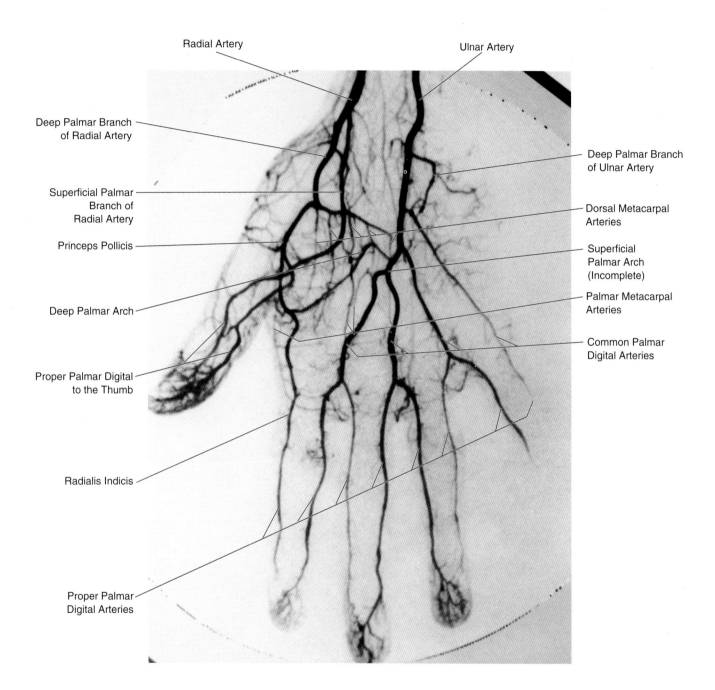

Figure 15.30. Right hand with incomplete superficial palmar arch and main branches.

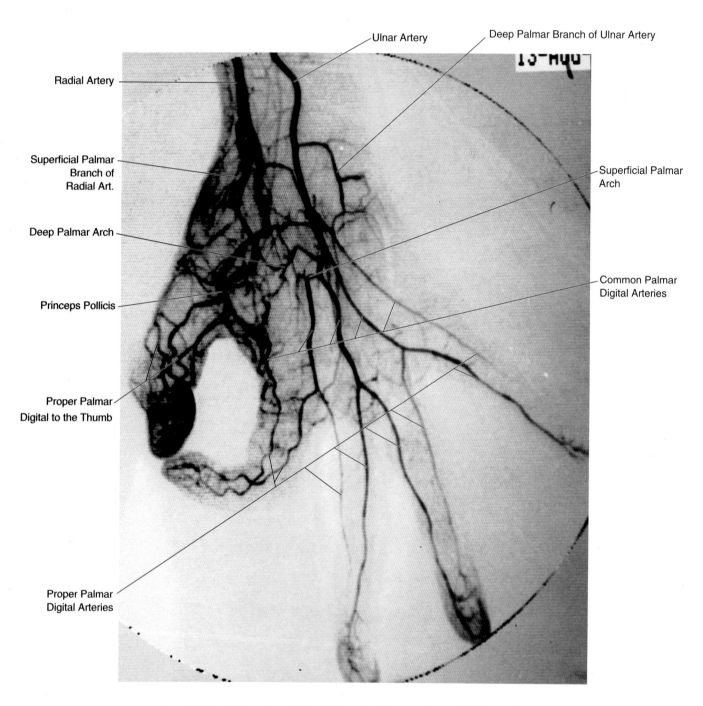

Figure 15.31. Oblique view of the right hand angiogram. Same as in Figure 15.29.

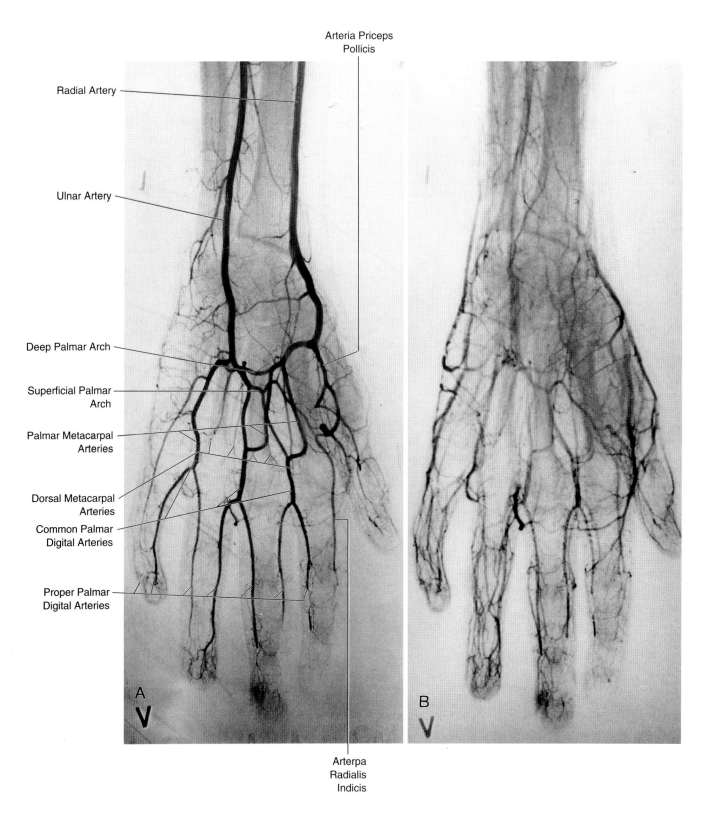

Arteria Priceps
Pollicis

Radial Artery

Ulnar Artery

Deep Palmar Arch

Superficial Palmar
Arch

Palmar Metacarpal
Arteries

Dorsal Metacarpal
Arteries

Common Palmar
Digital Arteries

Proper Palmar
Digital Arteries

A

B

Arterpa
Radialis
Indicis

Figure 15.32. A. Prone view of the left hand showing a complete superficial palmar arch. **B.** Later phase of the angiogram showing venous drainage. Note distal obstruction of the proper palmar digital arteries.

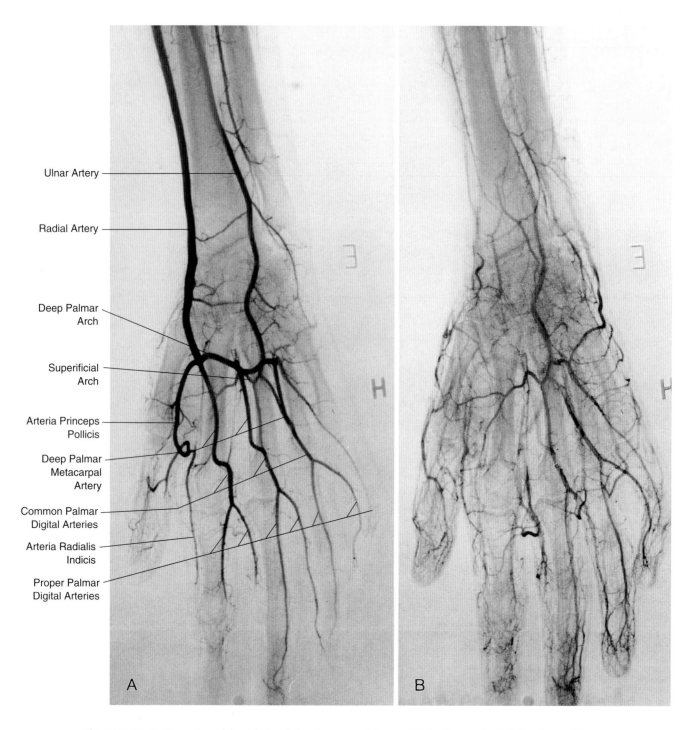

Ulnar Artery

Radial Artery

Deep Palmar Arch

Superificial Arch

Arteria Princeps Pollicis

Deep Palmar Metacarpal Artery

Common Palmar Digital Arteries

Arteria Radialis Indicis

Proper Palmar Digital Arteries

A

B

Figure 15.33. A. Prone view of the right hand showing a complete superficial palmar arch. **B.** Later phase of the angiogram showing the distal arteries and the beginning of the venous drainage. Note distal obstruction of the distal proper palmar digital arteries.

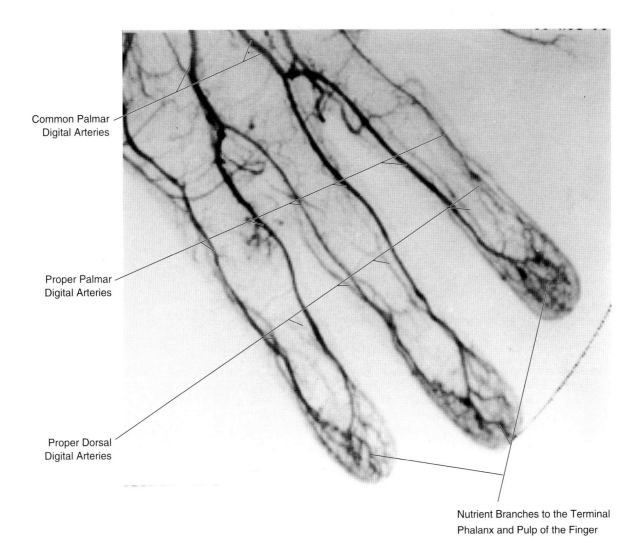

Common Palmar
Digital Arteries

Proper Palmar
Digital Arteries

Proper Dorsal
Digital Arteries

Nutrient Branches to the Terminal
Phalanx and Pulp of the Finger

Figure 15.34. Close up view of the tip of the second, third and fourth fingers of the right hand showing the rich anastomotic bed of the digital circulation and the digital tufts. The proper dorsal and palmar digital arteries are visible. Note that the dorsal arteries are attenuated.

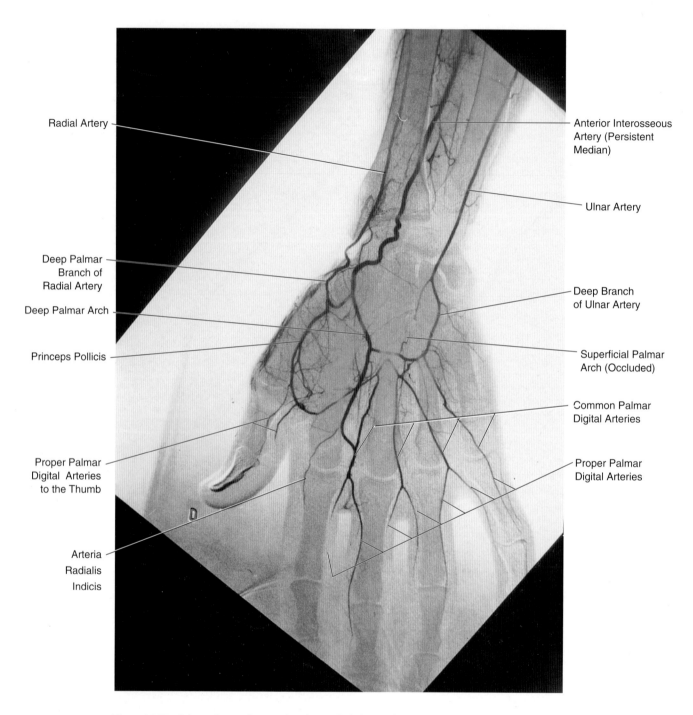

Radial Artery

Anterior Interosseous
Artery (Persistent
Median)

Ulnar Artery

Deep Palmar
Branch of
Radial Artery

Deep Palmar Arch

Deep Branch
of Ulnar Artery

Princeps Pollicis

Superficial Palmar
Arch (Occluded)

Common Palmar
Digital Arteries

Proper Palmar
Digital Arteries
to the Thumb

Proper Palmar
Digital Arteries

Arteria
Radialis
Indicis

Figure 15.35. Subtraction angiogram showing occluded superficial palmar arch. Note the persistent median
artery as part of the deep palmar arch.

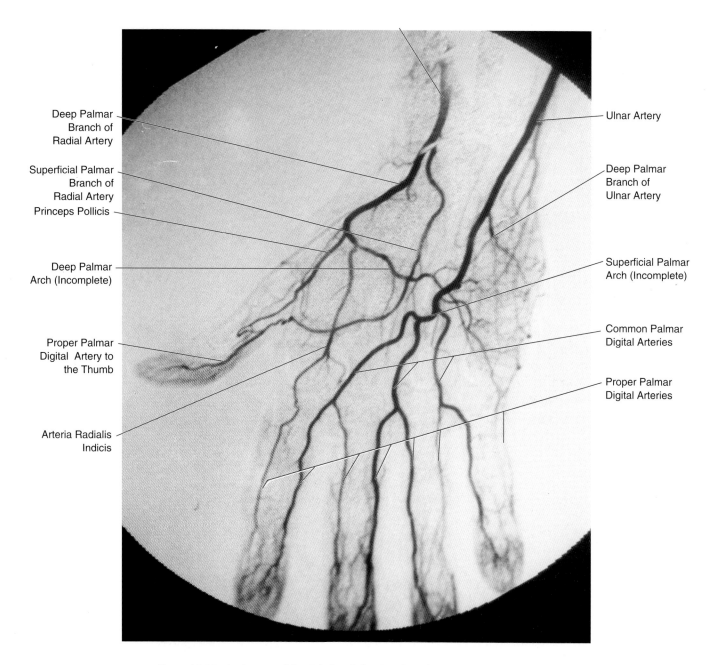

Deep Palmar
Branch of
Radial Artery

Superficial Palmar
Branch of
Radial Artery

Princeps Pollicis

Deep Palmar
Arch (Incomplete)

Proper Palmar
Digital Artery to
the Thumb

Arteria Radialis
Indicis

Ulnar Artery

Deep Palmar
Branch of
Ulnar Artery

Superficial Palmar
Arch (Incomplete)

Common Palmar
Digital Arteries

Proper Palmar
Digital Arteries

Figure 15.36. Angiogram of the right hand showing the palmar arch and distal arteries.

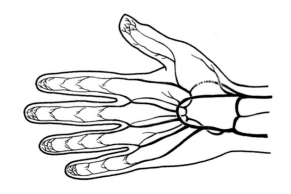

COMPLETE   ARCH

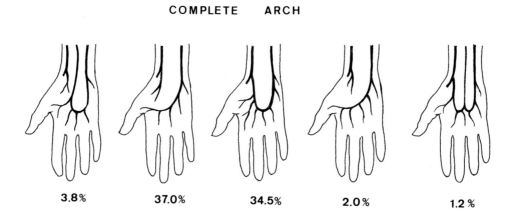

| 3.8% | 37.0% | 34.5% | 2.0% | 1.2% |

INCOMPLETE   ARCH

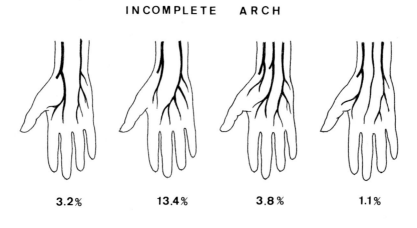

| 3.2% | 13.4% | 3.8% | 1.1% |

Figure 15.37. Schematic demonstration of the hand with complete arch and variations.

16

VEINS OF THE UPPER EXTREMITY

There are two groups of veins in the upper limb, the superficial and deep venous systems, with free anastomoses between them. The superficial veins are in the superficial fascia, immediately under the skin. The deep veins accompany the arteries.

SUPERFICIAL VEINS OF THE UPPER EXTREMITY

The superficial veins of the upper extremity are the cephalic, basilic, median antebrachial veins, and their tributaries (Fig. 16.1).

At the Hand (Figs. 16.2, 16.3, 16.4)

Dorsal digital veins
Three dorsal metacarpal veins
Dorsal venous network

Laterally the dorsal venous network is joined by the dorsal digital vein from the radial side of the index finger and both dorsal digital veins of the thumb, prolonged proximally as the cephalic vein.

Medially the network receives the dorsal digital vein of the ulnar side of the fifth finger and is continued upwards as the basilic vein.

Palmar digital veins
    Connected to the dorsal system by intercapitular veins
Palmar venous plexus
    Drain into the median vein of the forearm
Median vein of the forearm
    Connected to the basilic vein

At the Forearm (Fig. 16.1)

Cephalic Vein (Figs. 16.5, 16.6, 16.7)

This vein originates from the dorsal venous network and follows the radial border of the forearm. The median cubital vein is given in front of the elbow, which receives a communicating branch from the deep veins of the forearm, passing medially to communicate with the basilic vein. The cephalic vein ascends subcutaneously lateral to the biceps. The

infraclavicular fossa ends in the axillary vein just below the level of the clavicle. An accessory cephalic vein may be present.

Basilic Vein (Figs. 16.5, 16.6)

This vein originates from the ulnar aspect of the dorsal venous network of the hand, following a subcutaneous path in the dorsal side of the forearm but moves forward to the ventral surface. It is joined by the median cubital vein and ascends between the biceps and pronator teres muscles. At the shoulder level, it perforates the deep fascia continuing as the axillary vein.

Median Vein of the Forearm (Fig. 16.5)

This vein is formed by the superficial palmar venous plexus and ends in the basilic or median cubital vein.

DEEP VEINS OF THE UPPER EXTREMITY

These are the "Venae Comitans," companions of the arteries. Generally, in pairs, they follow the corresponding arteries. The deep veins are usually small.

At the Hand

Superficial and palmar arches are accompanied by venae comitans, superficial and deep palmar venous arches. The common palmar digital veins open in the superficial palmar venous arch. The palmar metacarpal veins end into the deep palmar venous arch.

At the Forearm (Fig. 16.8)

There are companion veins of the radial interosseous and ulnar arteries that join at the elbow level as the brachial veins.

Brachial Veins (Fig. 16.1)

These veins follow the brachial artery in pairs and receive tributaries. They join the axillary vein and occasionally the basilic vein.

Axillary Vein (Fig. 16.9)

This vein begins at the lower border of the teres major, as the continuation of the basilic vein, up to the outer border of the first rib; it lies medially to the axillary artery. Major tributary is the cephalic vein.

Subclavian Vein (Fig. 16.9)

This vein is the continuation of the axillary vein, extending from the outer border of the ribs to the medial border of the scalenus anterior, where it is joined by the internal jugular vein to form the brachiocephalic vein; it lies anterior and inferior to the subclavian artery.

Major tributaries: External jugular and dorsal scapular. They receive the thoracic duct in the left side, at the angle of junction with the internal jugular, and the right lymphatic duct on the right.

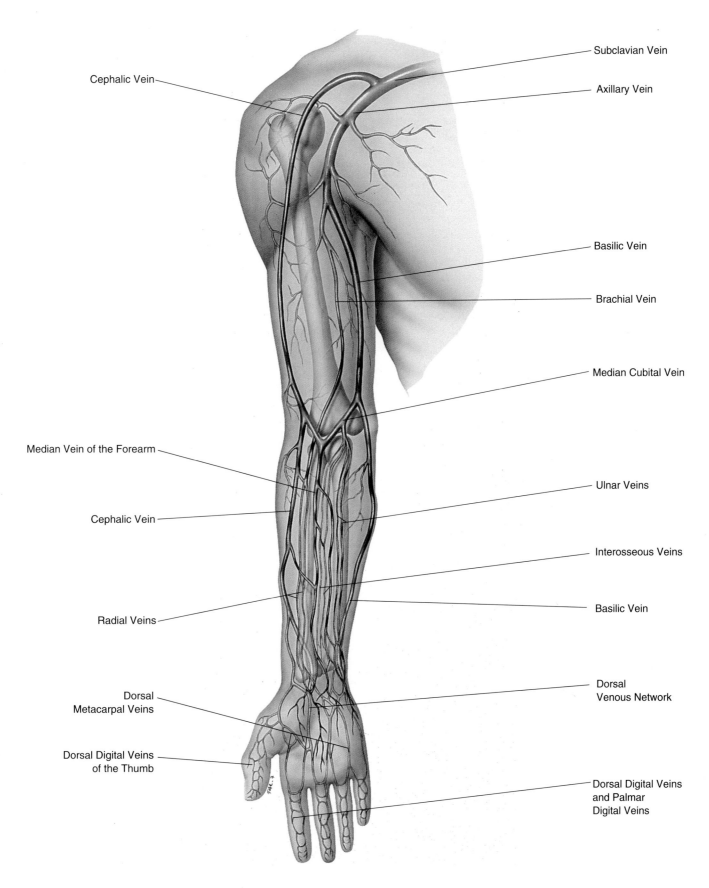

Figure 16.1. Venous anatomy of the right upper extremity.

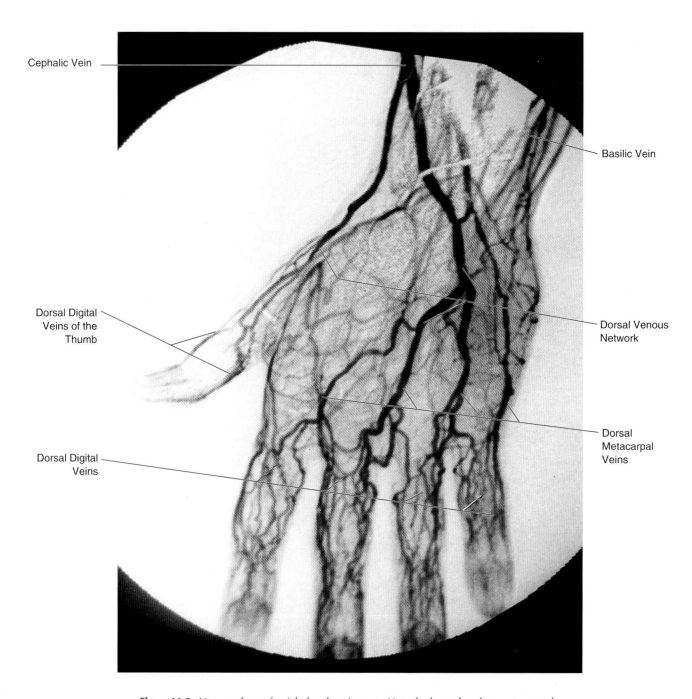

Cephalic Vein

Basilic Vein

Dorsal Digital
Veins of the
Thumb

Dorsal Venous
Network

Dorsal
Metacarpal
Veins

Dorsal Digital
Veins

Figure 16.2. Venous phase of a right hand angiogram. Note the large dorsal venous network.

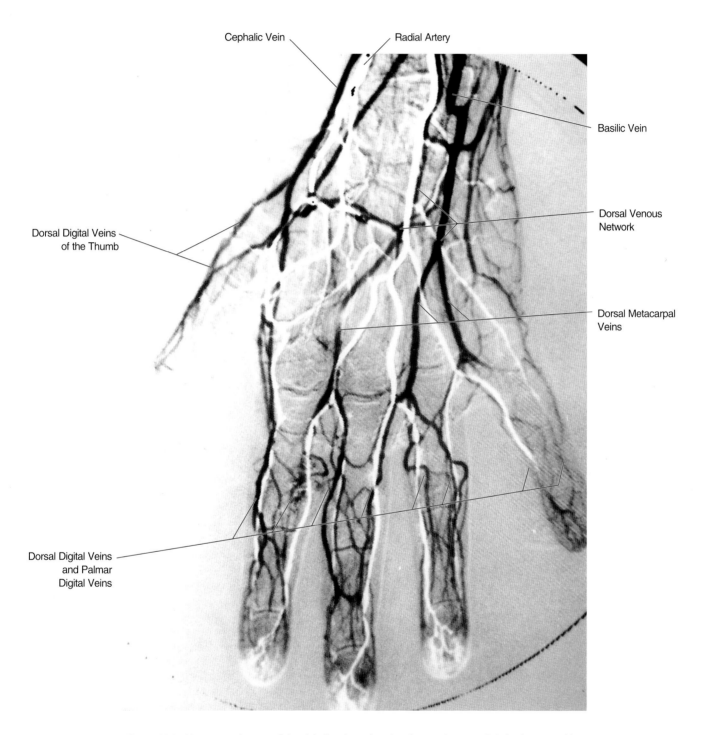

Figure 16.3. Venous angiogram of the right hand overlapping the arteries on a digital subtraction film.

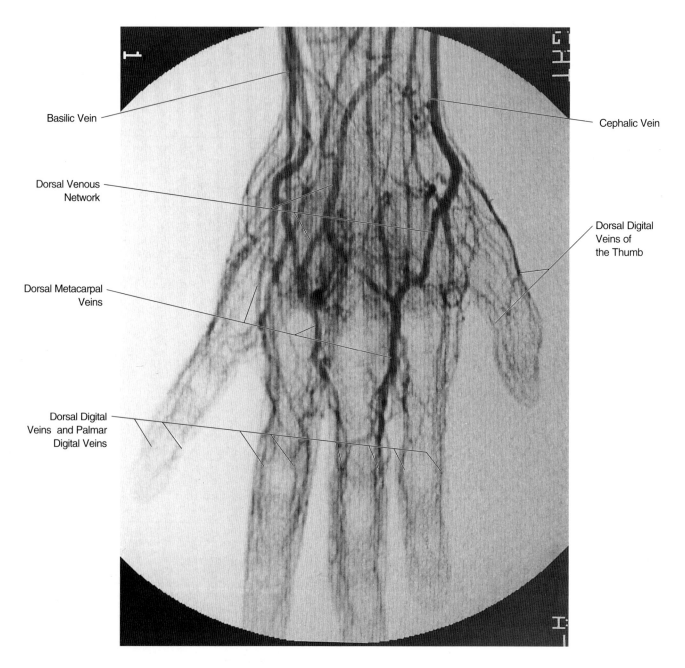

Basilic Vein

Cephalic Vein

Dorsal Venous
Network

Dorsal Digital
Veins of
the Thumb

Dorsal Metacarpal
Veins

Dorsal Digital
Veins and Palmar
Digital Veins

Figure 16.4. Late phase of an angiography of the right hand showing the venous anatomy of the right hand in
prone view.

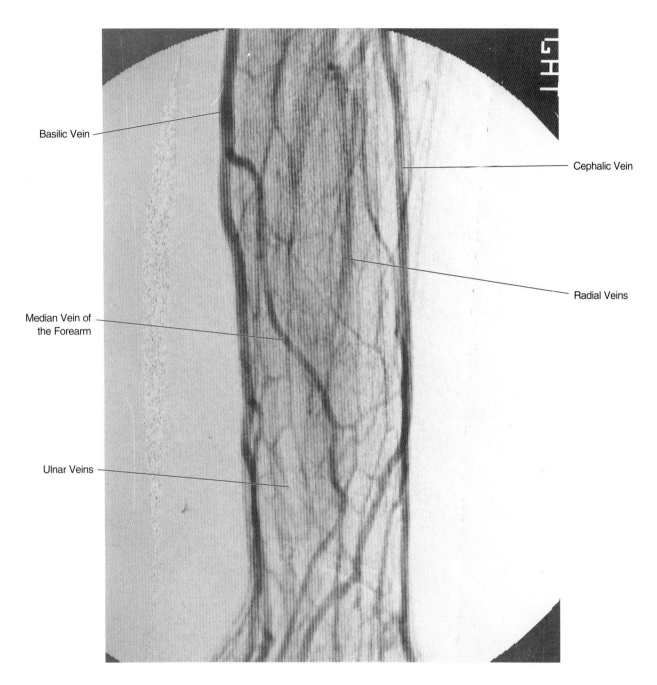

Basilic Vein

Cephalic Vein

Radial Veins

Median Vein of
the Forearm

Ulnar Veins

Figure 16.5. Venous anatomy of the right forearm.

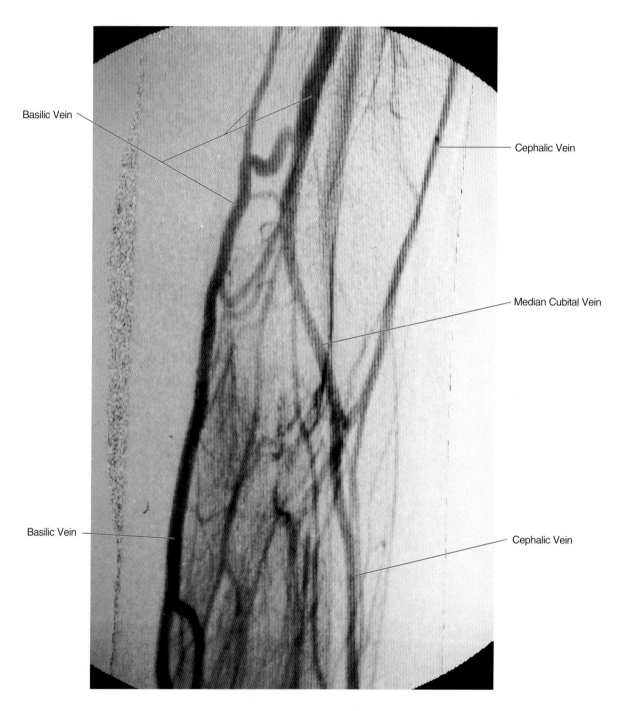

Basilic Vein

Cephalic Vein

Median Cubital Vein

Basilic Vein

Cephalic Vein

Figure 16.6. Venous anatomy at the right elbow region.

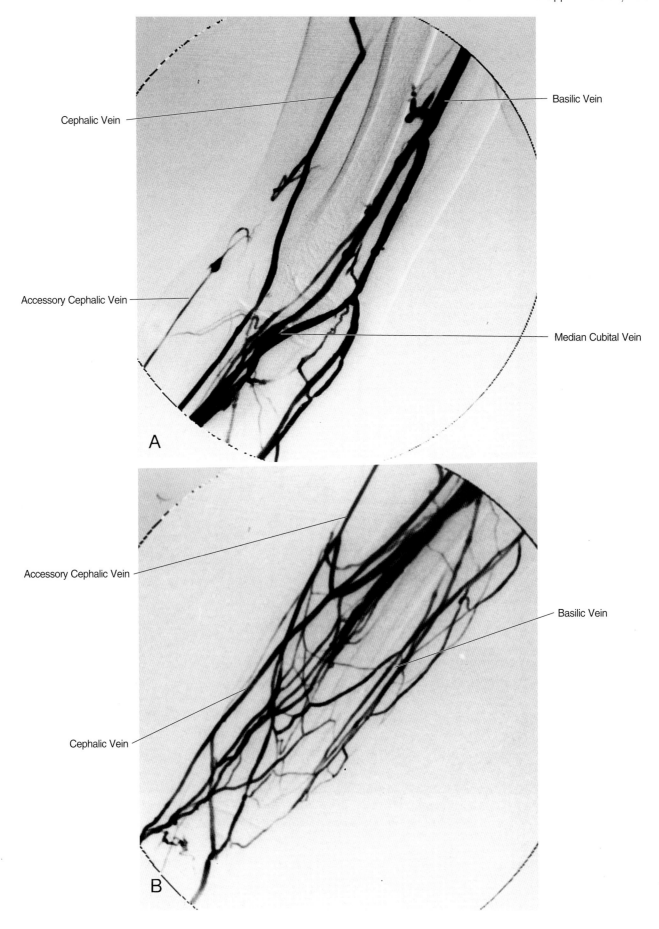

Cephalic Vein

Basilic Vein

Accessory Cephalic Vein

Median Cubital Vein

A

Accessory Cephalic Vein

Basilic Vein

Cephalic Vein

B

Figure 16.7. Phlebography of the right upper extremity. A. Forearm. B. Antecubital area.

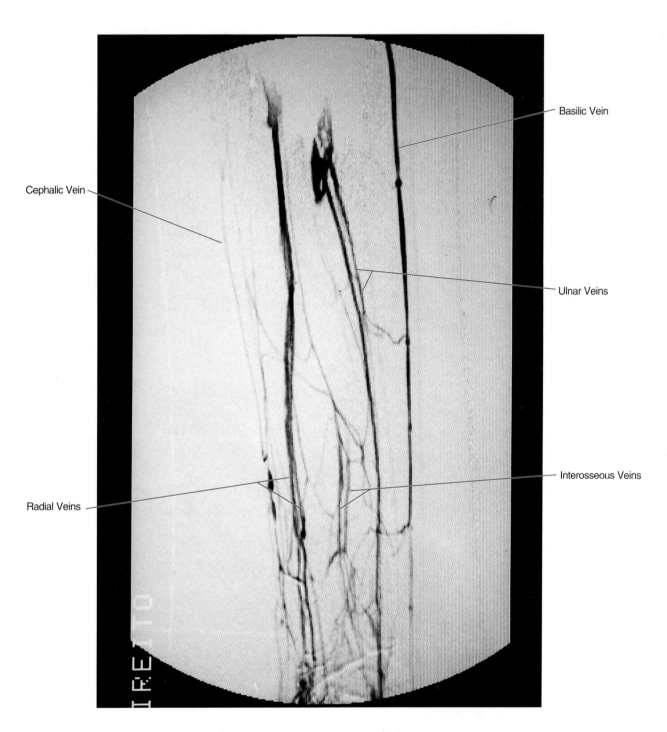

Figure 16.8. Deep venous system at the forearm.

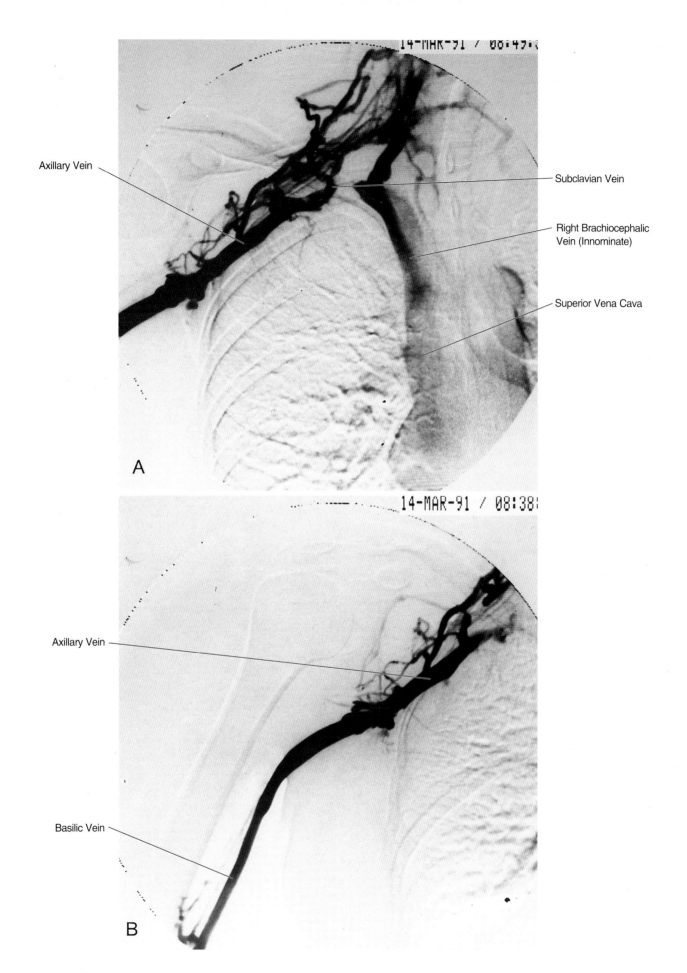

Axillary Vein

Subclavian Vein

Right Brachiocephalic
Vein (Innominate)

Superior Vena Cava

14-MAR-91 / 08:49

A

14-MAR-91 / 08:38

Axillary Vein

Basilic Vein

B

Figure 16.9. Right subclavian vein. Note the pathologic occlusion and collateral circulation.

17

LYMPHATIC DRAINAGE OF THE UPPER EXTREMITY

LYMPHATICS OF THE DEEP TISSUES

The lymphatic drainage of the deep tissues of the upper limb follows the main neurovascular bundles ending in the lateral axillary lymph nodes. Lymphatic vessels draining the deep tissues are internal to the deep fascia (Fig. 17.1).

LYMPHATICS OF THE SUPERFICIAL TISSUES

The superficial lymphatic drainage begins at the lymphatic plexuses in the skin and converges in the direction of the superficial veins following approximately the same direction towards the terminal group of axillary lymph nodes (Fig. 17.1).

At the Hand

The groups of lymphatic plexus are finer on the palmar than on the dorsal surface. The digital vessels run along the border of the fingers and join larger vessels at the palm, passing towards the dorsal aspect of the hand. The main palmar vessels pass toward the wrist joining vessels along the ulnar border of the hand and laterally joining the draining vessels of the thumb.

At the Forearm and Arm

In the forearm and arm the lymphatic vessels run together with the superficial veins. The ventral aspect of the forearm and arm display the largest number of vessels because they pass successively from behind to the front winding around the forearm and joining ventral larger vessels. At the arm level the vessels, above the elbow, crowd together and follow the medial aspect of the arm ending in the lateral group of the axillary lymph nodes. There are small isolated nodes along the radial, ulnar, and interosseous vessels, in the cubital fossa and in the arm, medial to the brachial vessels.

AXILLARY LYMPH NODES

This is the terminal group of nodes for the upper limb, varying from 20 to 30 in number, and are divided in five groups (Figs. 17.1, 17.2).

Lateral Group

Medial and behind the axillary vein. Drain most of the upper limb. Are connected to the central and apical groups and to the lower deep cervical nodes.

Anterior or Pectoral Group

Positioned along the lower border of the pectoralis minor. Receive the afferents from the skin and muscles of the lateral and anterior walls of the trunk and central and lateral parts of the mammary gland.

Posterior or Subscapular Group

Situated along the lower margin of the posterior wall of the axilla. Same course of the subscapular vessels. Receive afferents draining the posterior aspect of the trunk and lower part of the neck.

Central Group

Embedded in the fat of the axilla. Afferents from all the above described groups.

Apical Group

Situated in the apex of the axilla. Along the medial side of the axillary vein. Receive afferents from all the other groups. The efferent vessels of this group join and form the subclavian trunk opening directly into the junction of the internal jugular and subclavian veins. On the left side it may end in the thoracic duct.

Other Lymph Nodes of the Upper Limb

Supratrochlear group
Infraclavicular group
Isolated lymph nodes

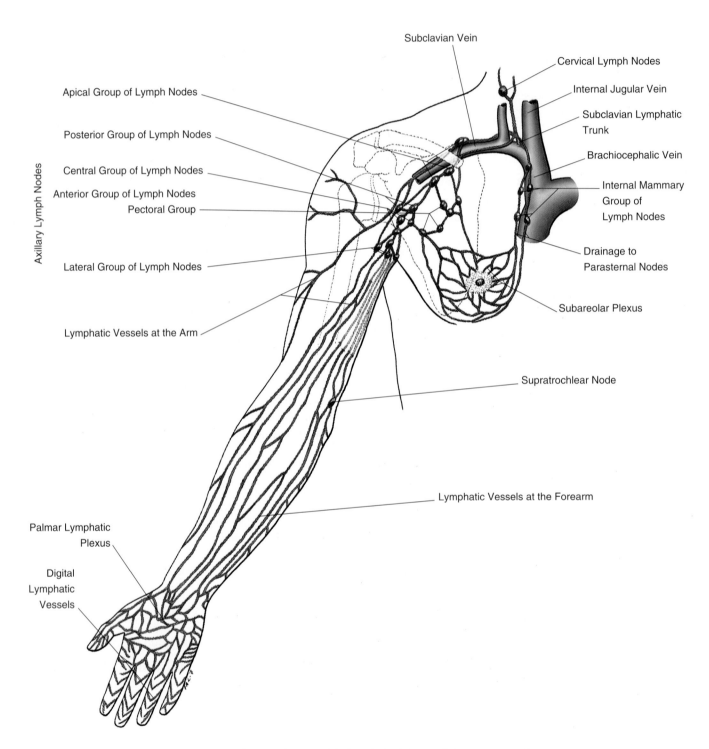

Subclavian Vein

Cervical Lymph Nodes

Internal Jugular Vein

Subclavian Lymphatic Trunk

Apical Group of Lymph Nodes

Brachiocephalic Vein

Posterior Group of Lymph Nodes

Central Group of Lymph Nodes

Anterior Group of Lymph Nodes

Internal Mammary Group of Lymph Nodes

Pectoral Group

Drainage to Parasternal Nodes

Axillary Lymph Nodes

Lateral Group of Lymph Nodes

Subareolar Plexus

Lymphatic Vessels at the Arm

Supratrochlear Node

Lymphatic Vessels at the Forearm

Palmar Lymphatic Plexus

Digital Lymphatic Vessels

Figure 17.1. Schematic drawing of the lymphatic drainage of the upper extremity.

Apical Group of Lymph Nodes

Pectoral Group of
Lymph Nodes

Central Group of Lymph
Nodes

Lateral Group of Lymph
Nodes

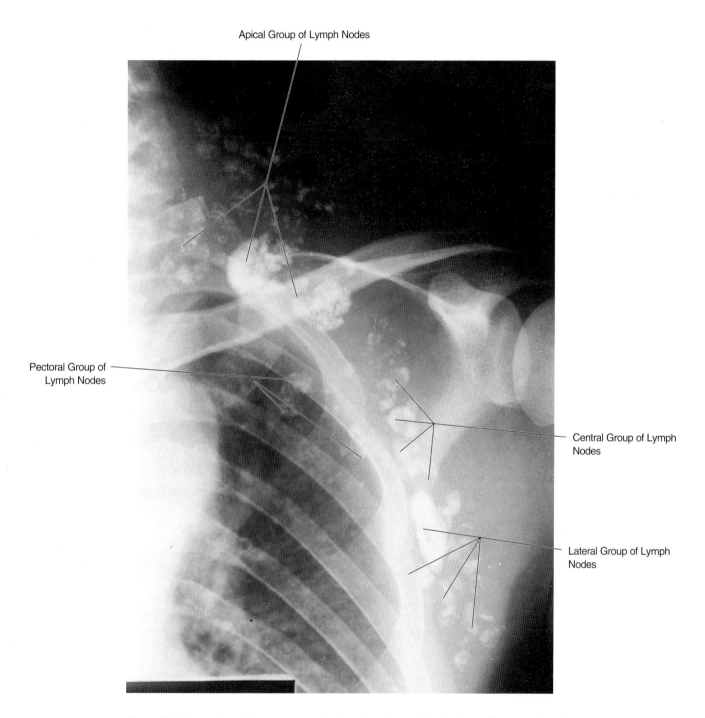

Figure 17.2. Late phase of an upper extremity lymphangiogram showing the Axillary Lymph Nodes.

18

ABDOMINAL AORTA AND BRANCHES

ABDOMINAL AORTA

The abdominal aorta begins at the aortic hiatus of the diaphragm, anterior and at the level of the lower portion of the 12th thoracic vertebra, descending slightly laterally to the middle line and in close relation to the vertebral bodies, ending at the 4th lumbar vertebra. At that point, it bifurcates into two common iliac arteries forming an angle of 37º. The abdominal aorta reduces the diameter rapidly because the branches are large and numerous (Figs. 18.1, 18.2).

The aorta is in contact, anteriorly with the celiac plexus and the lesser sac or omental bursa, and the pancreatic body with the splenic vein attached posteriorly. Behind the pancreas, between the superior mesenteric artery and the aorta, is the left renal vein in close relation with the anterior wall of the aorta. Below the pancreas is the horizontal part of the duodenum; further distally, it is covered by the posterior parietal peritoneum and crossed by the oblique parietal attachment of the mesentery. Laterally on the right, the aorta is in contact with the cisterna chyli, and thoracic duct, azygos vein and right crus of the diaphragm, which separates it from the inferior vena cava. Below the 2nd lumbar vertebra, the aorta is in contact with the inferior vena cava, all the way down. Laterally on the left, the aorta is in contact with the crus of the diaphragm and celiac ganglion. At the level of the 2nd lumbar vertebra, there is contact with the duodenojejunal flexure and sympathetic trunk, ascending duodenum and inferior mesenteric vessels. The bifurcation of the abdominal aorta is projected on the abdominal wall surface at the level of the umbilicus (Figs. 18.3–18.8).

Branches of the Abdominal Aorta

Ventral
    Celiac trunk
    Superior mesenteric artery
    Inferior mesenteric artery
Lateral
    Inferior phrenic artery
    Middle suprarenal artery
    Renal artery
    Testicular or ovarian artery (gonadal)

Dorsal
    Lumbar
    Median sacral
Terminal
    Common iliac

Celiac Trunk

It is the first wide ventral branch of the aorta, 1.5 cm long, arising just below the aortic diaphragmatic hiatus (Figs. 18.9, 18.10). It is generally horizontal and oriented forward, but may be caudally or cranially oriented (Figs. 18.11–18.15). It may give off the inferior phrenic arteries before the origin of the left gastric artery. In approximately 50% of the population, the celiac trunk follows the standard pattern.

Branches
    Left gastric artery
    Hepatic artery
        Common hepatic artery
    Gastroduodenal artery
    Pancreaticoduodenal arcades
    Right gastroepiploic artery
    Hepatic artery proper
    Right gastric artery
    Cystic artery
    Arteries of the liver
    Segmental branches
    Microscopic hepatic structure
    Terminal hepatic artery
    Hepatic arterial collaterals
    Variations of the hepatic artery

Splenic Artery

    Arteries of the pancreas
    Pancreaticoduodenal arcades
    Dorsal pancreatic artery
    Arteria pancreatica magna
    Arteria caudae pancreatis
    Short gastric arteries
    Posterior gastric artery
    Left gastroepiploic artery
    Terminal splenic branches
    Segmental splenic branches
    Variations of the celiac trunk

Left Gastric Artery

This is the smallest celiac branch. The origin of the LGA may be in the aorta, close to the celiac trunk, or at the cranial aspect of the celiac trunk, all the way, from the ostium to the bifurcation creating a real trifurcation. It ascends cranially to the left, behind the omental bursa, to the upper end of the stomach. After giving distal esophageal branches and branches to the gastric fundus, the artery turns anteroinferiorly into the left gastropancreatic fold, running along the gastric lesser curvature, reaching the pylorus, supplying both gastric walls (anterior and posterior) and ends with an anastomoses with the right gastric artery (Figs. 18.16, 18.17). The left gastric artery may give origin to the left hepatic artery, or an accessory left gastric artery may arise from the left hepatic artery (Figs. 18.18–18.20). At the gastric fundus, there are anastomoses with the splenic artery, through the short gastric arteries (Fig. 18.21).

Hepatic Artery

In the adult, the hepatic artery is smaller than the splenic artery, but larger than the left gastric artery. It originates from the bifurcation of the celiac trunk, directed forward and to the right, toward the porta hepatis, where it divides in the right and left branches to the hepatic lobes (Fig. 18.10). The artery is subdivided in common hepatic artery from the celiac trunk to the origin of the gastroduodenal artery and hepatic artery proper. It is called the hepatic artery proper, from the gastroduodenal artery to the bifurcation into right and left hepatic branches (Fig. 18.12). The common hepatic artery may be extremely short or not exist at all (Fig. 18.15). The proper hepatic artery may not exist at all (Fig. 18.11) and may be part of a trifurcation of the common hepatic artery. The hepatic artery may arise from the superior mesenteric artery (replaced hepatic artery). The right hepatic branch may arise from the superior mesenteric artery, whereas the left hepatic branch may originate from the left gastric artery. See Variations of the Hepatic Artery at the end of this section.

Common Hepatic Artery

Gastroduodenal Artery. The gastroduodenal artery arises from the hepatic artery, characterizing the beginning of the hepatic artery proper (Figs. 18.22, 18.23). It is short and large, descending between the duodenum and neck of the pancreas. It may be located at the left aspect or anteriorly to the bile duct. The gastroduodenal artery has three constant branches: the posterior and anterior pancreaticoduodenal arcades, the terminal branch, and the right gastroepiploic artery (Figs. 18.24, 18.25). The gastroduodenal artery may be duplicated, or the pancreaticoduodenal arcades may arise from the common hepatic artery (Fig. 18.26)

Posterior Pancreaticoduodenal Arcade. This artery arises 1 to 2 cm from the origin of the gastroduodenal artery. It is also called the retroduodenal artery or posterior superior pancreaticoduodenal artery. It gives branches to the duodenum (to the right) and the head of the pancreas (to the left). The pancreatic branches anastomoses freely with arteries in the head of the pancreas, anterior pancreaticoduodenal arcade, and dorsal pancreatic artery (Figs. 18.24, 18.25). The arcades are frequently multiple with two, three, and four branches. The lower part of the bile duct has the main blood supply from the posterior pancreaticoduodenal arcade.

Anterior Pancreaticoduodenal Arcade. Along with the right gastroepiploic artery, the anterior pancreaticoduodenal arcade is a terminal branch of the gastroduodenal artery. It is also called the superior pancreaticoduodenal or anterior superior pancreaticoduodenal artery and may give a pyloric branch and have a distal anastomoses with the superior mesenteric artery or the inferior pancreaticoduodenal artery. The anterior arcade has free communications with the posterior arcade and dorsal pancreatic and transverse pancreatic arteries (Figs. 18.24, 18.25, 18.27). The middle colic artery may also have anastomoses with the anterior pancreaticoduodenal arcade.

Right Gastroepiploic Artery. This artery is the terminal branch of the gastroduodenal artery, and is the main artery of the stomach (Figs. 18.28, 18.29). It follows a winding course along the greater curvature of the stomach and gives off an ascending pyloric branch and several ascending gastric branches, which anastomose with descending branches of the right and left gastric arteries. Several omental branches are also originated from the right gastroepiploic artery. The right and left omental branches form an anastomotic arcade at the greater omentum and have anastomoses with the posterior omental branches from the transverse mesocolon. The gastroepiploic artery reaches and anastomoses with the left gastroepiploic artery, where it ends (Figs. 18.30–18.33).

Other Branches. Less constant branches are occasionally seen, including the right gastric artery, the transverse pancreatic artery, accessory cystic artery, and supraduodenal artery.

Right Gastric Artery. This artery arises from any site at the hepatic artery, before or after the gastroduodenal artery. It anastomoses with the left gastric artery (Fig. 18.34).

Cystic Artery. This artery arises from the right branch of the hepatic artery. It divides into superficial and deep branches. It may originate from the hepatic artery itself or the gastroduodenal artery. An accessory cystic artery may be present (Figs. 18.35, 18.36).

Arteries of the Liver

Segmental Anatomy of the Liver

The intrahepatic arteries follow a segmental distribution (Figs. 18.37, 18.38). The division of the liver into segments is delineated by fissures and the distribution of the vascular and ductal structures. The three main hepatic veins divide the liver into four sectors, each of which receives a portal pedicle, with an alternation between hepatic veins and portal pedicles. Of the four fissures, only one is represented superficially — the portoumbilical fissure. The other three fissures are related to the three large hepatic veins, but not apparent in the liver surface.

Right Fissure

This fissure commences at the right margin of the inferior vena cava and follows the attachment of the right superior coronary ligament to about 3 to 4 cm from the junction of the latter with the right inferior layer. The fissure then curves anteriorly to a point on the inferior margin about midway between the gallbladder fossa and the right margin of the liver. Passing posteriorly, the fissure follows a line that runs parallel to the gallbladder fossa and crosses the caudate process to reach the right side of the inferior vena cava. Lying almost in the coronal plane, the fissure contains the right hepatic vein, with branches passing anteriorly to segments V and VIII and posteriorly to segments VI and VII (Figs. 18.37, 18.38).

Median Fissure (Main Portal Fissure, also called Cantlie's Line)

This fissure passes from the gallbladder fossa to the left margin of the inferior vena cava.

Posteroinferiorly, this fissure is represented by a line from the gallbladder fossa to the main bifurcation of the hepatic pedicle (portal triad) and, then, to the retrohepatic inferior vena cava (Figs. 18.37, 18.38).

Left Fissure (Left Portal Fissure)

This fissure runs from the left side of the inferior vena cava to a point between the dorsal one third and ventral two thirds of the left margin of the liver; it divides the left liver into two sectors: anterior and posterior, separating the segments III and II. It is not the umbilical fissure. Inferiorly, the fissure passes to the commencement of the ligamentum venosum (Figs. 18.37, 18.38).

Portoumbilical Fissure (or Umbilical Fissure)

This fissure is marked superficially by the attachment of the falciform ligament, which contains the ligamentum teres hepatis in its inferior border. Angled less generously than the right fissure, it meets the inferior margin of the liver at an angle of about 50º.

The liver is divided into right and left lobes, separated by the main portal fissure or median fissure (projection of the path of the middle hepatic vein upon the liver surface). The portal fissure runs from the medial side of the inferior vena cava to the middle of the gallbladder bed. The right lobe is vascularized by the right hepatic artery and the left lobe is fed by the left hepatic artery. The hepatic lobes are divided in sectors. The right lobe has an anterior and posterior sector (also called anteromedial and posterolateral), separated by the right portal fissure (projection of the path of the right hepatic vein upon the liver surface). The left lobe has a lateral (left) and a medial sector (right), separated by the falciform ligament and portoumbilical fissure (partial projection of the path of the involuted umbilical vein, called round ligament) (Figs 18.37, 18.38, 18.39).

Hepatic Segments

The caudate lobe is an independent segment, supplied by the right and left hepatic artery and portal vein. It is called segment I and has venous drainage directly into the inferior vena cava. It is also called lobule of Spiegel. It is considered to be part of the left hepatic lobe (segment I of the left lobe) for surgical purposes. The caudate lobe is connected to the right lobe by a narrow bridge called caudate process, behind the porta hepatis. Below and to the left, there is a small round appendage called papillary process, which sometimes covers completely the inferior vena cava bridging the caudate lobe to the right liver lobe (Fig. 18.40a–d).

The left hepatic lobe is further subdivided into three segments. The lateral sector is divided into segment II and segment III by the left portal fissure (projection of the path of the left hepatic vein upon the surface of the left lobe of the liver). Segment II is posterior and superior, and segment III is inferior and anterior (Figs. 18.41, 18.42). The medial sector of the left lobe is segment IV. It has a cuneiform format, with the base turned anteriorly. It may be subdivided in a cranial and a caudal part, also called segments IVa and IVb. Segment IVa is also called the quadrate lobe of the liver (Fig. 18.43).

The right hepatic lobe is subdivided into four segments. The anterior sector is divided in segment VIII and segment V. Segment VIII is superior and segment V is inferior (Figs. 18.44, 18.45). The posterior sector is divided in segment VI and segment VII. Segment VI is inferior and segment VII is superior. The posterior sector is posterior and more lateral than the anterior sector (Figs. 18.46, 18.47).

The segments of the liver, either at the left or the right hepatic lobes, follow a clockwise distribution. The hepatic artery, the bile ducts, and the portal vein branches run in the center of the hepatic segments, whereas the hepatic veins run within the fissures between the segments. The fissures of the liver can not be seen at the liver surface, except at the umbilical fissure, due to the presence of the falciform ligament and round ligament (ligamentum teres) (Figs. 18.37, 18.38, 18.39).

Microscopic Hepatic Structure

The classical hepatic lobules are polyhedral structures (hexagonal in histological sections), about 1 mm in diameter, with a small central vein as a central axis, surrounded by portal triads. Each triad contains a branch of the portal vein, a hepatic artery, a lymphatic vessel, and an interlobular biliary ductule. The portal triad is sheathed by connective tissue, called the portal canal or perivascular fibrous capsule, surrounded by the limiting plate, having in between the space of Mall. In humans, the idea of a functional unit has been proposed instead because the hepatic lobules are not readily perceptible. The functional unit is the portal lobule, consisting of parts of at least three neighboring classic lobules, bile from which drains into a biliary ductule in the portal canal between three such hepatic lobules. Again, the section shows a portal lobule as a polygonal area, centered on a portal triad, with boundaries passing through adjacent central veins. The concept of a portal acinus is more useful considering metabolic organization. The portal acinus is centered on a preterminal branch of an hepatic arteriole and includes the hepatic tissue served by this, with boundaries at the territory of other acini and by two adjacent central veins (Fig. 18.48). The acinus has been divided into three zones: zone 1 (periportal), zone 2, and zone 3 (close to the central venous drainage). Zone 3 (in the circulatory periphery and close to the central vein) suffer most from injury, developing bridging necrosis. Zone 1 close to the afferent vessels survives longer and may trigger the regeneration of the liver (Fig. 18.49).

Terminal Hepatic Artery

The hepatic artery ramifies parallel with the portal vein branches and bile ducts. Arterioles are released into the lobular parenchyma and terminate at different levels of the lobule, providing arterial blood flow to zone 1 of the acinus through anastomoses with the portal venule inlet (Fig. 18.50). Much like the bronchial arteries that provide bronchial circulation and pulmonary arterial anastomosis in the lungs, in the liver, the main circulatory arterial flow is provided to the periportal area by arterial branches directly to the peribiliary plexus and to the bile duct. Subsequently and to a much lesser extent, the artery provides nutrition to the acinus and to the liver parenchyma itself through the anastomosis of the arterioles with the portal inlet venule. In fact, due to importance of the hepatic artery to the bile ducts, the hepatic artery should be called biliary artery.

According to Lunderquist, there are four types of arterioportal communications: 1) the peribiliary plexus; 2) the terminal arterioloportal anastomosis connecting to the sinusoids; 3) the vasa vasorum on the wall of the portal vein; and 4) the direct arterio-portal communications. The vasa vasorum to the wall of the portal vein is provided by direct small branches from the hepatic artery. There are two concentric vascular layers within the wall of the larger bile duct, constituting the peribiliary plexus. The inner layer is a capillary plexus present in the submucosa, which drains into the outer adventitial venous plexus. The latter opens directly into the hepatic sinusoids via the lobular vein or into the portal vein via the interlobular vein (Fig. 18.51). The intrahepatic bile duct is supplied by the hepatic arterial branches, which form the peribiliary plexus, while the extrahepatic bile duct receives its arterial nutrition from various sources, but most commonly from branches of the gastroduodenal artery.

According to Ekataksin, unlike the portal vein which exclusively supplies sinusoids, the hepatic artery supplies five compartments: 1) peribiliary plexus, 2) portal tract interstitium, 3) portal venous vasa vasorum, 4) fibrous capsule of Glisson, and 5) central sublobular-hepatic venous vasa vasorum, which subsequently either secondarily flows through the lobules or directly drains into the hepatic vein.

Within the portal tract, the arterial beds form distinct collecting vessels, forming a portal system, the so-called hepatic artery-derived portal system, which anastomoses with and/or follows or joins the vein-venule to open at lobular periphery.

Outside the portal tract, the hepatic artery departs from the tract as an "isolated artery" directed toward the two compartments, the Glisson capsule and the central sublobular-hepatic venous vasa vasorum. The capsular arteriole that eventually drains into the local subcapsular lobules is likely to be misinterpreted as evidence of the hepatic artery being a primary feeder of sinusoids. The hepatic venous vasa vasorum that immediately drains into the respective hepatic vein without passing through lobular sinusoids is a hitherto unrecognized, but occasionally suspected, unusual pathway, a "bypass artery."

To facilitate description, the biliary duct has been divided in three segments, namely hilar (right and left ducts), supraduodenal (common hepatic duct and upper common bile duct), and retropancreatic (lower common bile duct).

The arterial supply of the hilar bile duct (right and left) is provided by direct numerous small branches from the right and left hepatic arteries that form a rich network on the surface of the ducts in continuity with the plexus around the supraduodenal duct (Fig. 18.52).

The arterial supply of the supraduodenal bile duct is essentially axial, and most arteries arise from named arteries related to its upper and lower ends. The main vessels run along the lateral aspects of the duct. These vessels are named 3 o'clock and 9 o'clock arteries and most commonly originated from the posterior pancreaticoduodenal arcade and gastroduodenal artery. About 60% of the vessels supplying the supraduodenal duct run upward from vessels below, whereas 38% run downward from the right hepatic and other arteries. Only 2% of the supply is non-axial arising from the common or proper hepatic artery. The 3 o'clock and 9 o'clock arteries give branches to the duct forming the pericholedocal plexus (Figs. 18.32, 18.52–18.55).

An additional supply to the supraduodenal bile duct may be the retroportal artery, arising from the celiac trunk or superior mesenteric artery close to the origin of these vessels from the aorta. This artery courses to the right, behind the portal vein and to the back of the head of the pancreas, reaching the lower end of the supraduodenal duct. This artery may end, joining the posterior pancreaticoduodenal arcade, close to the distal supraduodenal duct giving off small branches to the posterior surface of the duct (type I pattern). In one third of the cases, the retroportal artery passes upwards on the back of the supraduodenal duct reaching the right hepatic artery (type II pattern). The retroportal artery along its route give branches to join the pericholedocal plexus (Fig. 18.53).

The retropancreatic bile duct is supplied by direct small branches from the posterior pancreaticoduodenal artery or gastroduodenal artery, forming a mural plexus (Fig. 18.52).

Hepatic Arterial Collaterals

There are 26 known potential collateral pathways for the arterial supply of the liver. They may be classified as intrahepatic collaterals (Fig. 18.56) and extrahepatic collaterals (Fig. 18.57).

Intrahepatic Collaterals (Fig. 18.56)

Perivascular
Interlobar or intersegmental
Intralobar or intrasegmental
Vasa vasorum of the portal veins and hepatic veins
Peribiliary plexus

Extrahepatic Collaterals (Fig. 18.57)

Pancreaticoduodenal arcades
    Inferior pancreaticoduodenal artery
    Dorsal pancreatic artery
    Arc of Bühler (Fig. 18.58)
Periportal route
    Common bile duct collaterals
    Retroduodenal or supraduodenal artery
    Cystic artery
    Right branches of dorsal pancreatic artery
    Multiple unnamed branches in the porta hepatis

Left gastric route
    Left gastric to right gastric anastomosis
    Left gastric to left hepatic via lesser omentum
Inferior phrenic route
    Right inferior phrenic artery
    Left inferior phrenic artery
Right paracolic gutter route
    Branches from middle or right colic artery
    Direct adhesions to hepatic flexure
Omental branches
Internal mammary and superior epigastric artery
Intercostal and lumbar artery
Capsular branches of the right renal artery

Variations of the Hepatic Artery

In more than 40% of cases, the origin and course of the hepatic arteries (Fig. 18.59) vary. Two concepts must be defined. The "replaced" artery originates from a different vessel, related to the standard description and substitutes the typical vessel. The "accessory" artery is an additional vessel to the originated accordingly to the standard description.

Type 1

Type 1 is a replacement of the common hepatic artery, arising from the superior mesenteric artery. The replaced common hepatic artery passes through or behind the head of the pancreas (Figs. 18.59, 18.60).

Type 2

Type 2 is early bifurcation of a short common hepatic artery in right and left hepatic arteries. The right and left hepatic artery may originate separately from the celiac trunk. The gastroduodenal artery arises from the right hepatic artery (Fig. 18.59).

Type 3

Type 3 is a replaced right hepatic artery that originates from the superior mesenteric artery and the left hepatic artery taking origin from the celiac trunk (Figs. 18.59, 18.61).

Type 4

Type 4 is a replaced left hepatic artery that originates from the left gastric artery, whereas the right hepatic artery originates from the celiac trunk (Figs. 18.18, 18.19, 18.20, 18.59)

Type 5

The right and left hepatic arteries arise from the celiac trunk but there is an accessory right hepatic artery from the superior mesenteric artery. The accessory passes through or behind the head of the pancreas (Fig. 18.59).

Type 6

Type 6 is an accessory left hepatic artery arising from the left gastric artery (Fig. 18.59).

Type 7

Type 7 is an accessory left hepatic artery arising from the right hepatic artery (Fig. 18.59).

Type 8

Right hepatic artery passes anteriorly to the common hepatic bile duct, instead of posteriorly (Fig. 18.59).

Splenic Artery

The splenic artery gives branches to the pancreas, to the stomach, and to the spleen. It originates from the celiac trunk in more than 80% of cases. Most of the arteries feeding the body and tail of the pancreas originate from the splenic artery (Figs. 18.62, 18.63, 18.64).

Arteries of the Pancreas

The pancreas does not have a central hilum like other abdominal organs. It is situated between the celiac trunk and the superior mesenteric artery, receiving the blood supply from several arteries originated from those main trunks (Fig. 18.65). The arteries of the head of the pancreas originate from the gastroduodenal artery, and the arteries of the body and tail originate from the splenic artery, celiac trunk, or common hepatic artery.

Pancreaticoduodenal Arcades

The head of the pancreas is encircled by two arterial arcades, the posterior (retroduodenal artery) and anterior pancreaticoduodenal arcades, branches of the gastroduodenal artery. The posterior arcade is proximal on the gastroduodenal artery, while the anterior arcade is a terminal branch of the gastroduodenal artery, together with the right gastroepiploic artery. The anterior pancreaticoduodenal arcade joins the posterior arcade, behind the head of the pancreas, forming a common trunk, called inferior pancreaticoduodenal artery (or trunk), ending in an anastomosis with the superior mesenteric artery or the first jejunal artery. In a number of cases, there is an intermediary pancreaticoduodenal arcade, and in some cases, it is not a real arcade, but a terminal artery to the pancreatic head (Fig. 18.24–18.27)

Dorsal Pancreatic Artery

The main vessel to the neck and proximal body of the pancreas is the dorsal pancreatic artery (Figs. 18.22, 18.65) (also called superior pancreatic artery, or colli, or suprema, or propria, or media, or isthmi, or dorsalis, and less correctly arteria pancreatica magna). The dorsal pancreatic artery arises most commonly from the initial splenic artery, but also frequently from the celiac trunk bifurcation (Fig. 18.66) or from the common hepatic artery (Fig. 18.67). Less commonly, it originates from the superior mesenteric artery or from a branch of the superior mesenteric artery (Figs. 18.23, 18.68, 18.69). The dorsal pancreatic artery is commonly connected, in the right aspect, with the anterior pancreaticoduodenal arcade or other gastroduodenal artery branch by an anastomotic branch (prepancreatic arcade) and originates the transverse pancreatic artery in the left aspect (arteria transversa pancreatis), which crosses all along the pancreatic body and tail (Figs. 18.65, 18.66). The dorsal pancreatic artery may give rise to omental branches and also an actual or accessory middle colic artery (Fig. 18.70).

Arteria Pancreatica Magna

The body of the pancreas is supplied by the arteria pancreatica magna (arteria corporis pancreatica or great pancreatic artery) (Fig. 18.71). The arteria pancreatica magna may be single, but it is usually a group of comb-shaped branches, perpendicular to the splenic artery. It anastomoses with the transverse pancreatic artery.

Arteria Caudae Pancreatis (Caudal Pancreatic Artery)

The tail of the pancreas is supplied by multiple branches originated from the splenic artery, right gastroepiploic artery or splenic branches (Fig. 18.72). These branches anastomoses with the transverse pancreatic artery and branches of the arteria pancreatica magna.

Short Gastric Arteries

The short gastric arteries (rami gastrici breves) arise from the splenic artery, divisional branches, polar arteries for the spleen and splenic parenchyma (Figs. 18.21, 18.28). They supply the cranial part of the gastric greater curvature (Fig. 18.17). It varies in number from one to four. Up to nine arteries may be found. Anastomosis occurs with other gastric branches.

Posterior Gastric Artery

The posterior gastric artery arises from the splenic artery and supplies the posterior fundic portion of the stomach, passing through the gastrosplenic ligament. It may provide splenic branches for the upper pole of the spleen.

Left Gastroepiploic Artery

This artery is also called the left gastro-omental artery. It is most commonly a branch of the splenic artery and arises as a trunk together with the left gas-troepiploic artery and the inferior splenic branch. It may, however, arise from the splenic artery isolated. It reaches the greater gastric curvature in the middle and eventually anastomoses with the right gastroepi-ploic artery (Fig. 18.73). The left omental (epiploic) artery is a major branch of the left gastroepiploic artery and forms the omental arcade in a significant number of cases. Other branches are the omental (or epiploic) arteries and the posterior and anterior short gastric arteries along the gastric body and antrum (Figs. 18.21, 18.28, 18.64).

Terminal Splenic Branches

The splenic branches enter the hilum after division of the main splenic artery in five or more branches (Figs. 18.74, 18.75). The spleen arterial circulation consists of multiple separate segments, with adjacent compartments without arterial interconnections. Within the spleen, the finest arteriolar branches pass out of the trabeculae, their adventitia being replaced by a periarteriolar sheath. These sheaths constitute the white pulp with splenic lymphatic follicles. The arterioles divide into a series of straight vessels termed penicillary arterioles. These pass through the marginal zones of the white pulp, developing the ellipsoids by thickening of the sheath by aggregation of macrophages and fibroblasts. Beyond the ellip-soids, each vessel continues as a fine arteriole or divide in two. Eventually the blood passes into the red pulp and the venous sinusoids, venules, and small veins. The small veins form the larger veins and exit through the hilum.

Segmental Splenic Branches

In more than 80% of cases, there are only two seg-ments, the superior and the inferior. The superior segment is larger and heavier than the inferior seg-ment in more than 65% of cases. In fewer cases, there are three and four splenic segments (superior, inter-mediate, and inferior).

Variations of the Celiac Trunk

The celiac trunk divides into three branches in 55 to 65% of cases: the left gastric artery, the splenic artery, and common hepatic artery. In more than 55% of cases, the inferior phrenic arteries also arise from the celiac trunk either as a single trunk or separately. The rest of the population presents one or more replaced arteries in origin. The celiac trunk may be absent, and the three arteries arise independently from the aorta (Fig. 18.76).

Couinaud described the following eight different types of variations of the celiac trunk.

Type 1. Classic Celiac Trunk: Hepato-Gastro-Splenic Trunk

This is the classical configuration of the celiac trunk, with the hepatic, left gastric, and splenic artery arising as a trunk from the abdominal aorta (Fig. 18.77). Three subtypes are described: 1) hepato-splenic trunk with the left gastric artery arising from the trunk (Fig. 18.74); 2) hepato-gastro-splenic trunk, with the three arteries arising at the same time in a trifurcation (Fig. 18.77); and 3) gastrosplenic trunk, the splenic is dominant and the hepatic artery arises from the aplenic (Figs. 18.18, 18.78).

Type 2. Hepatosplenic Trunk

The hepatic and splenic arteries form a trunk, and the left gastric artery arises from the aorta (Fig. 18.16).

Type 3. Hepatogastric Trunk

The hepatic and left gastric arteries arise from a common trunk, and the splenic artery arises directly from the aorta (Fig. 18.63) or from the superior mesenteric artery, called splenic-mesenteric trunk.

Type 4. Hepato-Splenic-Mesenteric Trunk

The left gastric artery arises directly from the aorta and the hepatic, the splenic, and the mesenteric arteries form a single trunk (Figs. 18.79, 18.80).

Type 5. Gastrosplenic Trunk

This is the most complex configuration. The left gastric artery and the splenic artery form a common trunk. The middle hepatic artery, when present, may arise from the aorta or from the superior mesenteric artery. When the middle hepatic artery does not exist, it is replaced by the right or left or both at the same time.

Type 6. Celiac-Mesenteric Trunk

The superior mesenteric artery arises from the celi-ac trunk.

Type 7. Celiac-Colic Trunk

The left colic artery or the middle colic artery aris-es from the celiac trunk.

Type 8. Absent Celiac Trunk

The three main arteries arise directly from the abdominal aorta.

Superior Mesenteric Artery

This is the second ventral branch of the abdominal aorta. This artery supplies all the small intestine, the right colon, and most of the transverse colon (Figs.

18.81, 18.82). The origin of the superior mesenteric artery is about 1 cm below the origin of the celiac trunk, behind the pancreas and is crossed anteriorly by the splenic vein. The left renal vein crosses right behind the first centimeters of the superior mesenteric artery, followed by the uncinate process of the pancreas and the horizontal part of the duodenum.

Branches

Inferior pancreaticoduodenal artery
   Anterior branch
   Posterior branch
Jejunal and ileal branches
   Straight vessels (vasa recta)
Ileocolic artery
   Superior branch
   Inferior branch
   Ascending colic artery
   Anterior and posterior cecal artery
   Appendicular artery
   Ileal branch
Right colic artery
   Ascending branch
   Descending branch
Middle colic artery
   Right branch
   Left branch
Other replaced and accessory branches
Different origins of the superior mesenteric artery
Terminal arteries and intestinal villi

Inferior Pancreaticoduodenal Artery

This is the first right side branch of the SMA. It may have origin in the first jejunal branch. It divides in an anterior and a posterior branch. The anterior branch crosses anteriorly to the head of the pancreas joining the anterior pancreaticoduodenal arcade. The posterior branch crosses posteriorly to the head of the pancreas anastomosing with the posterior pancreaticoduodenal arcade (Fig. 18.83).

Jejunal and Ileal Branches

The jejunal and ileal branches arise from the left aspect of the superior mesenteric artery, varying in number from 12 to 15. These branches vascularize the jejunum and ileum, except for the terminal ileum, forming a series of arches and anastomoses in three or four levels. The straight arteries (vasa recta) and the short arteries (vasa brevia) arise from the 4th or 5th level arches and supply the intestinal wall and mucosa (Fig. 18.84).

Ileocolic Artery

This artery is the last branch on the right side of the superior mesenteric artery. It is oriented to right underneath the retroperitoneal layer and vascularizes the terminal ileum, the right colon, the cecum, and the appendix (Figs. 18.85, 18.86). Four major branches are identified: the ascending branch, to the right colon (with anastomoses to the right colic artery), the cecal branches (anterior and posterior) to the cecum, the ileal branch to the ileum, with anastomoses to the terminal superior mesenteric artery, and the appendicular artery of the appendix.

Right Colic Artery

This artery originates at the middle of the superior mesenteric artery, but may share a common origin with the ileocolic artery. It courses behind the parietal peritoneum reaching the right ascending colon. It presents two main branches, the descending and the ascending branches. The descending anastomoses with the ileocolic artery and the ascending with the middle colic artery (Figs. 18.87–18.91).

Middle Colic Artery

This artery arises from the superior mesenteric artery just after passing the pancreas, following a path at the transverse mesocolon. It has a right and left branch. The right anastomoses with the right colic artery, the left branch with the left colic artery, a branch of the inferior mesenteric artery through the marginal arteries. It may be replaced and arises from the dorsal pancreatic artery or from the celiac trunk (Figs. 18.92–18.95).

Other Replaced and Accessory Branches

The common hepatic artery, the gastroduodenal, an accessory right hepatic artery, an accessory pancreatic artery or splenic artery may arise from the superior mesenteric artery. The dorsal pancreatic artery arises from the superior mesenteric artery in 14% of cases (Figs. 18.23, 18.68). The replaced hepatic artery or accessory hepatic artery follows a path behind the head of the pancreas in intimate contact with the pancreas tissue, sometimes actually encircled by pancreatic parenchyma (Fig. 18.96). The arc of Bühler is an uncommon direct pathway between the celiac and superior mesenteric arteries, due to the remaining embryologic ventral anastomosis (Fig. 18.58).

Different Origins of the Superior Mesenteric Artery

The superior mesenteric artery most commonly arises from the abdominal aorta; it may, however, originate as a celiac mesenteric trunk. It may also originate together with the splenic artery (Fig. 18.76).

Terminal Arteries and Intestinal Villi

The intramural vessels of the bowel arise from both vasa recta and the vasa brevia and form the external muscular plexus (Fig. 18.97). After crossing the muscle, a rich submucosal plexus is formed, from which a few recurrent branches run backward into the muscle and may join the external muscular plexus. The submucosal plexus is found over the length of the bowel and is arranged in a coarse rectangular pattern. From the submucosal plexus arterioles spring the vertical arterioles reaching the villi and the mucous membrane. A mucosal plexus is also found in the small bowel (Fig. 18.98).

The circulation to the villus is supplied from a single arteriole originated from the submucosal plexus, with about 20 mm in diameter, which runs up to the villi stroma and becomes capillarized, loosing its smooth muscle coat. At the tip of the villus, the arteriole is arborescent and divides into a fine subepithelial channel system, which eventually drain into a central venule. There is also a central lymphatic channel. The arterial and venous loops in the villi are so close that there is evidence of a countercurrent exchange of oxygen and nutrients in the intestinal villus, aggravated in low flow states as in intestinal ischemia (Fig. 18.99).

There is evidence of arteriovenous anastomoses in the submucous plexus of the gut wall, better demonstrated in the stomach and colon rather than the small bowel.

The regulation of the blood flow reaching the intestine is complex and interdependent, playing an important role in the theory of vascular circuits running in parallel, with resistance in series (Fig. 18.100) among several other central and regional mechanisms.

Inferior Mesenteric Artery

The inferior mesenteric artery supplies the left third of the transverse colon, the descending colon, the sigmoid colon, and part of the rectum. It arises a few centimeters from the aortic bifurcation and is much smaller in diameter compared with the superior mesenteric artery. It follows a retroperitoneal path in the left colonic branches and enters the sigmoid mesocolon with the rectal arteries (Fig. 18.101, 18.102).

Branches

Left colic artery
    Ascending branch
    Descending branch
Sigmoid arteries (inferior left colic artery)
Superior rectal artery (superior hemorrhoidal artery)
Right branch
Left branch

Left Colic Artery

This artery courses a retroperitoneal route and divides into ascending and descending branches. The ascending branch reaches the transverse mesocolon where it anastomoses with the middle colic artery. Arches that originate from this ascending branch provide the blood supply of the distal transverse colon and descending left colon. The descending branch anastomoses with the highest sigmoid artery. From the anastomosis between these arteries, the continuous marginal artery near the colon wall originates; this artery is called the marginal artery of Drummond (Figs. 18.104, 18.105). The anastomosis of the marginal artery with the ascending branch of the left colic artery and the distal left middle colic artery is frequently made through an additional arcade, the arc of Riolan. When the arc of Riolan is not well developed, there will be a critical area of anastomosis, called Griffith's point, at the splenic flexure of the colon, which is important in the etiology of ischemia of the left colon when occlusion of one of the mesenteric arteries develop.

Sigmoid Arteries

There are two or three sigmoid arteries within the sigmoid mesocolon. Branches supply the left descending colon and the sigmoid colon. There is an upper anastomosis with the descending branch of the left colic artery and a lower anastomosis with the superior rectal artery (Fig. 18.105, 18.106).

Superior Rectal Artery

This artery descends into the pelvis in the sigmoid mesocolon and when it reaches the rectum divides in two lateral branches, right and left, dividing further into smaller branches reaching the sphincter ani internus, forming loops around the lower rectum (Fig. 18.107). There are communications with the middle rectal artery (branch of the internal iliac artery) and with the inferior rectal artery (branch from the internal pudendal artery) (Fig. 18.108).

Lateral Branches of the Abdominal Aorta

Inferior Phrenic Artery

The inferior phrenic arteries may arise together as a trunk or separately as independent vessels, just above or at the origin of the celiac trunk (Figs. 18.1, 18.4). These arteries ascend along the diaphragmatic crura (Fig. 18.109). Each artery divides into a medial and a lateral branch (Fig. 18.110). The medial curves forward and the lateral reaches the thoracic wall, having anastomosis with the posterior intercostal and musculophrenic arteries (Fig. 18.111). Each artery gives the small superior suprarenal branches to the upper portion of the adrenal glands (Figs. 18.112, 18.113). The inferior phrenic artery supplies the Glisson's capsule of the liver through anastomoses at the bare area of the liver within the triangular ligaments (Fig. 18.115).

Middle Suprarenal Artery

These are small arteries that arise laterally to the aorta, about the same level of the origin of the superior mesenteric artery, reaching the adrenal glands, and with anastomoses with the superior phrenic artery, and inferior suprarenal artery originated from the renal artery (Figs. 18.1, 18.4). The right middle suprarenal artery passes behind the inferior vena cava.

Arteries of the Adrenal Glands

The adrenal glands are vascular organs and are supplied by three groups of arteries (Fig. 18.116): the superior adrenal artery (Fig. 18.114), the middle adrenal artery (Fig. 18.117), and the inferior adrenal artery, originated from the inferior phrenic artery, the aorta and the renal artery, respectively.

The capsular arteries ramify extensively before entering the gland to form a subcapsular plexus, which extends into the zona glomerulosa as sinusoids. The sinusoids continue into the zona fasciculata as straight cortical sinusoids between columns of cells. These are followed by a deep plexus of sinusoids at the zona reticularis. At the internal aspect of the zona reticularis, there are muscle fibers, restricting or releasing the flow, acting as a dam at the corticomedullary junction. Some larger arterioles bypass the described route and connect the capsular artery with the medullary capillaries (Fig. 18.118). There is a medullary plexus that connects with the medullary vein, which emerges from the hilum to form the suprarenal vein, draining to the inferior vena cava in the right and to the renal vein in the left side.

Kidney Arterial Vascularization

Extrarenal Arteries

Each renal artery is described as a single vessel, emerging on each side of the vertebral column between the first and the second lumbar vertebra, immediately below (1–2 cm) of the superior mesenteric artery. The renal artery usually has a slightly oblique cranial-caudal course and close to the renal sinus, after giving off the inferior suprarenal artery, it divides into an anterior and a posterior branch. The aortic origin of the left renal artery is higher than the right renal artery origin; nevertheless, it is not a definitive rule.

Anatomic variations of the renal blood supply occur frequently. Multiplicity of renal arteries is more common than multiple veins and is more prevalent than any other arteries of the same size in other organs.

Material of Investigation

Renal pedicles (266) that were dissected from 133 formalin-fixed cadavers of adult patients, of both sexes, who died of causes not related to the urinary tract were analyzed.

Findings

Figures 18.119, 18.120, and 18.121 show schematic drawings with the frequency of each type of renal arterial supply that we have found. The current nomenclature used and that must be adopted to denominate the renal arteries is the following:

Hilar Artery

Aortic branch that penetrates the kidney in the hilar region (Fig. 18.119a).

Extrahilar Artery

Renal artery branch that has an extrahilar penetration (superior pole) in the kidney (Fig. 18.119b).

Superior Polar Artery

Aortic branch that penetrates the kidney in the superior pole (Fig. 18.119d).

Inferior Polar Artery

Aortic or common iliac artery branch that penetrates the kidney in the inferior pole (Fig. 18.120a).

Precocious Bifurcation

Renal artery in which the main trunk has less than 1 cm in length before branching off (Fig. 18.120c).

When variations in the renal arteries exist, these vessels shall be named multiple arteries; the words "extra," "aberrant," and "accessory," should be avoided because these vessels are normal segmental end arteries, without anastomoses between them. Even the term "supernumerary" should not be used because it might imply that these vessels are superfluous.

The presence of the superior pole extrahilar branch (Fig. 18.119b) should not be considered an anatomic variation because this vessel is a ramification of the main trunk of the renal artery. Variations in the kidney arterial supply in 81 of the 266 pedicles analyzed (30.5%) were found. There was no significant statistical difference in arterial variations between right and left kidneys. In 12 cases (4.5%), an individual presented bilateral variation; among these, in five cases (1.9%), the variation was the same on both sides (Fig. 18.121).

A low incidence of multiple renal arteries in black subjects (0.17%) has been reported. Also, in individual cases, the number of multiple arteries (when present) tends to be greater in black subjects than in white subjects.

Renal Ectopy

Ectopic kidneys are rare, about 0.1% of the population. It is assumed that caudal ectopic kidneys have multiple arteries, but it is not always the case. The most common type of fused kidney is the horseshoe kidney but a variety of ectopic kidneys exist, including crossed ectopia, fused presacral kidney, and pelvic kidney. The vascular supply of these malformations is unpredictable. Multiple arteries originating from the lower aorta or pelvic arteries are usually present to supply the ectopic kidney (Figs. 18.122, 18.123).

Intrarenal Arteries

The main renal artery divides into an anterior and a posterior branch after giving off the inferior suprarenal artery. Whereas the posterior branch (retropelvic artery) proceeds as the posterior segmental artery to supply the homonymous segment without further significant branching, the anterior branch of the renal artery provides three or four segmental arteries. The renal artery branches are terminal vessels, and there is no anastomosis between the segmental arteries. These segmental arteries divide before entering the renal parenchyma into interlobular arteries (infundibular arteries), which progress adjacent to the caliceal infundibula and the minor calices, entering the renal columns between the renal pyramids (Figs. 18.124, 18.125, 18.126).

As the interlobar arteries progress, they give origin (usually by dichotomous division) to the arcuate arteries (Figs. 18.124, 18.125, 18.126). The arcuate arteries give off the interlobular arteries, which run to the periphery giving off the afferent arterioles of the glomeruli (Fig. 18.125). The afferent arteriole invaginates into the glomerular capsule (Bowman's), forming the glomerulus, from which an efferent arteriole leaves (Fig. 18.127). The complex formed by the glomerulus invaginated into the capsule is called renal corpuscle (Malpighi). In the renal corpuscle, one may identify a vascular pole (site where the afferent and efferent arterioles are located) and, in a diametrically opposite position, a urinary pole (site where the glomerular capsule narrows into a tube) (Fig. 18.127).

Because the division branches of the renal artery and the intrarenal distribution of these vessels varies, study of the isolated vessels has a limited practical value. An analysis considering the anatomic relationship between the intrarenal arteries and the kidney collecting system, and considering these relationships in the specific kidney regions, is useful. Moreover, the anatomic relationships between the arteries and the collecting system have a fairly constant pattern in the different kidney regions. Also, these relationships are independent of both the number and the arrangement of the arterial segments.

Material of Investigation

Eighty-two three-dimensional endocasts of the renal collecting system together with the intrarenal arteries, obtained from 41 fresh cadavers, of both sexes, who died of causes not related to the urinary tract, were studied.

A yellow polyester resin was injected into the ureter to fill the kidney collecting system and a red resin was injected into the main trunk of the renal artery to fill

the renal arterial tree, according to the proportions and technique described previously. For this research, only the kidneys presenting a single main renal were used.

To study the intrarenal arteries and their anatomic relationships to the collecting system, the arterial tree was injected to its full capacity to preserve the same spatial associations as existed in vivo. Because the polyester resin has low viscosity and consequently high penetration power, the injection reached the interlobular arteries, the afferent arterioles, the glomerular tufts, the efferent arterioles, and even the vasa recta. Therefore, after organic matter corrosion and washing of the injected specimen, the cast looks like a sponge (Fig. 18.128). The aspect of a sponge corresponds to glomeruli filled with resin. If one examines the cast under magnification, it is easy to identify the microcirculation of the kidney (Figs. 18.129, 18.130). The fine vessels and glomerular tufts were removed by needle hand picking, allowing clear visualization of the targeted arteries and the underlying collecting system (Fig. 18.131).

Findings

The findings were presented in relation to the pelvicaliceal system and considering the specific kidney regions.

Superior Pole

The superior segmental artery (apical) can have different origins, but it usually arises from the anterosuperior segmental artery, being positioned in the medial midline and progressing to the uppermost region of the superior pole. This artery often has a proximal origin, passes far from the upper infundibulum to reach the superior segment (apical) (Figs. 18.132a, 18.133) and is not related to the collecting system.

In 86.6% of cases (71 of 82 casts), the arterial supply related to the upper caliceal group arose from two arteries: one originated from the anterior division and the other from the posterior division of the renal artery. The upper caliceal group was involved by these two arterial trunks, which coursed alongside the anterior and posterior surfaces of the caliceal infundibulum (Fig. 18.132a,b). In the remaining 13.4% of cases (11 casts), these two arteries originated only from the anterior division or only from the posterior division of the renal artery.

Midzone (Hilar)

In all cases, the arterial supply to the anterior surface of the kidney midzone arose from the anterior division of the renal artery. Two possibilities may be found: in 64.6% (53 of 82 casts), there was one artery that coursed horizontally in the mid-renal pelvis (Figs. 18.134a, 18.135); the mid-kidney receives secondary division branches from arteries of other regions (Figs. 18.134b, 18.136). The relationship between the calices and the anterior artery varied amply and followed the caliceal variations, which are typical and large in the mid-kidney. One may predict the mid-kidney arterial vascularization through an intravenous pyelogram: if the mid-kidney caliceal drainage is independent of the superior and inferior caliceal groups, the mid-kidney usually has an individualized artery; in contrary, when the caliceal drainage is dependent on the superior and the inferior caliceal groups, the mid-kidney usually receives secondary division branches from arteries of other regions (Fig. 18.14 referring to veins).

Inferior Pole

In the inferior pole, two possibilities of arterial distribution may be found. In 62.2% of the cases (51 of 82 casts) the arterial supply to the inferior pole, both front and back, arose from the inferior segmental artery (Figs. 18.137, 18.138). This vessel, which originates from the anterior division of the main renal artery, passes in front of the ureteropelvic junction, and, after entering the inferior pole, divides into an anterior and a posterior branch. The anterior branch is related to the anterior surface of the lower infundibulum (Fig. 18.137a). The posterior branch progresses under the neck of the lower calyx to reach the posterior aspect of the kidney (Fig. 18.137 a,b). In these cases, the posterior segmental artery does not reach the lower infundibulum, leaving its posterior surface free from arteries (Fig. 18.137b). In this situation, both anterior and posterior aspects of the inferior pole are supplied by a single anterior artery (inferior segmental artery).

In the other 37.8% of cases (31 of 82 casts), the anterior branch arose from the inferior segmental artery and the posterior branch was an extension of the posterior segmental artery (retropelvic artery) (Figs. 18.139a,b, 18.140). In these cases, the anterior aspect of the inferior pole is supplied by the anterior branch and its posterior aspect is supplied by the posterior branch.

Dorsal Kidney

The dorsal kidney is supplied by the posterior segmental artery (retropelvic artery), which is a direct extension of the posterior division of the main renal artery. Within the kidney substance, the retropelvic artery usually describes an arc and from its convexity three constant subdivision branches emerge and may be identified (superior, middle and inferior; Figs. 18.141, 18.142). The superior branch is in close relationship to the posterior surface of the upper caliceal infundibulum. In some instances, the posterior segmental artery may give off two or even three superior branches related to the dorsal aspect of the superior

pole (Fig. 18.141). The middle branch supplies the middle portion of the posterior segment and may interdigitate with the anterior branches of the midkidney. The inferior branch is an extension of the retropelvic artery itself (Fig. 18.141). Its course and arrangement is dependent on the inferior vascularization, as described previously (Figs. 18.137, 18.139).

The posterior segmental artery itself was in close relationship to the upper infundibulum or to the junction of the pelvis with the upper calyx in 57.3% of the cases (Fig. 18.143a). In this situation, this artery usually described an arc that contacted the upper infundibulum (Fig. 18.143b). In the other 42.7% of cases, the posterior segmental artery coursed in the middle posterior surface of the renal pelvis (Fig. 18.143c).

Relationships to the Ureteropelvic Junction

In 53.7% of cases (44 of 82 casts), a close relationship between the inferior segmental artery and the anterior surface of the ureteropelvic junction (UPJ) was found, when this vessel passed this region to enter the inferior pole (Fig. 18.144a). Among these cases, there was one artery anterior and another artery posterior to the UPJ, simultaneously (Fig. 18.145). In the remaining 46.3% of cases (38 of 82 casts), the UPJ was not related to the arteries, either anteriorly or posteriorly (Figs. 18.144b, 18.146, 18.147).

Arterial Segmental Analysis

The independence between portions of an organ (segments) may be based on different structures, according to their specifically functional importance. Concerning the kidney, no branch of the renal artery anastomoses with another. Some of the primary and secondary branches of the renal artery have been called segmental arteries, and the zone supplied by these arteries being named renal segments. Since the intrarenal veins have no segmental organization and anastomoses freely, the segmentation of the kidney is mainly based on the arterial supply.

Besides a study of the arterial segmental arrangement, it is presented an analysis of the surface proportional area of each segment as measured on polyester resin endocasts of the kidney arterial vasculature.

Material of Investigation

Forty-nine three-dimensional endocasts of the intrarenal arterial tree obtained from 33 fresh cadavers of both sexes (cause of death not related to the urinary tract) were analyzed. In 16 subjects, the kidneys were studied bilaterally, and in 17 subjects, only one side was studied. For this study, only kidneys with a single renal artery were considered.

It is defined as a segmental artery a primary or a secondary branch of the main renal artery that can be identified and isolated outside the renal hilum. It is considered as posterior segmental artery (retropelvic artery) the posterior branch of the renal artery, not considering the subdivisions (branches) inside the renal parenchyma as segmental arteries.

A polyester resin (volume ranging from 2.0 to 6.0 ml) was injected into each segmental branch as just defined previously. The segments were injected with resins of different colors, corresponding to the following:

Posterior segment: red
Superior (apical) segment: brown
Anterosuperior segment: blue
Anteroinferior segment: white
Inferior segment: yellow

Two other possibilities existed: First, when the main artery to the apex of the kidney (superior segment) was a branch of the posterior segmental artery (retropelvic artery) the superior segment was injected with the same color as the posterior segment (red), because in these cases, both anatomically and functionally, the arterial supply of the kidney apex is dependent on the posterior segmental artery. Second, when the mid-kidney has only one segmental artery, the anterosuperior and the anteroinferior segments were fused in the anterior segment (this segment was injected with blue resin).

The possibilities of segmental arrangement are shown in Figures 18.148 and 18.149.

After the endocasts were obtained, they were positioned horizontally and their anterior and posterior sides were photographed (Fig. 18.150). A B-100 translucent Weuibel grid 11 was placed over the photographs to evaluate the surface area of each segment by using the "point-counting planimetry method" (Fig. 18.150). The B-100 grid presents 100 points, and each point is the geometric center of a square (Fig. 18.150c). If a B-100 translucent grid is superimposed on a photograph of a cast, one may evaluate the number of points that correspond to one surface of the cast (Fig. 18.150d). Because individual segments are injected with different colors, it is also possible to evaluate the number of points that correspond to each segment. Performing this technique for both sides and adding the results, one may achieve an estimated evaluation concerning the proportional area that each arterial segment represents in the whole kidney.

In this work, just the absolute values in percentage were used, that is, the number of points on each side of the cast (anterior and posterior) were evaluated. After adding these results, the number of points that represent the whole kidney (100.0%) was obtained. Afterward, the number of points for each segment on both sides was evaluated by using a single rule of three. The proportional area of each segment was determined.

For example: The whole kidney (anterior and posterior surfaces) corresponds to 85 points. The inferior segment (anterior and posterior surfaces) corresponds to 27 points.

Thus:

85 points (whole kidney) = 100.0%
27 points (inferior segment) = X

$$X = \frac{100 \times 27}{85} = 31.8\% \text{ (inferior segment)}$$

Findings: The bifurcation of the main renal artery into an anterior and a posterior branch was found in all cases of kidneys with a single artery. The anterior branch usually had greater caliber than the posterior branch.

In 61.2% of cases (30 of 49 casts), kidneys with five arterial segments (Fig. 18.151a,b) were found; and in 38.8% of cases (19 of 49 casts), we found kidneys with four arterial segments (Fig. 18.151c,d).

Superior Segment (Apical)

The superior segmental artery usually has an extrahilar origin. In 73.5% of cases (36 of 49 casts), this artery arose from the anterior division of the main renal artery and in 26.5% of the cases (13 of 49 casts) from its anterior division (posterior segmental artery). When the main artery to the apex of the kidney (superior segment) was a branch of the posterior segmental artery (retropelvic artery), we did not consider the superior segment as independent and it was included with the posterior segment. When the superior segment existed independently (Fig. 18.151) its area varied from 1.84 to 27.02% of the total kidney area (mean: 13.02%).

Anterosuperior Segment

In 61.2% of cases (30 of 49 casts), an anterosuperior segment (Fig. 18.151a,b) was found. Its area varied from 5.17 to 34.22% of the total kidney area (mean: 21.36%).

Anteroinferior Segment

The anteroinferior segment (Fig. 18.151a,b) was also found in 61.2% of cases (30 of 49 casts), and its area varied from 1.29 to 25.8% of the total kidney area (mean: 17.18%).

Anterior Segment

In 38.8% of cases (19 of 49 casts), there was only one segmental artery to the mid-kidney; the anterosuperior and the anteroinferior segments being fused as the anterior segment (Fig. 18.151c,d). When the anterior segment existed, its area varied from 16.57 to 42.95% of the total kidney area (mean: 28.44%).

Inferior Segment

The inferior segment was found in 100.0% of the cases (Fig. 18.151). Its area varied from 7.42 to 38.18% of the total kidney area (mean: 22.65%).

Posterior Segment

Just as with the inferior segment, the posterior segment was found in 100.0% of the specimens studied (Fig. 18.152). Its area varied from 14.57 to 52.93% of the total kidney area (mean: 33.76%).

The posterior segment, supplied by the posterior segmental artery (called retropelvic artery), presented the greatest median value of proportional area (33.76%) and also the greatest maximum value of proportional area, comprehending up to 52.93% of the total kidney area (Fig. 18.152b). This knowledge is important because it demonstrates the significance of the posterior segmental artery.

Capsular and Perirenal Collateral Circulation

The renal capsular arterial system is composed of three basic pathways: superior, medial, and inferior capsular arteries (Figs. 18.153, 18.154). These vessels usually arise from or together with the adrenal arteries. It may also originate from the main renal artery or from the gonadal artery.

The superior capsular artery usually arises from the inferior adrenal artery, or from the main renal artery or a branch. It may also originate from the inferior phrenic artery, from the aorta or a superior polar artery.

The middle capsular artery arises from the renal artery or its main branches at the renal hilum.

The inferior capsular artery is uncommonly observed, but usually arises from the gonadal artery or from an inferior polar artery.

There is a number of perforating capsular arteries arising from arcuate and interlobular arteries, connecting the intrarenal circulation with the larger capsular arteries. The perforating capsular arteries are usually small and enlarge only when advanced nephropathy or arterial occlusion is encountered.

The pelvic arteries are small and difficult to observe either angiographically or at dissection. When there is renal artery occlusive disease, they may enlarge and may be observed as tortuous small vessels. The ureteric and pelvicoureteric arteries are also small and originate from the main renal artery or from its main branches. It may also arise from the gonadal artery.

Testicular and Ovarian Artery

The testicular and ovarian arteries arise anterolaterally from the abdominal aorta (Fig. 18.1), following a descending path, anterior to the inferior vena cava and parallel to the gonadal vein, anteriorly to the ureter in the right side, and posterior to the left gonadal vein at the beginning, but anterior to the left ureter (Figs. 18.153, 18.155). The gonadal artery may arise from an inferior polar renal artery (Fig. 18.156) and may send branches to the ureter. Both testicular arteries pass the deep inguinal ring to enter the sper-matic cord, traversing the inguinal canal into the scrotum. At the posterosuperior aspect of the testis, two branches are found on its medial and lateral surfaces, which form the tunica vasculosa after ramifying (Fig. 18.157). The ureter, the perirenal fat and iliac lymph nodes, and the cremaster muscle are arterialized by the testicular artery. The ovarian arteries correspond to the testicular arteries, but follow a different path in the pelvis, to supply the ovaries, reaching the uterine broad ligament. Some branches of the gonadal artery supply the ureters, the uterine tubes and have anastomoses with the uterine artery.

DORSAL BRANCHES

Lumbar Arteries

There are usually four lumbar arteries in each side, arising from the posterior aspect of the abdominal aorta. A smaller 5th pair of lumbar arteries may arise from the middle sacral artery, but lumbar branches of the iliolumbar arteries are usually in their place. These arteries follow a posterior path over the lumbar vertebral bodies, continuing in the posterior abdominal wall (Fig. 18.1). They anastomose with one another (Fig. 18.158) and with the lower posterior intercostal, subcostal, iliolumbar, deep circumflex iliac and inferior epigastric arteries (Figs. 18.159, 18.160, 18.161).

Branches

Dorsal ramus
Spinal branches
Muscular branches

The dorsal ramus of the lumbar arteries supply the dorsal muscles, joints, and skin (Figs. 18.159, 18.160).

The spinal branches of the dorsal ramus enter the spinal canal to supply its structures and adjacent vertebras. They anastomose with arteries from above and from below, crossing the midline. The spinal branch of the 1st lumbar artery supplies the terminal spinal cord, the others the cauda equina, meninges and the vertebral canal.

Muscular branches of the dorsal rami supply the adjacent muscles, fascia, bones, red marrow, ligaments, and joints (Fig. 18.161).

Median Sacral Artery

This is a small posterior branch of the abdominal aorta, arising from the aorta above its bifurcation, that descends in the middle line, anterior to the 4th and 5th lumbar vertebra, sacrum and coccyx. There are anastomoses with the rectum, lumbar branches of the iliolumbar artery, and the lateral sacral arteries (Fig. 18.160).

TERMINAL BRANCHES

Common Iliac Arteries

The abdominal aorta bifurcates at the level of the 4th lumbar vertebra, into two arteries, called right and left common iliac arteries, that supply the pelvis and lower extremities. The common iliac arteries divide into the external iliac artery, which is in straight line with the axis of the common iliac artery, and the internal iliac artery, which is a posteromedial branch.

In addition to the terminal branches, the common iliac arteries give branches to the surrounding tissues, peritoneum, psoas muscle, ureter and nerves. Occasional branches are the iliolumbar and accessory renal arteries for topic or ectopic kidneys.

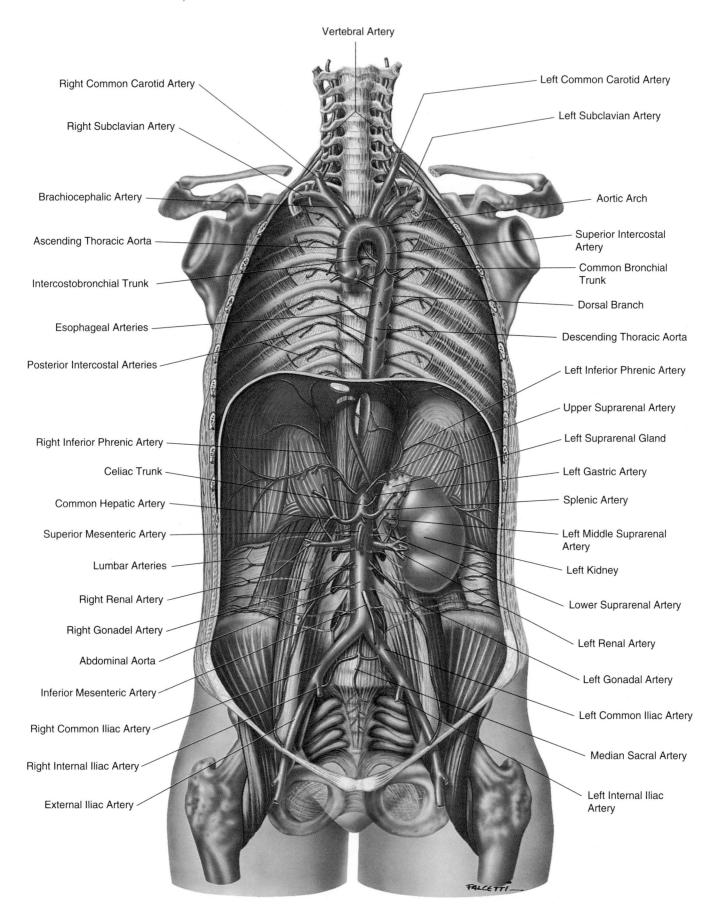

Vertebral Artery

Right Common Carotid Artery

Right Subclavian Artery

Brachiocephalic Artery

Ascending Thoracic Aorta

Intercostobronchial Trunk

Esophageal Arteries

Posterior Intercostal Arteries

Right Inferior Phrenic Artery

Celiac Trunk

Common Hepatic Artery

Superior Mesenteric Artery

Lumbar Arteries

Right Renal Artery

Right Gonadel Artery

Abdominal Aorta

Inferior Mesenteric Artery

Right Common Iliac Artery

Right Internal Iliac Artery

External Iliac Artery

Left Common Carotid Artery

Left Subclavian Artery

Aortic Arch

Superior Intercostal Artery

Common Bronchial Trunk

Dorsal Branch

Descending Thoracic Aorta

Left Inferior Phrenic Artery

Upper Suprarenal Artery

Left Suprarenal Gland

Left Gastric Artery

Splenic Artery

Left Middle Suprarenal Artery

Left Kidney

Lower Suprarenal Artery

Left Renal Artery

Left Gonadal Artery

Left Common Iliac Artery

Median Sacral Artery

Left Internal Iliac Artery

Figure 18.1. Schematic drawing of the thoracic and abdominal aorta and branches.

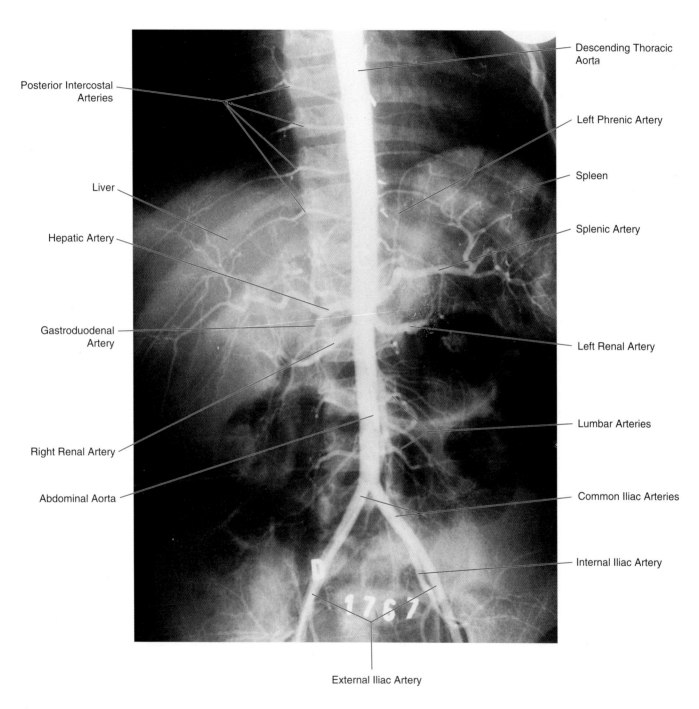

Posterior Intercostal
Arteries

Liver

Hepatic Artery

Gastroduodenal
Artery

Right Renal Artery

Abdominal Aorta

Descending Thoracic
Aorta

Left Phrenic Artery

Spleen

Splenic Artery

Left Renal Artery

Lumbar Arteries

Common Iliac Arteries

Internal Iliac Artery

External Iliac Artery

Figure 18.2. Angiography of the thoracoabdominal aorta and the main branches.

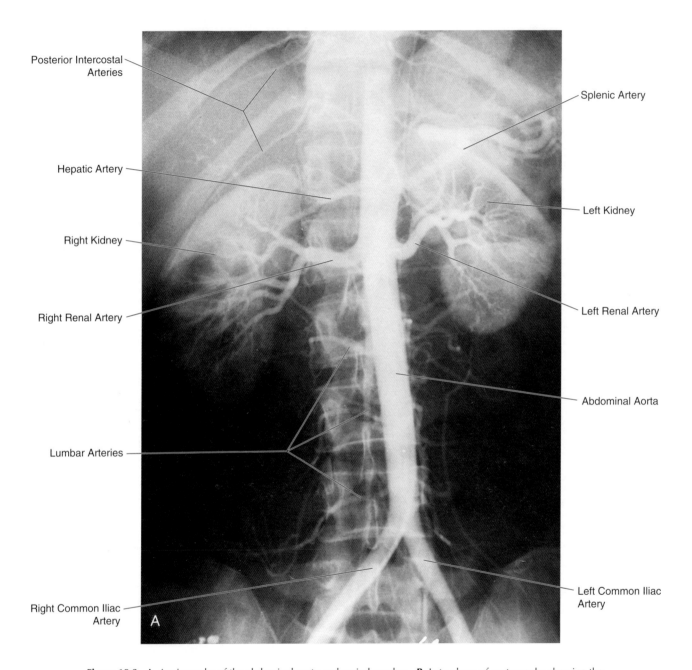

Posterior Intercostal Arteries

Splenic Artery

Hepatic Artery

Left Kidney

Right Kidney

Right Renal Artery

Left Renal Artery

Abdominal Aorta

Lumbar Arteries

Left Common Iliac Artery

Right Common Iliac Artery

A

Figure 18.3. A. Angiography of the abdominal aorta and main branches. **B.** Late phase of aortography showing the bilateral nephrogram and contrast enhancement of the adrenal glands.

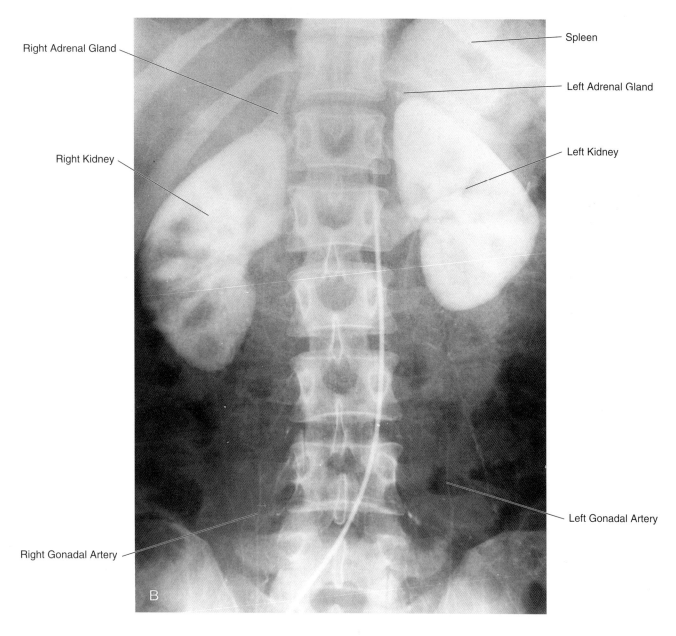

Figure 18.3. *Continued*

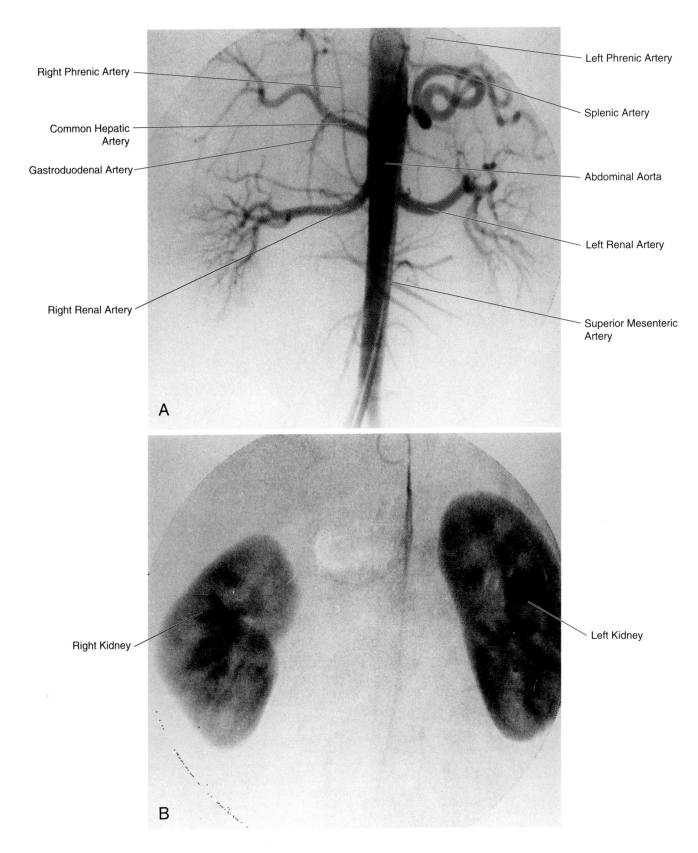

Right Phrenic Artery

Common Hepatic Artery

Gastroduodenal Artery

Right Renal Artery

Left Phrenic Artery

Splenic Artery

Abdominal Aorta

Left Renal Artery

Superior Mesenteric Artery

A

Right Kidney

Left Kidney

B

Figure 18.4. A. Angiography of the abdominal aorta on digital subtraction. Note the relationship of the renal arteries and the origin of the celiac trunk and superior mesenteric artery. **B.** Late phase of the aortography showing bilateral nephrogram.

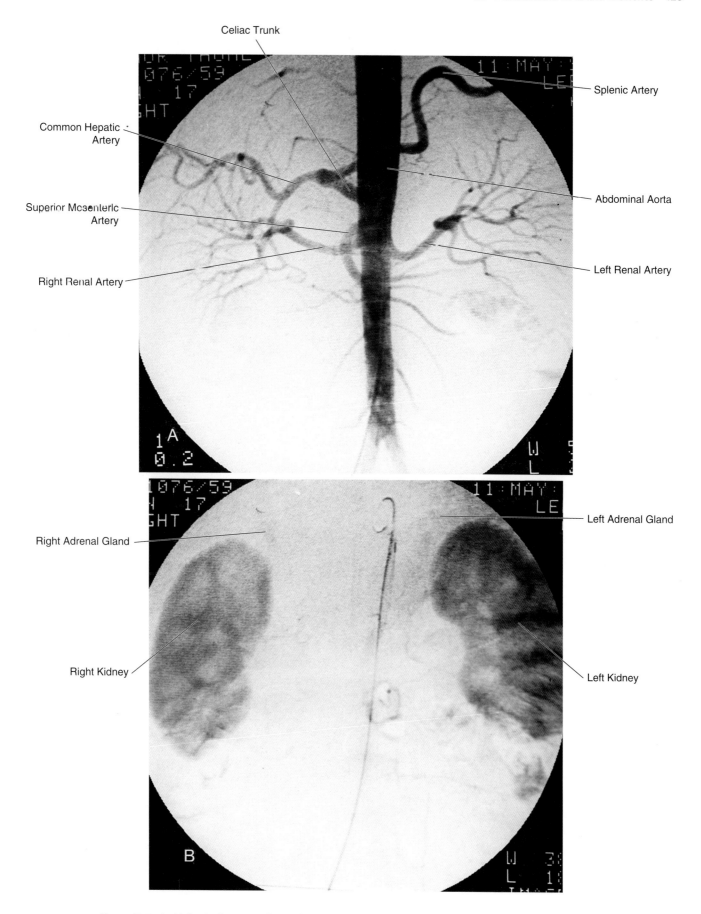

Figure 18.5. A. Abdominal aortography on digital subtraction. **B.** Late phase showing the bilateral nephrogram.

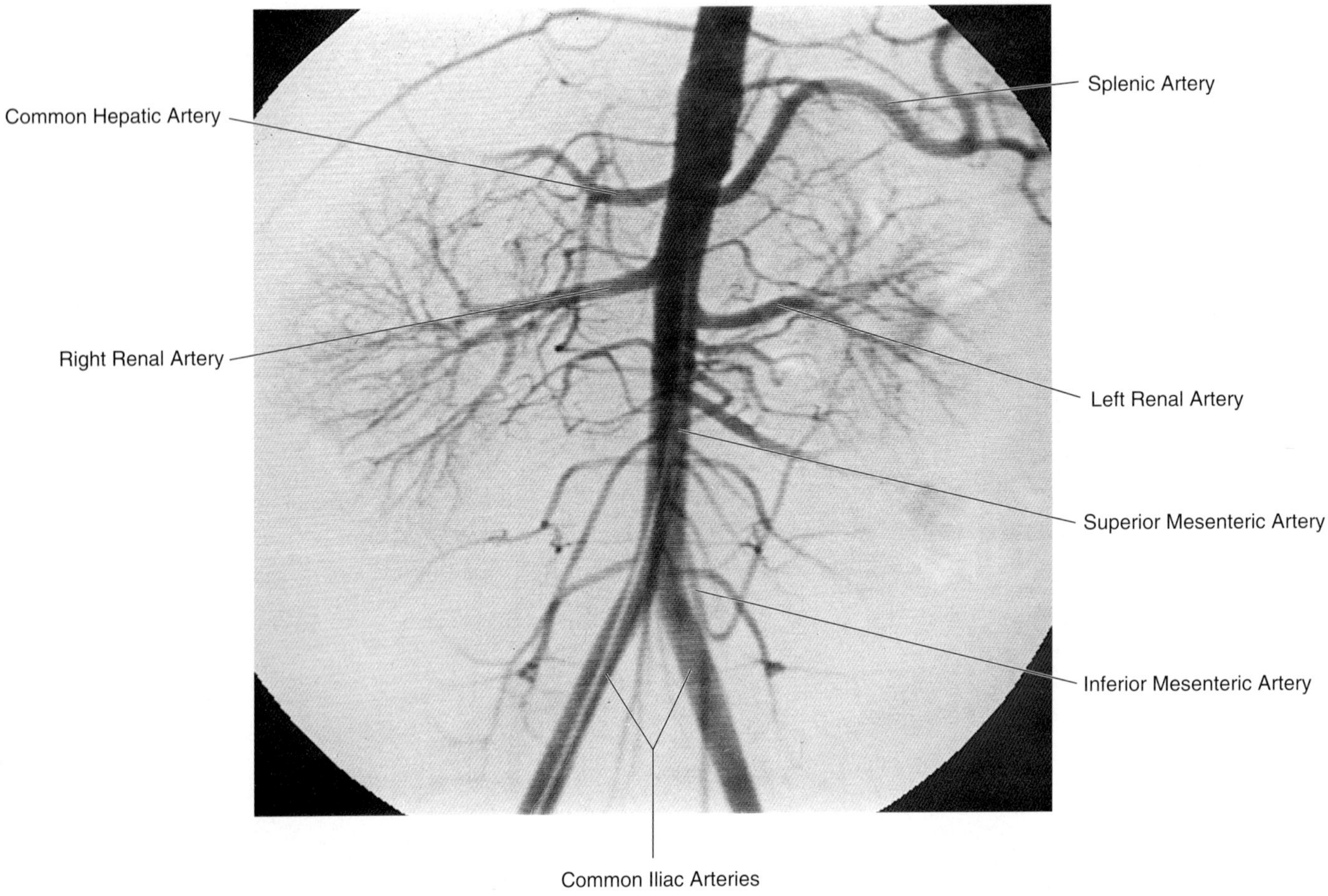

Common Hepatic Artery

Right Renal Artery

Splenic Artery

Left Renal Artery

Superior Mesenteric Artery

Inferior Mesenteric Artery

Common Iliac Arteries

Figure 18.6. Abdominal aortography.

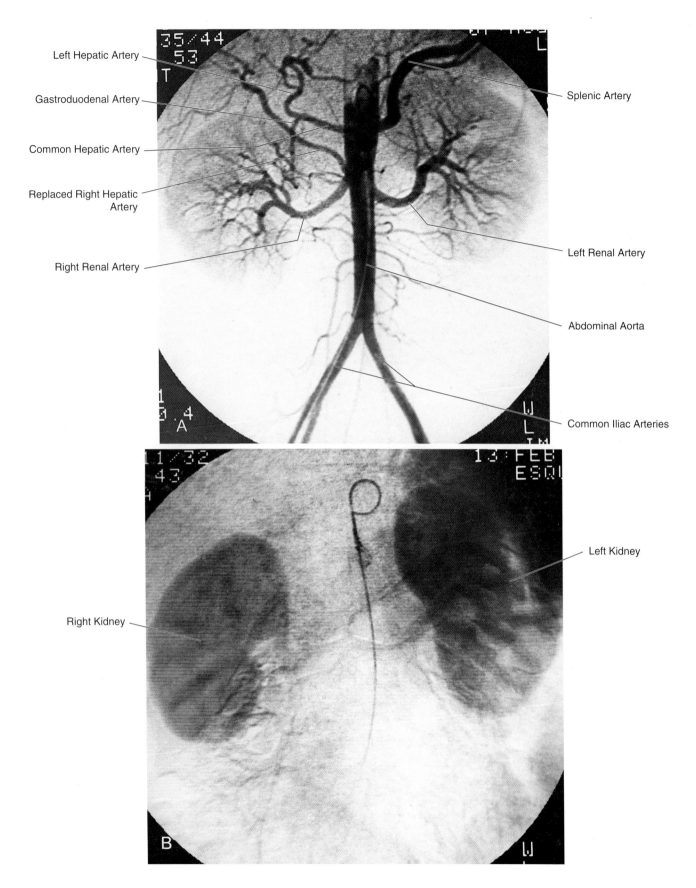

Left Hepatic Artery

Gastroduodenal Artery

Common Hepatic Artery

Replaced Right Hepatic Artery

Right Renal Artery

Splenic Artery

Left Renal Artery

Abdominal Aorta

Common Iliac Arteries

Right Kidney

Left Kidney

Figure 18.7. A. Abdominal aortography. **B.** Late phase showing the bilateral nephrogram.

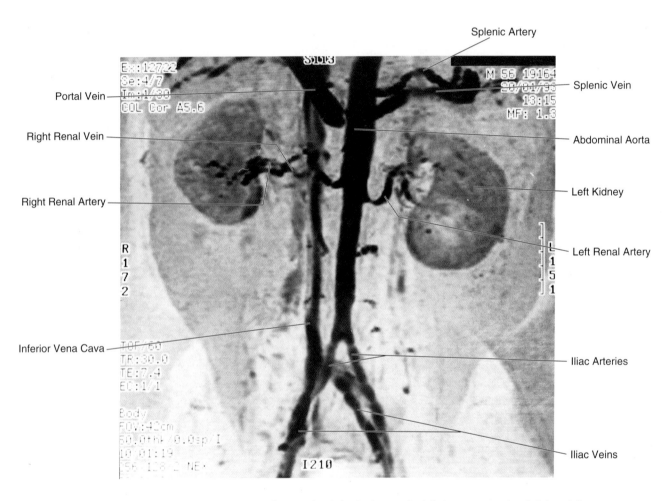

Figure 18.8. Magnetic resonance imaging showing the abdominal aorta, the inferior vena cava (partially), and the portal and splenic veins.

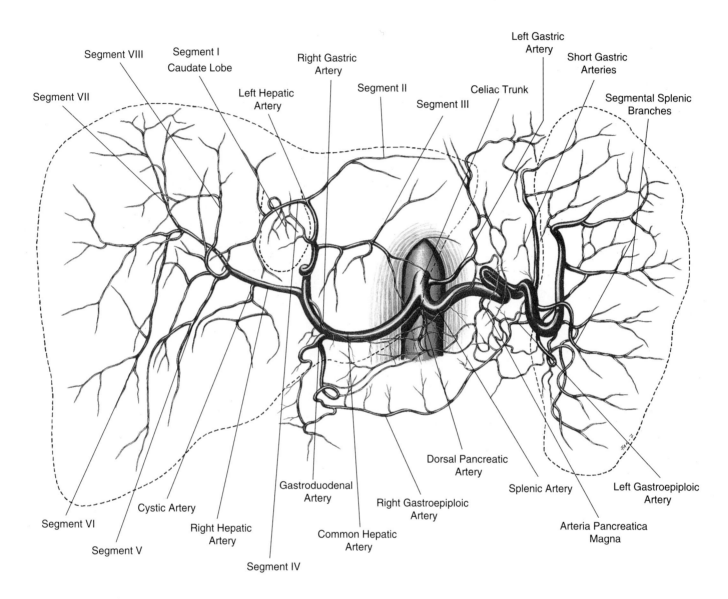

Figure 18.9. Schematic drawing of the celiac trunk, showing the hepatic arteries, segments (Couinaud), gastric and splenic circulation. Based on a real angiogram.

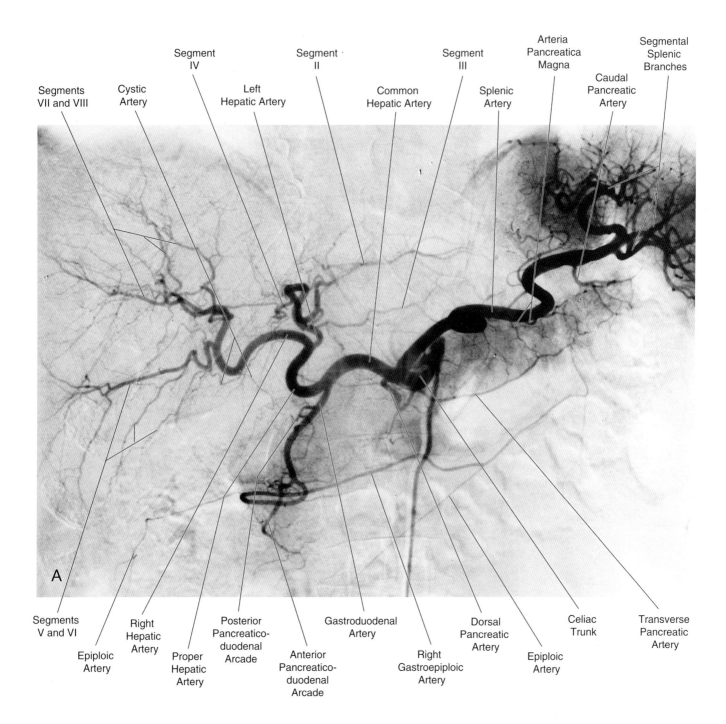

Figure 18.10. A. Selective angiogram of the celiac trunk, showing the hepatic circulation, gastric, pancreatic and splenic circulation. The pattern presented here is the most common and present in about 40 to 50% of the population. **B.** Late phase of the angiogram showing the splenic and portal veins, as well as the splenic blush and the hepatic blush.

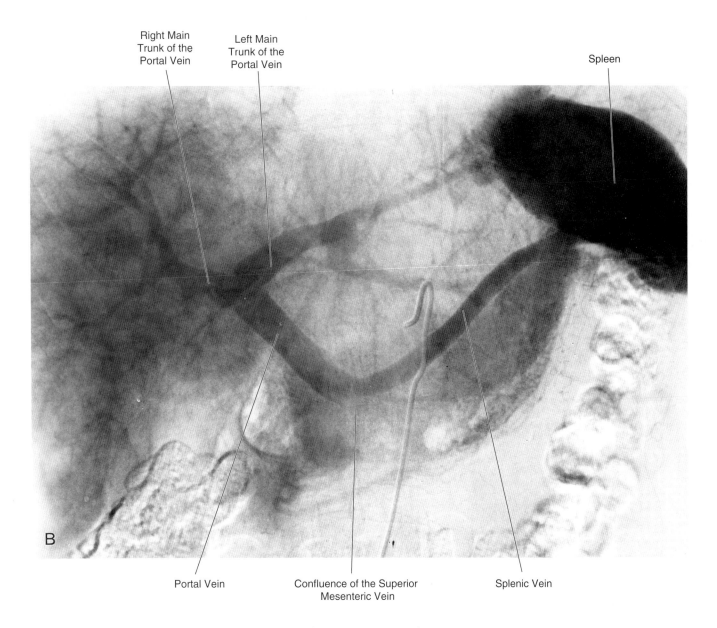

Right Main
Trunk of the
Portal Vein

Left Main
Trunk of the
Portal Vein

Spleen

B

Portal Vein

Confluence of the Superior
Mesenteric Vein

Splenic Vein

Figure 18.10. *Continued*

Left Hepatic Artery   Left Gastric Artery   Splenic Artery

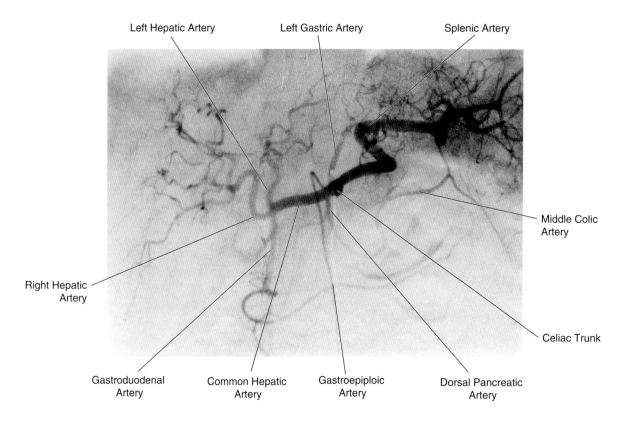

Right Hepatic
Artery

Middle Colic
Artery

Celiac Trunk

Gastroduodenal
Artery

Common Hepatic
Artery

Gastroepiploic
Artery

Dorsal Pancreatic
Artery

Figure 18.11. Selective angiogram of the celiac trunk, showing absence of the proper hepatic artery, due to the tri-furcation of the common hepatic artery into the right and left hepatic arteries and the gastroduodenal artery. Note that the dorsal pancreatic artery originates the middle colic artery.

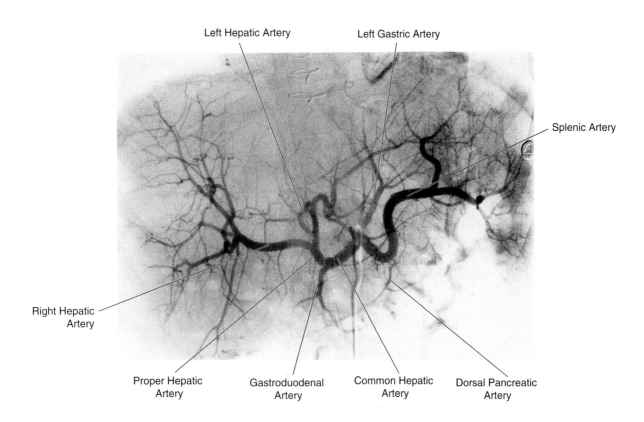

Figure 18.12. Selective angiogram of the celiac trunk, showing normal distribution of the hepatic and splenic arteries. This is an example of a horizontal celiac trunk.

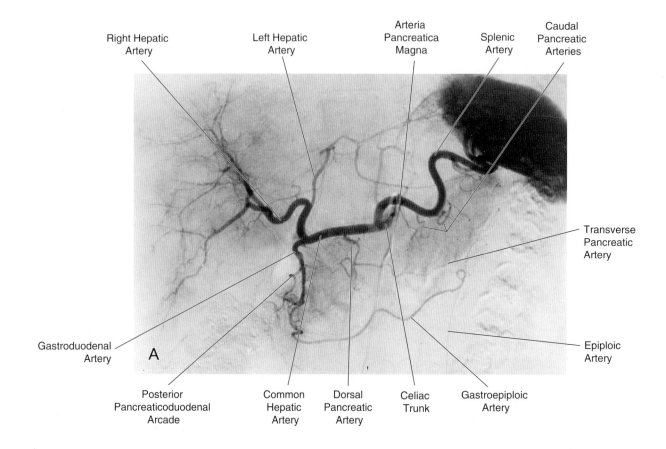

Right Hepatic Artery

Left Hepatic Artery

Arteria Pancreatica Magna

Splenic Artery

Caudal Pancreatic Arteries

Transverse Pancreatic Artery

Gastroduodenal Artery

A

Epiploic Artery

Posterior Pancreaticoduodenal Arcade

Common Hepatic Artery

Dorsal Pancreatic Artery

Celiac Trunk

Gastroepiploic Artery

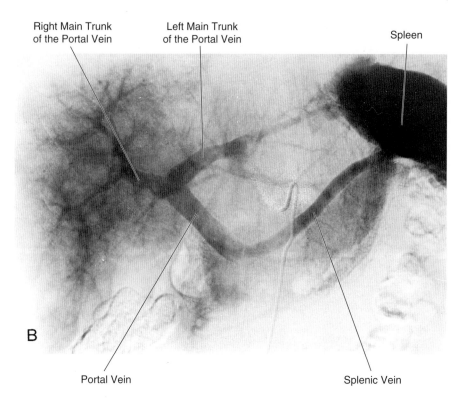

Right Main Trunk of the Portal Vein

Left Main Trunk of the Portal Vein

Spleen

B

Portal Vein

Splenic Vein

Figure 18.13. A. Selective angiogram of the celiac trunk, showing normal distribution of the arteries. The celiac artery is caudally oriented. **B.** Normal splenic and portal vein.

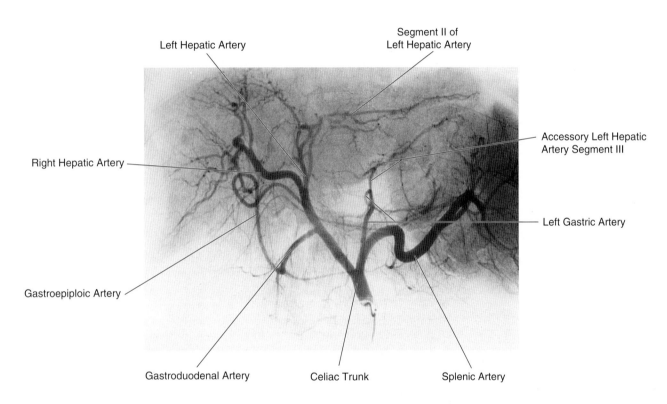

Left Hepatic Artery

Segment II of
Left Hepatic Artery

Right Hepatic Artery

Accessory Left Hepatic
Artery Segment III

Left Gastric Artery

Gastroepiploic Artery

Gastroduodenal Artery

Celiac Trunk

Splenic Artery

Figure 18.14. Selective angiogram of the celiac trunk, showing a cranial orientation. The distribution of the
arteries is of the most common pattern.

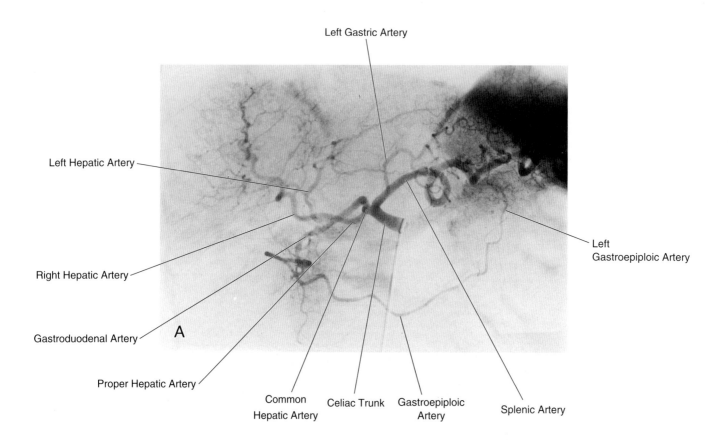

Left Gastric Artery

Left Hepatic Artery

Right Hepatic Artery

Gastroduodenal Artery

Left
Gastroepiploic Artery

A

Proper Hepatic Artery

Common
Hepatic Artery

Celiac Trunk

Gastroepiploic
Artery

Splenic Artery

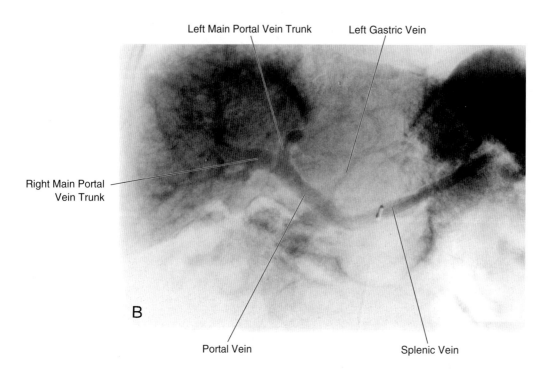

Left Main Portal Vein Trunk

Left Gastric Vein

Right Main Portal
Vein Trunk

B

Portal Vein

Splenic Vein

Figure 18.15. A. Angiogram of the celiac trunk, showing absence of the common hepatic artery. The gastroduodenal artery arises directly from the bifurcation of the celiac trunk. The proper hepatic artery divides into the right and left hepatic arteries. **B.** Late phase of the angiogram showing the normal splenic and hepatic veins.

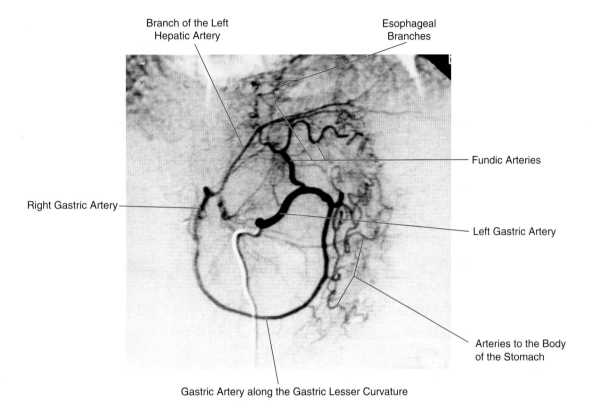

Branch of the Left
Hepatic Artery

Esophageal
Branches

Fundic Arteries

Right Gastric Artery

Left Gastric Artery

Arteries to the Body
of the Stomach

Gastric Artery along the Gastric Lesser Curvature

Figure 18.16. Selective injection at the left gastric artery. Note the gastric arteries at the fundus and body of the stomach. The left gastric artery anastomoses with the right hepatic artery and courses along the lesser curvature of the stomach. Note partial filling of the left hepatic artery.

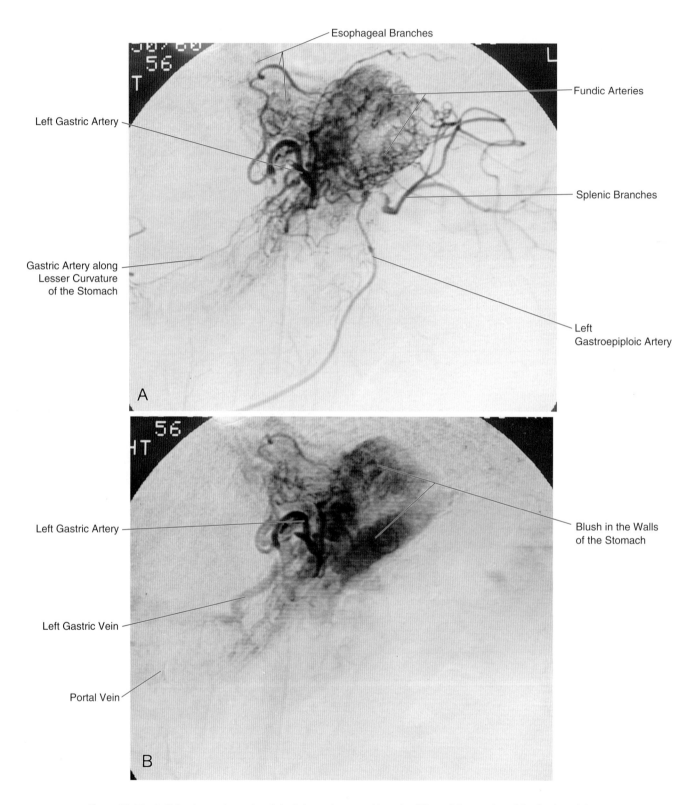

Esophageal Branches

Fundic Arteries

Left Gastric Artery

Splenic Branches

Gastric Artery along
Lesser Curvature
of the Stomach

Left
Gastroepiploic Artery

A

Left Gastric Artery

Blush in the Walls
of the Stomach

Left Gastric Vein

Portal Vein

B

Figure 18.17. A. Selective angiography of the left gastric artery. Note the filling of the arteries of the fundus of the
stomach and the anastomoses with the splenic arteries, as well as filling of the left gastroepiploic artery. **B.** Later
phase of the left gastric artery injection, showing blush at the gastric wall and filling of the drainage veins,
especially the left gastric vein.

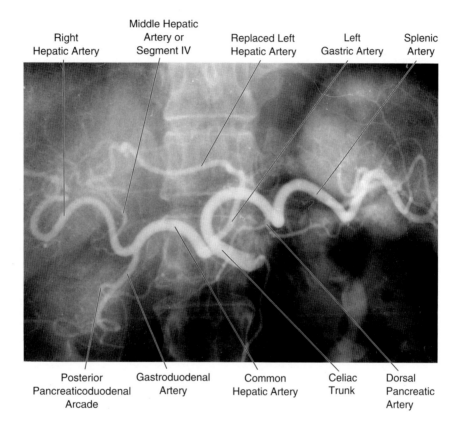

Right
Hepatic Artery

Middle Hepatic
Artery or
Segment IV

Replaced Left
Hepatic Artery

Left
Gastric Artery

Splenic
Artery

Posterior
Pancreaticoduodenal
Arcade

Gastroduodenal
Artery

Common
Hepatic Artery

Celiac
Trunk

Dorsal
Pancreatic
Artery

Figure 18.18. Selective injection on the celiac trunk showing the normal bifurcation, with distal origin of the left gastric artery giving rise to the left hepatic
artery. There is a "middle hepatic artery" or the artery to segment IV arising
from the proximal right hepatic artery. The splenic artery is long and tortuous.
There is no visible dorsal pancreatic artery and the circulation of the body and
tail of the pancreas is done mainly by the arteria pancreatica magna.

Replaced Left
Hepatic Artery

Left Gastric Artery

Splenic Artery

Right Hepatic Artery

Gastroduodenal Artery

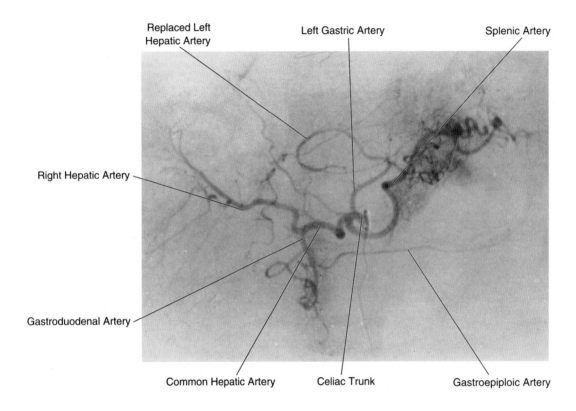

Common Hepatic Artery

Celiac Trunk

Gastroepiploic Artery

Figure 18.19. Injection at the celiac trunk, showing normal bifurcation, but with an enlarged left gastric artery giving origin to the left hepatic artery. The artery to the segment IV originates from the right hepatic artery. The splenic artery is long and tortuous. The pancreatic tail is partially stained by the contrast.

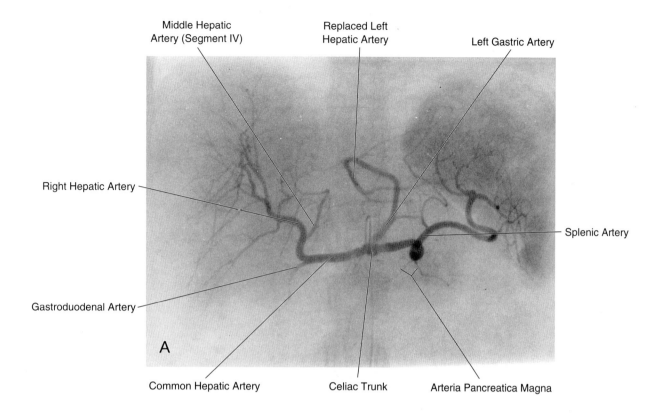

Middle Hepatic
Artery (Segment IV)

Replaced Left
Hepatic Artery

Left Gastric Artery

Right Hepatic Artery

Splenic Artery

Gastroduodenal Artery

A

Common Hepatic Artery

Celiac Trunk

Arteria Pancreatica Magna

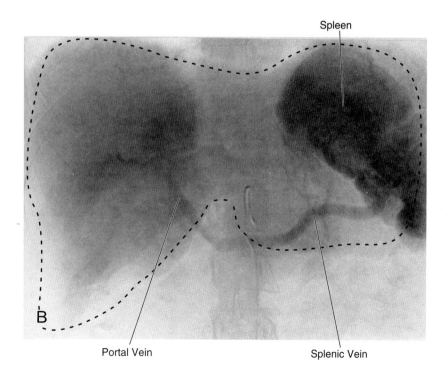

Spleen

B

Portal Vein

Splenic Vein

Figure 18.20. A. Selective injection at the celiac trunk showing an horizontal celiac trunk, with the left hepatic artery arising from the left gastric artery. The artery to segment IV is a branch of the right hepatic artery. **B.** Late phase of the celiac injection showing the patent splenic and portal vein. Note the laminar flow into the portal vein. **C.** Late phase of a SMA injection showing the superior mesenteric vein and the intrahepatic portal vein. The segments can be individualized. The segment V has a specific branch originating from the main portal vein.

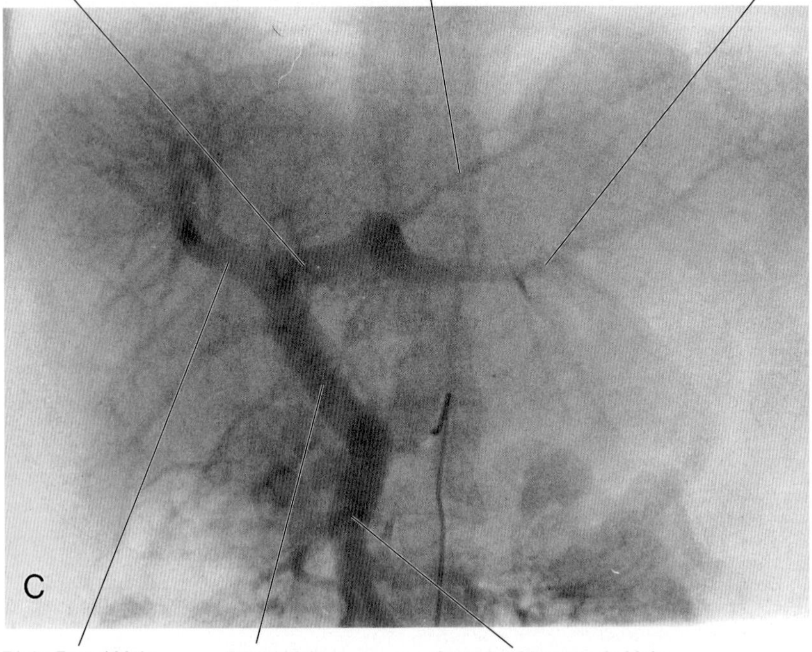

Figure 18.20. *Continued*

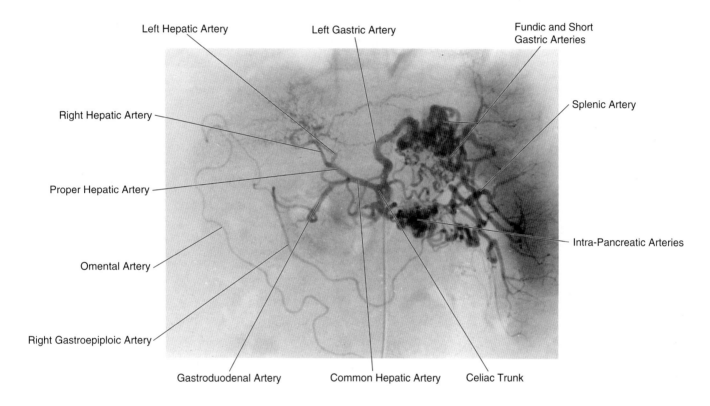

Figure 18.21. Celiac injection showing occlusion of the splenic artery and development of the collateral circulation through the Left gastric artery, gastric fundus arteries, short gastric arteries and with filling of the splenic artery at the hilum. There are some collateralization through pancreatic arteries on the tail and body of the pancreas, through the dorsal pancreatic artery.

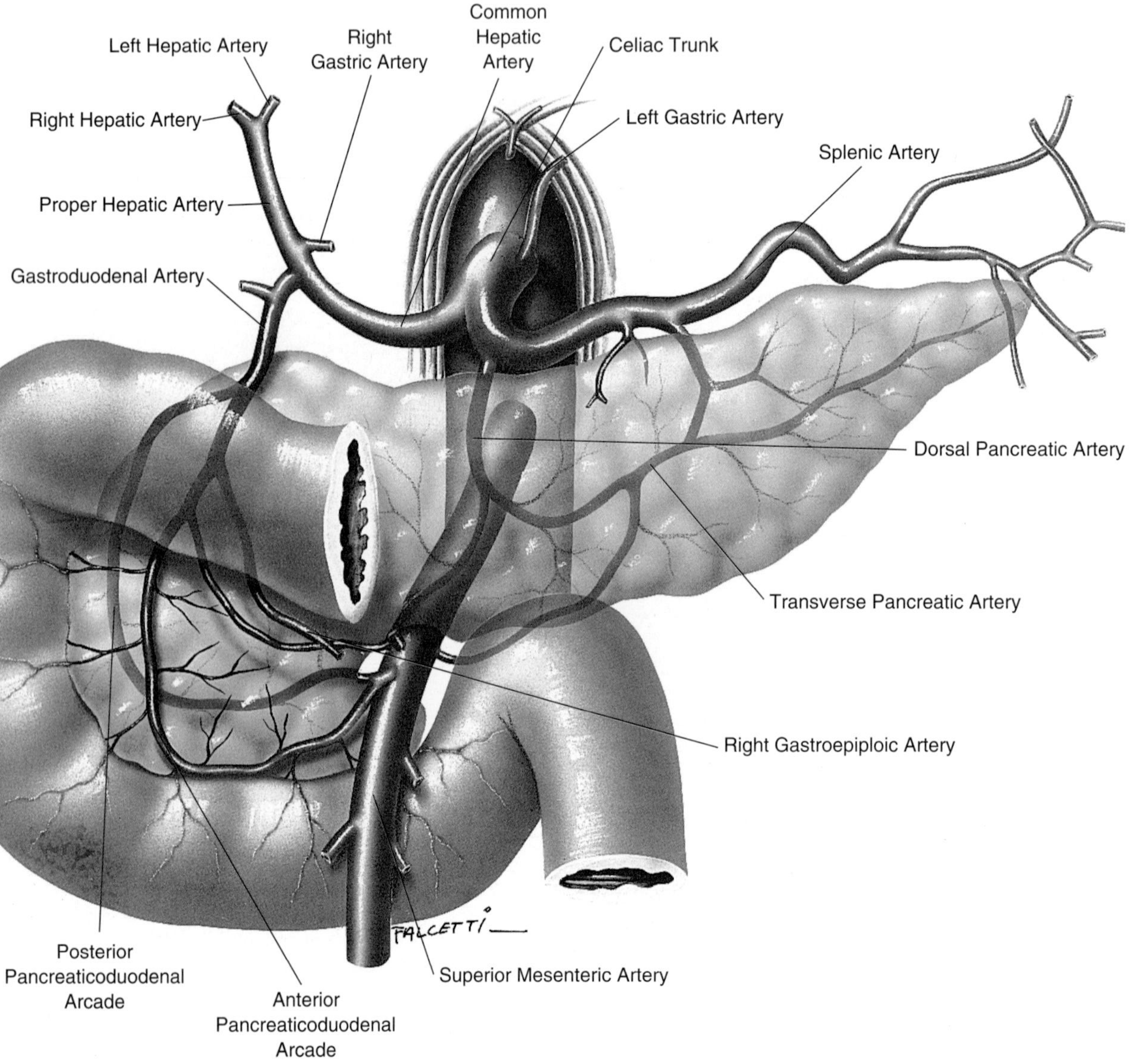

Figure 18.22. Schematic drawing of the celiac artery and branches to the duodenum, pancreas and connections with the superior mesenteric artery.

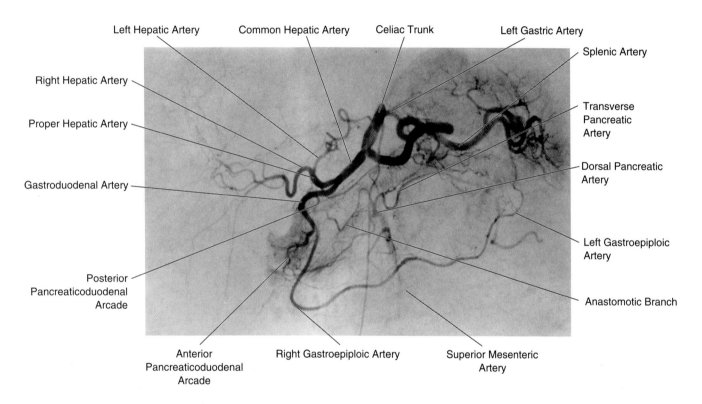

Figure 18.23. Celiac artery angiography showing the normal distribution of the main branches, the pancreatic branches and the gastric and duodenal branches.

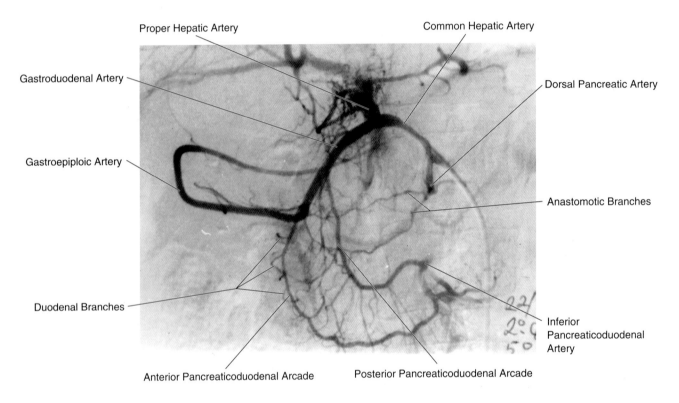

Proper Hepatic Artery

Common Hepatic Artery

Gastroduodenal Artery

Dorsal Pancreatic Artery

Gastroepiploic Artery

Anastomotic Branches

Duodenal Branches

Inferior Pancreaticoduodenal Artery

Anterior Pancreaticoduodenal Arcade

Posterior Pancreaticoduodenal Arcade

Figure 18.24. Selective injection at the gastroduodenal artery, showing the duodenal and pancreatic head branches. The proper hepatic artery is occluded. The dorsal pancreatic artery is a branch of the common hepatic artery and is retrograde filled.

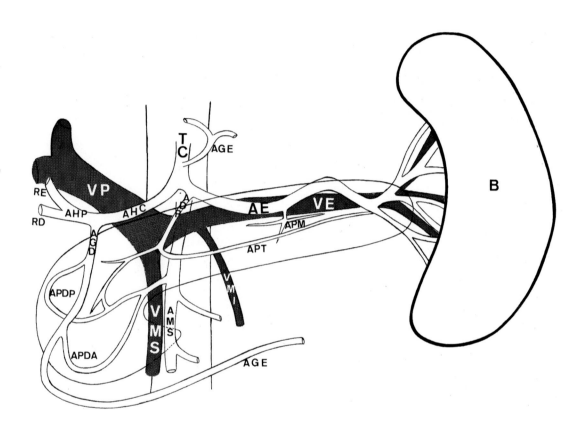

Figure 18.25. Schematic drawing of the pancreatic and celiac branches.

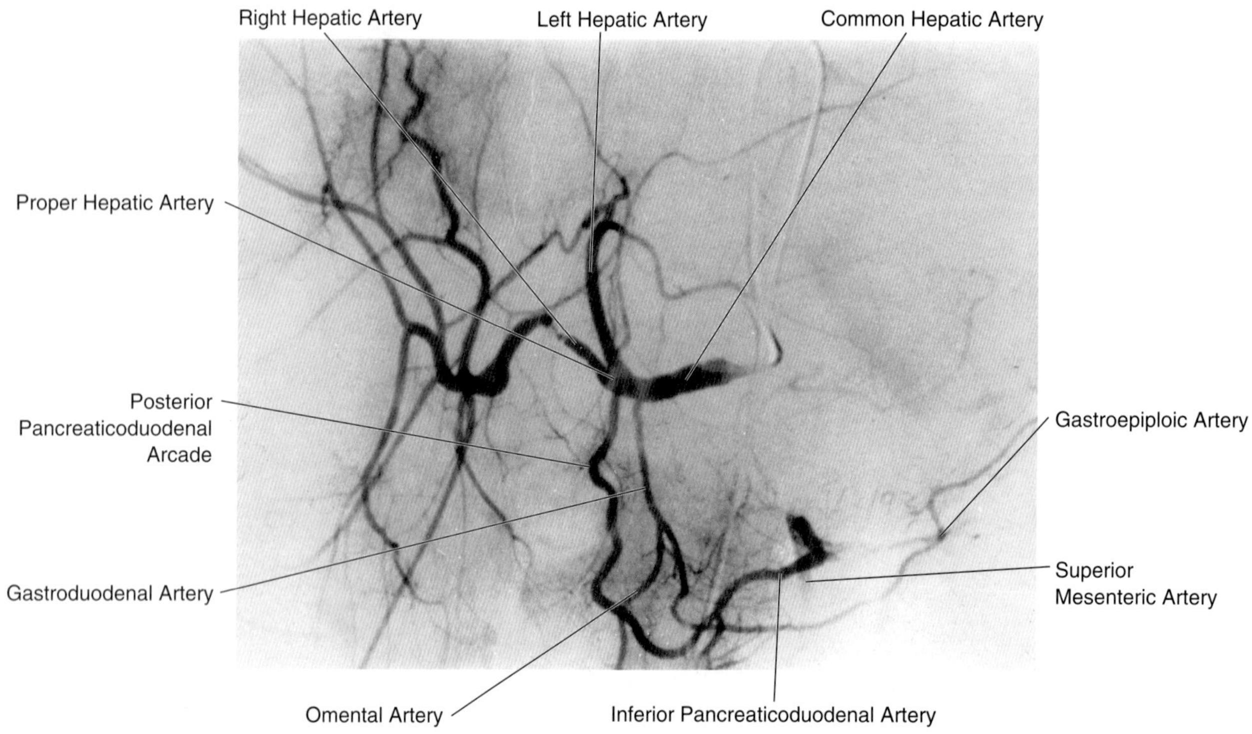

Figure 18.26. Selective angiography of the common hepatic artery showing the duplicated gastroduodenal artery of direct origin of the pancreaticoduodenal arcades from the common hepatic artery. Note significant spasm of the right hepatic artery. There is filling of the inferior pancreatic artery and a small part of the superior mesenteric artery.

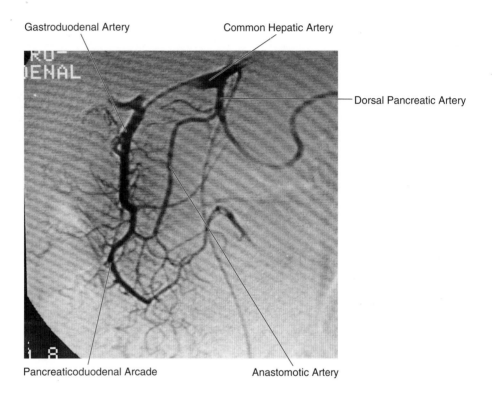

Figure 18.27. Selective angiography at the gastroduodenal artery, showing the pancreaticoduodenal arcades and the anastomosis with the dorsal pancreatic artery and filling of the inferior pancreatic artery.

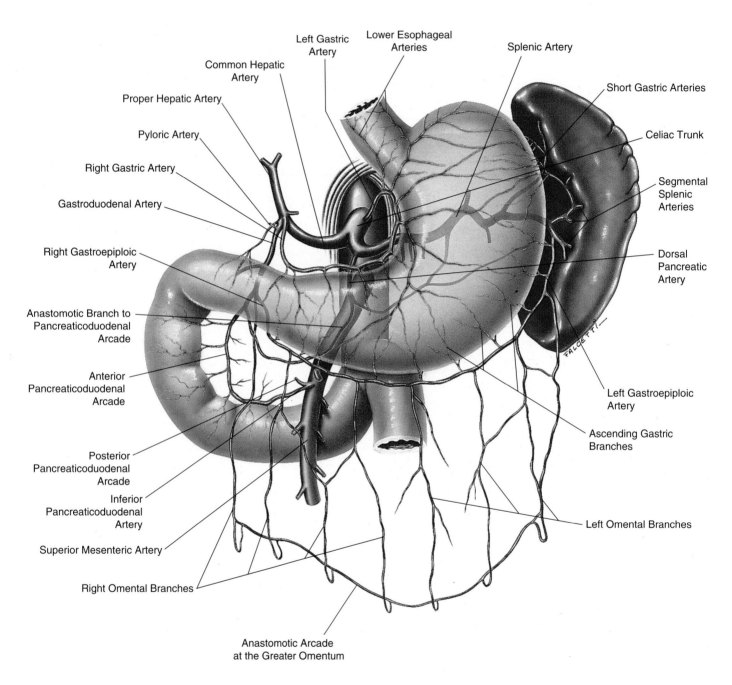

Left Gastric
Artery

Lower Esophageal
Arteries

Splenic Artery

Common Hepatic
Artery

Short Gastric Arteries

Proper Hepatic Artery

Celiac Trunk

Pyloric Artery

Segmental
Splenic
Arteries

Right Gastric Artery

Gastroduodenal Artery

Dorsal
Pancreatic
Artery

Right Gastroepiploic
Artery

Anastomotic Branch to
Pancreaticoduodenal
Arcade

Left Gastroepiploic
Artery

Anterior
Pancreaticoduodenal
Arcade

Ascending Gastric
Branches

Posterior
Pancreaticoduodenal
Arcade

Inferior
Pancreaticoduodenal
Artery

Left Omental Branches

Superior Mesenteric Artery

Right Omental Branches

Anastomotic Arcade
at the Greater Omentum

Figure 18.28. Schematic drawing showing the arterial circulation of the duodenum, stomach, spleen and greater
omentum, as well as the anastomotic collaterals.

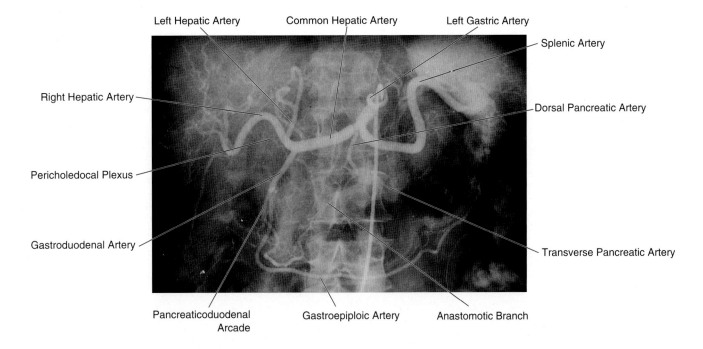

Left Hepatic Artery

Common Hepatic Artery

Left Gastric Artery

Splenic Artery

Right Hepatic Artery

Dorsal Pancreatic Artery

Pericholedocal Plexus

Gastroduodenal Artery

Transverse Pancreatic Artery

Pancreaticoduodenal
Arcade

Gastroepiploic Artery

Anastomotic Branch

Figure 18.29. Selective injection at the celiac trunk with a normal distribution of the branches. Note the dorsal pancreatic artery arising from the bifurcation of the celiac artery. Note that most of the arterial circulation of the pancreas arises from the dorsal pancreatic artery. Only one major artery in the head of the pancreas is visualized.

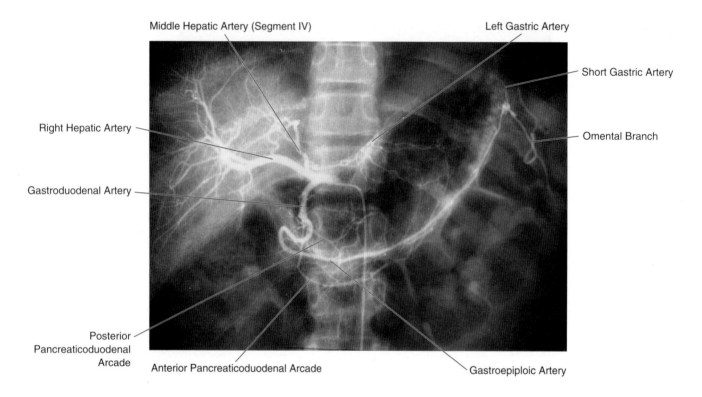

Middle Hepatic Artery (Segment IV)

Left Gastric Artery

Short Gastric Artery

Right Hepatic Artery

Omental Branch

Gastroduodenal Artery

Posterior Pancreaticoduodenal Arcade

Anterior Pancreaticoduodenal Arcade

Gastroepiploic Artery

Figure 18.30. Selective angiogram of the gastroduodenal artery shows the right and left gastric arteries, as well as the gastroepiploic and the hepatic arteries. Note the left omental branches and anastomose with the splenic circulation.

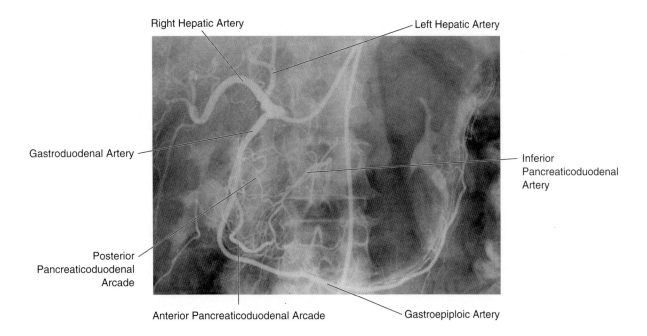

Right Hepatic Artery

Left Hepatic Artery

Gastroduodenal Artery

Inferior
Pancreaticoduodenal
Artery

Posterior
Pancreaticoduodenal
Arcade

Anterior Pancreaticoduodenal Arcade

Gastroepiploic Artery

Figure 18.31. Selective angiogram of the gastroduodenal artery showing the pancreaticoduodenal arcades and the gastroepiploic arteries. There is dominance of one of the pancreaticoduodenal arcades.

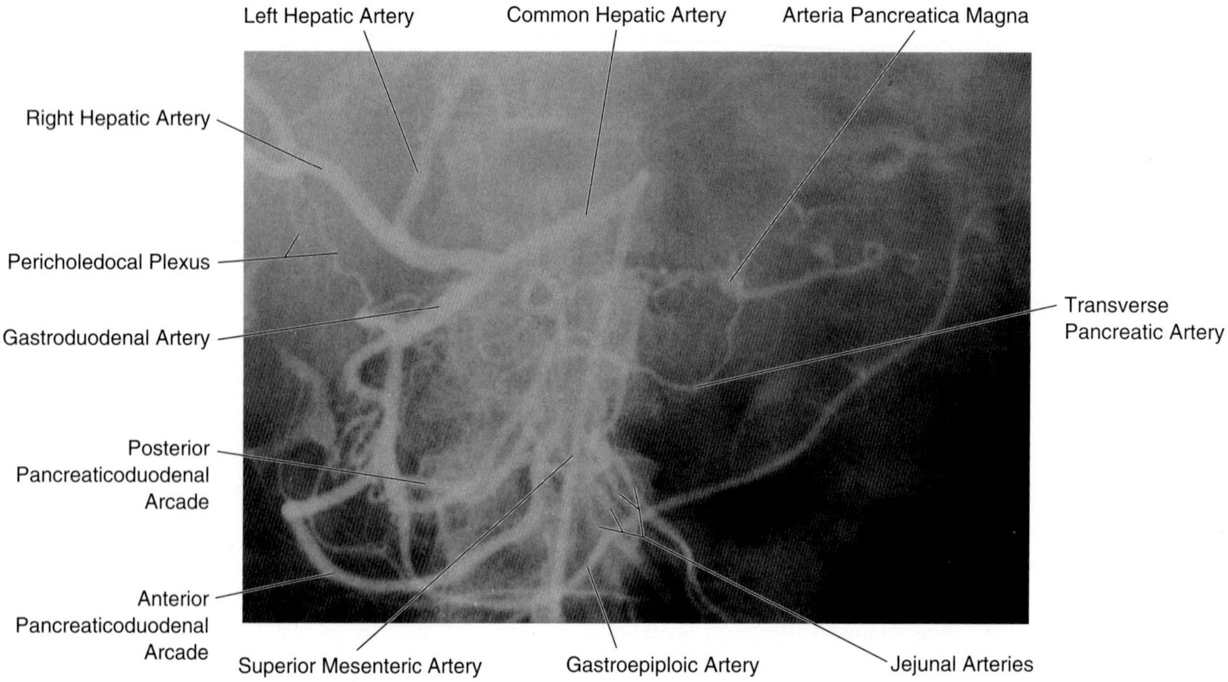

Figure 18.32. Selective angiogram of the gastroduodenal artery showing the arteries for the pancreatic head and the anastomoses within the pancreas. Note filling of the arteria pancreatica magna and opacification of the gastroepiploic artery.

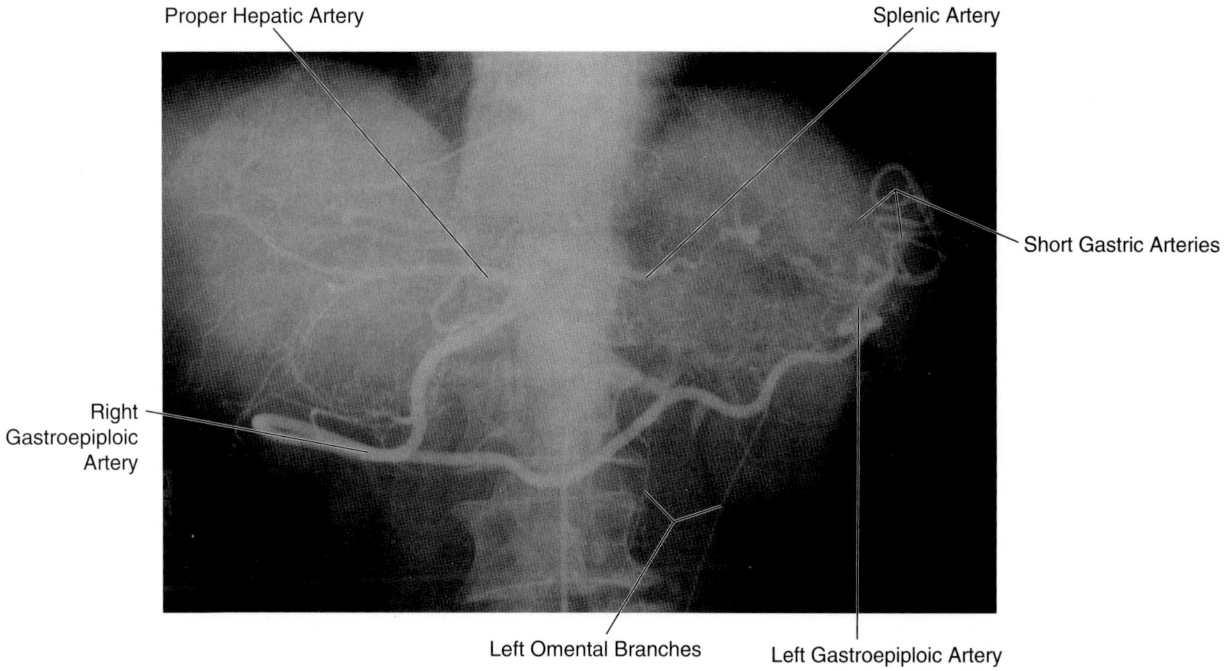

Figure 18.33. Selective angiogram of the celiac trunk. Note the enlargement of the gastroepiploic artery and the anastomosis with the splenic circulation, due to the partial occlusion of the splenic artery by a pancreatic tumor.

Lower Esophageal Arteries

Gastric Fundic Arteries

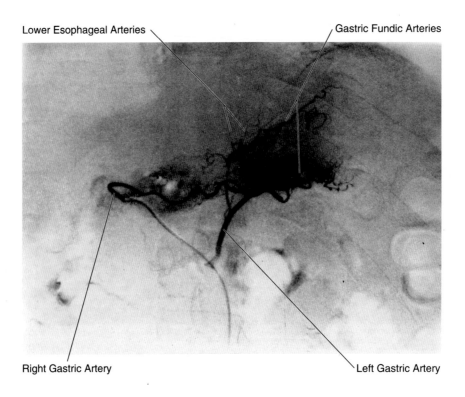

Right Gastric Artery

Left Gastric Artery

Figure 18.34. Selective angiogram of the right gastric artery showing the anastomosis with the left gastric artery and the filling of the gastric wall circulation at the fundus.

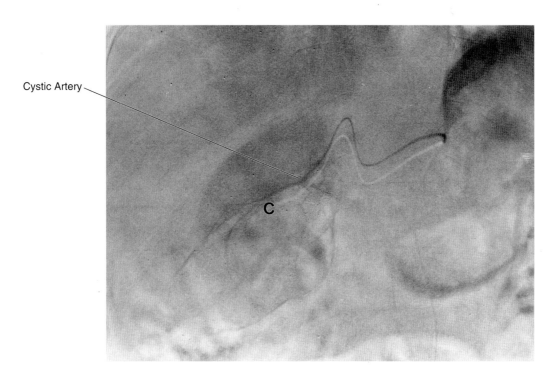

Figure 18.35. Selective injection at the cystic artery. Note the small size of the arteries and the bulging of the arteries around the gallbladder.

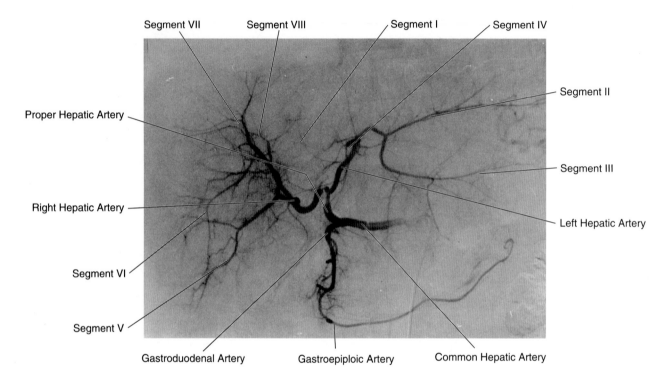

Figure 18.36. Selective injection of the proper hepatic artery showing the intrahepatic circulation, the gastroduodenal artery and the gastroepiploic artery. The left lobe of the liver is enlarged. There is spasm of the hepatic arteries at the bifurcation.

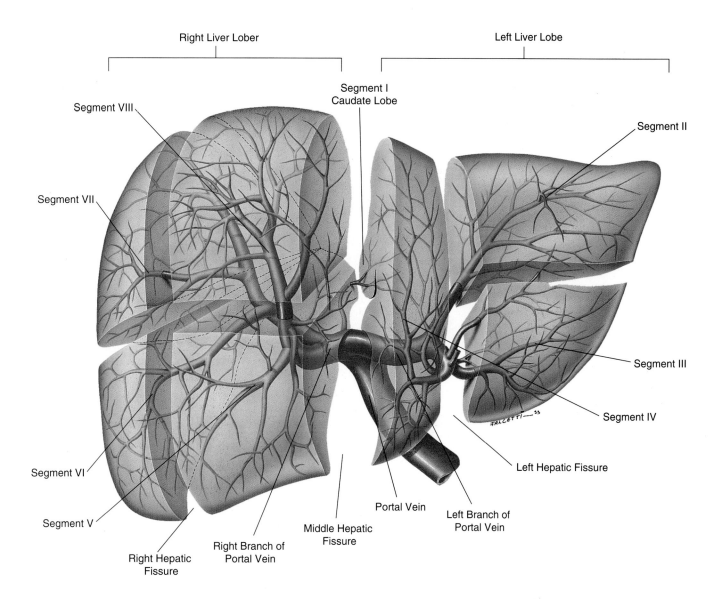

Right Liver Lober

Left Liver Lobe

Segment I
Caudate Lobe

Segment VIII

Segment II

Segment VII

Segment III

Segment IV

Left Hepatic Fissure

Segment VI

Portal Vein

Segment V

Left Branch of
Portal Vein

Middle Hepatic
Fissure

Right Hepatic
Fissure

Right Branch of
Portal Vein

Figure 18.37. Schematic drawing of the hepatic segments accordingly to the Couinaud description, showing the portal vein distribution, the hepatic lobar division and hepatic fissures.

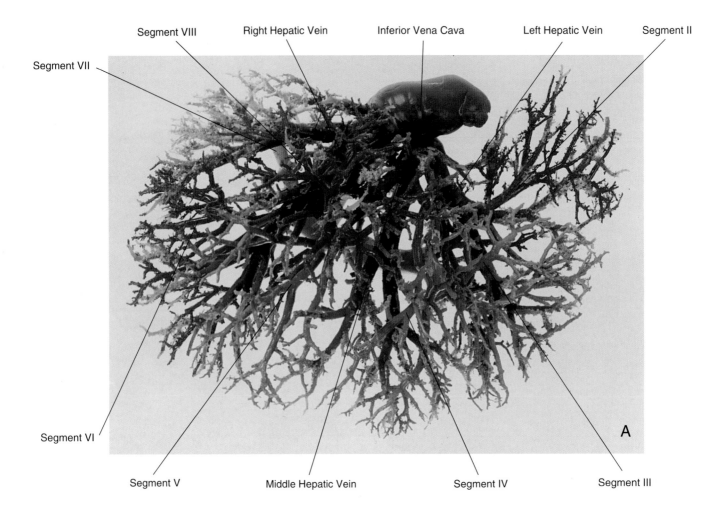

Segment VII

Segment VIII   Right Hepatic Vein   Inferior Vena Cava   Left Hepatic Vein   Segment II

A

Segment VI

Segment V   Middle Hepatic Vein   Segment IV   Segment III

Figure 18.38. Anterior view **(A)** and posterior view **(B)** of a liver cast with injections in the hepatic veins and portal vein, showing the liver segments in different colors. Navy blue is the IVC and hepatic veins, light blue is the caudate lobe or segment I, red is segment II, darker blue is segment III, green is segment V, light red is segment VI, white is segment VII, and brown is segment VIII.

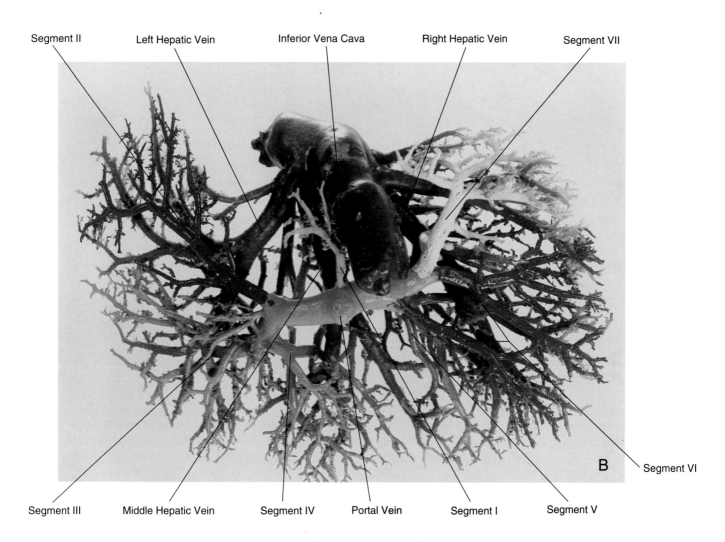

Segment II

Left Hepatic Vein

Inferior Vena Cava

Right Hepatic Vein

Segment VII

Segment III

Middle Hepatic Vein

Segment IV

Portal Vein

Segment I

Segment V

Segment VI

B

Figure 18.38. *Continued*

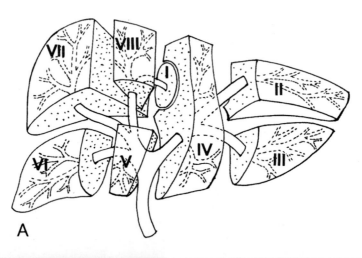

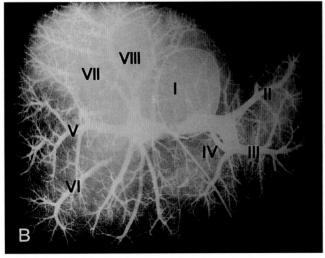

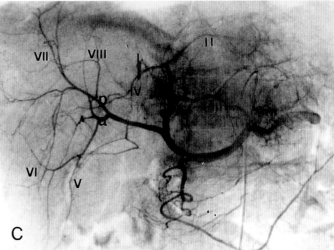

Figure 18.39. **A.** Schematic drawing of the liver segments according to Couinaud description. **B.** Specimen injection in the portal vein depicting the liver segments I through VIII. **C.** Arterial angiogram of the liver showing the hepatic segments in the hepatic artery branches. Note the presence of a large tumoral mass in the left lobe of the liver.

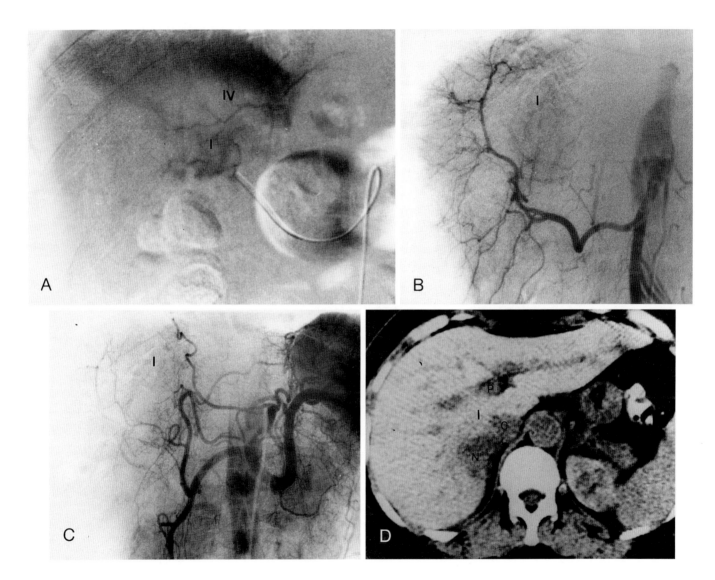

Figure 18.40. A. Hepatic arteriography. Selective injection at the segment I (caudate lobe). Note that segment IV is also opacified. **B.** Replaced right hepatic artery showing some contrast stain at segment I with arterial feeders from the right hepatic artery. **C.** Same patient as in B, showing feeders from the left hepatic artery to segment I. Note the liver stain at the same place due to the tumoral lesion observed in the CT of the liver. **D.** CT of the liver showing the metastatic tumoral lesion at the segment I, adjacent to the IVC.

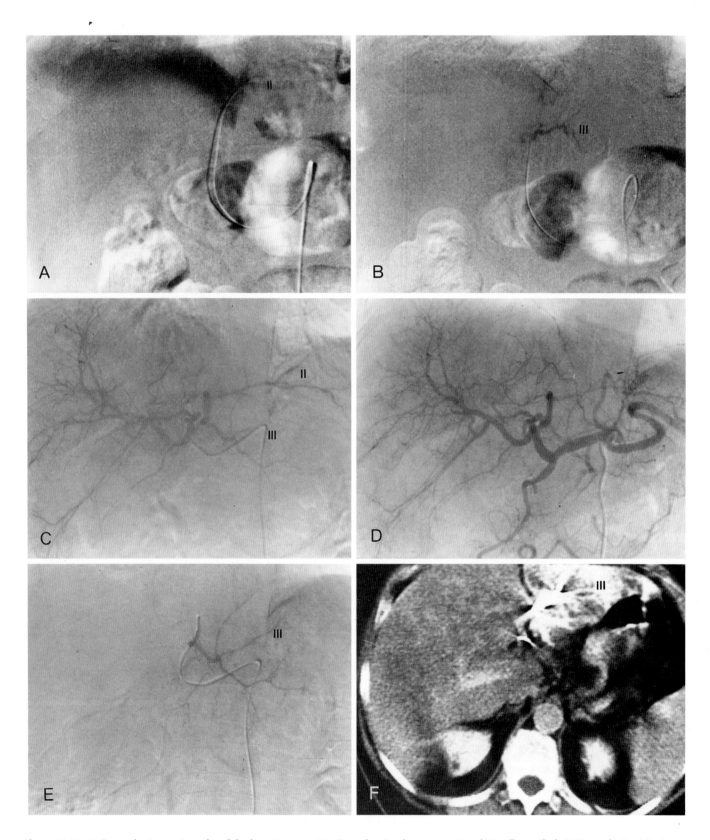

Figure 18.41. A. Superselective angiography of the hepatic segment II. **B.** Superselective angiography of hepatic segment III. **C.** Celiac angiography showing the liver arterial segments. **D.** Superselective hepatic angiography showing the segments II and III well opacified. **E.** Superselective injection at the hepatic segment III. **F.** CT of the liver showing selective stain of the hepatic segment III. Note the medial limit of segment III by the falciform ligament.

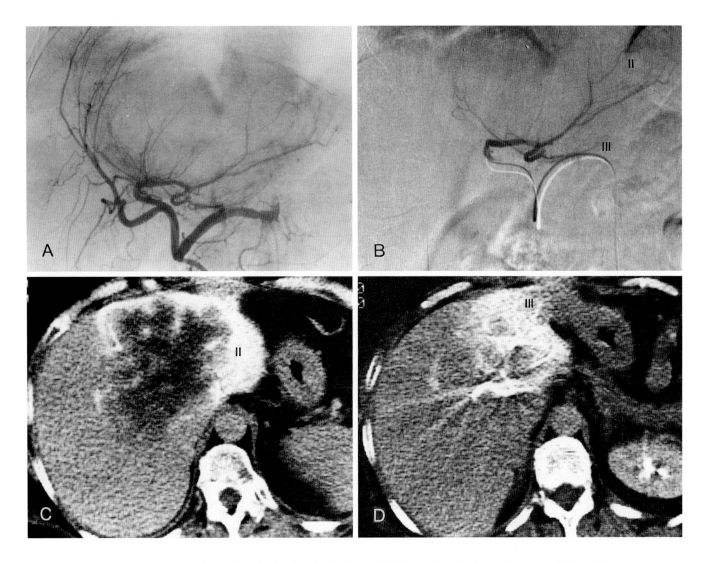

Figure 18.42. A. Hepatic angiography showing the left lobe of the liver enlarged and with the arteries displaced by a metastatic lesion, but showing the segments II and III. **B.** Selective injection in the left hepatic artery showing segments II and III. **C.** CT of the liver showing selective stain of the segment II. **D.** CT of the liver showing selective stain of the segment III.

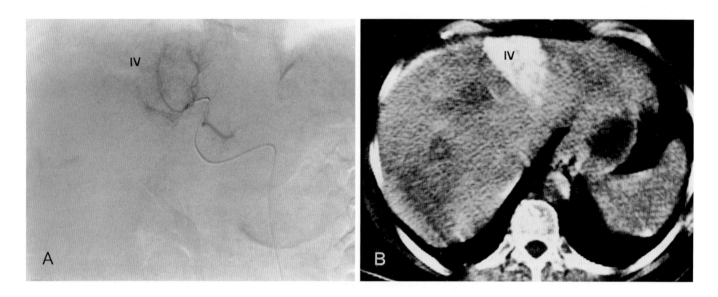

Figure 18.43. A. Superselective angiography of the segment IV. **B.** CT of the liver showing the segment IV with the typical appearance of a wedge with the base turned ventrally.

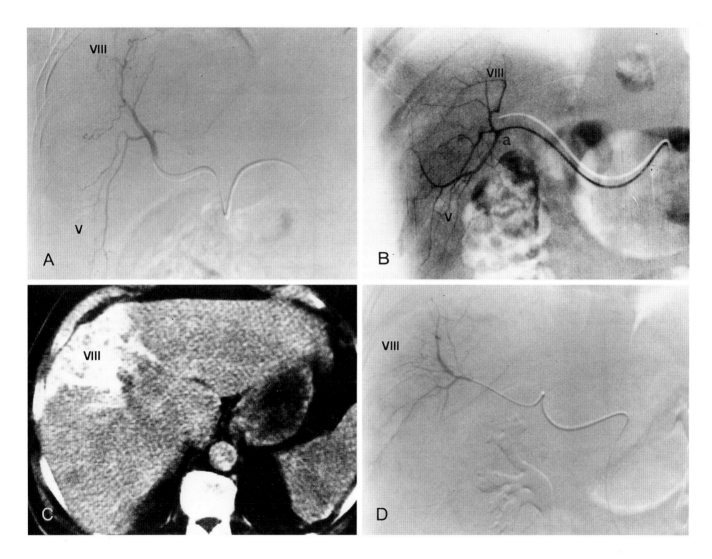

Figure 18.44. A. Superselective angiography of the segments V and VIII (sector anteromedial of the right lobe of the liver). **B.** Superselective angiography of the segments V and VIII in another patient. **C.** CT of the liver showing segment VIII with a dense stain due to the selective injection. **D.** Superselective angiography of the segment VIII of the liver used to perform the CT shown in part C of the figure.

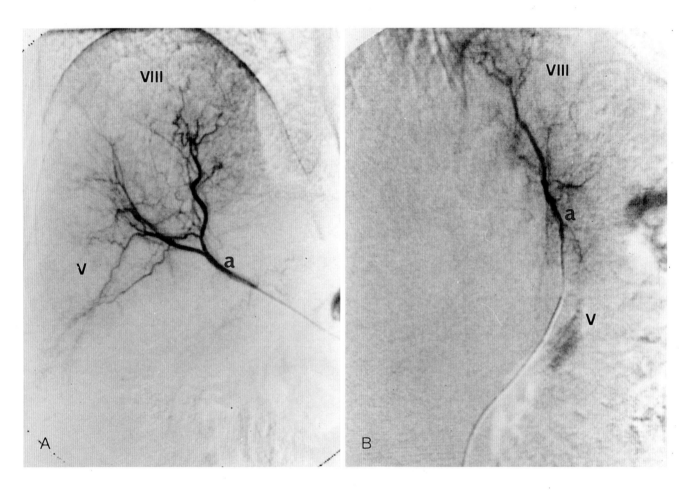

Figure 18.45. A. Anterior view of a selective injection of the anterior branch of the right hepatic artery showing segments V and VIII. **B.** Lateral view of the selective injection of the anterior branch of the right hepatic artery depicting segments V and VIII.

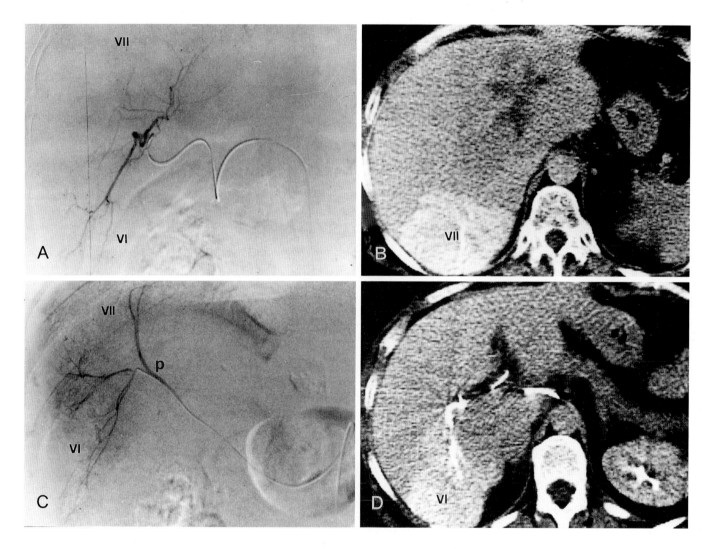

Figure 18.46. A. Anterior view of a selective injection of the posterior branch of the right hepatic artery showing segments VI and VII (sector posterolateral of the right lobe of the liver). **B.** CT of the liver showing the stain at the segment VII. **C.** Selective angiography at the posterior branch of the right hepatic artery, showing segments VI and VII. **D.** CT of the liver showing the stain at the segment VI.

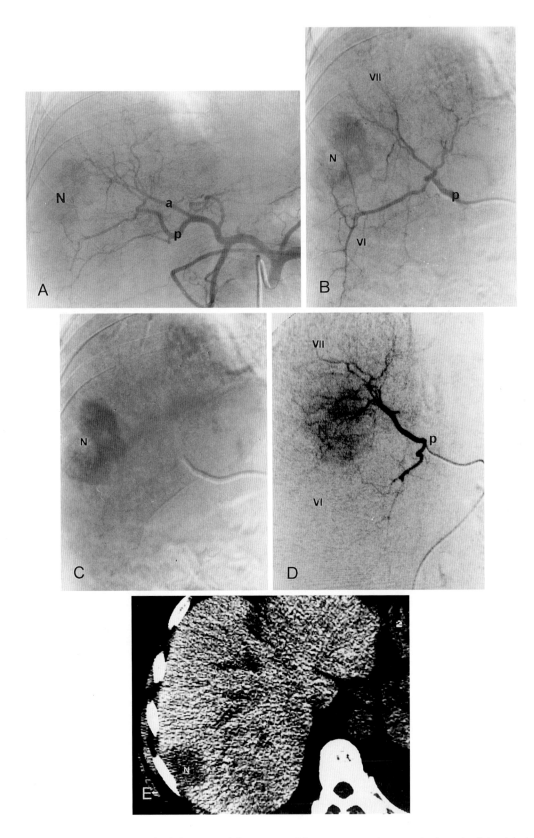

Figure 18.47. A. Celiac artery injection showing the bifurcation of the right hepatic artery in anterior and posterior branches. N denotes a tumoral nodule. **B.** Superselective angiography of the right posterior branch of the hepatic artery. Segments VI and VII are clearly visualized. N denotes the tumoral lesion with nutrient arteries from both segments. **C.** Later phase of the angiogram showing the tumoral nodule (N). **D.** Lateral view of the injection at the posterior branch of the right hepatic artery, showing the segments VI and VII. Note the tumor nodule stain. The selective injection at the anterior branch of the right hepatic artery of the same patient is seen on Figure 18.45 A and B. **E.** CT of the liver showing the lesion (N) between the segments VI and VII, at the posterolateral sector of the right lobe of the liver.

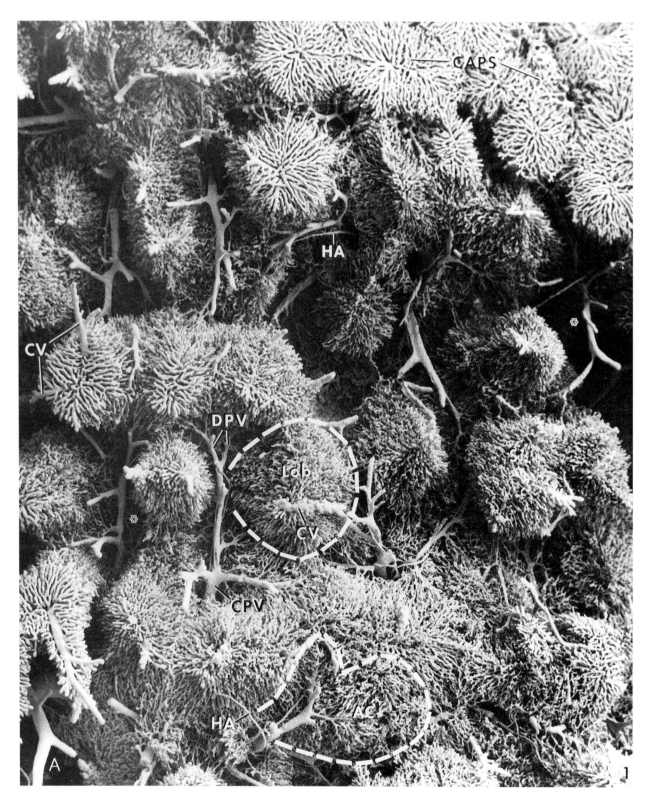

Figure 18.48. **A.** SEM of casted hepatic microcirculation in both capsular (CAPS) and subcapsular regions. The capsular surface is shown in upper right, of figure and the adjacent regions of the cast are from areas underlying this plane. Zone one (1), two (2), and three (3) of the liver acinus are denoted at the bottom of the figure. Adjacent areas also contain: sinusoids (Si), the arrangement of which corresponds to a lobular (Lob) parenchymal organization, conducting portal vein (CPV), distributing portal vein (DPV), collecting venule (CV), hepatic arteriole (HA), and non casted areas in portal tracts (*) (X 65). **B.** The left side of Figure 18.48 B is an enlargement of the lower portion of Figure 18.48 A (X 75), and the right side is an enlargement of the area enclosed by the rectangle (X 200). The approximate boundary of zone 1 of the liver acinus is denoted by broken lines in the figure on the right. Conducting portal vein (CPV), terminal divisions of the distributing portal vein (DPV), hepatic arteriole (HA), collecting venule (CV), blind-ends of portal vein (*), and anastomoses of sinusoids (arrows). The hepatic arteriole in the Figure 18.48 B on the right extends into acinar zones 2 and 3. Reprinted with permission from Kardon RH, Kessel RG. Gastroenterology 1980;79:72-81.

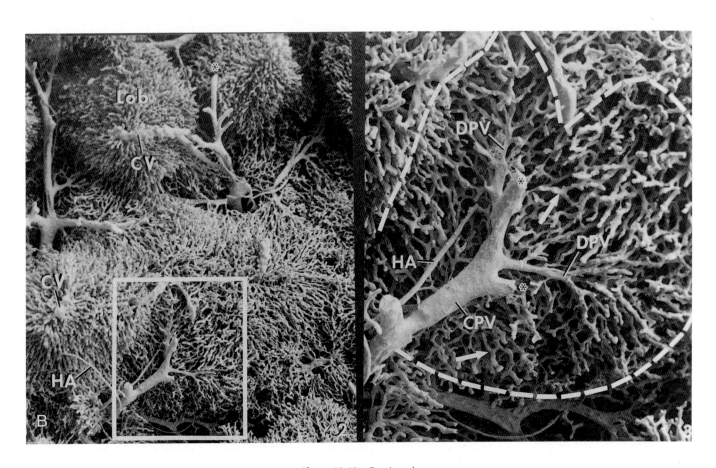

Figure 18.48. *Continued*

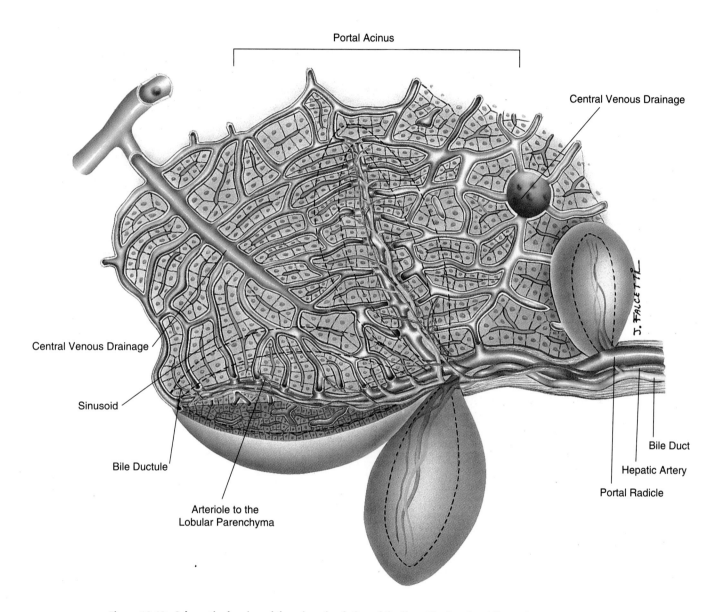

Figure 18.49. Schematic drawing of the microcirculation of the liver. The functional liver acinus zone 1, zone 2 and zone 3 are denoted by the broken line. The acinar 3D dimension is showed by the pear like structures. Zone 3 represents everything on the liver parenchyma around zone 2 till the draining vein. The artery, the portal radicle and the bile duct are in the center of the acinus, surrounded by sinusoids.

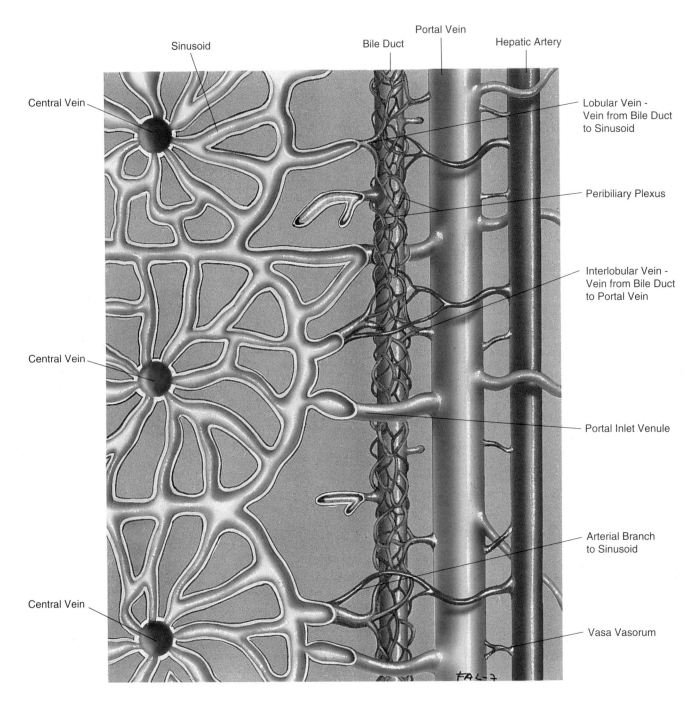

Figure 18.50. Schematic diagram showing the vascular plexus and venous drainage of the bile duct (peribiliary plexus). The hepatic artery gives off its branches to the sinusoid, the bile duct, and the portal vein (vasa vasorum). The venous plexus of the bile duct (blue vessels around the bile duct) is drained into the portal vein via the interlobular vein and into the sinusoids via the lobular vein. Note that there are four types of arterioportal communications: the peribiliary plexus (1), the terminal arterioportal anastomosis (2), the vasa vasorum on the wall of the portal vein (3), and direct arterioportal connections (4). Modified from Cho YJ, Lunderquist A. Radiology 1983;147:357-364.

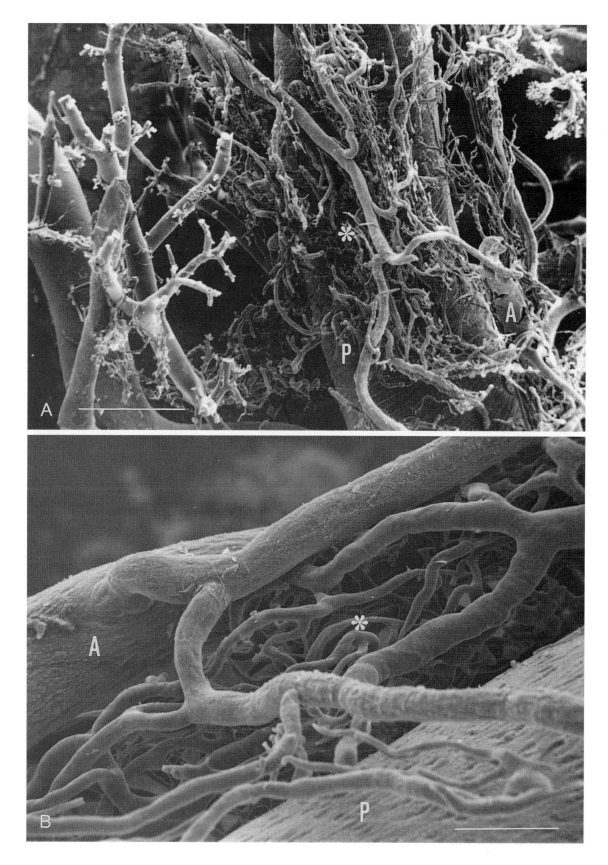

Figure 18.51. A. Scanning electron micrograph of the intrahepatic microvasculature .3 hours after hepatic artery embolization with Gelfoam particles. The hepatic artery (A) has about 290 mm in diameter and is occluded (arrow). The peribiliary plexus around the occluded artery (*) is well filled with the casting medium. Portal vein (P). Bar = 1,000 mm. **B.** Scanning electron micrograph of the intrahepatic vasculature in a normal rat. The peribiliary plexus (*) consists of two layers. The hepatic artery (A) supplies the peribiliary plexus (*). Portal vein (P). Bar = 100 mm.

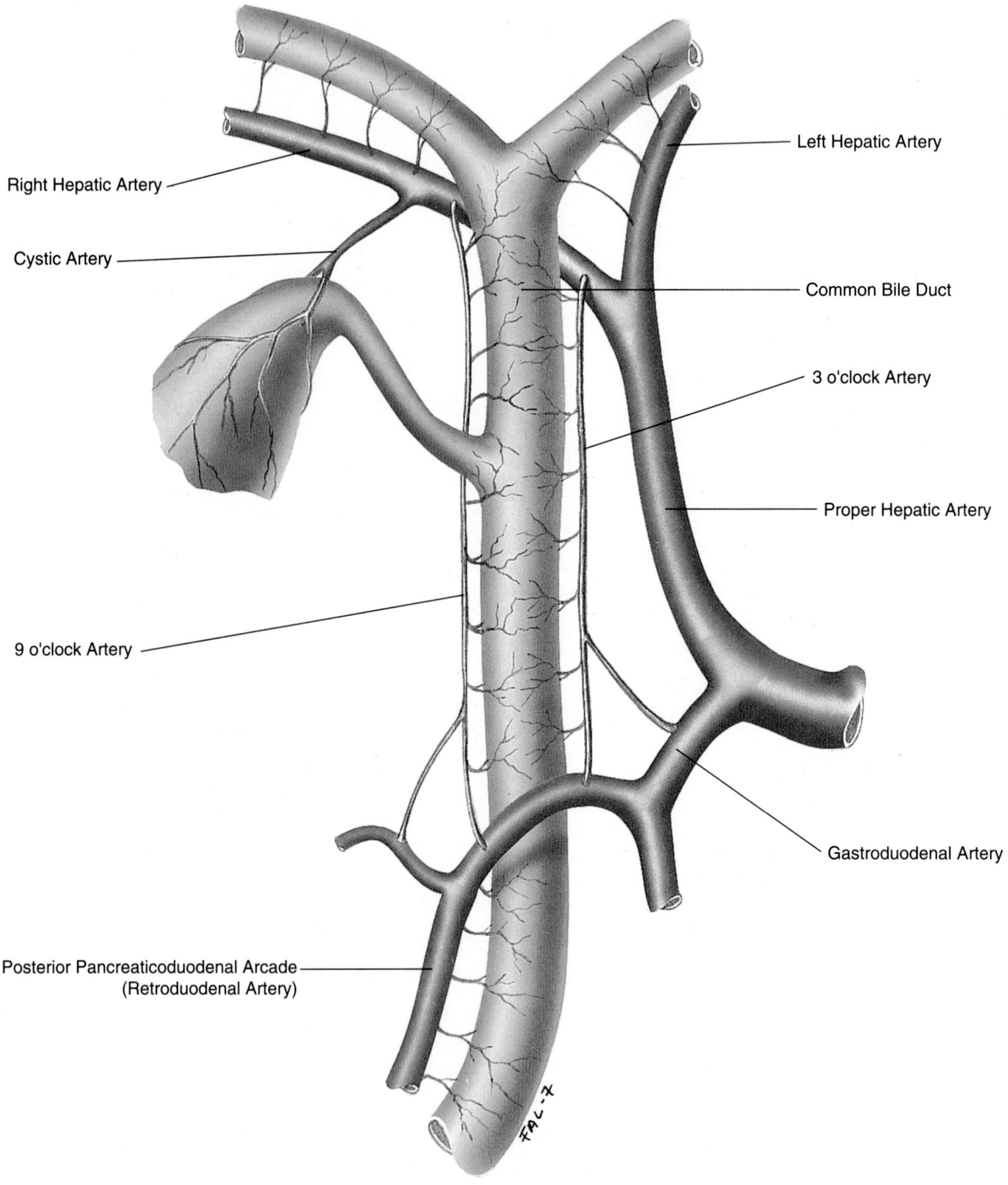

Right Hepatic Artery

Cystic Artery

9 o'clock Artery

Posterior Pancreaticoduodenal Arcade
(Retroduodenal Artery)

Left Hepatic Artery

Common Bile Duct

3 o'clock Artery

Proper Hepatic Artery

Gastroduodenal Artery

Figure 18.52. Schematic diagram showing the arterial supply of the main bile ducts. The right hepatic duct is supplied by small branches from the right hepatic artery, while the left duct is supplied by small branches from the left hepatic artery. The common bile duct (supraduodenal segment) is supplied by the 9 o'clock and 3 o'clock arteries. The common bile duct (infraduodenal segment) is supplied by direct small branches of the pancreaticoduodenal arcade.

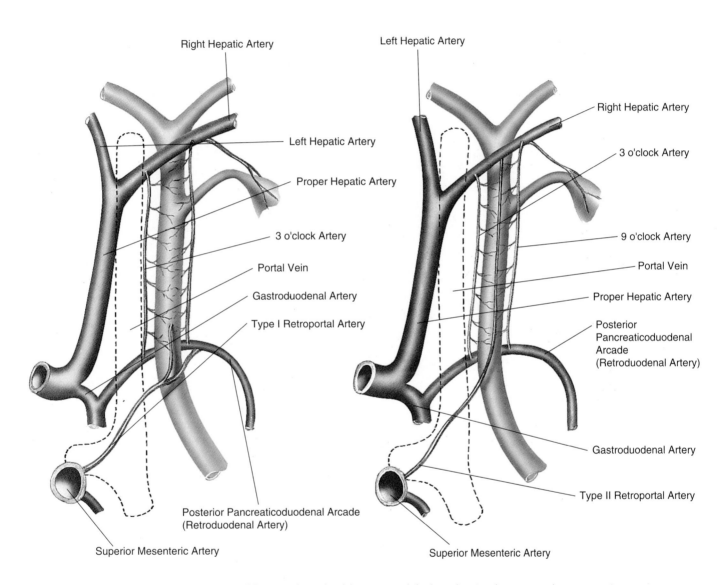

Figure 18.53. Posterior view of the arterial supply of the common bile duct, showing the retroportal artery, type I and type II. Type II retroportal artery increases the supply of the common bile duct.

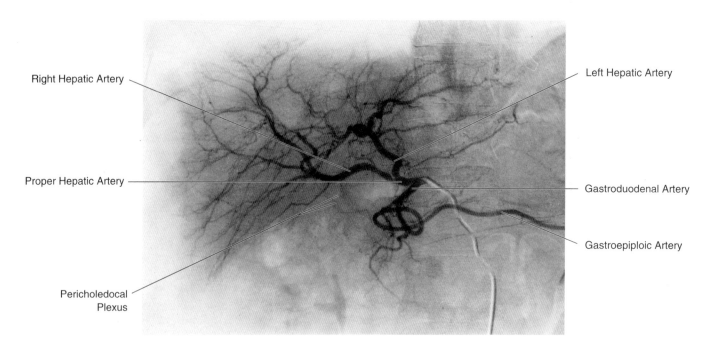

Right Hepatic Artery

Proper Hepatic Artery

Pericholedocal
Plexus

Left Hepatic Artery

Gastroduodenal Artery

Gastroepiploic Artery

Figure 18.54. Common hepatic arteriography, arterial phase. The peribiliary arteries are filled from the pancreatic arcade and reach the hepatic arterial branches at the hilus. The 3 o'clock and 9 o'clock arteries are seem. There is an early bifurcation of the proper hepatic artery.

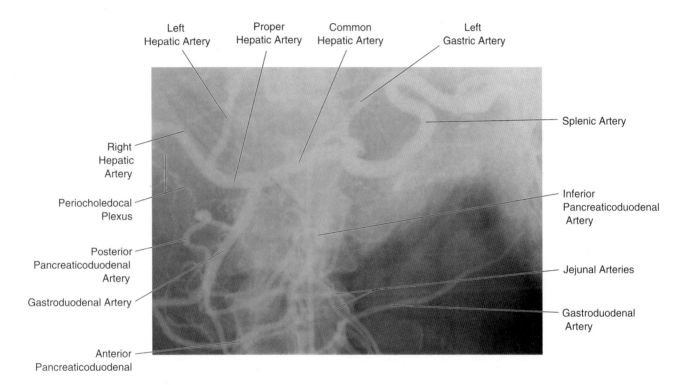

Left
Hepatic Artery

Proper
Hepatic Artery

Common
Hepatic Artery

Left
Gastric Artery

Splenic Artery

Right
Hepatic
Artery

Periocholedocal
Plexus

Posterior
Pancreaticoduodenal
Artery

Gastroduodenal Artery

Anterior
Pancreaticoduodenal

Inferior
Pancreaticoduodenal
Artery

Jejunal Arteries

Gastroduodenal
Artery

Figure 18.55. Celiac artery injection showing the peribiliary arteries parallel to the main bile duct, arising from the pancreatic arcade.

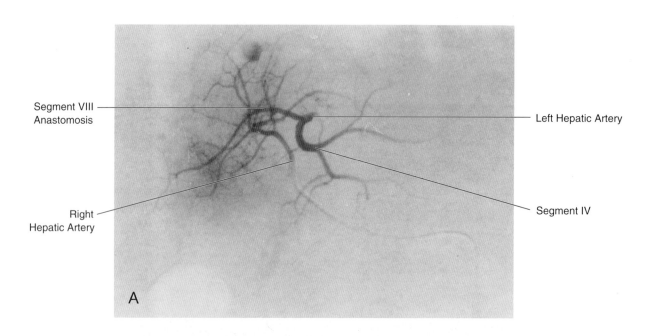

Segment VIII Anastomosis

Left Hepatic Artery

Right Hepatic Artery

Segment IV

A

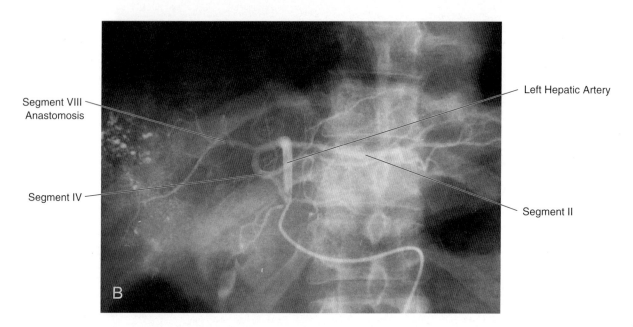

Segment VIII Anastomosis

Left Hepatic Artery

Segment IV

Segment II

B

Figure 18.56. Interlobar intrahepatic arterial collaterals. A. Selective injection in the right hepatic artery shows simultaneous filling of the left hepatic artery, segments IV and III. **B.** Selective injection in the left hepatic artery shows no filling of the right hepatic artery.

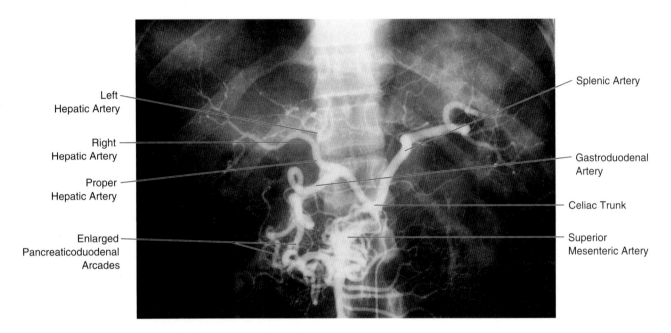

Figure 18.57. Extrahepatic arterial collaterals. Superior mesenteric arteriogram shows development of collateral circulation through the pancreaticoduodenal arcades. There is occlusion of the origin of the celiac trunk.

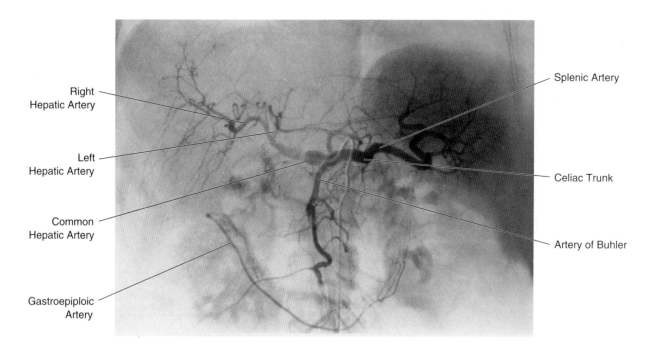

Right
Hepatic Artery

Left
Hepatic Artery

Common
Hepatic Artery

Gastroepiploic
Artery

Splenic Artery

Celiac Trunk

Artery of Buhler

Figure 18.58. Extrahepatic arterial collaterals. Celiac artery angiogram showing opacification of the Arc of Bühler, connecting to the superior mesenteric artery.

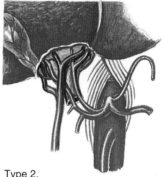

Type 1.
Total Replacement of CHA

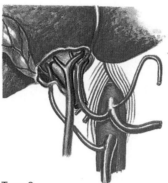

Type 2.
Early Bifurcation of CHA

Type 3.
Replaced Right HA

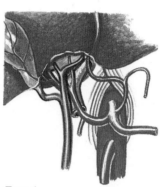

Type 4.
Replaced Left HA

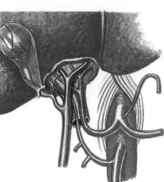

Type 5.
Right and Left HA from CT
Accessory Right HA

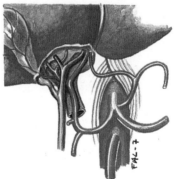

Type 6.
Accessory Left HA from
Left Gastric Artery

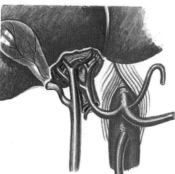

Type 7.
Accessory Left HA from Right HA

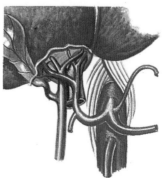
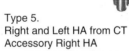

Type 8.
Right HA Passes Anteriorly to
the Common Bile Duct

Figure 18.59. Variations of the hepatic artery. Types 1 through 8. The most frequent variation is replacement of the hepatic artery. There are variations in about 40% of the population.

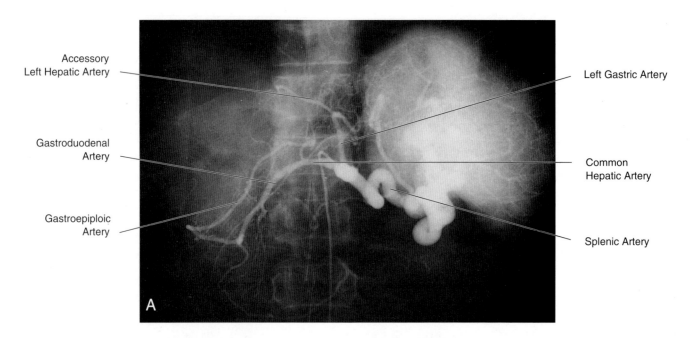

Accessory
Left Hepatic Artery

Gastroduodenal
Artery

Gastroepiploic
Artery

Left Gastric Artery

Common
Hepatic Artery

Splenic Artery

A

Figure 18.60. Variation of the hepatic artery. Type 1. Total replacement of the common hepatic artery. **A.** Celiac injection shows only the gastroduodenal artery, left gastric artery and splenic artery. This patient may have a very small accessory left hepatic artery, originated from the left gastric artery. **B.** Superior mesenteric artery injection shows the totally replaced hepatic artery.

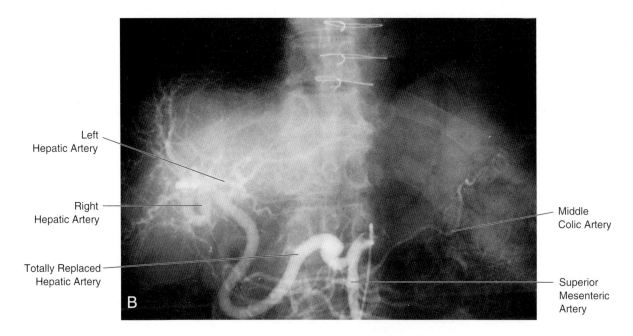

Left
Hepatic Artery

Right
Hepatic Artery

Totally Replaced
Hepatic Artery

Middle
Colic Artery

Superior
Mesenteric
Artery

Figure 18.60. *Continued*

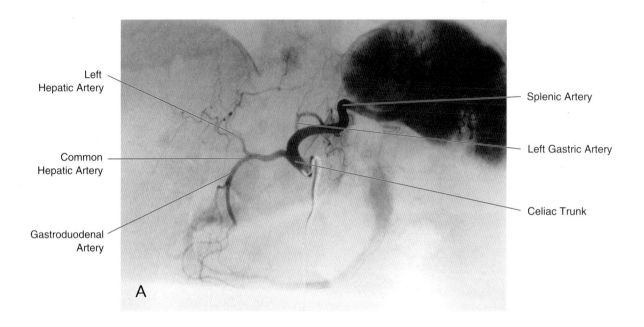

Left Hepatic Artery

Common Hepatic Artery

Gastroduodenal Artery

Splenic Artery

Left Gastric Artery

Celiac Trunk

A

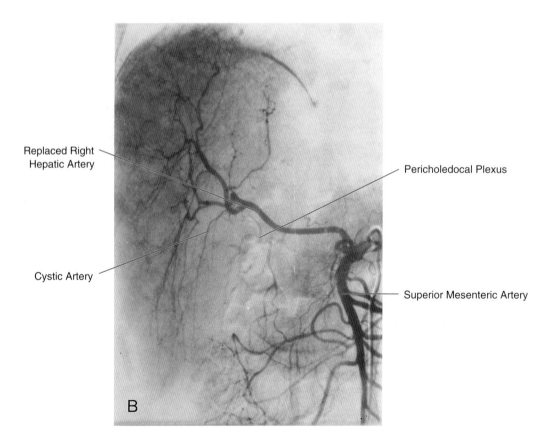

Replaced Right Hepatic Artery

Cystic Artery

Pericholedocal Plexus

Superior Mesenteric Artery

B

Figure 18.61. Variation of the hepatic artery. Type 3. Replaced right hepatic artery. **A.** Celiac trunk injection shows the left gastric artery originated from the common hepatic artery. **B.** Superior mesenteric artery injection giving origin to the right replaced hepatic artery.

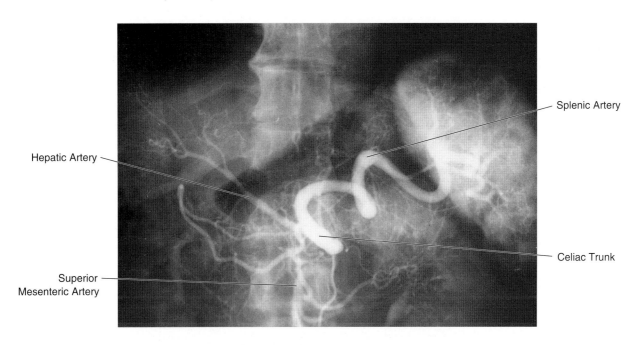

Hepatic Artery

Superior
Mesenteric Artery

Splenic Artery

Celiac Trunk

Figure 18.62. Splenic artery. Celiac trunk injection shows the large and convoluted splenic artery. Note the several pancreatic branches and the bifurcation of the splenic artery in the splenic hilus.

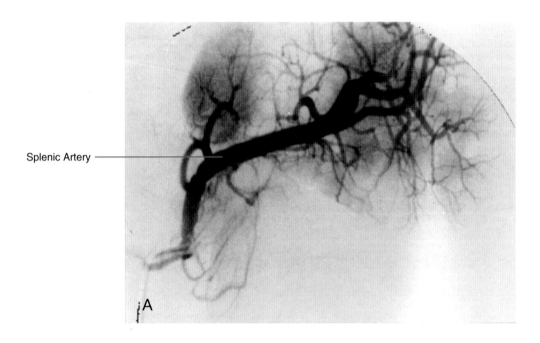

Splenic Artery ———

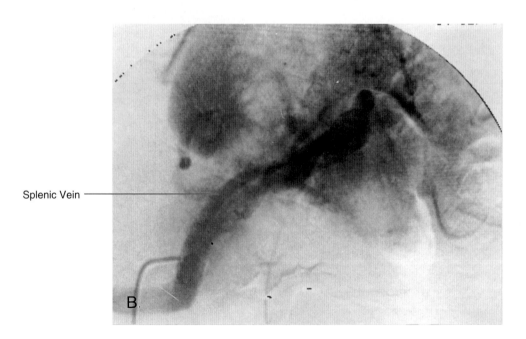

Splenic Vein ———

Figure 18.63. A. Selective splenic artery injection shows the intrasplenic circulation as well as the pancreatic arteries originated from the splenic artery. **B.** Late angiographic phase shows the splenic venous drainage, with dense opacification of the splenic vein.

Common Hepatic Artery

Pancreatic Blush

Gastroduodenal Artery

Gastroepiploic Artery

Splenic Artery

Celiac Trunk

Omental Branch

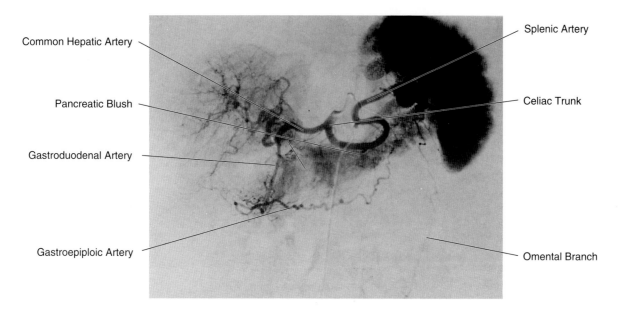

Figure 18.64. Celiac trunk injection shows a long and sinuous splenic artery. Note the dense stain of the pancreas by the injection and the close relationship of the splenic artery and the tail of the pancreas. The gastroepiploic artery is long and tortuous. The left epiploic artery is easily visualized.

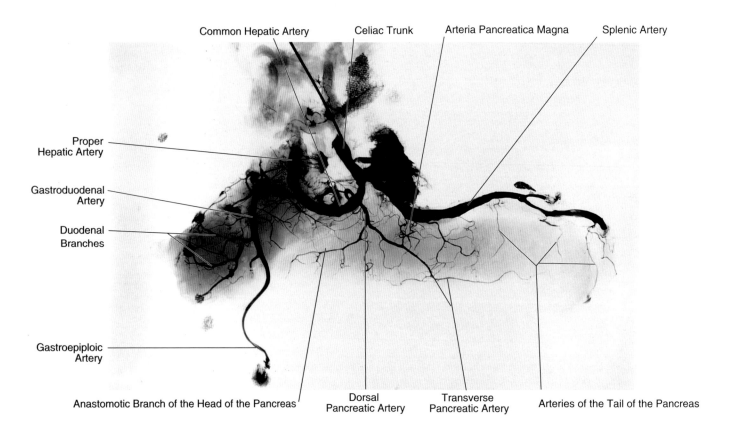

Common Hepatic Artery   Celiac Trunk   Arteria Pancreatica Magna   Splenic Artery

Proper
Hepatic Artery

Gastroduodenal
Artery

Duodenal
Branches

Gastroepiploic
Artery

Anastomotic Branch of the Head of the Pancreas   Dorsal
Pancreatic Artery   Transverse
Pancreatic Artery   Arteries of the Tail of the Pancreas

Figure 18.65. Necropsy specimen injection of contrast media showing the pancreatic arteries. There are artifacts
due to extravasation of contrast.

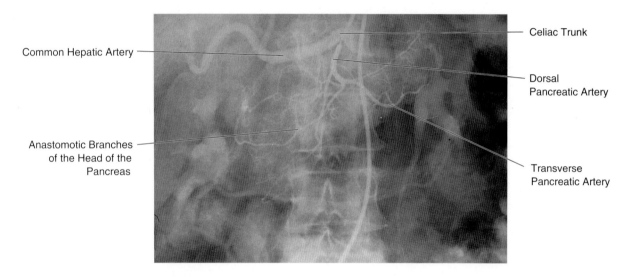

Common Hepatic Artery

Anastomotic Branches
of the Head of the
Pancreas

Celiac Trunk

Dorsal
Pancreatic Artery

Transverse
Pancreatic Artery

Figure 18.66. Selective angiography of the dorsal pancreatic artery arising from the bifurcation of the celiac trunk. Note the communications with the pancreaticoduodenal arcades and with the transverse pancreatic artery.

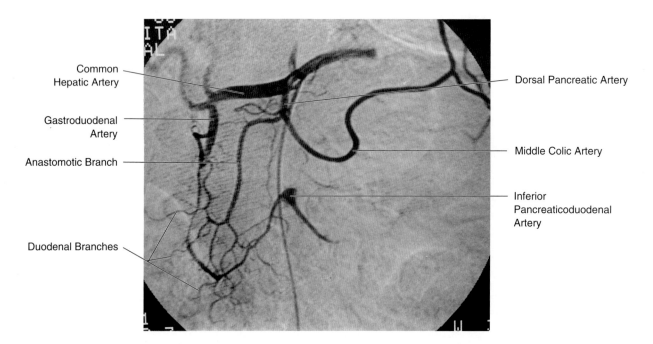

Common Hepatic Artery

Gastroduodenal Artery

Anastomotic Branch

Duodenal Branches

Dorsal Pancreatic Artery

Middle Colic Artery

Inferior Pancreaticoduodenal Artery

Figure 18.67. Selective angiography of the common hepatic artery shows the origin of the dorsal pancreatic artery from the common hepatic artery, in this case, it anastomoses with the pancreaticoduodenal arcade. Note that the middle colic artery originates from the dorsal pancreatic artery.

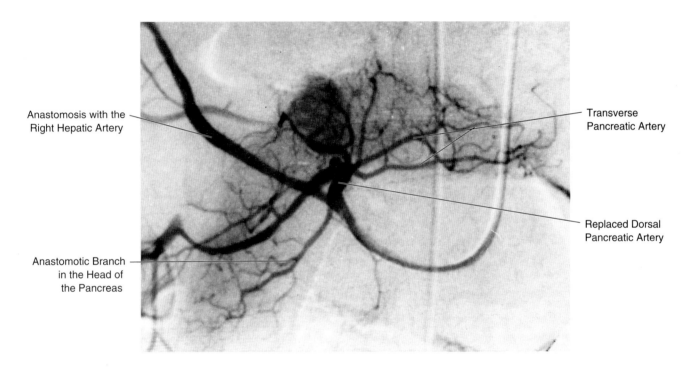

Anastomosis with the
Right Hepatic Artery

Anastomotic Branch
in the Head of
the Pancreas

Transverse
Pancreatic Artery

Replaced Dorsal
Pancreatic Artery

Figure 18.68. Variation of the origin of the dorsal pancreatic artery. Selective angiography of the dorsal pancreatic artery, in this case originated from the superior mesenteric artery. Incidentally a hypervascular lesion (insulinoma) is observed. Note that there is an anastomose with the right hepatic artery directly from the dorsal pancreatic artery.

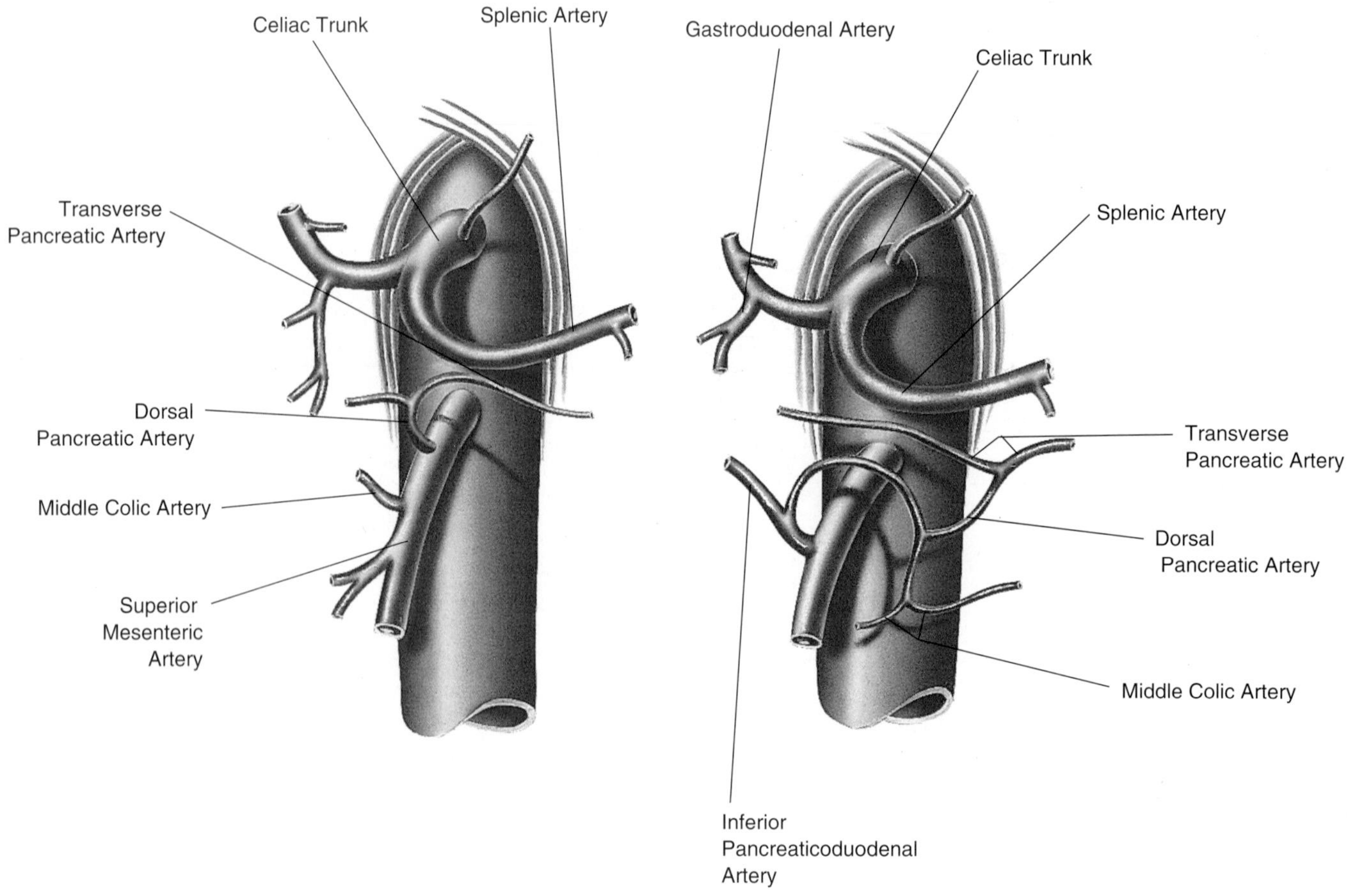

Figure 18.69. Schematic diagram showing variations in origin of the dorsal pancreatic artery. Note that the middle colic artery and the dorsal pancreatic artery may have a common origin.

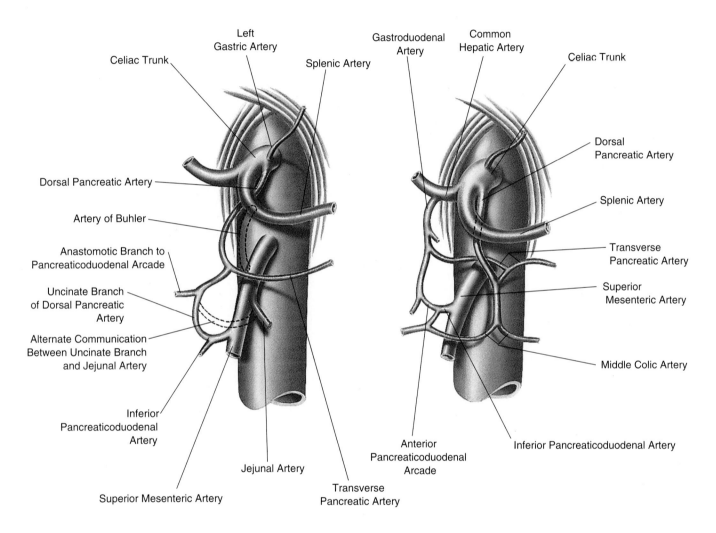

Figure 18.70. Schematic diagram shows possible connections between the celiac trunk and superior mesenteric artery through the dorsal pancreatic artery and the artery of Bühler.

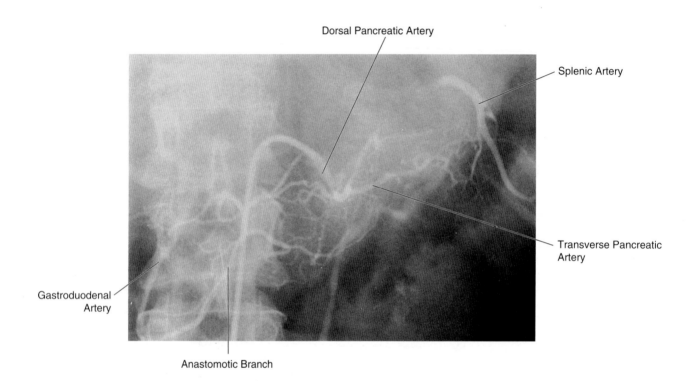

Dorsal Pancreatic Artery

Splenic Artery

Transverse Pancreatic Artery

Gastroduodenal Artery

Anastomotic Branch

Figure 18.71. Selective arteriography injection at the arteria pancreatica magna (great pancreatic artery) branch of the splenic artery. Note the connections with the arteries in the neck and head of the pancreas and the arteries in the tail of the pancreas with filling of the transverse pancreatic artery and smaller branches.

Arteria Pancreatica Magna   Splenic Artery

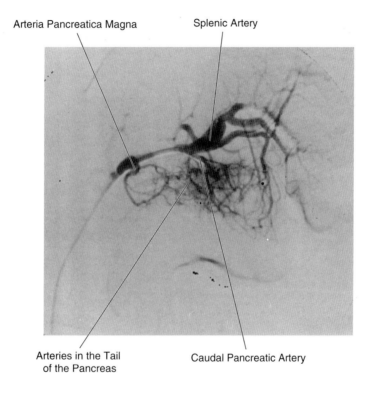

Arteries in the Tail   Caudal Pancreatic Artery
of the Pancreas

Figure 18.72. Selective arteriography of the caudal pancreatic artery, branch of the splenic artery. Note partial filling of the splenic arteries and smaller branches in the distal tail of the pancreas.

Right Hepatic Artery

Gastroduodenal
Artery

Right Gastroepiploic
Artery

Anterior
Pancreaticoduodenal
Arcade

Left Gastroepiploic
Artery

Left Hepatic
Artery

Common Hepatic
Artery

Posterior
Pancreaticoduodenal
Arcade

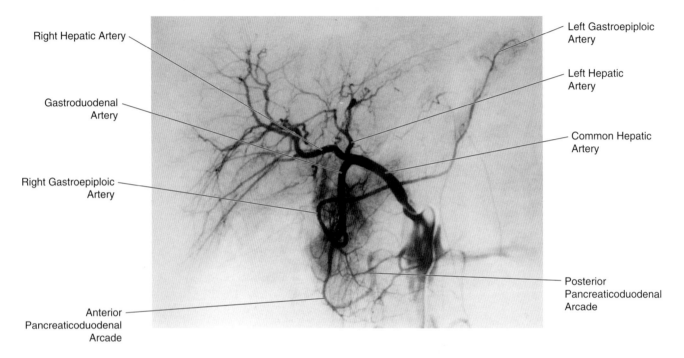

Figure 18.73. Selective injection in the common hepatic artery showing filling of the gastroduodenal artery, as well as the pancreaticoduodenal arcades and intrahepatic arteries and the right gastroepiploic artery. The right gastroepiploic artery is a continuation of the gastroduodenal artery and vascularizes the stomach wall and originates the omental branches (epiploic arteries).

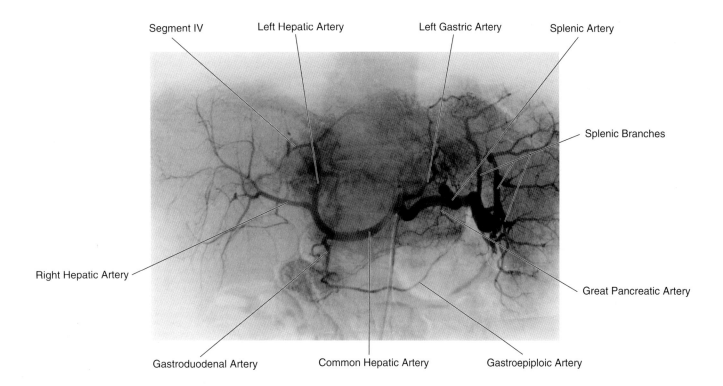

Segment IV   Left Hepatic Artery   Left Gastric Artery   Splenic Artery

Splenic Branches

Right Hepatic Artery

Great Pancreatic Artery

Gastroduodenal Artery   Common Hepatic Artery   Gastroepiploic Artery

Figure 18.74. Celiac trunk injection showing the large splenic artery and the intrasplenic circulation. Note the presence of an arterial bifurcation at the hilus making at least three independent segments in the spleen. In this specific case the spleen is enlarged.

Left Gastric Artery   Splenic Branches

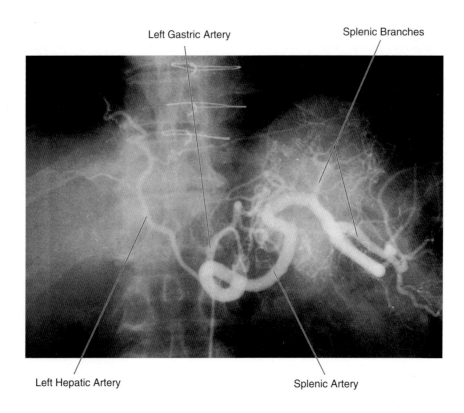

Left Hepatic Artery   Splenic Artery

Figure 18.75. Splenic artery angiography shows a tortuous splenic artery with bifurcation in at least three segments in the spleen.

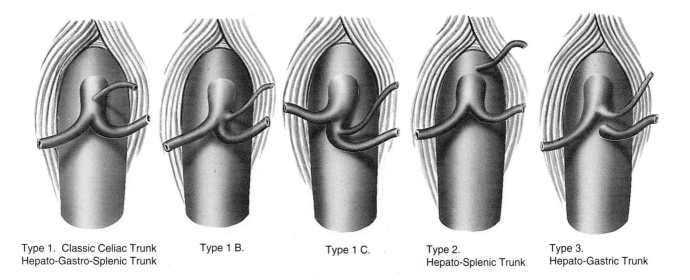

Type 1. Classic Celiac Trunk
Hepato-Gastro-Splenic Trunk

Type 1 B.

Type 1 C.

Type 2.
Hepato-Splenic Trunk

Type 3.
Hepato-Gastric Trunk

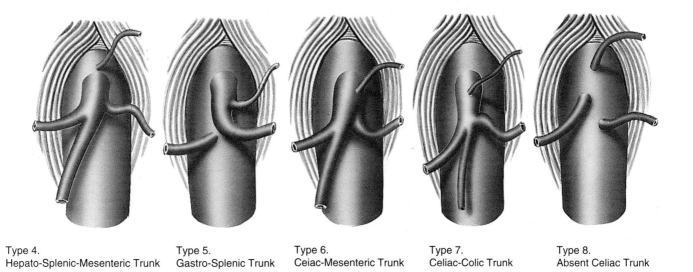

Type 4.
Hepato-Splenic-Mesenteric Trunk

Type 5.
Gastro-Splenic Trunk

Type 6.
Ceiac-Mesenteric Trunk

Type 7.
Celiac-Colic Trunk

Type 8.
Absent Celiac Trunk

Figure 18.76. Schematic drawing showing the variations in the configuration of the celiac trunk.

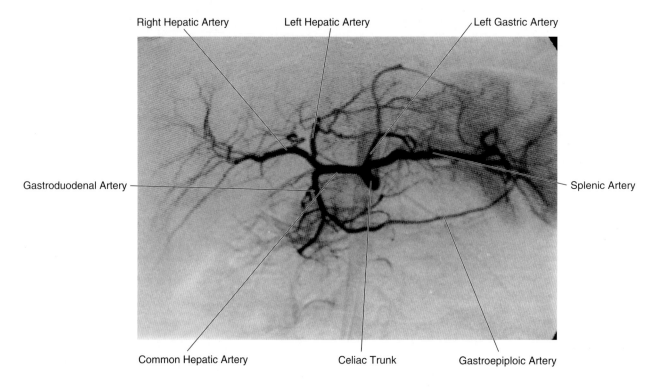

Figure 18.77. Celiac angiography shows the classical configuration of the celiac trunk also called Type 1, hepato-gastro-splenic trunk.

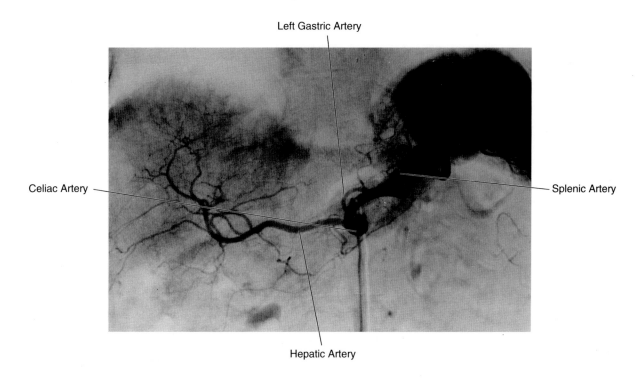

Figure 18.78. Celiac angiography shows the Type 1c celiac trunk, also called gastrosplenic trunk. The splenic artery is dominant and the hepatic artery arises from the splenic artery.

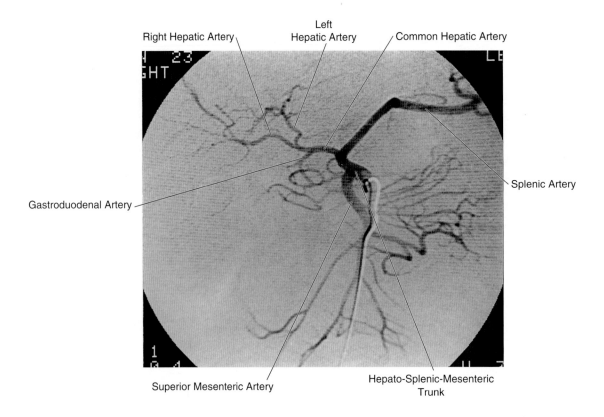

Figure 18.79. Celiac angiography shows a hepato-splenic-mesenteric trunk. The left gastric artery arises directly from the aorta. The hepatic, splenic and mesenteric arteries form a single trunk.

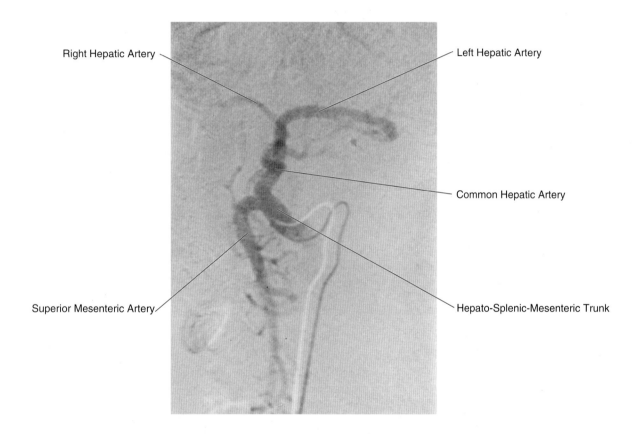

Figure 18.80. Celiac angiography shows a hepato-splenic-mesenteric trunk. The hepatic, splenic and mesenteric arteries have common origin from a single trunk.

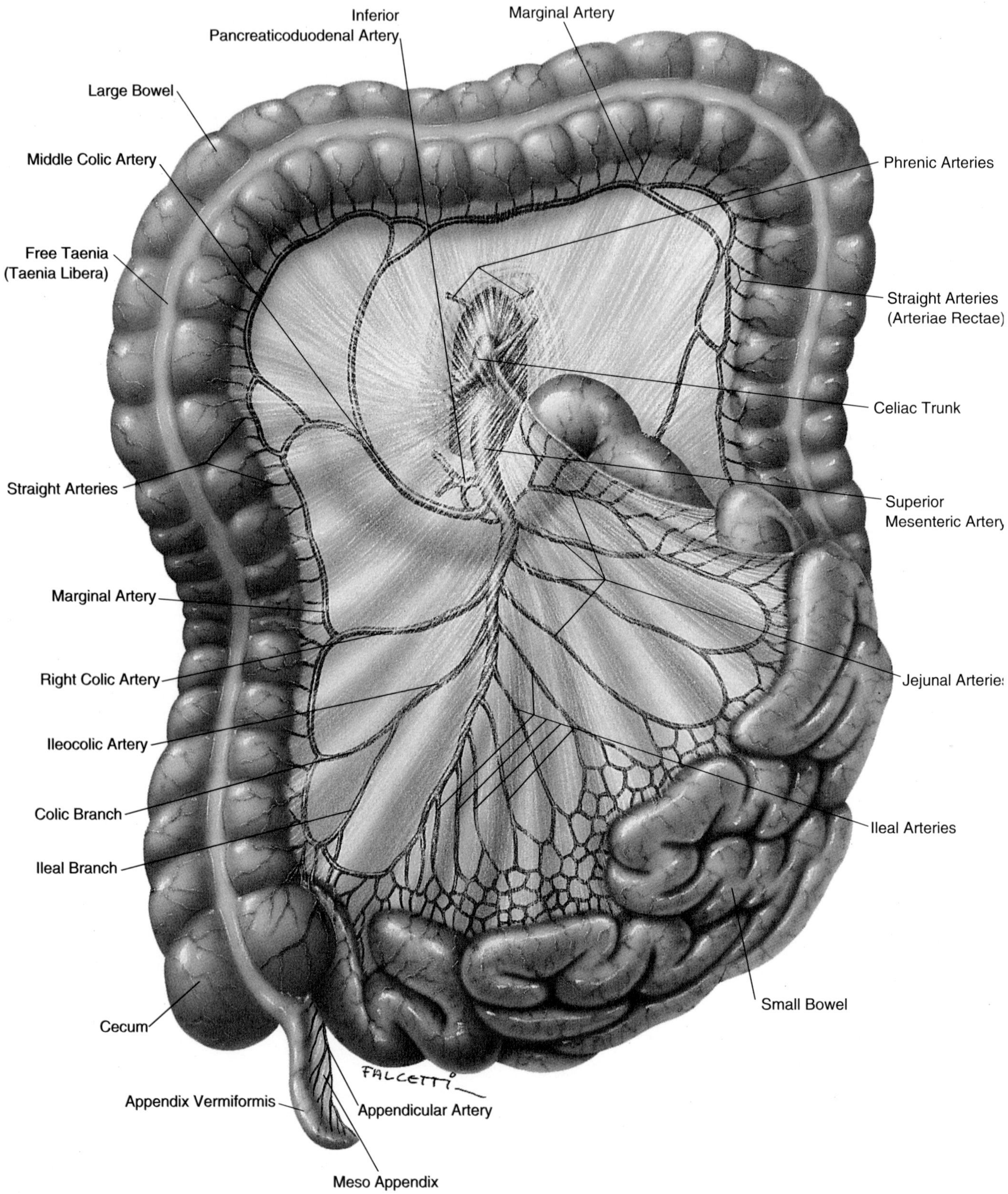

Inferior
Pancreaticoduodenal Artery

Marginal Artery

Large Bowel

Middle Colic Artery

Phrenic Arteries

Free Taenia
(Taenia Libera)

Straight Arteries
(Arteriae Rectae)

Celiac Trunk

Straight Arteries

Superior
Mesenteric Artery

Marginal Artery

Right Colic Artery

Jejunal Arteries

Ileocolic Artery

Colic Branch

Ileal Arteries

Ileal Branch

Cecum

Small Bowel

Appendix Vermiformis

Appendicular Artery

Meso Appendix

FALCETTI

Figure 18.81. Schematic drawing of the superior mesenteric artery and main branches to the large bowel and to the small bowel.

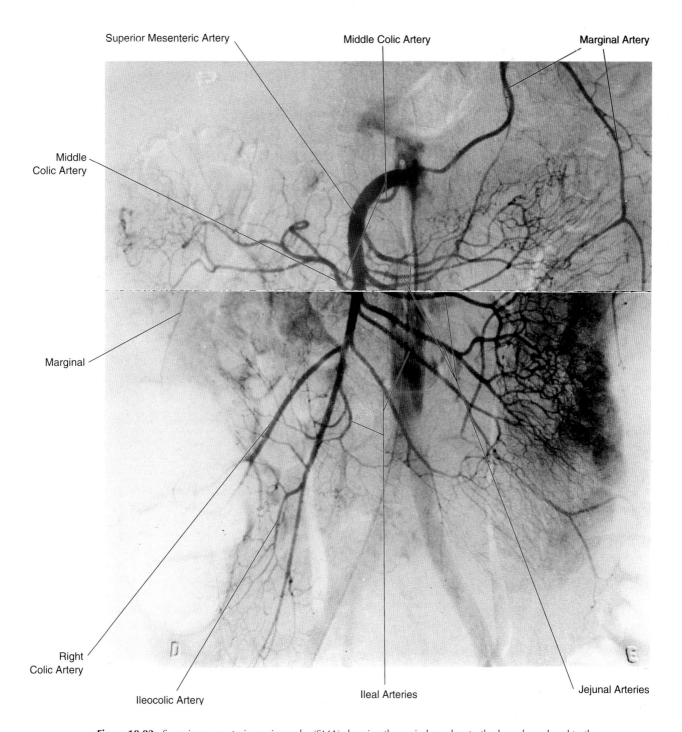

Figure 18.82. Superior mesenteric angiography (SMA) showing the main branches to the large bowel and to the small bowel. The middle colic artery has two separate origins from the SMA.

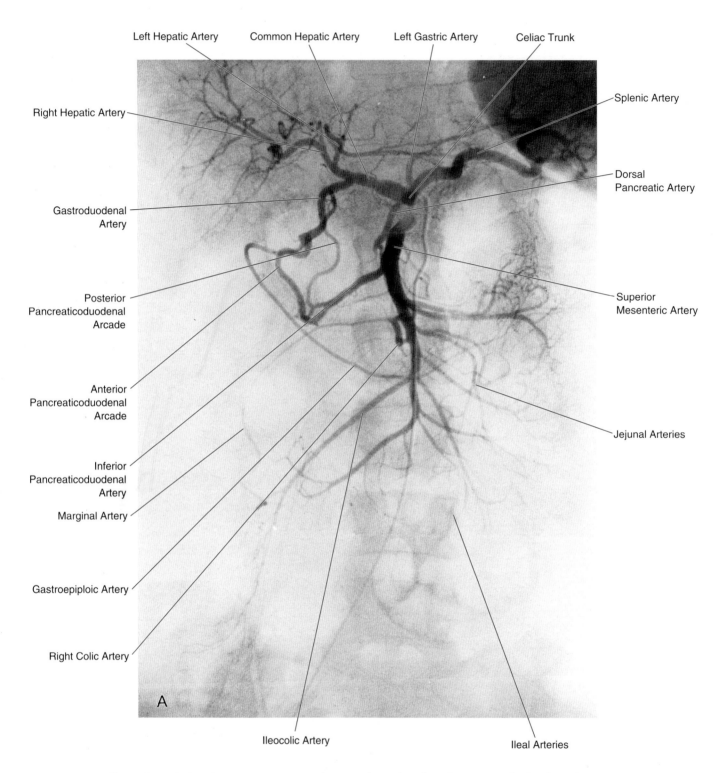

Left Hepatic Artery

Common Hepatic Artery

Left Gastric Artery

Celiac Trunk

Right Hepatic Artery

Splenic Artery

Dorsal Pancreatic Artery

Gastroduodenal Artery

Posterior Pancreaticoduodenal Arcade

Superior Mesenteric Artery

Anterior Pancreaticoduodenal Arcade

Inferior Pancreaticoduodenal Artery

Marginal Artery

Jejunal Arteries

Gastroepiploic Artery

Right Colic Artery

A

Ileocolic Artery

Ileal Arteries

Figure 18.83. A. Superior mesenteric angiography (SMA) shows the enlarged pancreaticoduodenal arcades communicating the SMA with the common hepatic artery through the inferior pancreaticoduodenal artery and gastroduodenal artery. There is severe stenosis of the celiac trunk. **B.** Late phase of the SMA angiogram showing the superior mesenteric vein, the colic veins and the jejunal and ileal veins, as well as the portal and splenic veins.

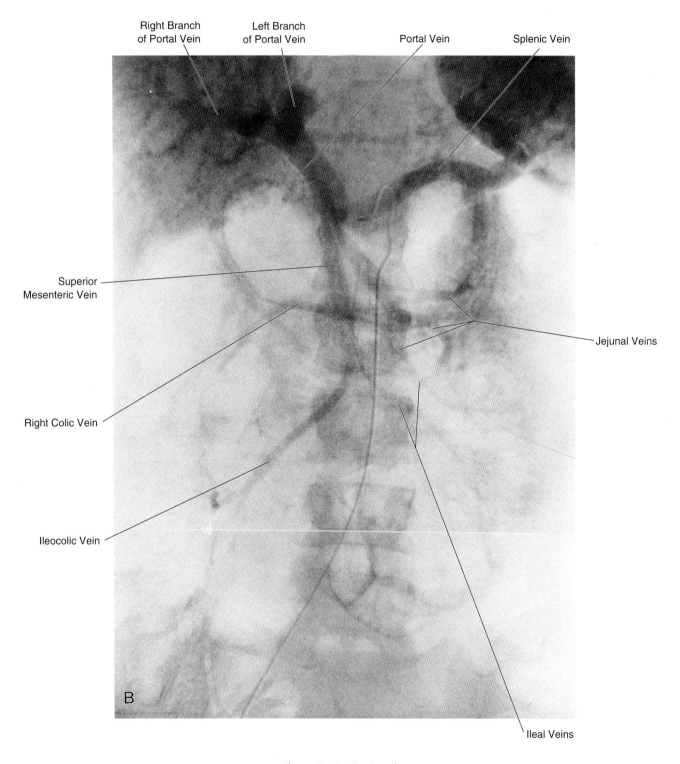

Figure 18.83. *Continued*

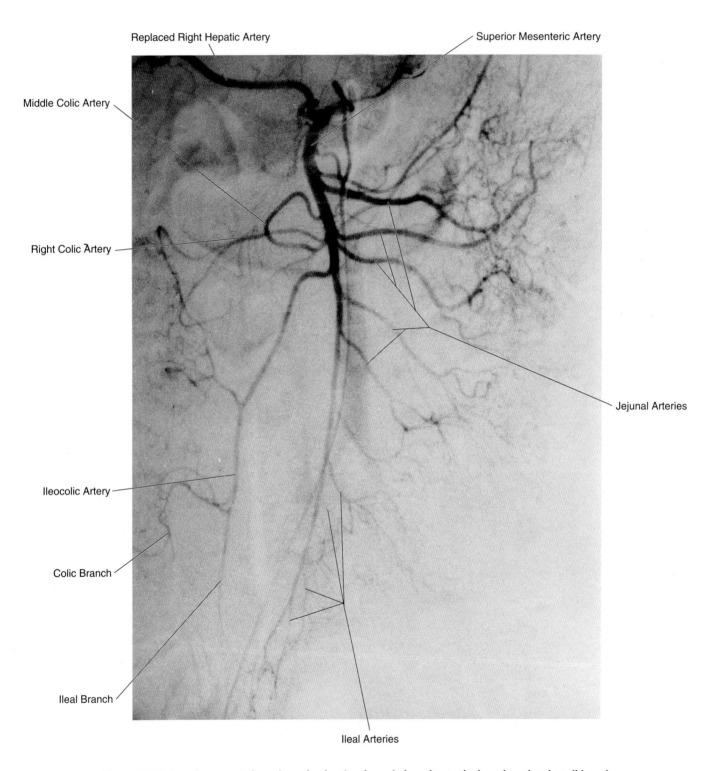

Replaced Right Hepatic Artery

Superior Mesenteric Artery

Middle Colic Artery

Right Colic Artery

Jejunal Arteries

Ileocolic Artery

Colic Branch

Ileal Branch

Ileal Arteries

Figure 18.84. Superior mesenteric angiography showing the main branches to the large bowel and small bowel.
Note the replaced right hepatic artery.

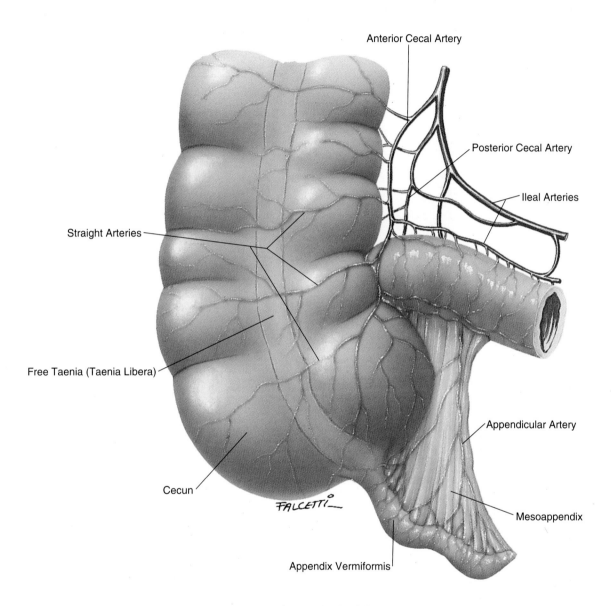

Anterior Cecal Artery

Posterior Cecal Artery

Ileal Arteries

Straight Arteries

Free Taenia (Taenia Libera)

Appendicular Artery

Cecun

Mesoappendix

Appendix Vermiformis

FALCETTI

Figure 18.85. Schematic drawing showing in close up the distal ileal arteries and the cecal arteries, as well as the appendicular artery.

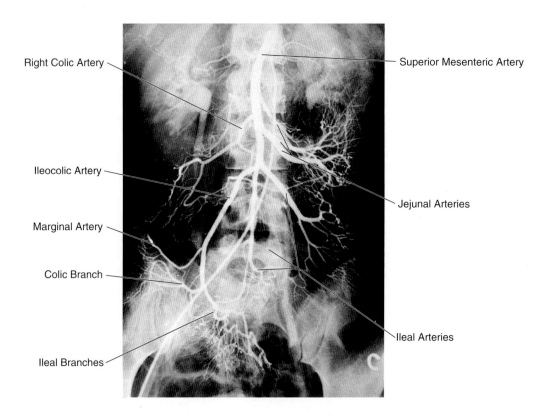

Right Colic Artery

Ileocolic Artery

Marginal Artery

Colic Branch

Ileal Branches

Superior Mesenteric Artery

Jejunal Arteries

Ileal Arteries

Figure 18.86. Superior mesenteric angiography showing the branches to the small bowel and large bowel.

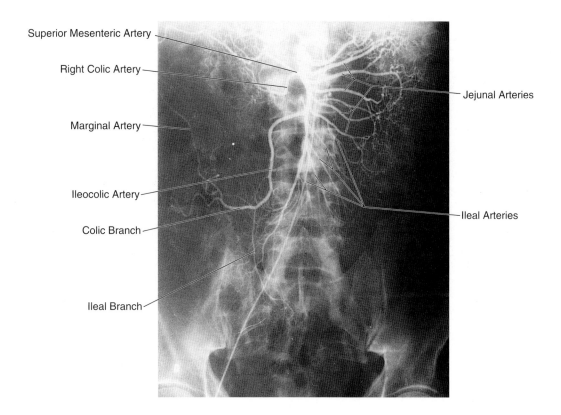

Superior Mesenteric Artery

Right Colic Artery

Marginal Artery

Ileocolic Artery

Colic Branch

Ileal Branch

Jejunal Arteries

Ileal Arteries

Figure 18.87. Superior mesenteric angiography showing the branches to the small bowel and large bowel.

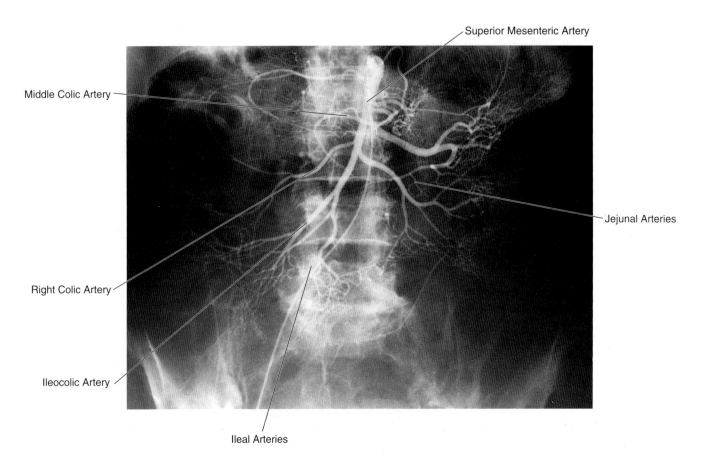

Figure 18.88. Superior mesenteric angiography showing the branches to the small bowel and large bowel.

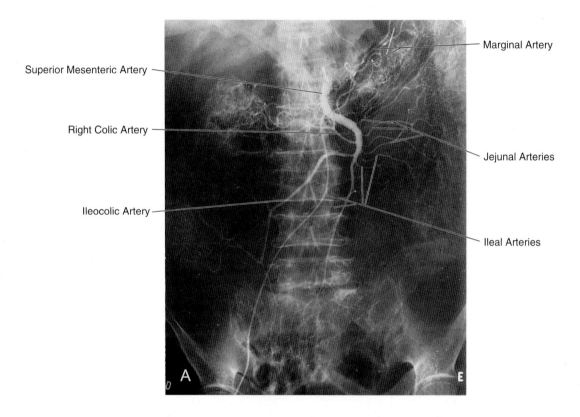

Figure 18.89. A. Early phase of the superior mesenteric angiography (SMA) showing the branches to the small bowel and large bowel. **B.** Late phase of the SMA angiography showing the superior mesenteric vein, the colic and jejunal and ileal veins.

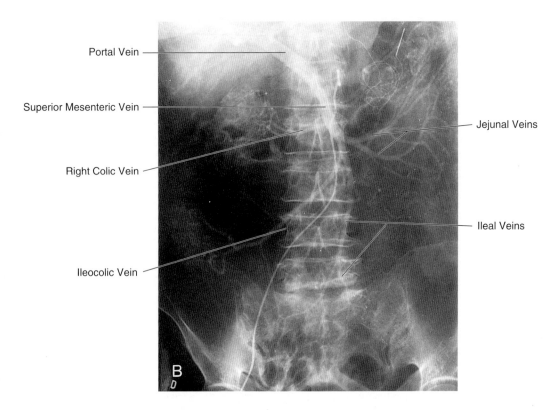

Portal Vein

Superior Mesenteric Vein

Right Colic Vein

Ileocolic Vein

Jejunal Veins

Ileal Veins

Figure 18.89. *Continued*

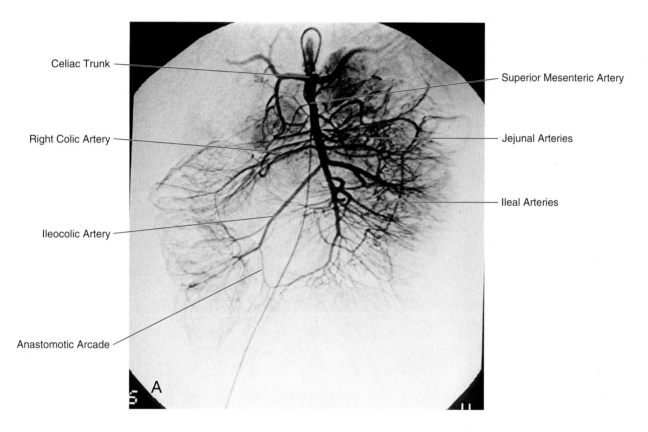

Figure 18.90.   A. SMA showing the branches to the small bowel and large bowel.   **B.** Later phase of the SMA angiography showing the superior mesenteric, jejunal and ileal veins, as well as the portal vein.

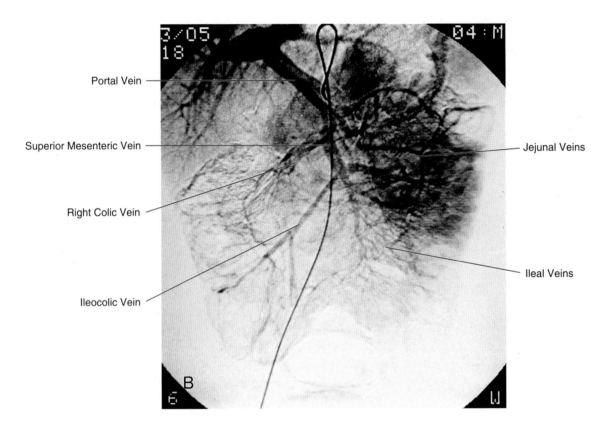

Figure 18.90. *Continued*

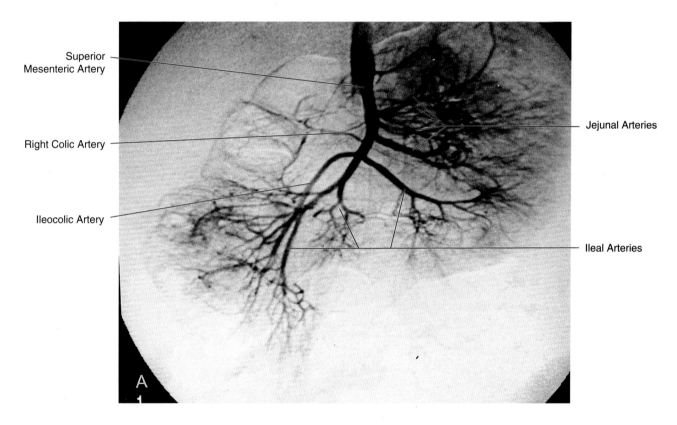

Figure 18.91. A. SMA angiography showing the arteries to the small bowel and large bowel. **B.** Later phase of the SMA angiography showing the bowel veins and the portal vein.

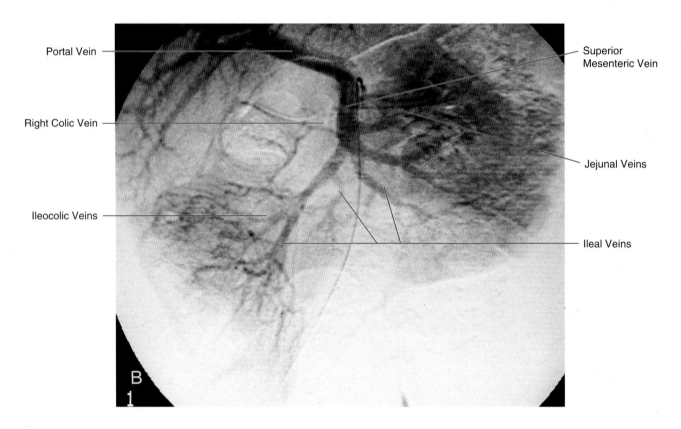

Portal Vein

Right Colic Vein

Ileocolic Veins

Superior
Mesenteric Vein

Jejunal Veins

Ileal Veins

Figure 18.91. *Continued*

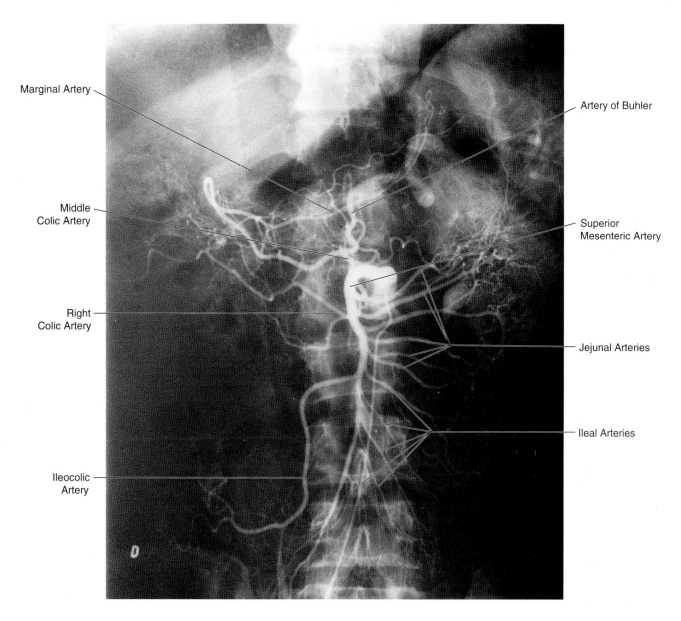

Figure 18.92. Superior mesenteric arteriogram shows the branches to the small and large bowel. Note the artery of Bühler connecting the middle colic artery to the celiac trunk. The splenic artery is faintly seen.

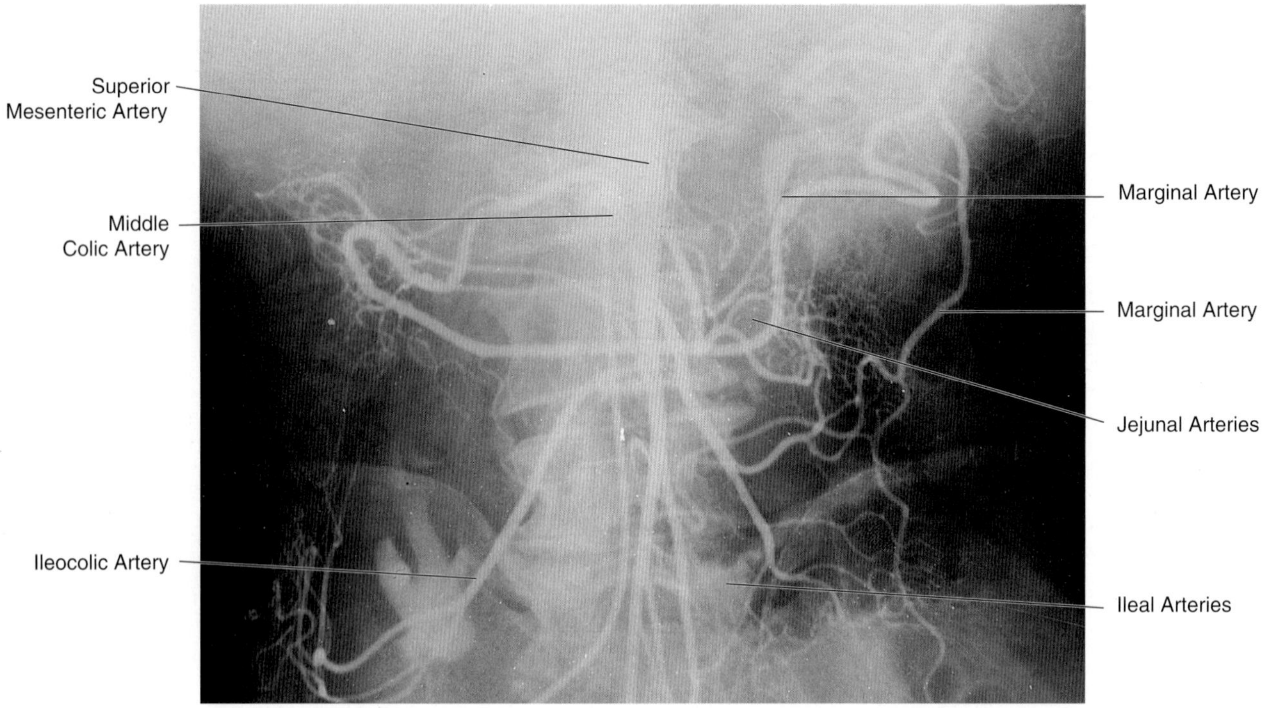

Figure 18.93. Superior mesenteric angiogram showing the enlarged marginal artery, branch of the middle colic artery.

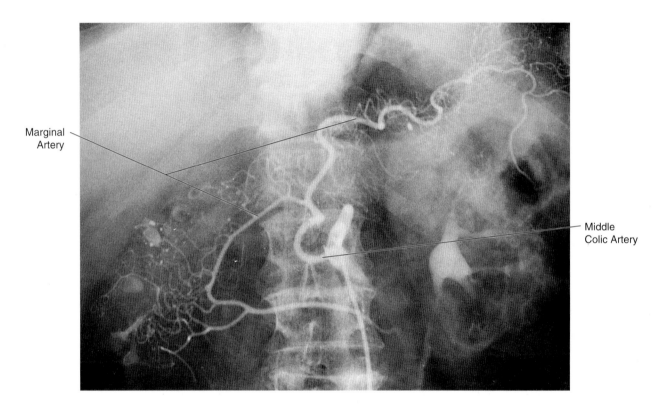

Figure 18.94. Selective injection at the middle colic artery. Note the marginal artery at the transverse colon.

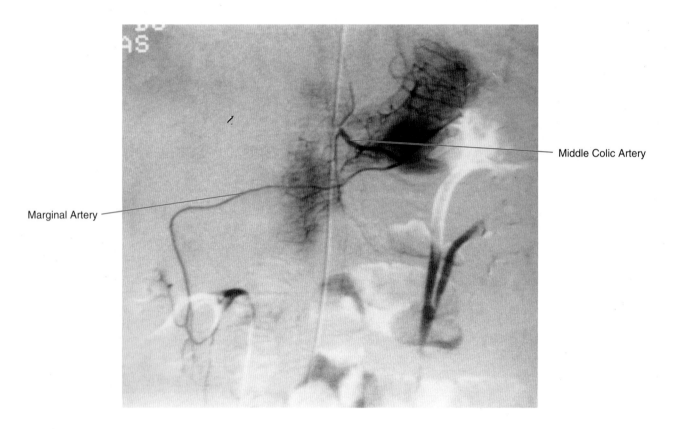

Middle Colic Artery

Marginal Artery

Figure 18.95. Selective injection at the middle colic artery.

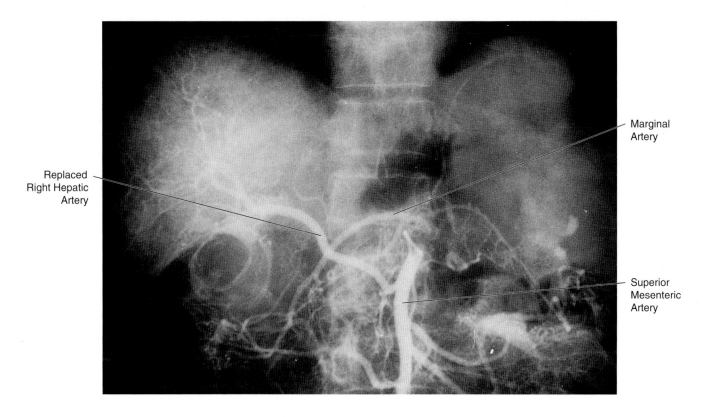

Figure 18.96. Selective angiogram of the superior mesenteric artery. Note the replaced right hepatic artery.

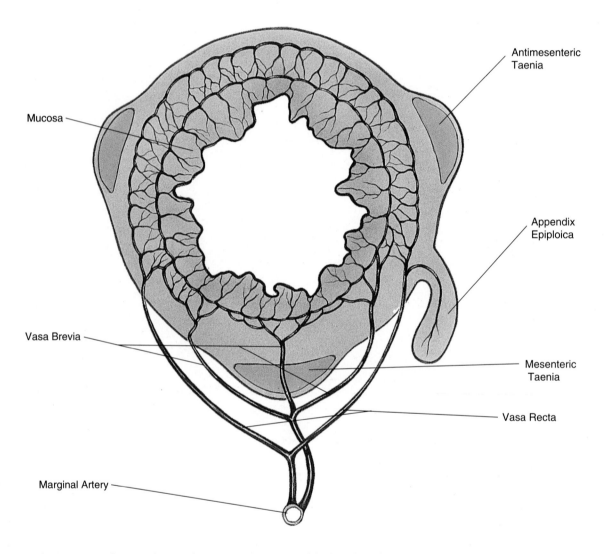

Figure 18.97. Schematic drawing showing a transverse cut of the large bowel with demonstration of the mucosal arteries, from the vasa brevia and the muscular arteries, from the vasa recta.

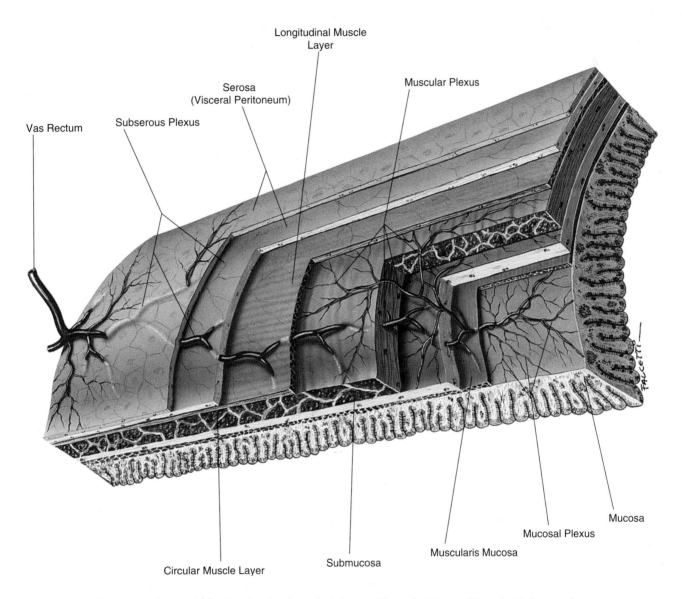

Figure 18.98. Schematic drawing showing the multiple layers of the wall of the small bowel with the vascular distribution from the peritoneum to the mucosa.

Villus

Arborization of Capillaries ⎯⎯⎯⎯⎯⎯

Capillaries

Subepithelial Channels ⎯⎯⎯⎯⎯⎯

Lymphatic Vessel

Arteriole

Venule

Submucosal Plexus

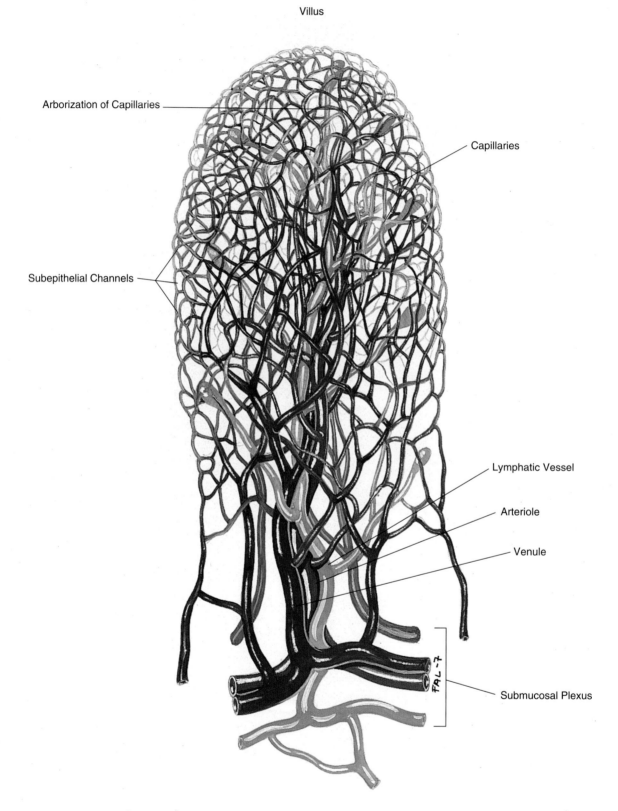

Figure 18.99. Schematic drawing of an intestinal villus showing the venules in blue, the arterioles in red and the lymphatic vessels in brown. Note the close relationship of the vessels in the center of the villus, being responsible for the counter current mechanism of O2 exchange between the arteriole and venule.

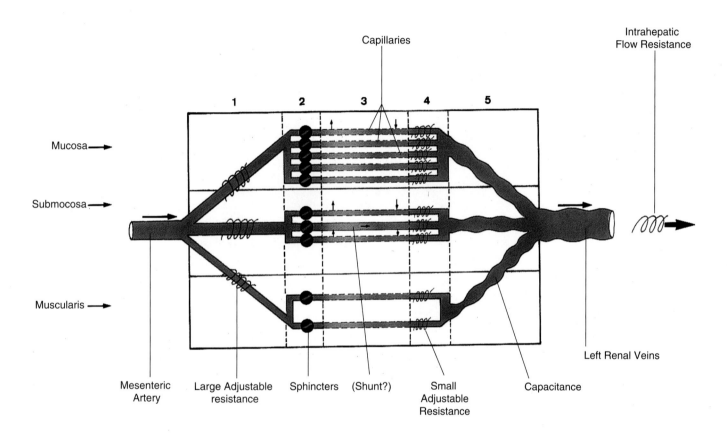

Figure 18.100. Schematic drawing of the intestinal wall compartments with the three layers. Mucosa, submucosa and muscularis mucosa. The regulation of the flow is done by the large adjustable resistance at the arterial side, sphincteric mechanisms and small adjustable resistance at the venous side. The intrahepatic flow resistance also plays a role the regulation of the flow.

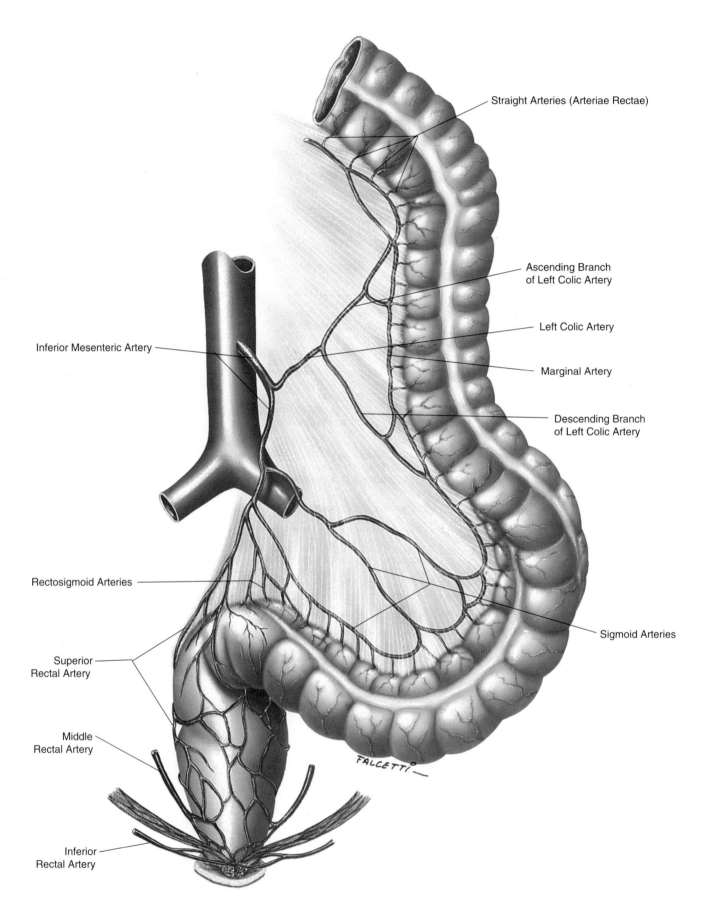

Straight Arteries (Arteriae Rectae)

Ascending Branch
of Left Colic Artery

Left Colic Artery

Marginal Artery

Descending Branch
of Left Colic Artery

Inferior Mesenteric Artery

Rectosigmoid Arteries

Sigmoid Arteries

Superior
Rectal Artery

Middle
Rectal Artery

Inferior
Rectal Artery

FALCETTI

Figure 18.101. Schematic drawing of the inferior mesenteric artery circulation.

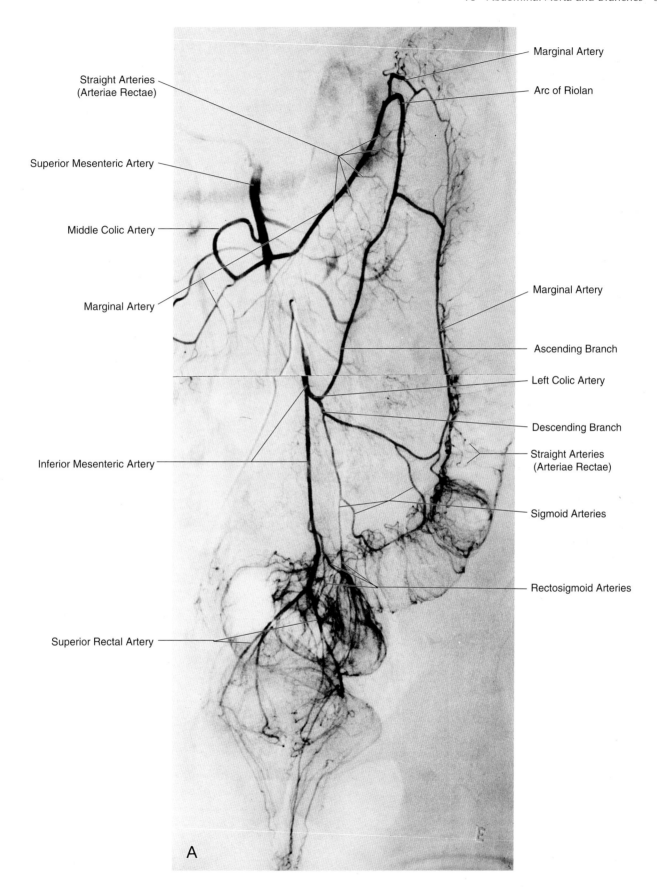

Straight Arteries
(Arteriae Rectae)

Superior Mesenteric Artery

Middle Colic Artery

Marginal Artery

Inferior Mesenteric Artery

Superior Rectal Artery

Marginal Artery

Arc of Riolan

Marginal Artery

Ascending Branch

Left Colic Artery

Descending Branch

Straight Arteries
(Arteriae Rectae)

Sigmoid Arteries

Rectosigmoid Arteries

A

Figure 18.102. A. Selective angiogram of the inferior mesenteric artery. Note the filling of the superior mesenteric artery through the middle colic artery. The arc of Riolan is the main connection of the ascending branch of the left colic artery and the marginal artery of the middle colic artery in this case. **B.** Late phase of the inferior mesenteric angiography showing the hypoplastic inferior mesenteric vein. The marginal vein along the left colon is the main via of drainage of the inferior mesenteric arterial venous system directly into the middle colic vein. The venous companion of the arc of Riolan is also depicted.

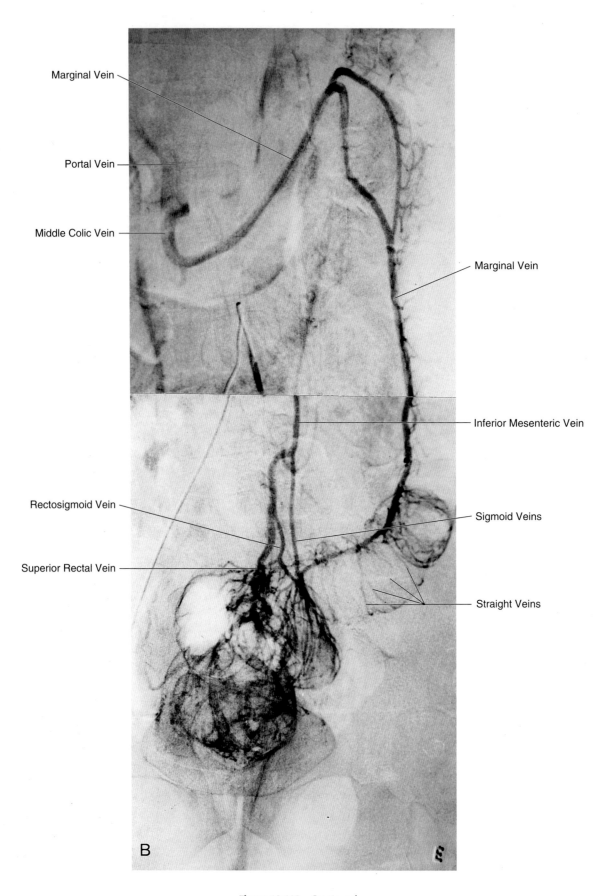

Figure 18.102. *Continued*

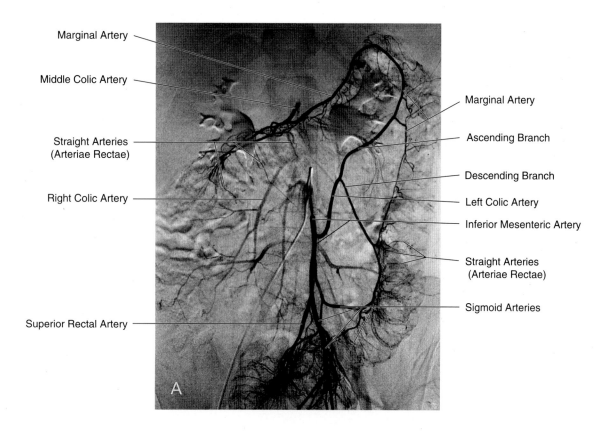

Marginal Artery

Middle Colic Artery

Straight Arteries
(Arteriae Rectae)

Right Colic Artery

Superior Rectal Artery

Marginal Artery

Ascending Branch

Descending Branch

Left Colic Artery

Inferior Mesenteric Artery

Straight Arteries
(Arteriae Rectae)

Sigmoid Arteries

A

Figure 18.103. A. Selective inferior mesenteric angiogram showing the superior rectal, the sigmoid, the left colic and marginal arteries. Note the communication between the left colic and the middle colic artery. **B.** Late phase of the angiogram showing the venous drainage of the left and transverse colon through the inferior mesenteric vein into the portal vein.

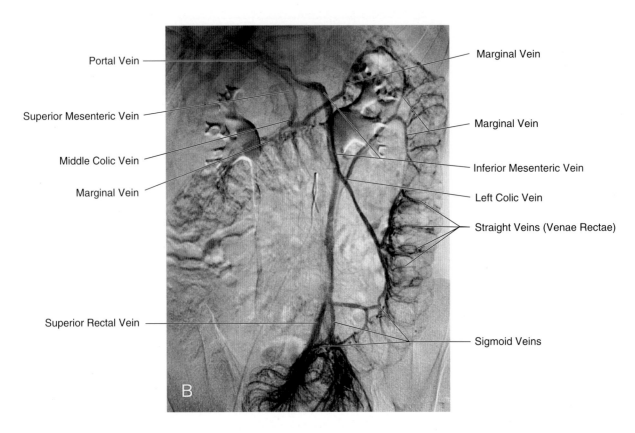

Portal Vein

Superior Mesenteric Vein

Middle Colic Vein

Marginal Vein

Superior Rectal Vein

Marginal Vein

Marginal Vein

Inferior Mesenteric Vein

Left Colic Vein

Straight Veins (Venae Rectae)

Sigmoid Veins

Figure 18.103. *Continued*

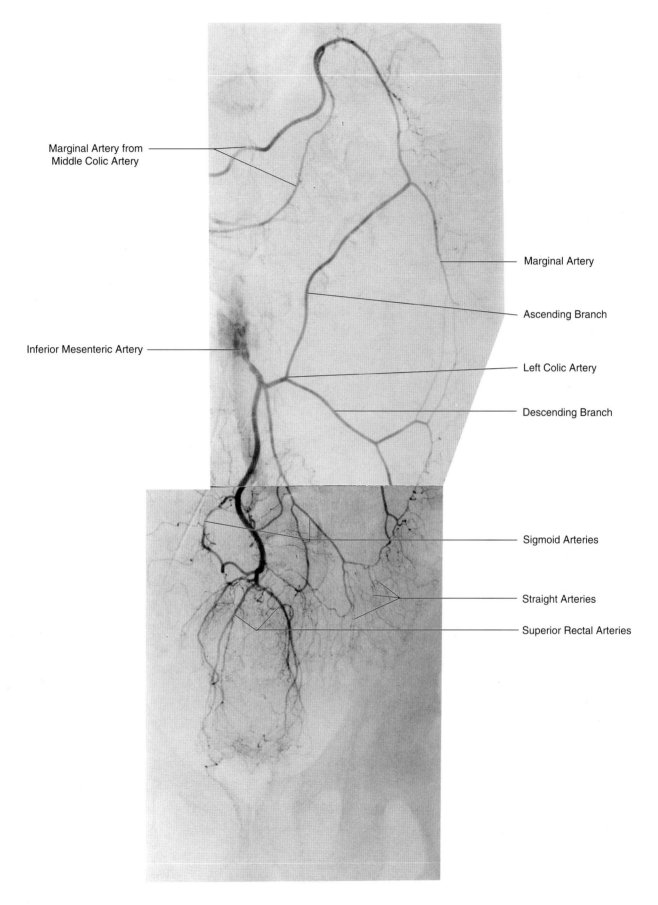

Marginal Artery from
Middle Colic Artery

Marginal Artery

Ascending Branch

Inferior Mesenteric Artery

Left Colic Artery

Descending Branch

Sigmoid Arteries

Straight Arteries

Superior Rectal Arteries

Figure 18.104. Selective angiogram of the inferior mesenteric artery, showing the circulation to the sigmoid, the rectum, the left colon and the transverse colon.

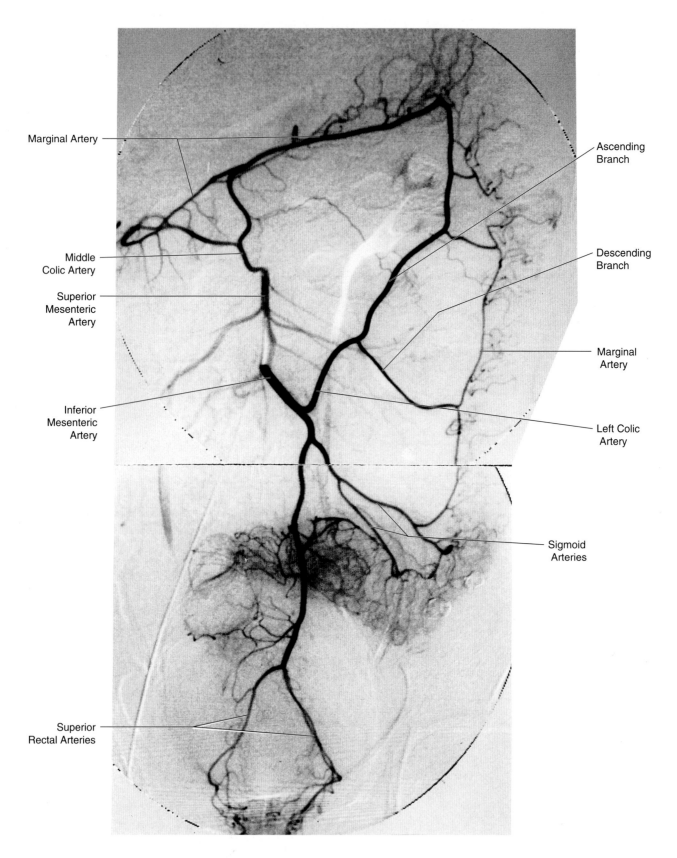

Marginal Artery

Middle
Colic Artery

Superior
Mesenteric
Artery

Inferior
Mesenteric
Artery

Superior
Rectal Arteries

Ascending
Branch

Descending
Branch

Marginal
Artery

Left Colic
Artery

Sigmoid
Arteries

Figure 18.105. Selective angiogram of the inferior mesenteric artery showing the arterial circulation to the colon and rectum. Note filling of the superior mesenteric artery through the connections through the middle colic artery.

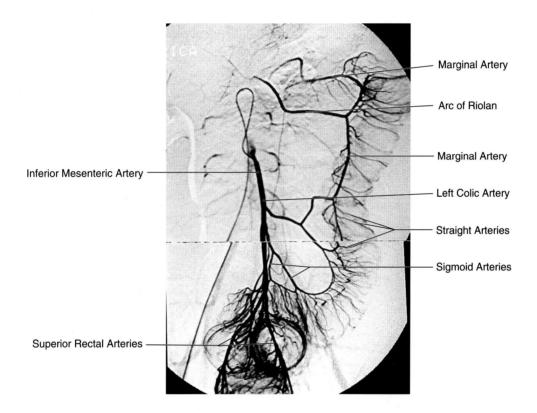

Figure 18.106. Selective angiogram of the inferior mesenteric artery showing the arterial circulation to the colon and rectum. Note the arc of Riolan as a large collateral vessel.

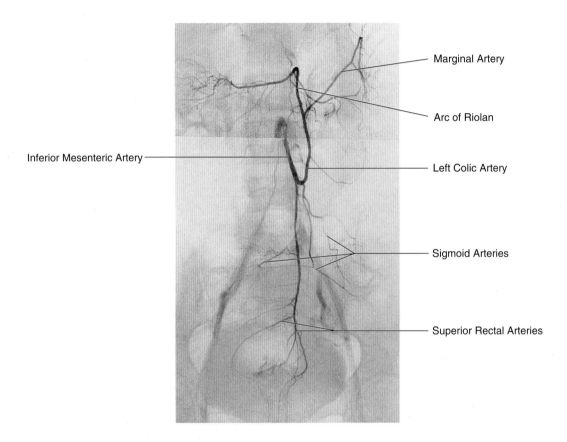

Marginal Artery

Arc of Riolan

Inferior Mesenteric Artery

Left Colic Artery

Sigmoid Arteries

Superior Rectal Arteries

Figure 18.107. Selective angiogram of the inferior mesenteric artery.

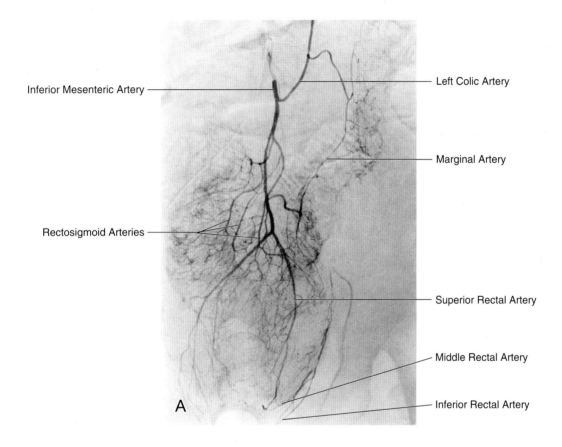

Inferior Mesenteric Artery

Left Colic Artery

Marginal Artery

Rectosigmoid Arteries

Superior Rectal Artery

Middle Rectal Artery

Inferior Rectal Artery

A

Figure 18.108. A. Selective angiogram of the inferior mesenteric artery showing the anastomosis of the superior rectal arteries with the middle rectal and inferior rectal arteries. **B.** Late phase of the angiogram showing the venous drainage of the rectum.

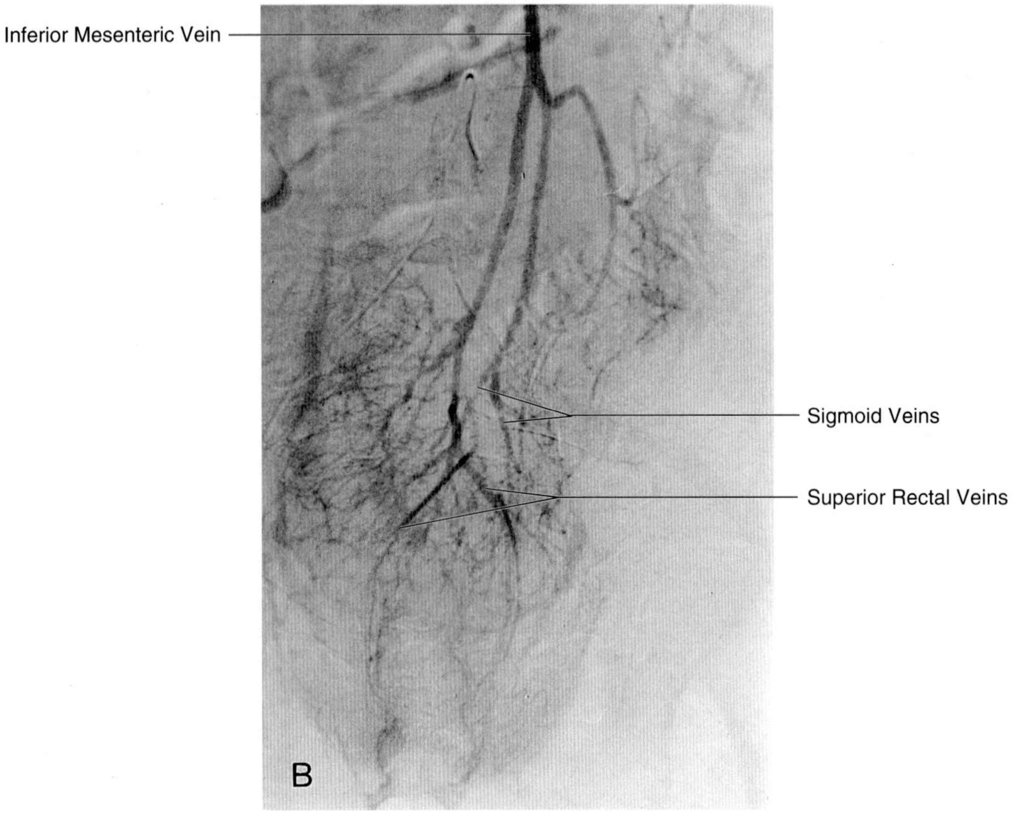

Inferior Mesenteric Vein

Sigmoid Veins

Superior Rectal Veins

B

Figure 18.108. *Continued*

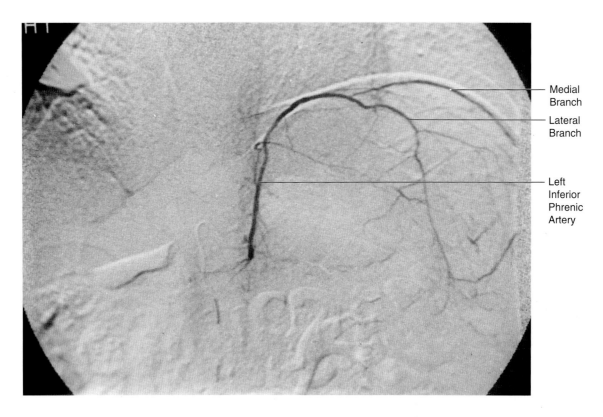

Medial
Branch

Lateral
Branch

Left
Inferior
Phrenic
Artery

Figure 18.109. Selective angiogram of the left inferior phrenic artery. Note the lateral and medial branches.

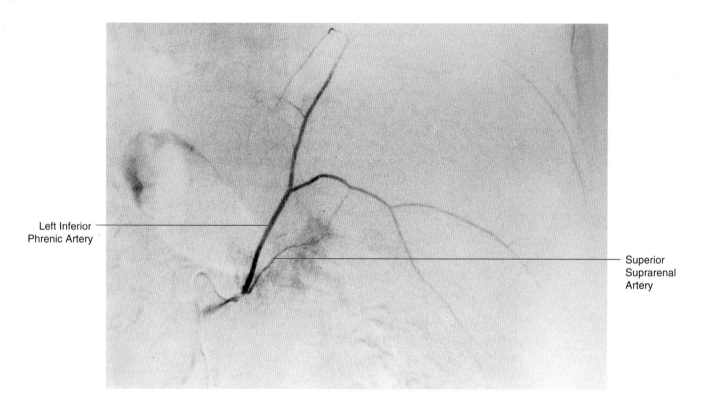

Left Inferior
Phrenic Artery

Superior
Suprarenal
Artery

Figure 18.110. Selective angiogram of the left inferior phrenic artery. The superior suprarenal artery is the first branch. Note the adrenal blush.

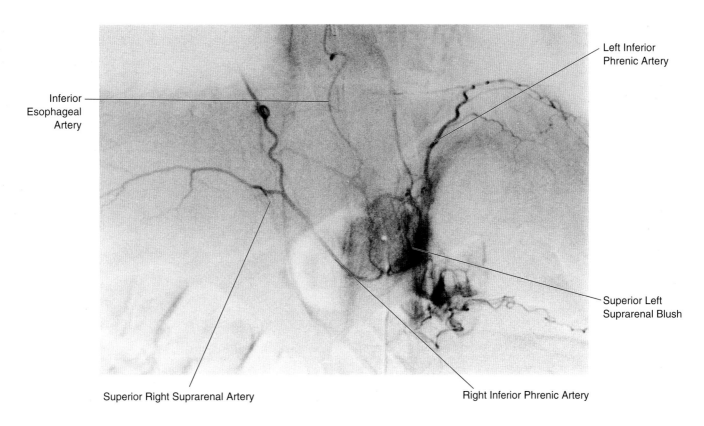

Inferior Esophageal Artery

Left Inferior Phrenic Artery

Superior Left Suprarenal Blush

Superior Right Suprarenal Artery

Right Inferior Phrenic Artery

Figure 18.111. Selective angiogram of the inferior phrenic artery, presented as a common trunk with branches to the left and right side. The superior suprarenal arteries are filled. Note the adrenal blush on the left. Some inferior esophageal arteries are also noted.

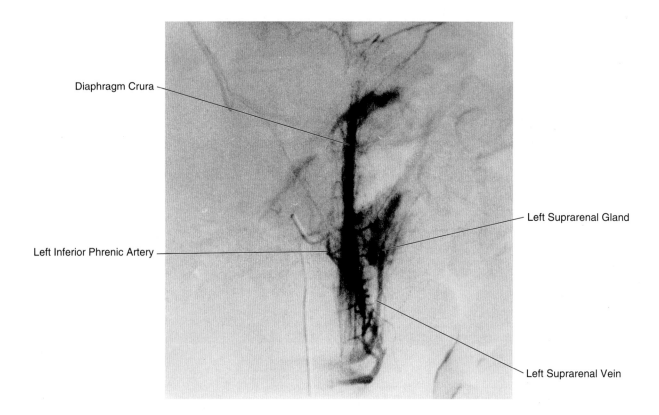

Diaphragm Crura

Left Inferior Phrenic Artery

Left Suprarenal Gland

Left Suprarenal Vein

Figure 18.112. Selective angiogram of the left inferior phrenic artery. Note the diaphragmatic crura stain. The left adrenal blush is observed as well as the left suprarenal vein draining into the left renal vein.

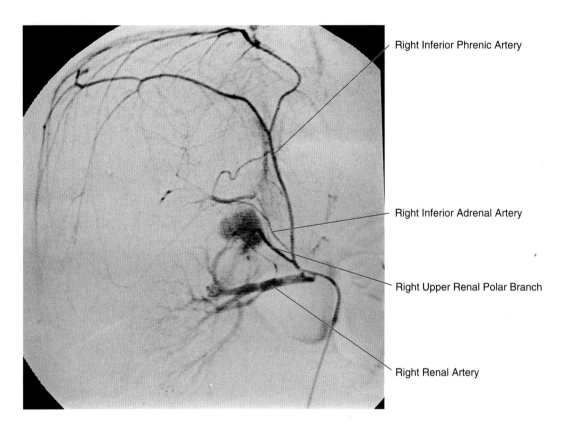

Right Inferior Phrenic Artery

Right Inferior Adrenal Artery

Right Upper Renal Polar Branch

Right Renal Artery

Figure 18.113. Selective injection at the right inferior phrenic artery arising as a common trunk with the right inferior adrenal artery as well as a upper renal polar branch. The right main renal artery is partially filled. Note a ill-defined right adrenal blush.

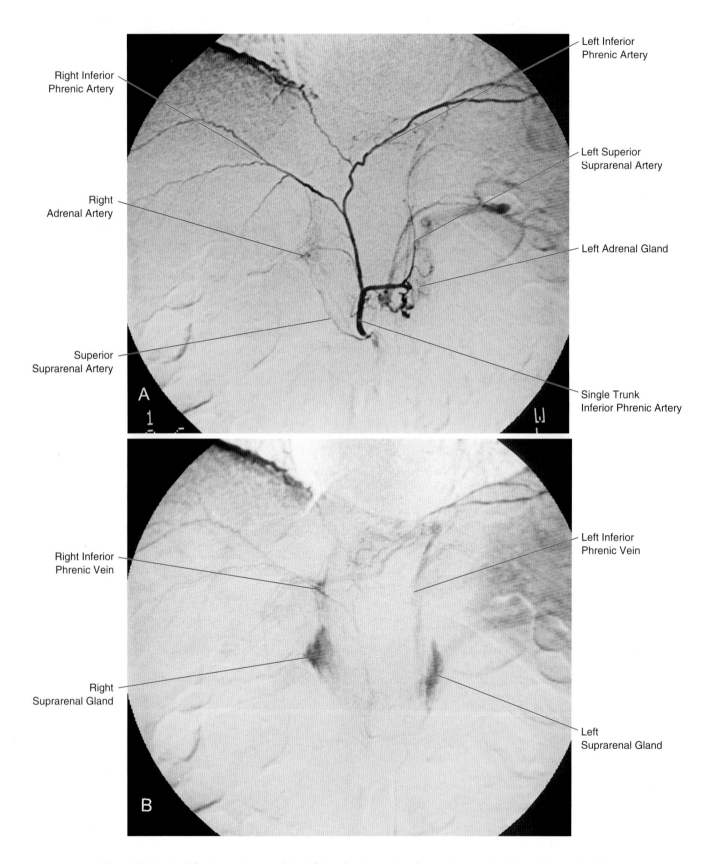

Right Inferior
Phrenic Artery

Right
Adrenal Artery

Superior
Suprarenal Artery

Left Inferior
Phrenic Artery

Left Superior
Suprarenal Artery

Left Adrenal Gland

Single Trunk
Inferior Phrenic Artery

A

Right Inferior
Phrenic Vein

Right
Suprarenal Gland

Left Inferior
Phrenic Vein

Left
Suprarenal Gland

B

Figure 18.114. A. Selective angiogram of the inferior phrenic arteries observed as a trunk giving origin to the right
and left inferior phrenic arteries. Note the origin of the right and left superior suprarenal arteries. The adrenal blush
is ill-defined in both sides. The right superior suprarenal artery is hardly visible. **B.** Late phase angiogram shows
the right and left adrenal blush and the right and left inferior phrenic veins.

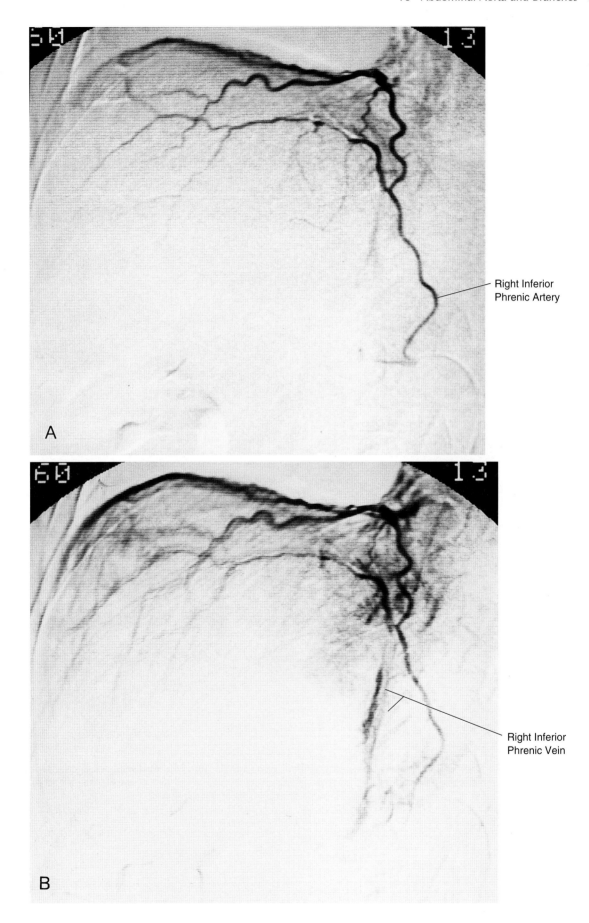

Figure 18.115. A. Right inferior phrenic artery angiogram. **B.** Late phase of the angiogram shows the venous drainage parallel to the arteries and the right inferior phrenic vein.

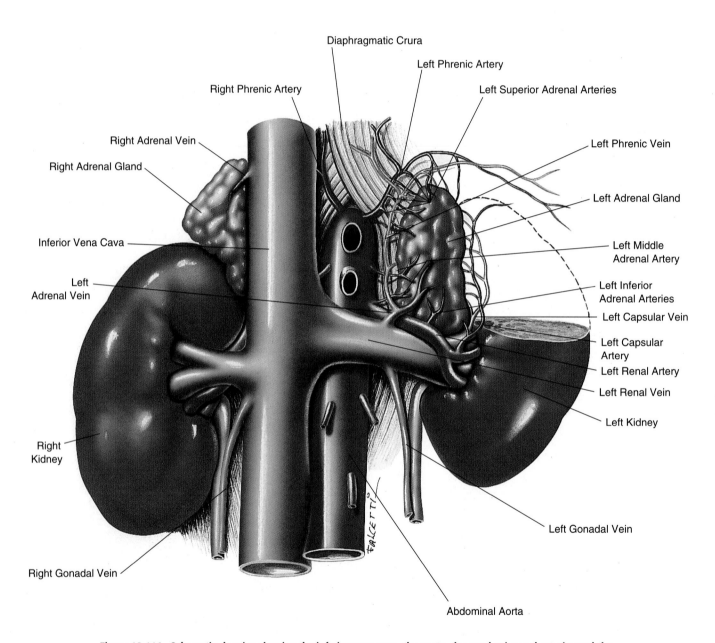

Figure 18.116. Schematic drawing showing the inferior vena cava, the aorta, the renal veins and arteries and the relationship of these structures with the adrenal glands. Note the arterial and venous supply of the left adrenal gland. Only the vein of the right adrenal gland is shown.

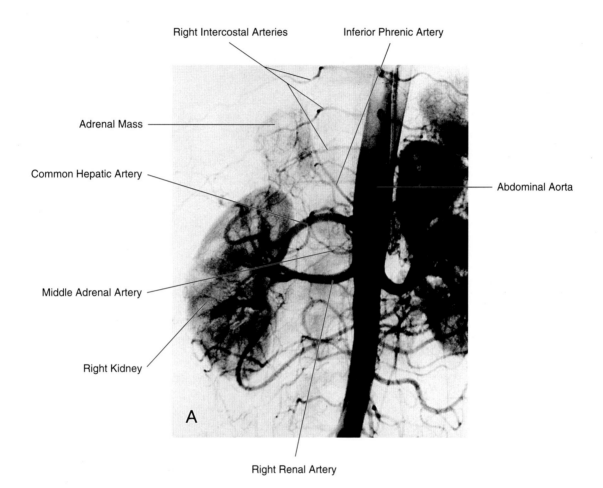

Right Intercostal Arteries

Inferior Phrenic Artery

Adrenal Mass

Common Hepatic Artery

Middle Adrenal Artery

Right Kidney

Abdominal Aorta

A

Right Renal Artery

Figure 18.117. A. Aortogram of the abdomen, showing the arteries to the right kidney and to the right adrenal gland. A vascular mass (pheochromocytoma) is demonstrated replacing the right adrenal gland. **B.** Selective injection into the middle adrenal artery shows retrograde filling of the inferior phrenic artery via the superior adrenal artery.

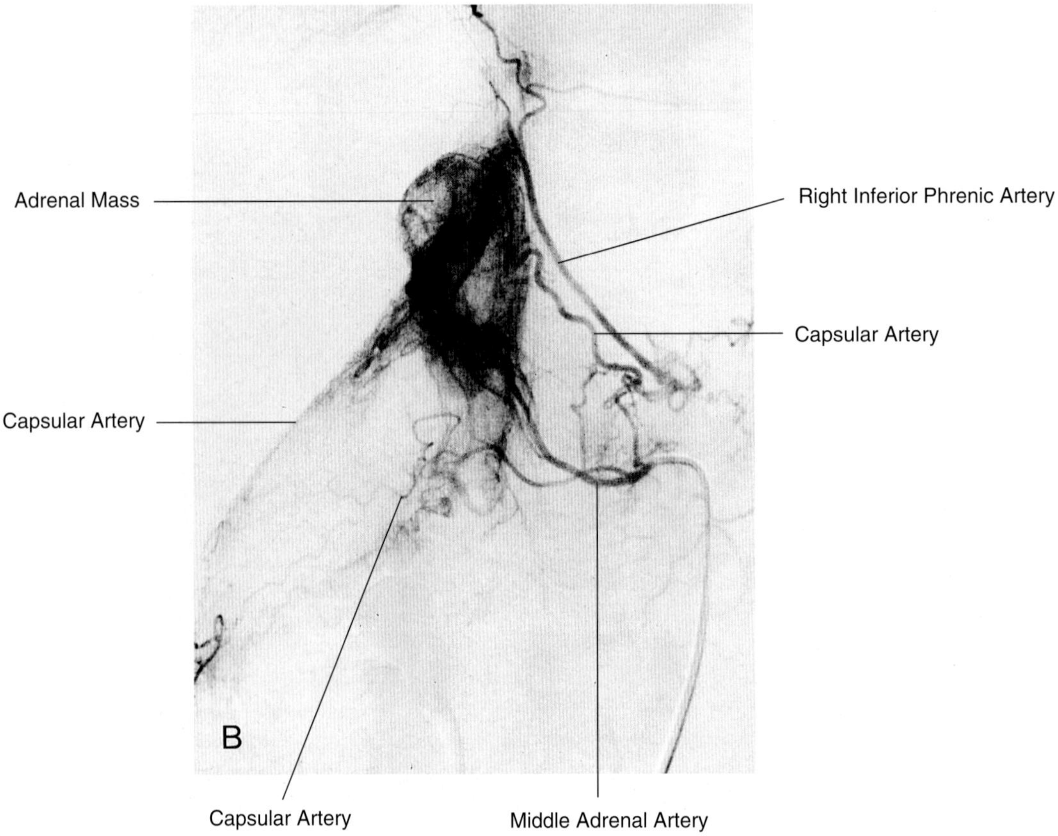

Figure 18.117. *Continued*

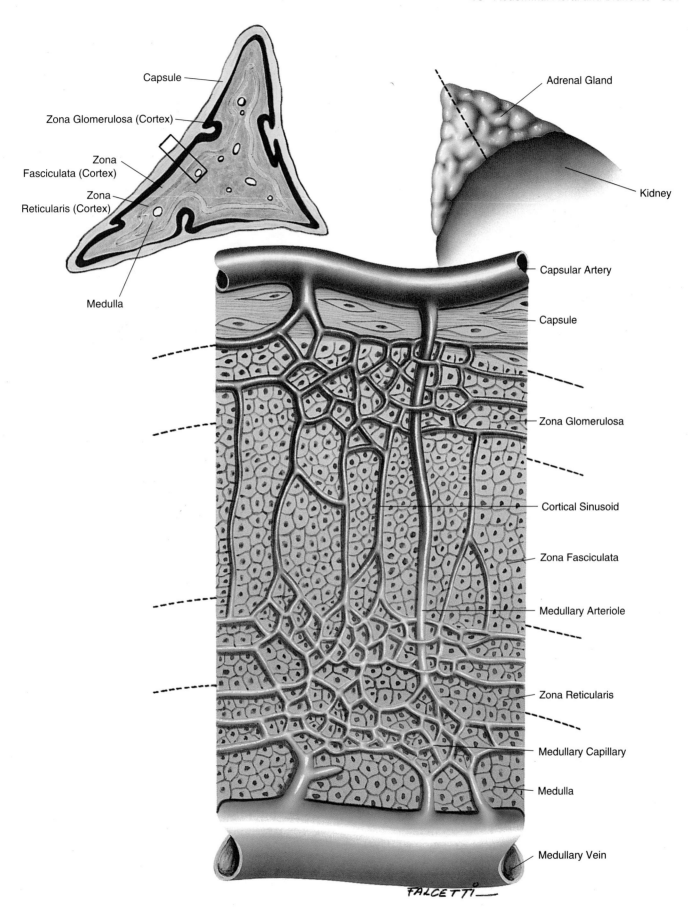

Capsule

Zona Glomerulosa (Cortex)

Zona Fasciculata (Cortex)

Zona Reticularis (Cortex)

Medulla

Adrenal Gland

Kidney

Capsular Artery

Capsule

Zona Glomerulosa

Cortical Sinusoid

Zona Fasciculata

Medullary Arteriole

Zona Reticularis

Medullary Capillary

Medulla

Medullary Vein

FALCETTI

Figure 18.118. Schematic drawing of the left adrenal gland showing the microstructure of the gland on a transverse cut. Note the capsular circulation and the connections through the sinusoids to the medullary vein.

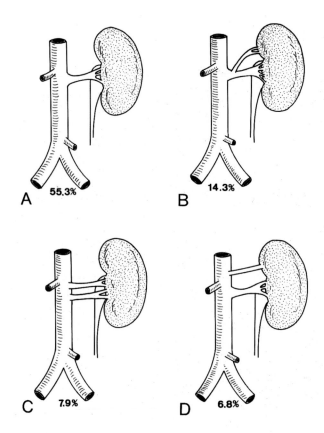

Figure 18.119. Types and incidence of renal arterial supply. A. One hilar artery, 55.3% (147 of 266 pedicles). **B.** One hilar artery with one superior pole extrahilar branch, 14.3% (38 of 266 pedicles). **C.** Two hilar arteries, 7.9% (21 of 266 pedicles). **D.** One hilar artery with one superior polar artery, 6.8% (18 of 266 pedicles).

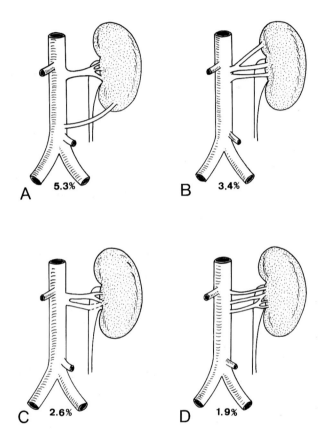

Figure 18.120. Types and incidence of renal arterial supply. A. One hilar artery with one inferior polar artery, 5.3% (14 of 266 pedicles). **B.** Two hilar arteries with one superior pole extrahilar branch, 3.4% (9 of 266 pedicles). **C.** One hilar artery with a precocious bifurcation, 2.6% (7 of 266 pedicles). **D.** Three hilar arteries, 1.9% (5 of 266 pedicles).

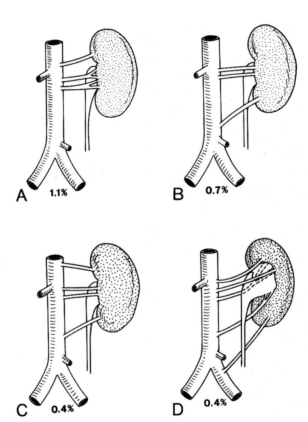

Figure 18.121. Types and incidence of renal arterial supply. A. Two hilar arteries with one superior polar artery, 1.1% (3 of 266 pedicles). **B.** Two hilar arteries with one inferior polar artery, 0.7% (2 of 266 pedicles). **C.** Two hilar arteries with one superior polar artery and one inferior polar artery, 0.4% (1 of 266 pedicles). **D.** Three hilar arteries with one superior polar artery and one inferior polar artery, 0.4% (1 of 266 pedicles).

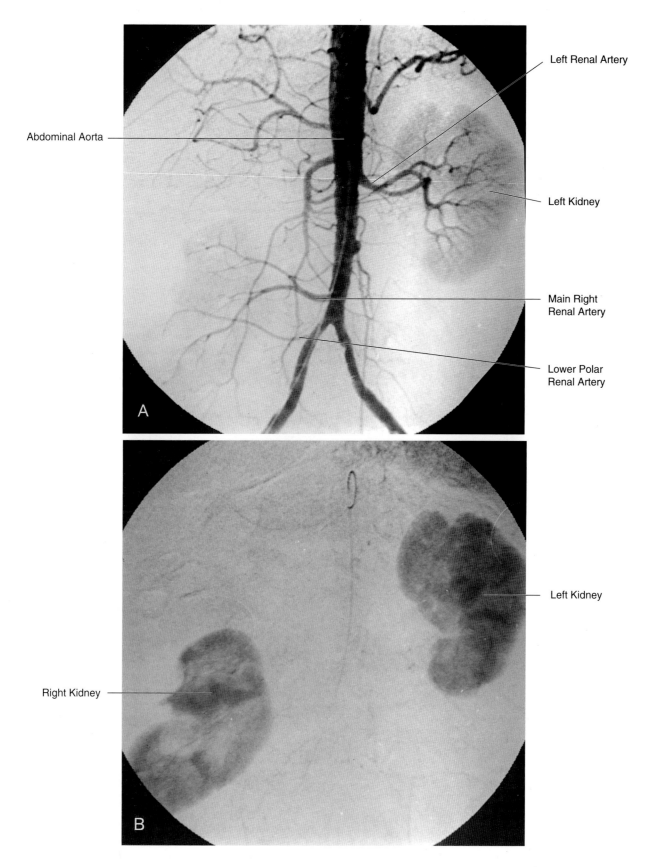

Figure 18.122. A. Abdominal aortogram. Normal positioned left kidney. The main renal artery on the right side originates from the distal aorta, close to the bifurcation. Note the smaller renal branch arising from the right common iliac artery. **B.** Late phase of the aortogram showing the bilateral nephrogram. Note the caudal position of the right kidney.

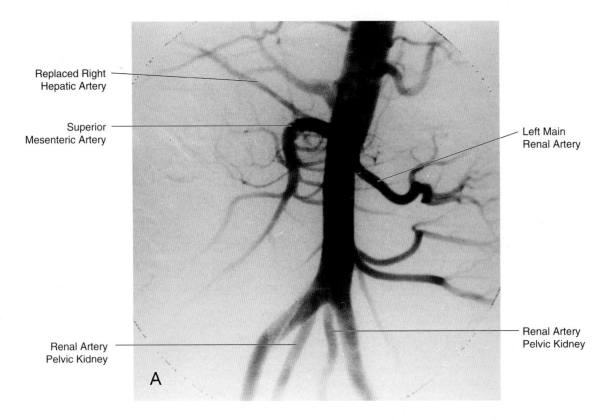

Replaced Right
Hepatic Artery

Superior
Mesenteric Artery

Left Main
Renal Artery

Renal Artery
Pelvic Kidney

Renal Artery
Pelvic Kidney

A

Figure 18.123. A. Abdominal aortogram showing a topic left kidney with the origin of the left main renal artery
in the abdominal aorta. Note the vessels arising from the bifurcation of the aorta and common iliac arteries.
B. Angiography of the iliac vessels shows the three renal arteries supplying the intrapelvic kidney. Two of
the main arteries arise from the common iliac arteries while a small artery arises from the distal aorta.

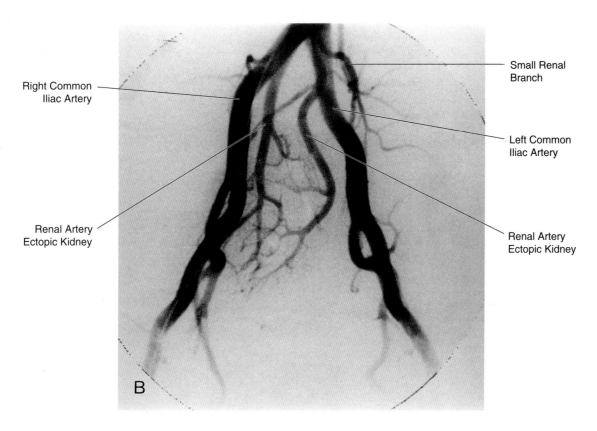

Right Common
Iliac Artery

Small Renal
Branch

Renal Artery
Ectopic Kidney

Left Common
Iliac Artery

Renal Artery
Ectopic Kidney

B

Figure 18.123. *Continued*

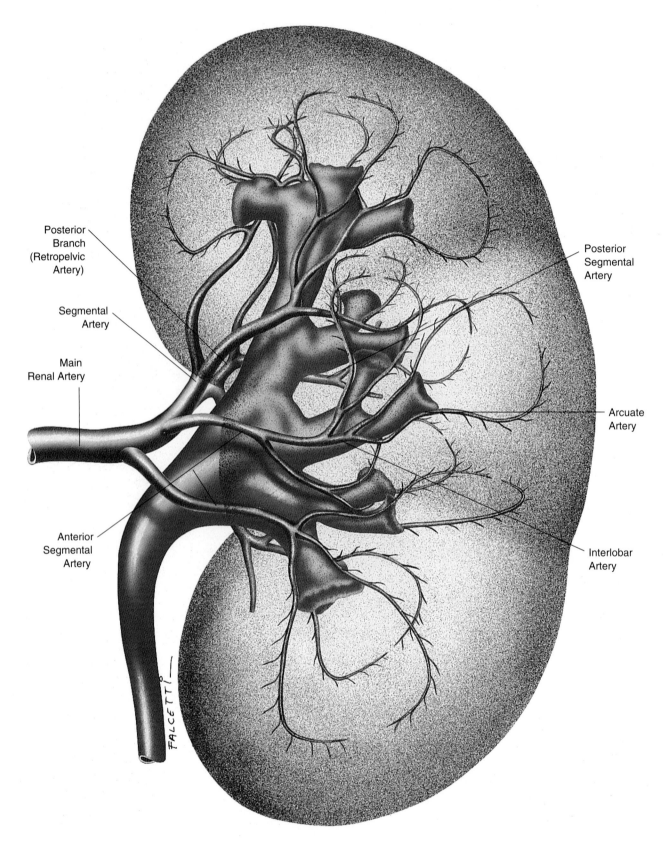

Posterior
Branch
(Retropelvic
Artery)

Segmental
Artery

Main
Renal Artery

Anterior
Segmental
Artery

Posterior
Segmental
Artery

Arcuate
Artery

Interlobar
Artery

FALCETTI

Figure 18.124. Schematic drawing of an anterior view from a left kidney shows the branching of the renal arteries and their official nomenclature according to kidney regions. Renal artery; segmental artery; interlobar artery (Infundibular) and arcuate artery.

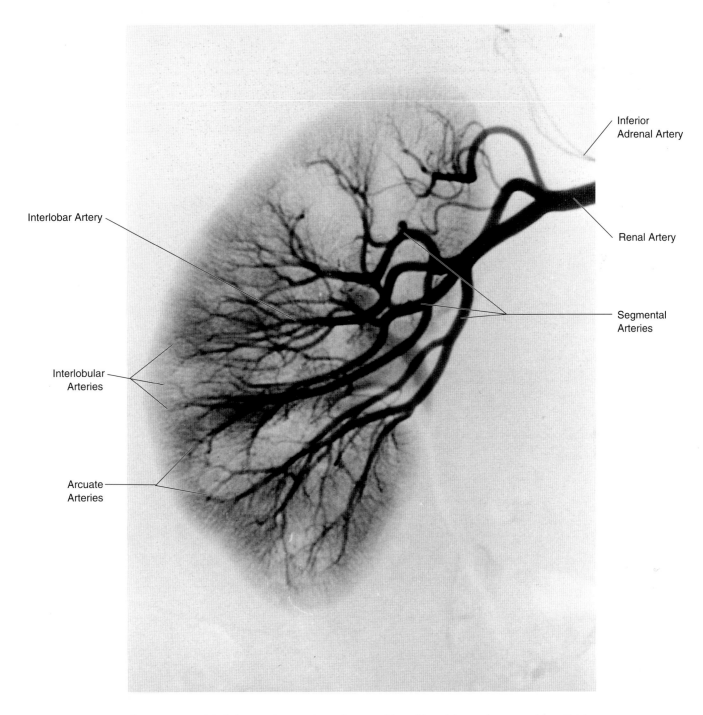

Figure 18.125. Right kidney angiogram shows the normal branching of the renal artery and the official nomenclature according to the kidney regions.

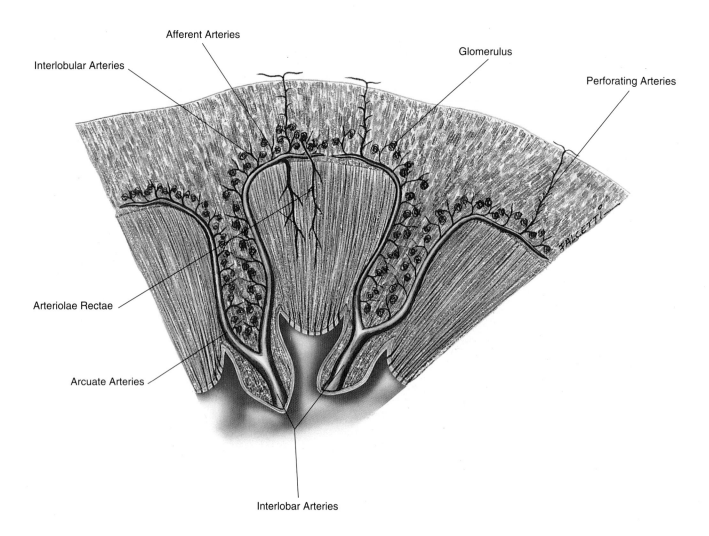

Figure 18.126. Schematic diagram of two adjacent pyramids and minor calices, depicts the vasculature of the renal parenchyma from the level of the interlobar arteries to the glomerular level.

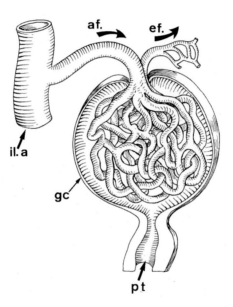

Figure 18.127. Schematic drawing representing the renal corpuscle (of Malpighi). il.a: interlobular artery; af.: afferent arterioles; ef.: efferent arterioles; gc: glomerular capsule (Bowman); pt: proximal tubule.

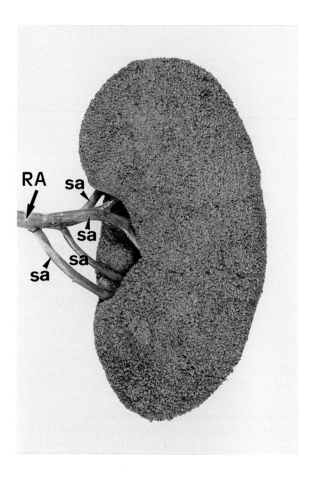

Figure 18.128. Anterior view of a left kidney polyester resin endocast of the renal arterial vasculature. Note the "sponge-like" appearance of the endocast, which represents the glomeruli filled with the polyester resin. RA: main trunk of the renal artery. sa: anterior segmental arteries. Reprinted with permission from Sampaio FJB.

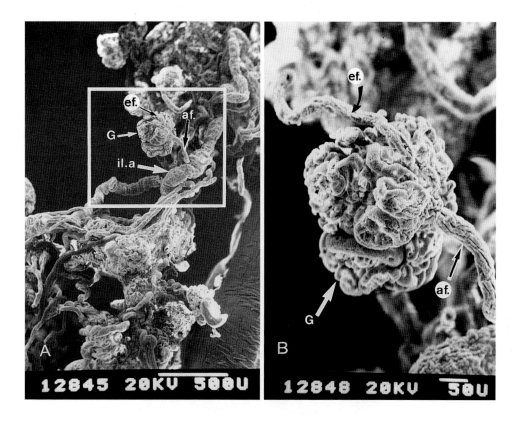

Figure 18.129. A. Scanning electron microscopy (SEM) of a polyester resin endocast of the renal arterial vasculature reveals an interlobular artery (il.a) giving off an afferent arteriole (af.) which forms a glomerulus (G). The efferent arteriole (ef.) of the glomerulus is also indicated (X 40). **B.** Magnified SEM view of the same region demarcated in A, details the afferent arteriole (af.), the efferent arteriole (ef.), and the glomerulus itself (G) (X 300). (From Sampaio FJB).

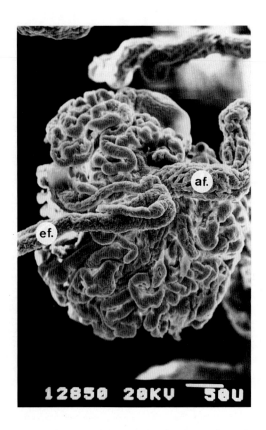

Figure 18.130. Scanning electron microscopy close-up view of a glomerular endocast reveals the vascular pole with the afferent (af.) and efferent (ef.) arterioles. This figure demonstrates that the afferent arteriole has a greater caliber than the efferent arteriole (X 300). Reprinted with permission from Sampaio FJB.

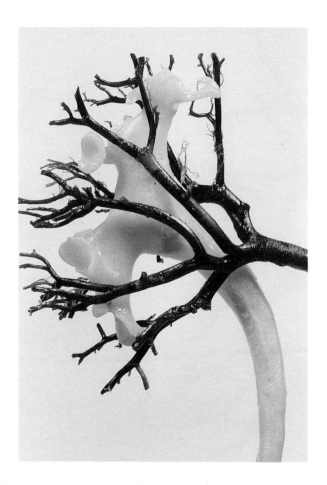

Figure 18.131. Anterior view of endocast (pelvicaliceal system and arteries) from a right kidney. This cast shows that the fine arterial vessels and the glomerular tufts were removed by needle hand picking, allowing a clear visualization of the major intrarenal arteries and the underlying collecting system. Reprinted with permission from Sampaio FJB.

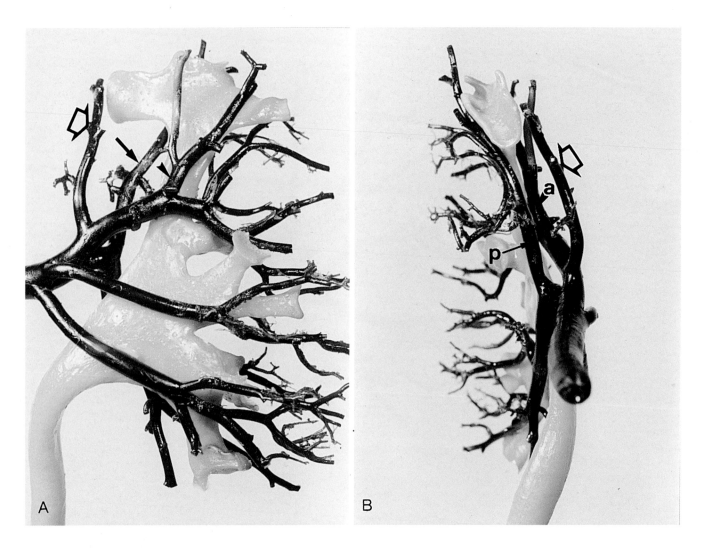

Figure 18.132. A. Anterior view of an endocast (pelvicaliceal system and arteries) from a left kidney shows arterial supply related to the superior pole: the superior (apical) segmental artery (open arrow), the artery related to the anterior surface of the upper infundibulum (arrowhead) and the branch of the posterior segmental artery related to the posterior surface of the upper infundibulum (arrow). **B.** Oblique posterior view of the same endocast shown in A, reveals the artery related to the anterior surface (a) and the artery related to the posterior surface (p) of the upper infundibulum. The open arrow points to the superior (apical) segmental artery, which is not related to the upper infundibulum. The asterisk marks the posterior segmental artery (retropelvic artery). Reprinted with permission from Sampaio FJB.

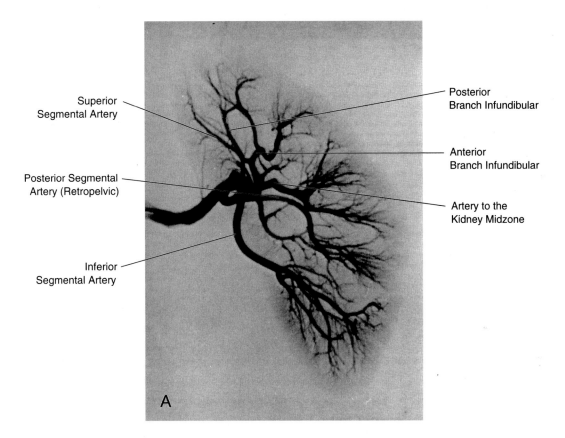

Superior
Segmental Artery

Posterior
Branch Infundibular

Anterior
Branch Infundibular

Posterior Segmental
Artery (Retropelvic)

Artery to the
Kidney Midzone

Inferior
Segmental Artery

A

Figure 18.133. A. Anterior view of a left renal angiogram shows the arterial supply related to the superior pole: the superior segmental artery, the artery related to the anterior surface of the upper infundibulum and the branch of the posterior segmental artery related to the posterior surface of the upper infundibulum. **B, C** and **D.** Later phase of the renal angiogram showing the progressive filling of the peripheral vessels, including the interlobar arteries, the arcuate arteries and the interlobular arteries. In D, the nephrogram is more prominent.

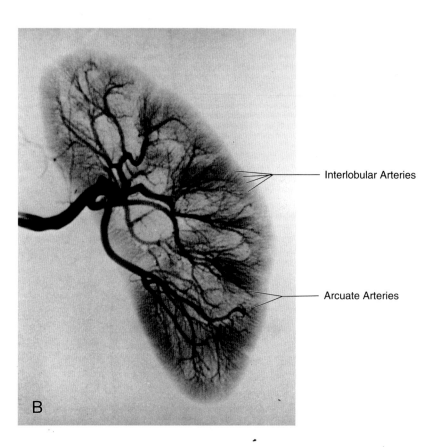

Interlobular Arteries

Arcuate Arteries

B

Figure 18.133. Continued

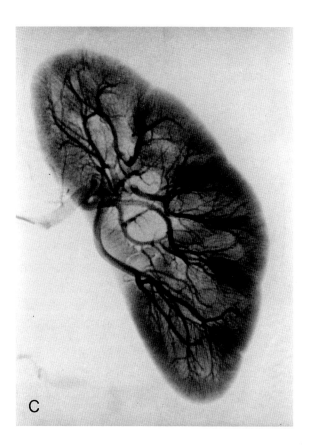

Figure 18.133. *Continued*

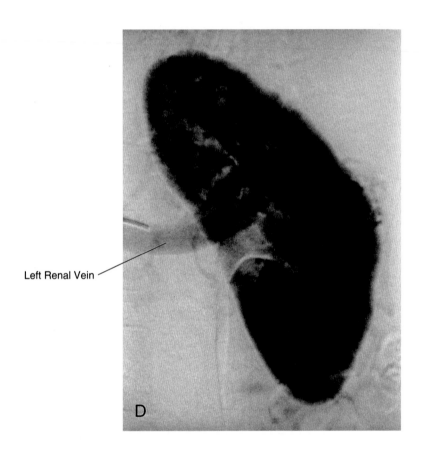

Left Renal Vein

D

Figure 18.133. *Continued*

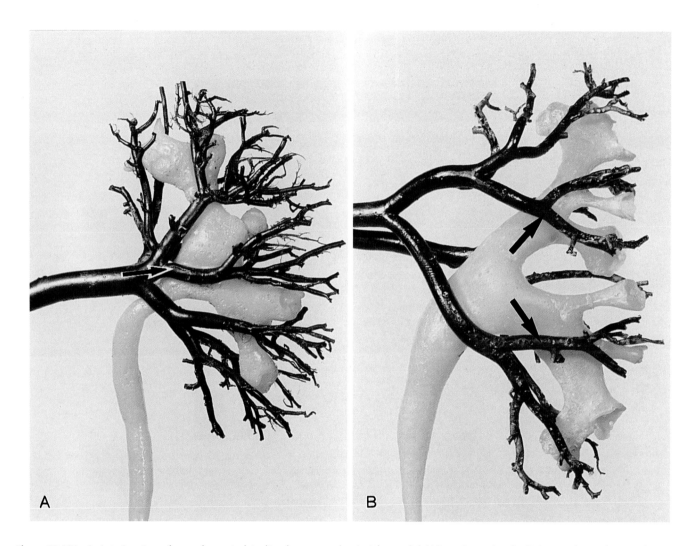

Figure 18.134. A. Anterior view of an endocast (pelvicaliceal system and arteries) from a left kidney shows an individualized artery to the kidney midzone coursing horizontally on the anterior surface of the renal pelvis (arrow). **B.** Anterior view of an endocast (pelvicaliceal system and arter-ies) from a left kidney shows that the kidney midzone does not have an individualized artery and receives vascular supply from secondary division branches of arteries of other regions (arrows). Reprinted with permission from Sampaio FJB.

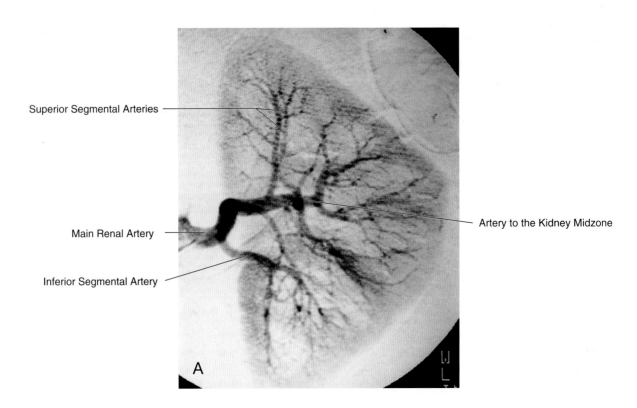

Figure 18.135. A. Anterior view of a left renal angiogram showing the artery to the kidney midzone, as well as the superior and inferior segmental arteries. **B.** Late angiographic phase shows the renal nephrogram and the drainage vein.

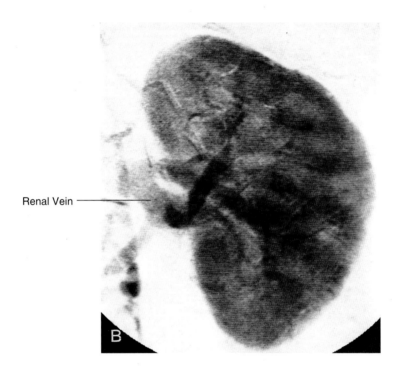

Renal Vein

Figure 18.135. *Continued*

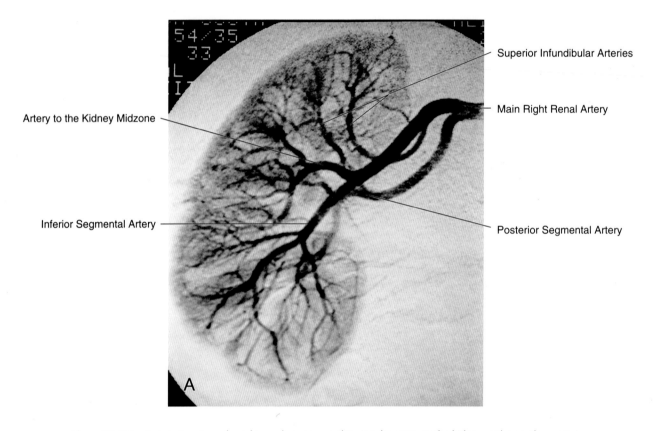

Artery to the Kidney Midzone

Inferior Segmental Artery

Superior Infundibular Arteries

Main Right Renal Artery

Posterior Segmental Artery

A

Figure 18.136. A. Anterior view of a right renal angiogram showing the artery to the kidney midzone, the posterior segmental artery and the superior and inferior segmental arteries. **B.** Later phase of the angiogram shows the more peripheral arteries.

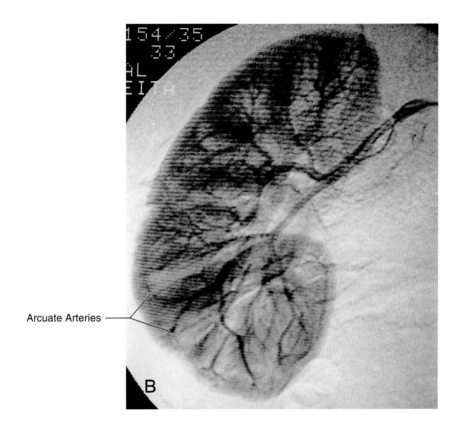

Figure 18.136. *Continued*

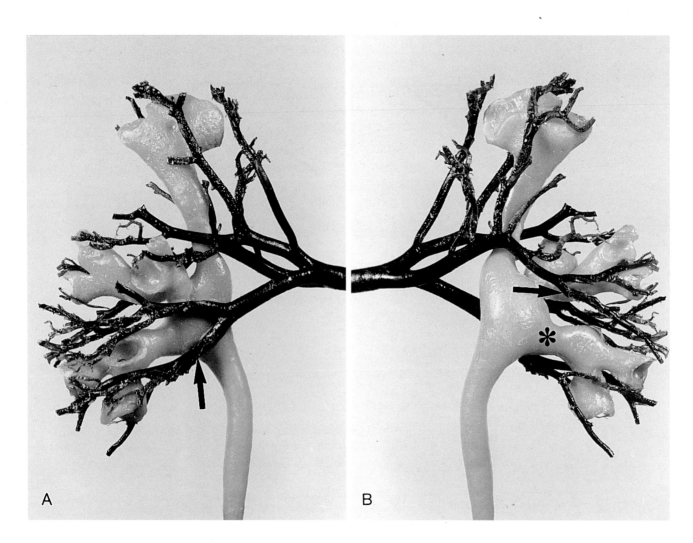

Figure 18.137. **A.** Anterior view of an endocast (pelvicaliceal system and arteries) from a right kidney demonstrates front and back arterial supply to inferior pole (arrow) arising from the anterior division of the renal artery (inferior segmental artery). **B.** Posterior view of the same cast shown in A demonstrates that the posterior segmental artery (retropelvic artery) does not reach the lower infundibulum (arrow). The posterior aspect of the lower infundibulum is free of arteries (asterisk). Reprinted with permission from Sampaio FJB.

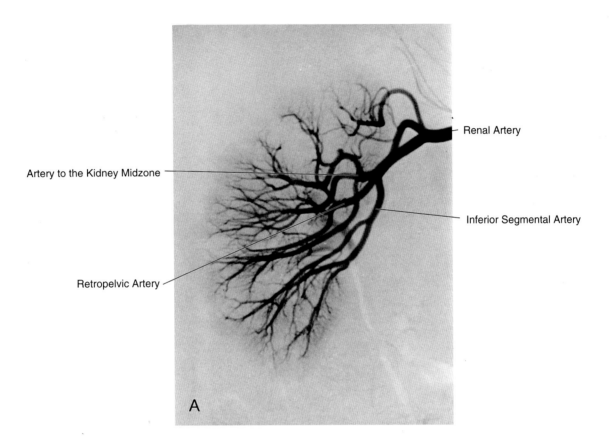

Renal Artery

Artery to the Kidney Midzone

Inferior Segmental Artery

Retropelvic Artery

A

Figure 18.138. A. Selective right kidney angiogram shows the arteries to the lower infundibulum arising from the Inferior Segmental Artery. The Artery to the Midzone of the Kidney is also seem. The Retropelvic Artery is also observed. **B.** Later arterial phase shows the Interlobar and Interlobular Arteries. **C.** Nephrographic phase shows the renal cortex and the drainage vein.

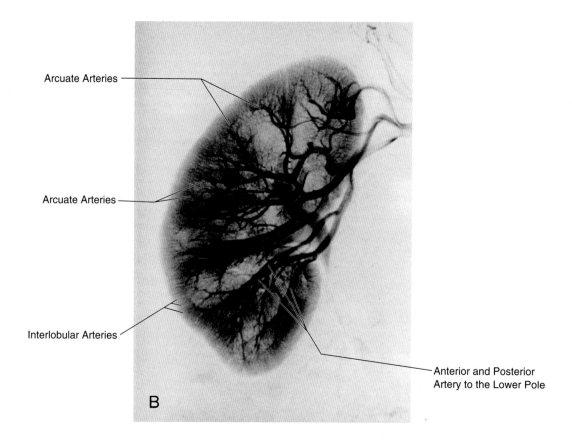

Arcuate Arteries

Arcuate Arteries

Interlobular Arteries

Anterior and Posterior
Artery to the Lower Pole

B

Figure 18.138. *Continued*

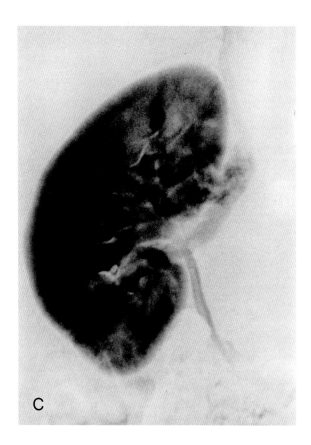

Figure 18.138. *Continued*

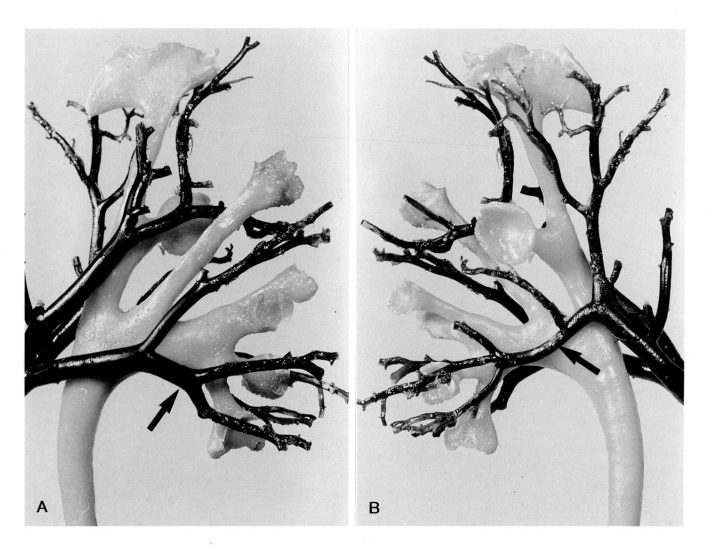

Figure 18.139. A. Anterior view of an endocast (pelvicaliceal system and arteries) from a left kidney shows the artery to the anterior surface of the lower infundibulum arising from the inferior segmental artery (arrow). **B.** Posterior view of the same cast shown in A reveals the posterior aspect of the lower infundibulum supplied by the inferior branch of the posterior segmental artery (arrow). Reprinted with permission from Sampaio FJB.

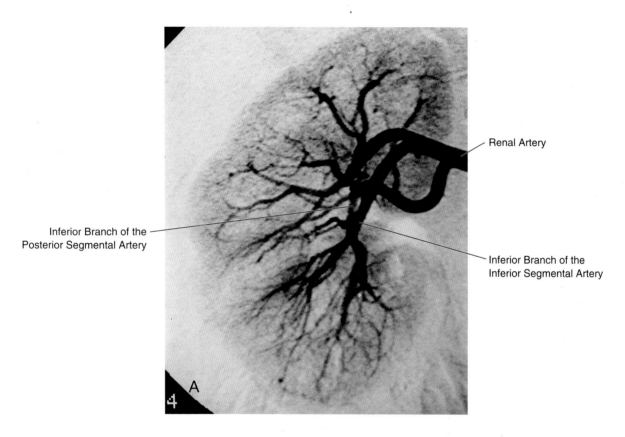

Renal Artery

Inferior Branch of the
Posterior Segmental Artery

Inferior Branch of the
Inferior Segmental Artery

A

Figure 18.140. A. Anterior view of a right renal angiogram. The artery to the anterior surface of the lower infundibulum arises from the inferior segmental artery. The inferior branch of the lower infundibulum arises from the posterior segmental artery. **B.** Nephrographic phase of the kidney. The vein is ill-defined.

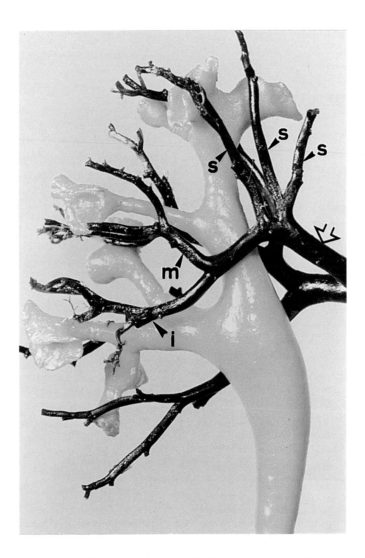

Figure 18.141. Posterior view of an endocast from a left kidney shows the posterior segmental artery (retropelvic artery) (open arrow). This cast also reveals the subdivision branches of the posterior segmental artery. In this case, there are three superior branches related to the posterior aspect of the upper infundibulum. s: superior subdivision branches; m: middle subdivision branch; i: inferior subdivision branch. Reprinted with permission from Sampaio FJB.

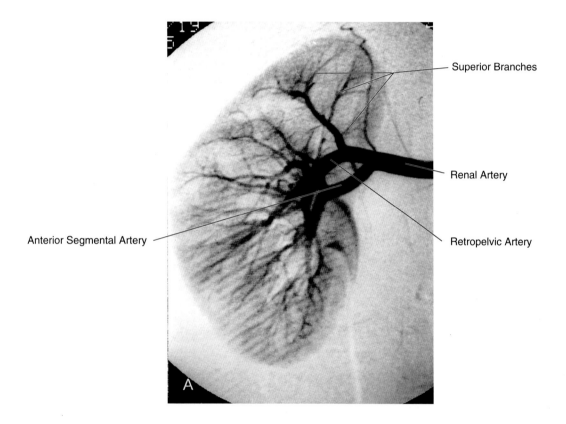

Figure 18.142. A. Anterior view of a right renal angiogram showing subdivisions branches of the retropelvic artery. **B.** Nephrographic phase. No vein is visible at that phase.

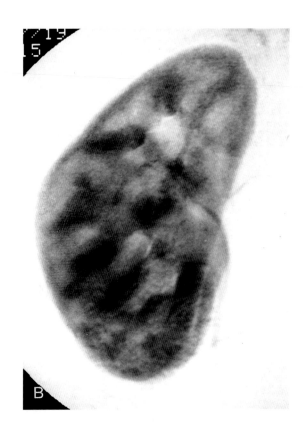

Figure 18.142. *Continued*

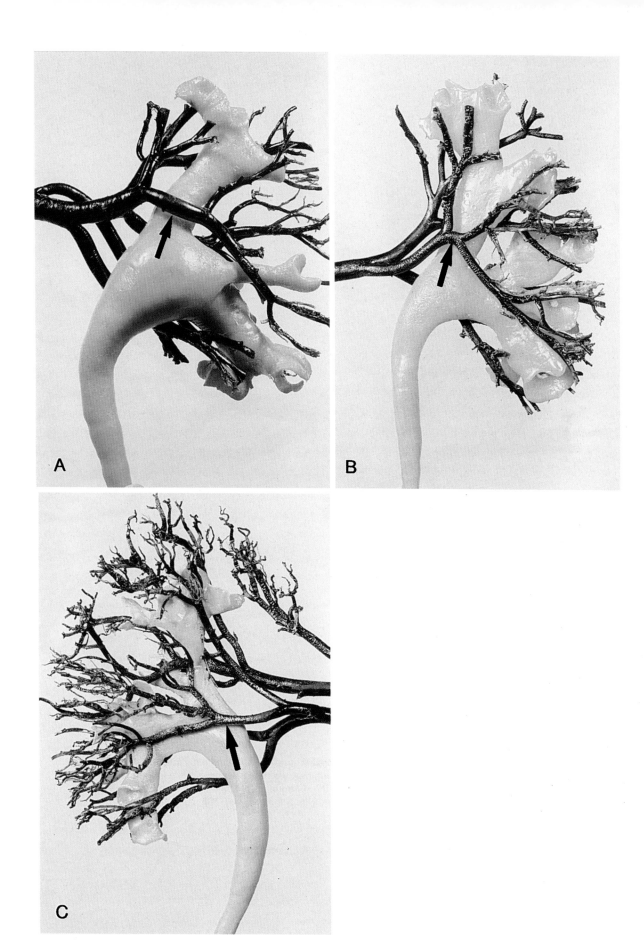

Figure 18.143. A. Posterior view of an endocast (pelvicaliceal system and arteries) from a right kidney shows the posterior segmental artery (retropelvic artery) crossing the dorsal surface of the upper infundibulum (arrow). **B.** Posterior view of an endocast (pelvicaliceal system and arteries) from a right kidney shows the posterior segmental artery (retropelvic artery) describing an arc and in close relationship to the upper infundibulum (arrow). **C.** Posterior view of an endocast (pelvicaliceal system and arteries) from a left kidney shows the posterior segmental artery (retropelvic artery) coursing in the middle posterior surface of the renal pelvis (arrow). Reprinted with permission from Sampaio FJB.

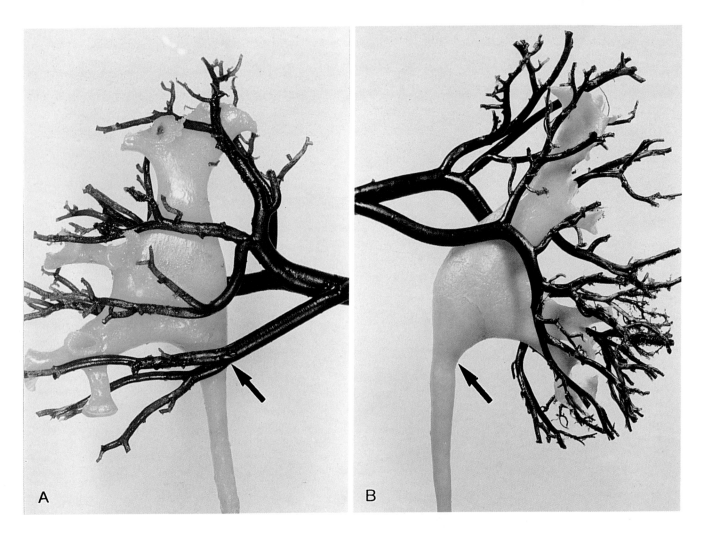

Figure 18.144. Anatomic relationships between ureteropelvic junction (UPJ) and renal arteries. A. Anterior view of an endocast from a right kidney shows a close relationship between the inferior segmental artery and the anterior aspect of the UPJ (arrow). **B.** Posterior view of an endocast from a right kidney shows the UPJ free of arteries (nonvascular area), (arrow). Reprinted with permission from Sampaio FJB.

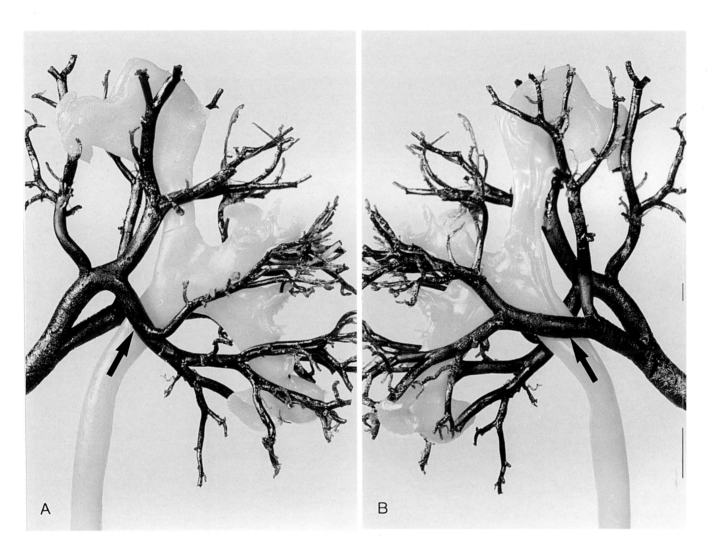

Figure 18.145. Anatomic relationships between ureteropelvic junction (UPJ) and renal arteries. A. Anterior view of an endocast from a left kidney shows a close relationship between an anterior segmental artery and the UPJ (arrow). **B.** Posterior view of the endocast shown in A reveals the UPJ in close relationship to a retropelvic artery (arrow).

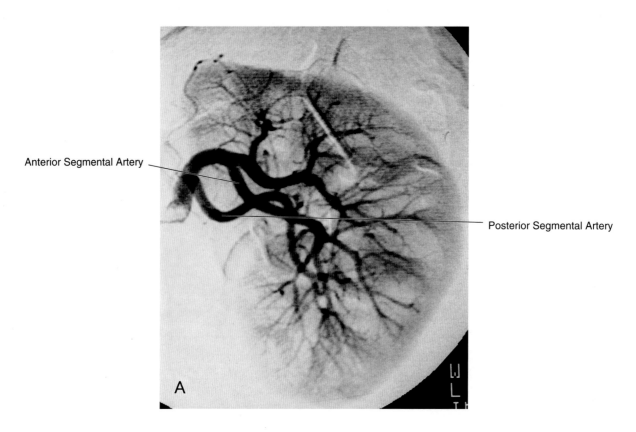

Figure 18.146. A. Left renal angiogram shows the relationship of the anterior segmental artery with the UPJ.
B. Late nephrographic phase.

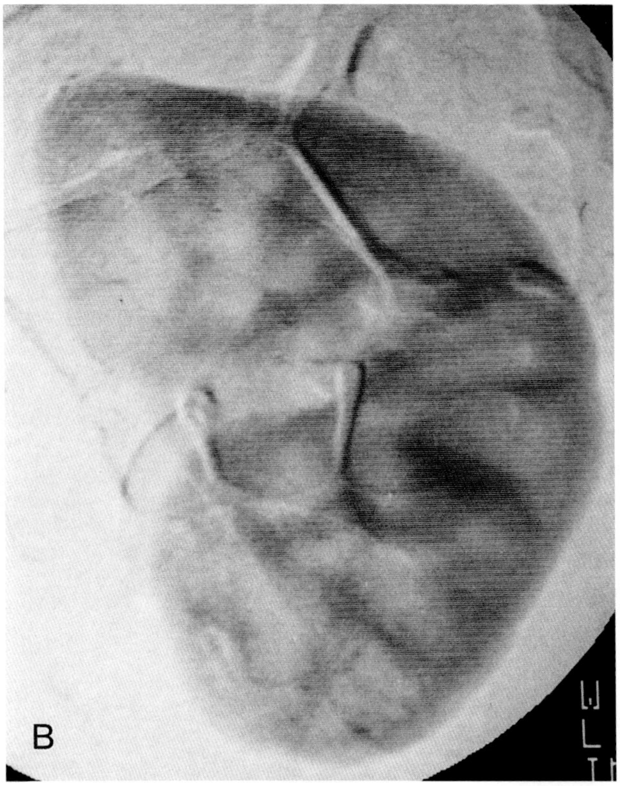

Figure 18.146. *Continued*

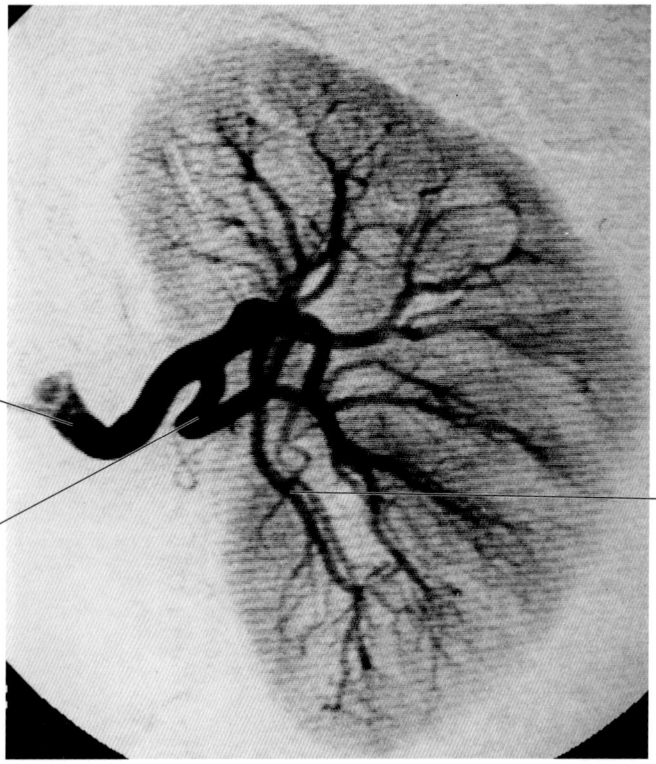

Figure 18.147. Left renal angiogram shows the relationship between the ureteropelvic junction and the renal arteries.

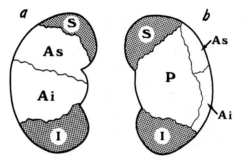

Figure 18.148. Schematic drawing depicts the more frequent kind of renal arterial segments distribution (five segments). A. Anterior view. **B.** Posterior view: S: Superior segment; As: Anterosuperior segment; Ai: Anteroinferior segment; P: Posterior segment.

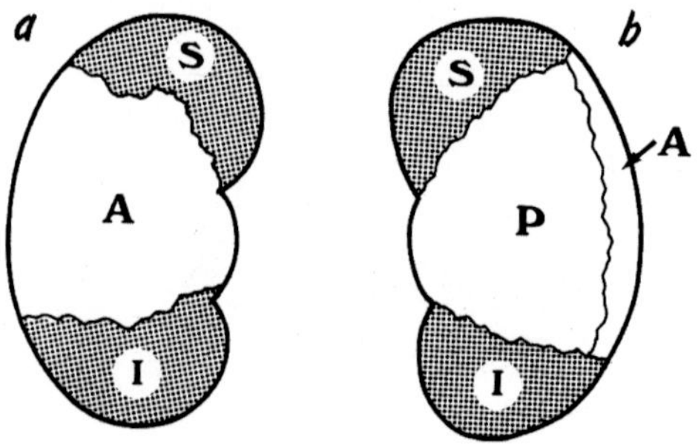

Figure 18.149. Schematic drawing depicts a kidney with four arterial segments. A. Anterior view. **B.** Posterior view. S: Superior segment; A: Anterior segment; I: Inferior segment; P: Posterior segment.

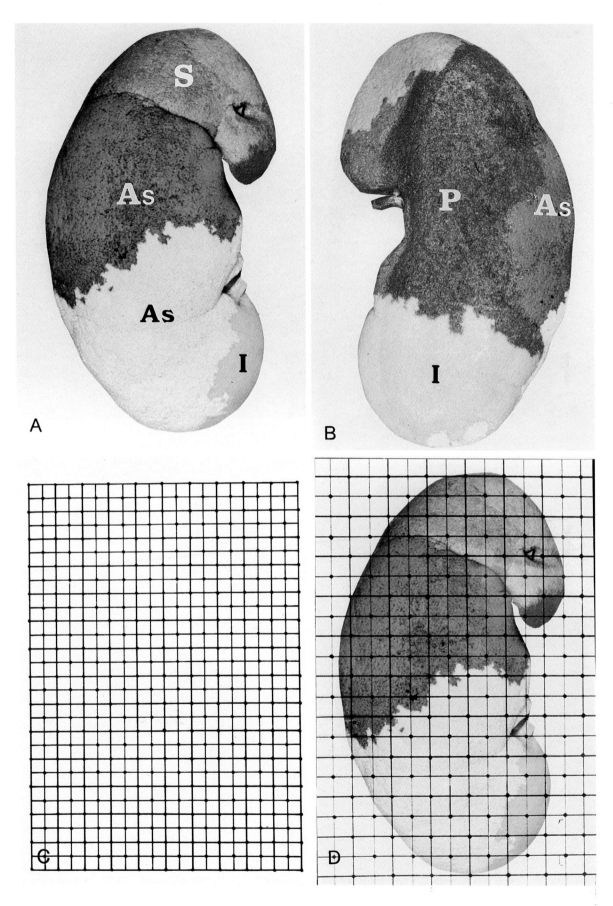

Figure 18.150. This figure shows an example of a polyester resin endocast obtained from a right kidney and illustrates the evaluation of the surface segmental area by using the "point-counting planimetry method." **A.** Anterior view of a right kidney endocast presenting five arterial segments that were injected with different colors. **B.** Posterior view of the same endocast shown in A. S: superior segment (brown); As: anterosuperior segment (blue); Ai: anteroinferior segment (white); I: inferior segment (yellow); P: posterior segment (red). **C.** The B-100 grid of planimetry used in the "point-counting method." **D.** The B-100 grid of planimetry placed over a photograph of the endocast shown in A depicts the evaluation of the surface segmental area by using the "point-counting method." Reprinted with permission from Sampaio FJB.

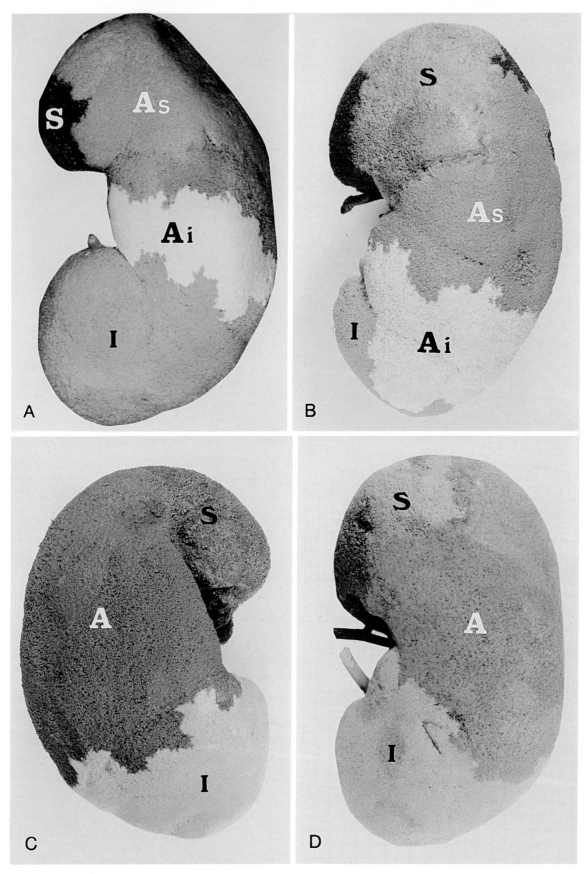

Figure 18.151. Anterior view of kidney endocasts exemplifies the different possibilities of arterial segment arrangements. A. Anterior view of a left kidney endocast presenting five arterial segments. The area of superior segment (S) corresponds to 1.84% of the total kidney area. The anterosuperior segment (As) corresponds to 28.16%; the anteroinferior segment (Ai) corresponds to 18.95%, and the inferior segment (I) corresponds to 30.0% of the total kidney area. **B.** Anterior view of a left kidney endocast presenting five segments. The area of the superior segment (S) corresponds to 16.59% of the total kidney area. The anterosuperior segment (As) corresponds to 19.75%; the anteroinferior segment (Ai) corresponds to 16.04%; the inferior segment (I) corresponds to 16.49% of the total kidney area. **C.** Anterior view of a right kidney endocast presenting four arterial segments. The area of superior segment (S) corresponds to 12.20% of the total kidney area. The anterior segment (A) corresponds to 37.28% and the inferior segment (I) corresponds to 23.21% of the total kidney area. **D.** Anterior view of a left kidney endocast presenting four arterial segments. The area of the superior segment (S) corresponds to 19.71% of the total kidney area. The anterior segment (A) corresponds to 34.90% and the inferior segment (I) corresponds to 27.39% of the total kidney area. Reprinted with permission from Sampaio FJB.

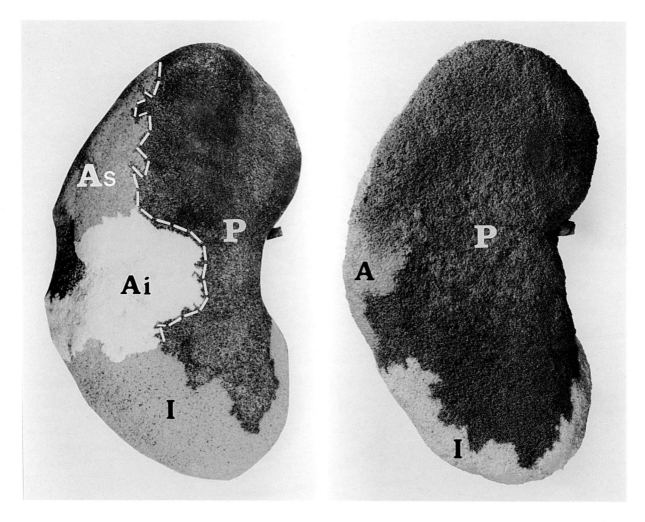

Figure 18.152. Posterior view of endocasts shows different types of posterior arterial segment arrangements. A. Posterior view of a left kidney endocast shows the limit between posterior (P) and anterior segments (Brodel's line) far from the lateral kidney margin (dashed white line). **B.** Posterior view of a left kidney endocast reveals a posterior segment (P) in red, corresponding to 49.36% of the total kidney area. In this case, the limit between posterior and anterior segments is located close to the lateral kidney margin. As = anterosuperior segment; Ai = anteroinferior segment; A= anterior segment; I = inferior segment. Reprinted with permission from Sampaio FJB.

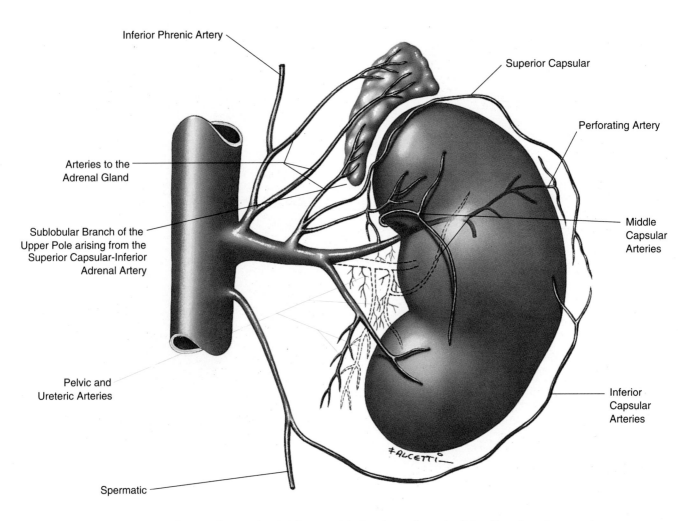

Figure 18.153. Schematic diagram showing the potential adrenal capsular and pelvic collateral arteries around and inside the kidney, most frequently observed in angiograms.

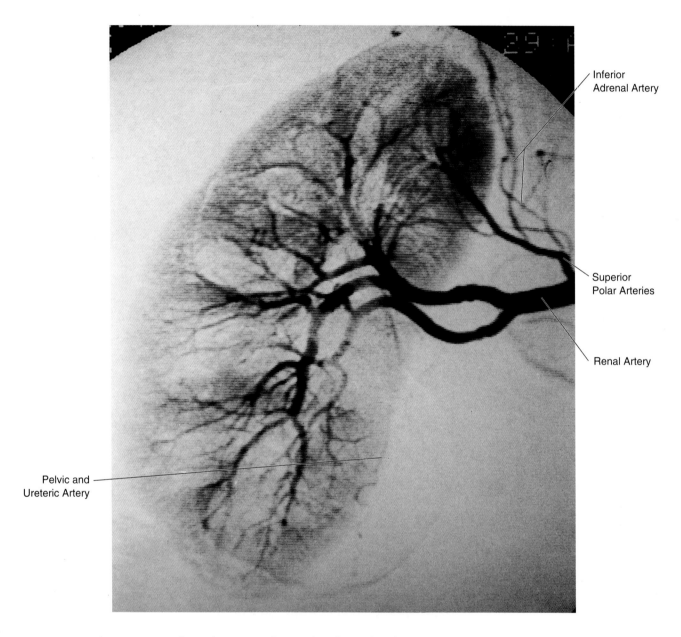

Inferior
Adrenal Artery

Superior
Polar Arteries

Renal Artery

Pelvic and
Ureteric Artery

Figure 18.154. Right renal angiogram showing the Inferior Adrenal Artery as the origin of the superior capsular arteries. Note the pelvic and ureteric artery.

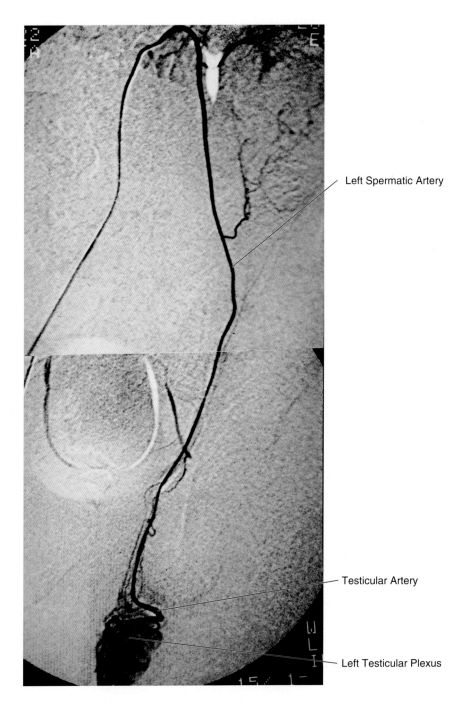

Left Spermatic Artery

Testicular Artery

Left Testicular Plexus

Figure 18.155. Selective angiogram of the left spermatic artery, arising from the abdominal aorta, and descending to the testis. Note the collaterals and the plexus at the testis.

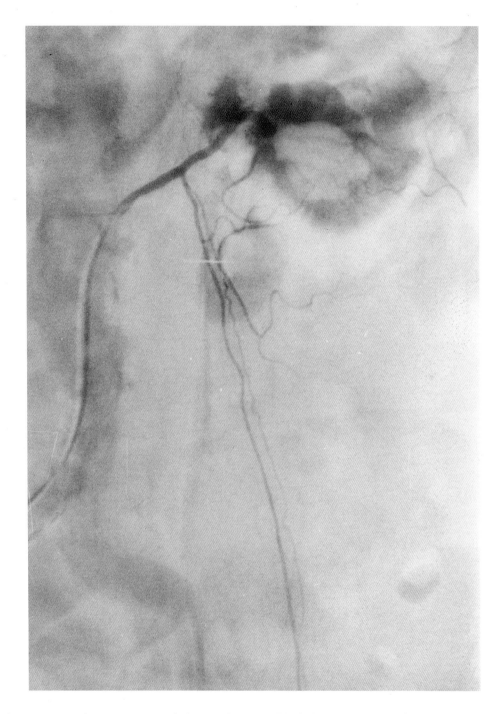

Figure 18.156. Selective angiogram of a lower polar artery of the kidney, given origin to the left spermatic artery. Note the collaterals and anastomosis with the capsular arteries.

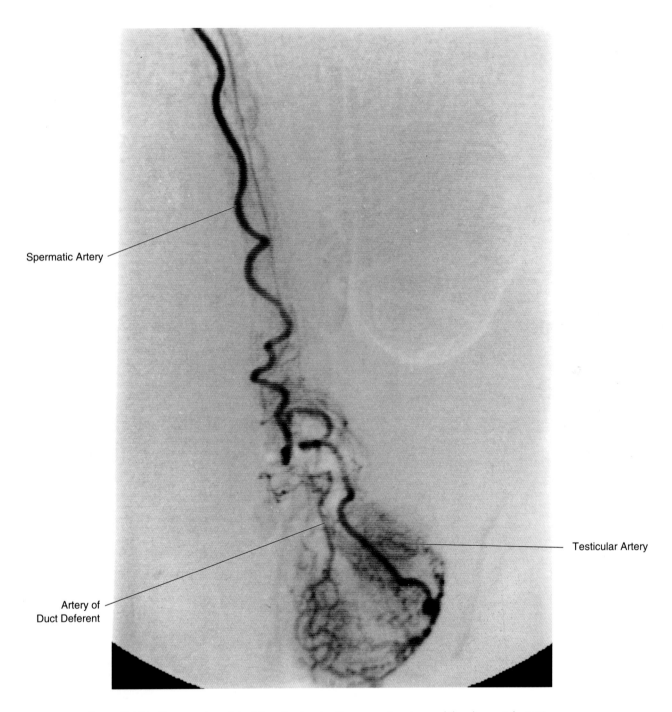

Figure 18.157. Close-up view of the left testis, showing the spermatic artery and the plexus at the testis.

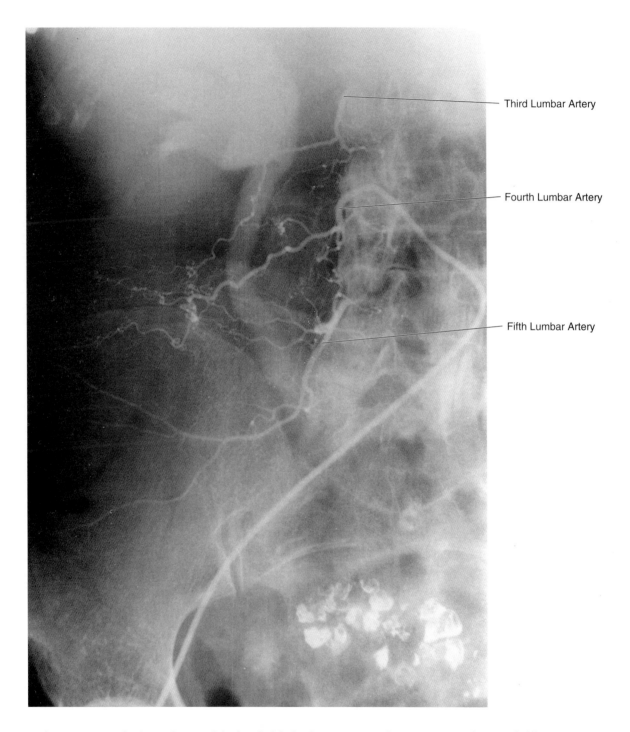

— Third Lumbar Artery

— Fourth Lumbar Artery

— Fifth Lumbar Artery

Figure 18.158. Selective angiogram of the fourth right lumbar artery. Note the anastomosis and retrograde filling of the third and fifth right lumbar arteries.

Third Lumbar Artery

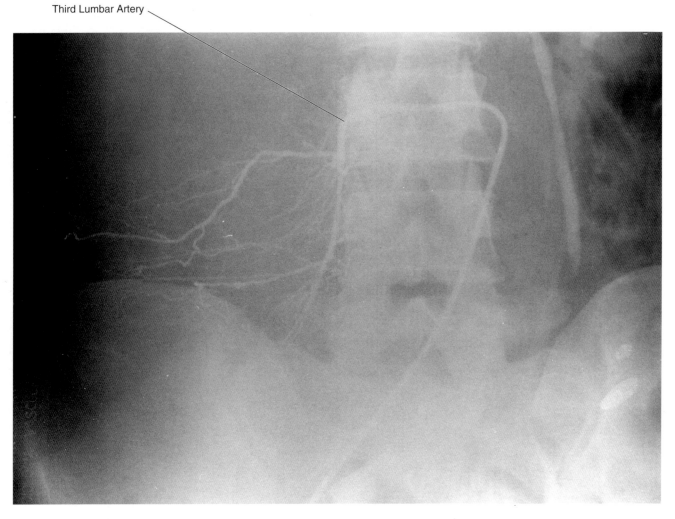

Figure 18.159. Selective angiogram of the third right Lumbar Artery and the muscular branches, as well as the anastomosis.

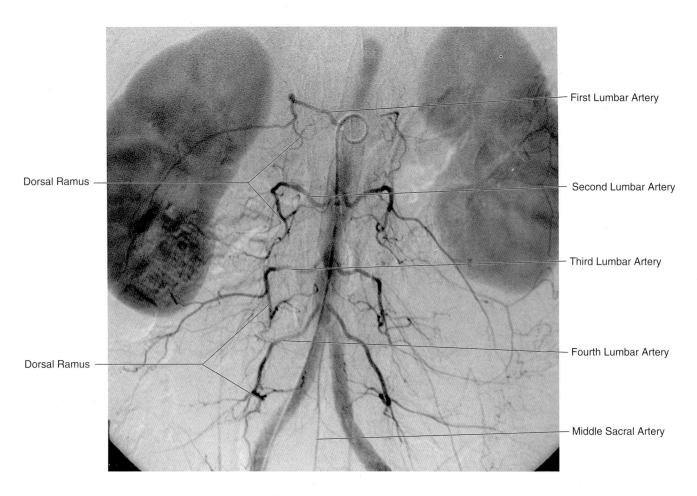

First Lumbar Artery

Dorsal Ramus

Second Lumbar Artery

Third Lumbar Artery

Dorsal Ramus

Fourth Lumbar Artery

Middle Sacral Artery

Figure 18.160. Late phase angiogram of the abdominal aorta, showing the lumbar arteries and normal branches.

Fifth Lumbar Artery

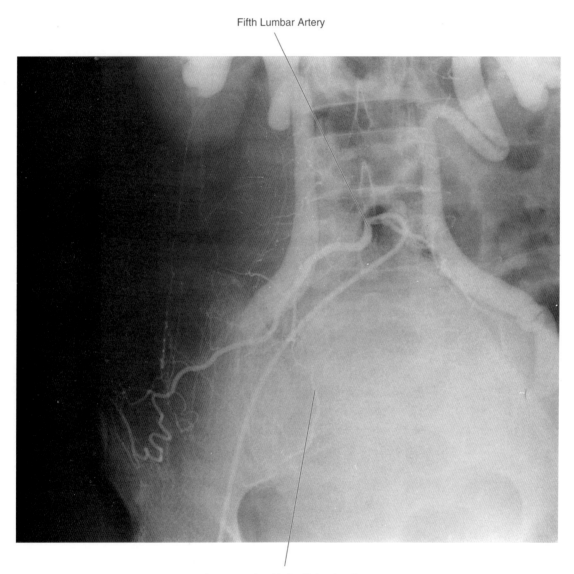

Anastomosis with the Iliolumbar Artery

Figure 18.161. Selective angiogram of the fifth right lumbar artery. Note the anastomosis with the iliolumbar artery.

19
ARTERIES OF THE PELVIS

COMMON ILIAC ARTERIES

The right and left iliac arteries have been described as the terminal branches of the abdominal aorta (Fig. 19.1).

INTERNAL ILIAC ARTERIES (HYPOGASTRIC ARTERIES)

These are about 4 cm long arteries, resulting from the bifurcation of the common iliac arteries, dividing into an anterior trunk and a posterior trunk (Figs. 19.1, 19.2).

Branches of the Anterior Trunk
(Figs. 19.3, 19.4, 19.5, 19.6)

Superior Vesical Artery (Fetal Umbilical Artery)

Supplies
  Vesical Fundus
  Ductus Deferens
  Ureteral Arteries

Inferior Vesical Artery (May Arise with the Middle Rectal Artery)

Supplies
  Vesical fundus
  Prostate (prostatic branches communicate
    across the midline)
  Seminal vesicle
  Lower ureter
  Ductus deferens

Middle Rectal Artery

Anastomoses with the superior and inferior rectal arteries
  Supplies
    Lower Rectum
    Seminal Vesicle
    Prostate
    Vesical Walls

Uterine Artery (Fig. 19.7)

This artery crosses above the ureter and the later

al vaginal fornix and ascends laterally to the body of the uterus, joining the ovarian artery. It anastomoses with the vaginal arteries, forming the azygos artery of the vagina (Fig. 19.7).

Supplies
  Ureter
  Vagina
  Uterus
  Broad ligament of uterus
  Round ligament of uterus
  Uterine tube
  The tortuous terminal branches in the uterus
    are called helicine arteries.

Vaginal Artery

The vaginal artery may be two or three arteries and corresponds to the inferior vesical artery in males.

Supplies
  Vagina
  Vesical fundus
  Rectum

Obturator Artery

This artery leaves the pelvis through the obturator canal and has an anterior and a posterior branch (Figs. 19.1, 19.4, 19.5).

Branches

Inside the Pelvis
  Iliac branches
  Vesical branch
  Pubic branch
Outside the Pelvis
  Anterior and posterior branches encircle the
    foramen
  Anterior branches supplies various muscles and
    anastomoses with the medial circumflex
    femoral artery
  Posterior branches supplies various muscles and
    anastomoses with the inferior gluteal artery;
    give an acetabular branch that supplies the

acetabular fossa and the femoral head
through the ligament of the femoral head

The obturator artery may be replaced by a pubic branch of the inferior epigastric artery. It may be a branch either of the anterior or posterior trunk of the internal iliac artery and may also be a branch of the superior or inferior gluteal artery.

Internal Pudendal Artery (Figs. 19.1, 19.5, 19.8, 19.9)

The internal pudendal artery is the smaller branch of the anterior trunk of the internal iliac artery. Supplies the external genitalia.

Branches

Inferior rectal artery (anastomoses with the contralateral inferior rectal artery and with the superior and middle rectal arteries)
    Perineal artery (Figs. 19.8, 19.9)
      Transverse branch
      Scrotal arteries
      Muscular branches
    Artery of the penis (Figs. 19.8, 19., 19.10)
      Name of the internal pudendal artery beyond the perineal artery
    Artery to the bulb of the penis (Fig. 19.9)
      Corpus spongiosum
      Bulb urethral gland
    Urethral artery (Figs. 19.8, 19.9, 19.10)
      Urethra and erectile tissue (Corpus Spongiosum)
    Deep penile artery (Cavernosal Artery) (Figs. 19.8, 19.9)
      One of the two terminal branches of the internal pudendal artery. Enters the crus penis and transverses the corpus cavernosum longitudinally, supplying the erectile tissue on each side; runs their entire length.
    Dorsal penile artery (Figs. 19.8, 19.9, 19.11, 19.12)
      The terminal branch of the internal pudendal artery. Ascends between the crus of the penis and the pubis, running along the dorsum reaching the glans; anastomoses with the deep artery of the penis and supplies the skin and fascia of the penis
    Erectile tissue (Fig. 19.13)
      The penis contains the corpus spongiosum, corpora cavernosa and glans penis, made of erectile tissue. Erection results from parasympathetic stimulation via the pudendal nerves, with contraction of the smooth muscles enlarging the sinusoids and the intersinusoidal connections, with simultaneous closure of the venous outflow and increase of the arterial inflow.
    Transverse root communication (Figs. 19.14, 19.15)
      There are constant anastomosis between the right and left arterial circulation through transverse root communication at the pubic

area, either from branches of the obturator artery or from the internal pudendal.

Inferior Gluteal Artery

The largest terminal branch of the anterior trunk of the internal iliac artery, the inferior gluteal artery supplies the muscles of the buttock and thigh (Figs. 19.4, 19.5, 19.7). It anastomoses distally with branches of the perforating arteries in the thigh.

Branches

Inside the pelvis
    Muscular (piriformis, coccygeus and levator ani)
    Perirectal fat
    Vesical fundus, seminal vesicles, and prostate
Outside the pelvis
Muscular branches
    Anastomoses with superior gluteal, internal pudendal, obturator, and medial circumflex femoral arteries
Coccygeal branches
Artery of the sciatic nerve
Anastomotic branch
    Join the cruciate anastomosis (perforating arteries)
Articular branch
Cutaneous branch

Branches of the Posterior Trunk

Iliolumbar Artery (Figs. 19.1, 19.16)

This artery ascends laterally anterior to the sacroiliac joint and lumbosacral trunk, posterior to the obturator nerve and external iliac vessels, dividing into the lumbar and iliac branches.

Branches

Lumbar branch (psoas and quadratus lumborum)
    Anastomoses with the 4th lumbar artery and sends a small spinal branch to the cauda equina
Iliac branch (Iliac bone through a nutrient branch)
    Anastomoses with the superior gluteal, circumflex iliac, and lateral circumflex femoral arteries

Lateral Sacral Arteries (Figs. 19.1, 19.17)

Branches

Superior lateral sacral branch (1st and 2nd sacral foramen) Supplies the sacral vertebras, sacral canal, and the skin and muscles dorsal to the sacrum
    Inferior lateral sacral branch
      Anastomoses with the median sacral artery, anterior to the coccyx and enters the sacral canal through the anterior sacral foramina

Superior Gluteal Artery (Figs. 19.1, 19.17)

This is the largest branch of the internal iliac artery and the continuation of the posterior trunk.

Leaves the pelvis through the greater sciatic foramen above the piriformis and dividing in superficial and deep branches.

Branches

Superficial branch
Supplies the gluteus maximus; anastomoses with the inferior gluteal artery and posterior branches of the lateral sacral arteries
Deep branch
Divides into superior and inferior rami. The superior ramus anastomoses with the deep circumflex iliac artery and the ascending branch of the lateral circumflex femoral artery. The inferior ramus anastomoses with the lateral circumflex femoral, inferior gluteal, and ascending branch of the medial circumflex femoral artery.

EXTERNAL ILIAC ARTERIES
(FIG. 19.1, 19.2, 19.6)

These arteries are the natural continuation of the common iliac artery. Larger than the internal iliac arteries, they descend laterally along the medial border of the psoas major, entering the thigh posteriorly to the inguinal ligament, becoming the femoral artery.

Branches

Inferior Epigastric Artery (Figs. 19.1, 19.2)

The inferior epigastric artery arises medially from the distal external iliac artery just above the inguinal ligament, ascending behind the rectus abdominis muscle. It anastomoses with the superior epigastric and lower posterior intercostal arteries.

Branches

Cremasteric artery
Pubic branch
Muscular branches
Cutaneous branches

Deep Circumflex Iliac Artery (Fig. 19.1)

This artery arises laterally from the external iliac

artery, opposite of the inferior epigastric artery. It anastomoses with the ascending branch of the lateral circumflex femoral artery and the iliolumbar and superior gluteal arteries and has a large ascending branch.

COLLATERAL PATHWAYS (FIG. 19.18)

There is a large number of potential pathways of collateral circulation, connecting the abdominal aorta and thoracic aorta with the pelvic arteries that may be developed in the case of aortoiliac femoral occlusive disease. The potential collateral circulation connectors are the superior epigastric, intercostal, subcostal, lumbar, middle sacral, common iliac, external iliac, iliolumbar, superior gluteal, lateral sacral, obturator, internal pudendal, external pudendal, deep iliac circumflex, superficial iliac circumflex, medial femoral circumflex, lateral femoral circumflex, lateral ascending branch, lateral descending branch, profunda femoris, superficial femoral, and inferior epigastric arteries.

It is important to be aware of the terminology employed in discussing collateral circulation. An affluent vessel is a collateral branch that arises from a patent main vessel above the obstruction or from a patent contralateral mate. An effluent vessel is a branch below the obstruction that receives blood from the effluent vessel and allows it to flow retrogradely to reconstitute the occluded artery.

The effluent vessel may pass blood into the effluent vessel as a continuous line, a phenomenon called inosculation, or may be connected to the effluent vessel by a network of fine vessels forming what is called retiform anastomosis. Inosculation keeps a good flow through the anastomosis, with a heavy head of pressure, leading to refilling of the main vessels distal to the occlusion. Retiform anastomosis allows passage of blood with decrease in flow and pressure. An example of retiform anastomosis is the communication between the lumbar and iliolumbar arteries or the Winslow's pathway (i.e., from the intercostal and internal mammary arteries to the external iliac arteries via the epigastric arteries).

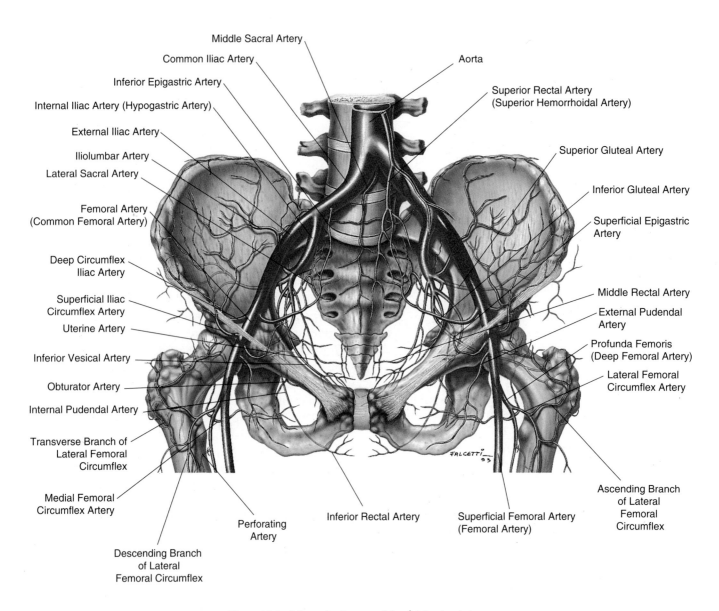

Middle Sacral Artery

Common Iliac Artery

Inferior Epigastric Artery

Internal Iliac Artery (Hypogastric Artery)

External Iliac Artery

Iliolumbar Artery

Lateral Sacral Artery

Femoral Artery
(Common Femoral Artery)

Deep Circumflex
Iliac Artery

Superficial Iliac
Circumflex Artery

Uterine Artery

Inferior Vesical Artery

Obturator Artery

Internal Pudendal Artery

Transverse Branch of
Lateral Femoral
Circumflex

Medial Femoral
Circumflex Artery

Descending Branch
of Lateral
Femoral Circumflex

Perforating
Artery

Inferior Rectal Artery

Aorta

Superior Rectal Artery
(Superior Hemorrhoidal Artery)

Superior Gluteal Artery

Inferior Gluteal Artery

Superficial Epigastric
Artery

Middle Rectal Artery

External Pudendal
Artery

Profunda Femoris
(Deep Femoral Artery)

Lateral Femoral
Circumflex Artery

Ascending Branch
of Lateral
Femoral
Circumflex

Superficial Femoral Artery
(Femoral Artery)

FALCETTI
93

Figure 19.1. Schematic diagram of the pelvic circulation.

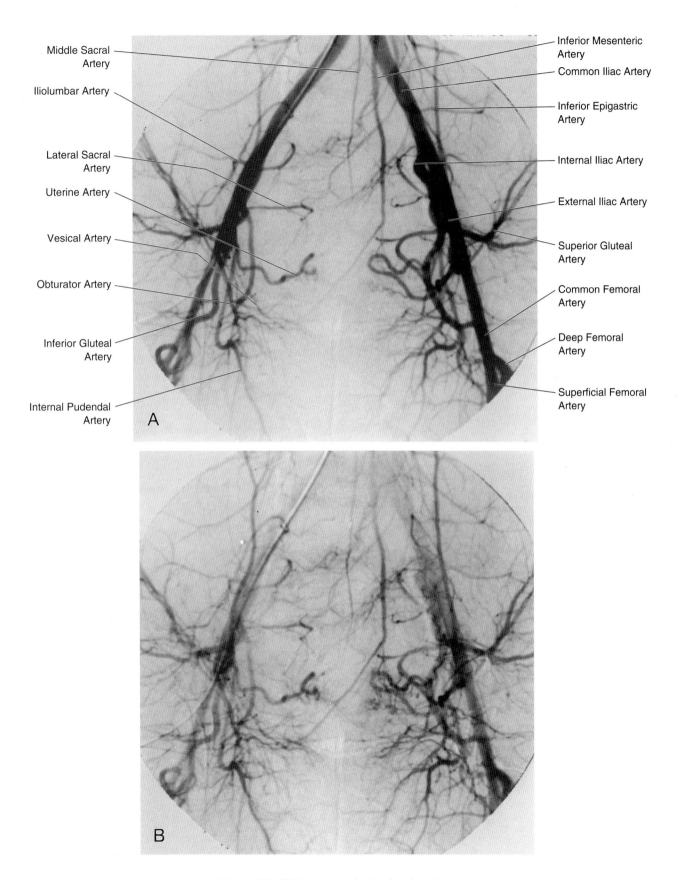

Middle Sacral Artery

Iliolumbar Artery

Lateral Sacral Artery

Uterine Artery

Vesical Artery

Obturator Artery

Inferior Gluteal Artery

Internal Pudendal Artery

Inferior Mesenteric Artery

Common Iliac Artery

Inferior Epigastric Artery

Internal Iliac Artery

External Iliac Artery

Superior Gluteal Artery

Common Femoral Artery

Deep Femoral Artery

Superficial Femoral Artery

A

B

Figure 19.2. Pelvic angiography in a female patient.

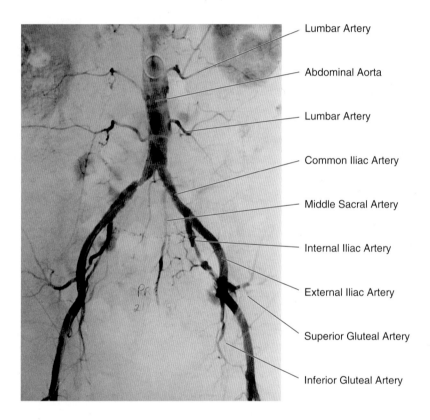

Lumbar Artery

Abdominal Aorta

Lumbar Artery

Common Iliac Artery

Middle Sacral Artery

Internal Iliac Artery

External Iliac Artery

Superior Gluteal Artery

Inferior Gluteal Artery

Figure 19.3. Pelvic angiography in a male patient with severe obstructive disease.

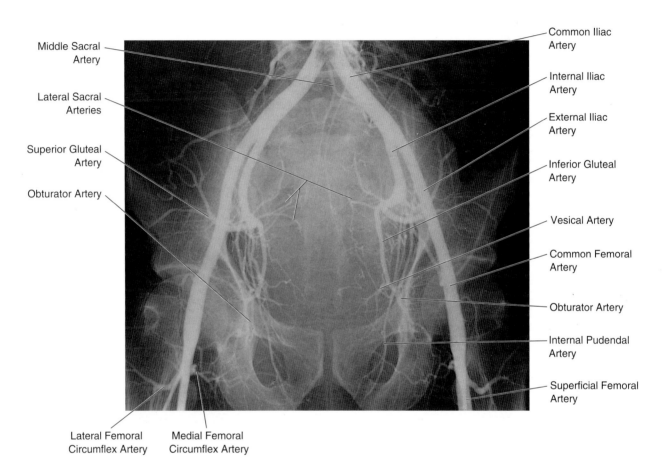

Middle Sacral Artery

Lateral Sacral Arteries

Superior Gluteal Artery

Obturator Artery

Common Iliac Artery

Internal Iliac Artery

External Iliac Artery

Inferior Gluteal Artery

Vesical Artery

Common Femoral Artery

Obturator Artery

Internal Pudendal Artery

Superficial Femoral Artery

Lateral Femoral Circumflex Artery

Medial Femoral Circumflex Artery

Figure 19.4. Pelvic angiography in a normal patient.

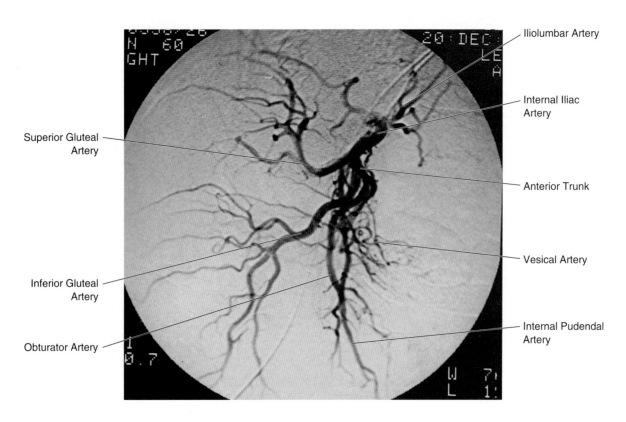

Figure 19.5. Selective arteriography of the right internal iliac artery in an elderly patient showing the gluteal arteries.

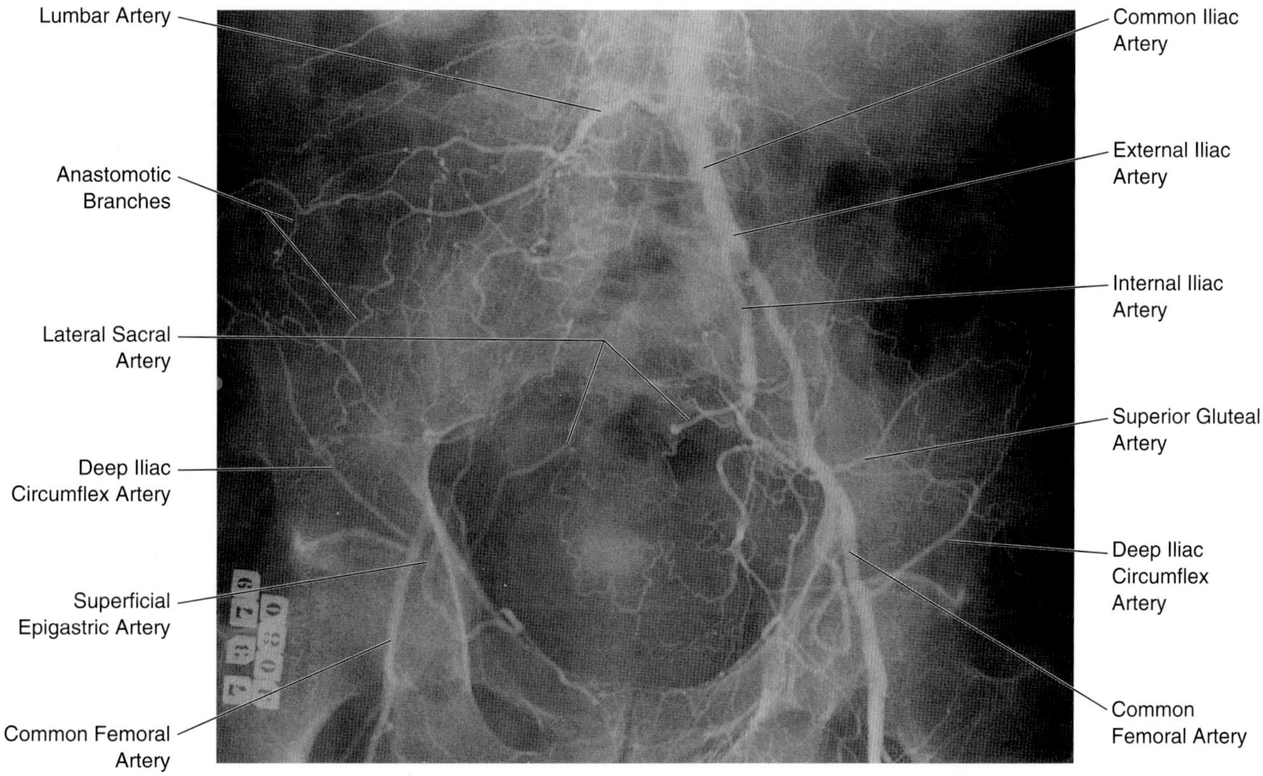

Figure 19.6. Pelvic angiography in a patient with occlusive disease, showing the development of the collateralization in the pelvis.

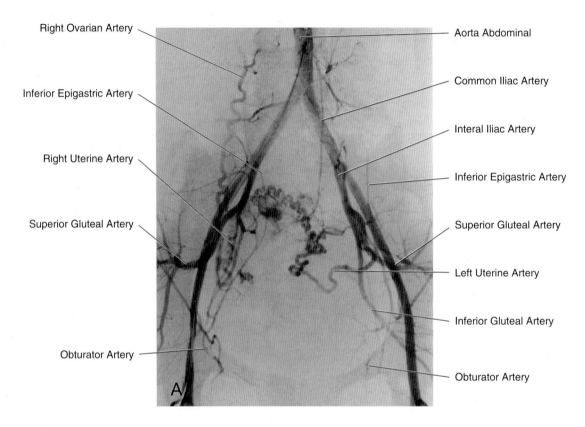

Right Ovarian Artery

Inferior Epigastric Artery

Right Uterine Artery

Superior Gluteal Artery

Obturator Artery

Aorta Abdominal

Common Iliac Artery

Interal Iliac Artery

Inferior Epigastric Artery

Superior Gluteal Artery

Left Uterine Artery

Inferior Gluteal Artery

Obturator Artery

A

Figure 19.7. A. Pelvic angiography in a patient with a uterine lesion showing the enlargement of the uterine arteries. **B, C.** Later phase of the angiogram shows contrast stain in the uterus. **D.** Selective angiography of the right internal iliac artery shows the pelvic circulation, mainly the uterine artery. **E.** Selective injection at the left uterine artery, shows the typical vascular pattern of the enlarged uterus.

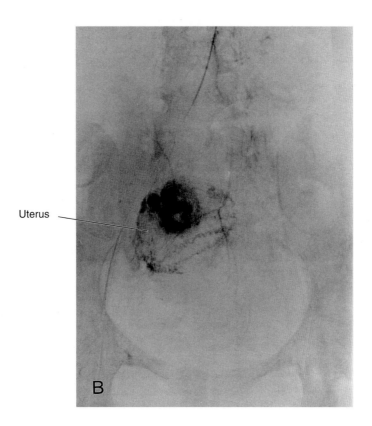

Uterus

Figure 19.7. *Continued*

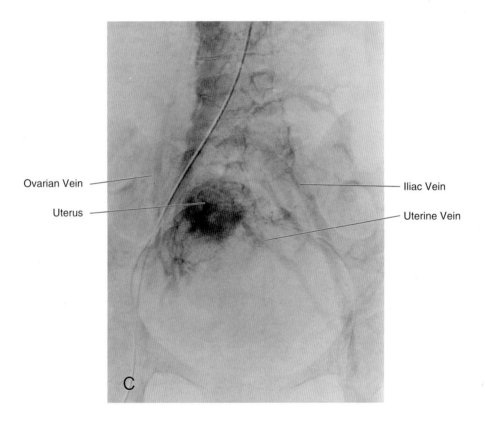

Ovarian Vein ——

—— Iliac Vein

Uterus ——

—— Uterine Vein

C

Figure 19.7. *Continued*

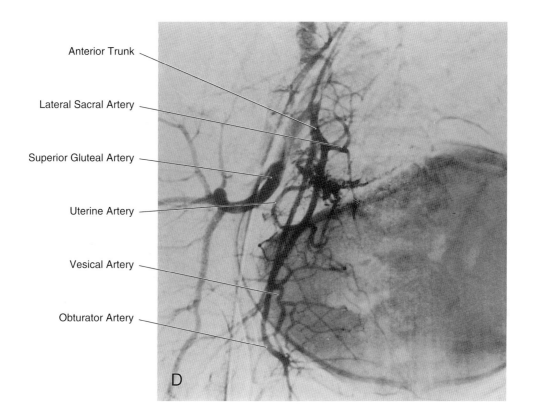

Anterior Trunk

Lateral Sacral Artery

Superior Gluteal Artery

Uterine Artery

Vesical Artery

Obturator Artery

D

Figure 19.7. *Continued*

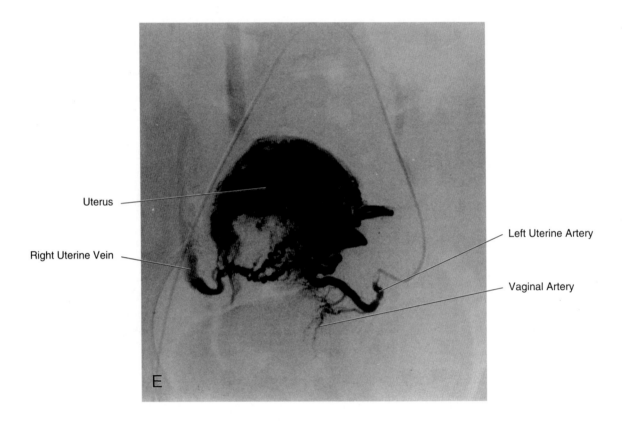

Uterus

Right Uterine Vein

Left Uterine Artery

Vaginal Artery

E

Figure 19.7. *Continued*

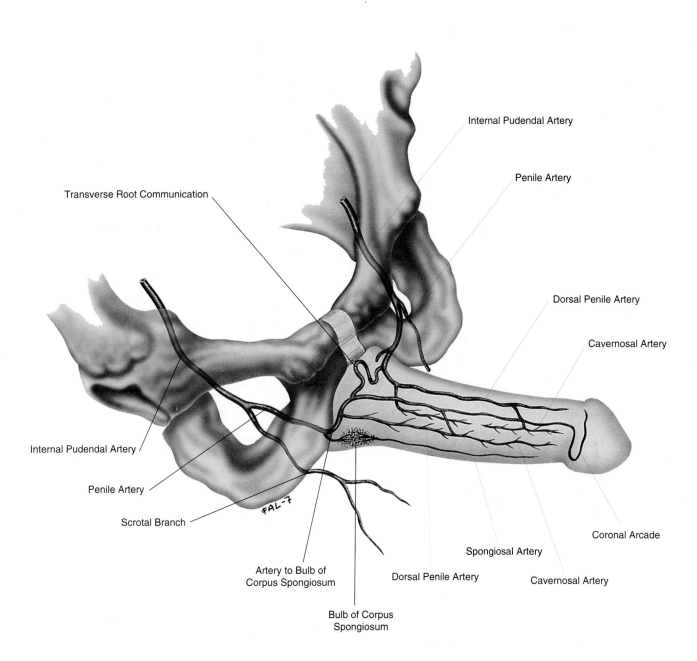

Figure 19.8. Schematic diagram of the penile arterial anatomy in an oblique projection. Not all arteries are always visible in the angiograms. The cavernosal artery is also called the deep penile artery. Branches of the cavernosal artery are the helicine arteries. The spongiosal artery is not always visible and the interruption at the bulb of the corpus spongiosum is an angiographic artifact. Sometimes the spongiosal artery arises independently from the bulbar artery.

Internal Pudendal Artery   Prostatic Artery   Dorsal Penile Artery

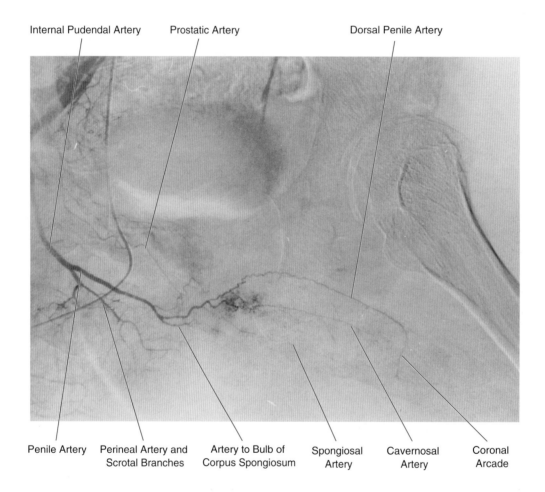

Penile Artery   Perineal Artery and   Artery to Bulb of   Spongiosal   Cavernosal   Coronal
                 Scrotal Branches   Corpus Spongiosum   Artery   Artery   Arcade

Figure 19.9. Selective right internal pudendal angiogram showing the classic arterial anatomy of the penis. Left posterior projection. The penile artery is the continuation of the internal pudendal artery after it gives origin to the perineal artery, and scrotal branches. Dorsal penile artery is large and long along the dorsum of the penis. Note the coronal arcade. Cavernosal artery is thinner and follow a path inside the corpus cavernosum. The artery to bulb of corpus spongiosum is the first branch of the penile artery.

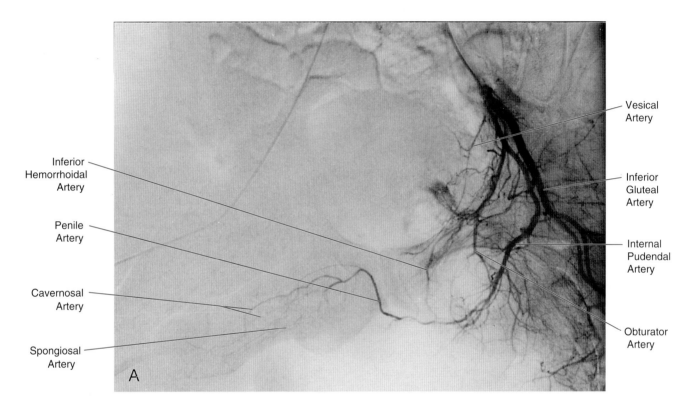

Vesical
Artery

Inferior
Hemorrhoidal
Artery

Inferior
Gluteal
Artery

Penile
Artery

Internal
Pudendal
Artery

Cavernosal
Artery

Obturator
Artery

Spongiosal
Artery

A

Figure 19.10. A. Selective left internal iliac angiogram showing the penile arterial anatomy. Right posterior projection. Note small size of the dorsal penile artery in this patient. The cavernosal artery is larger than usual and freely anastomose with segments of the dorsal penile artery. **B.** Late phase of the angiogram showing the corpus cavernosum and corpus spongiosum.

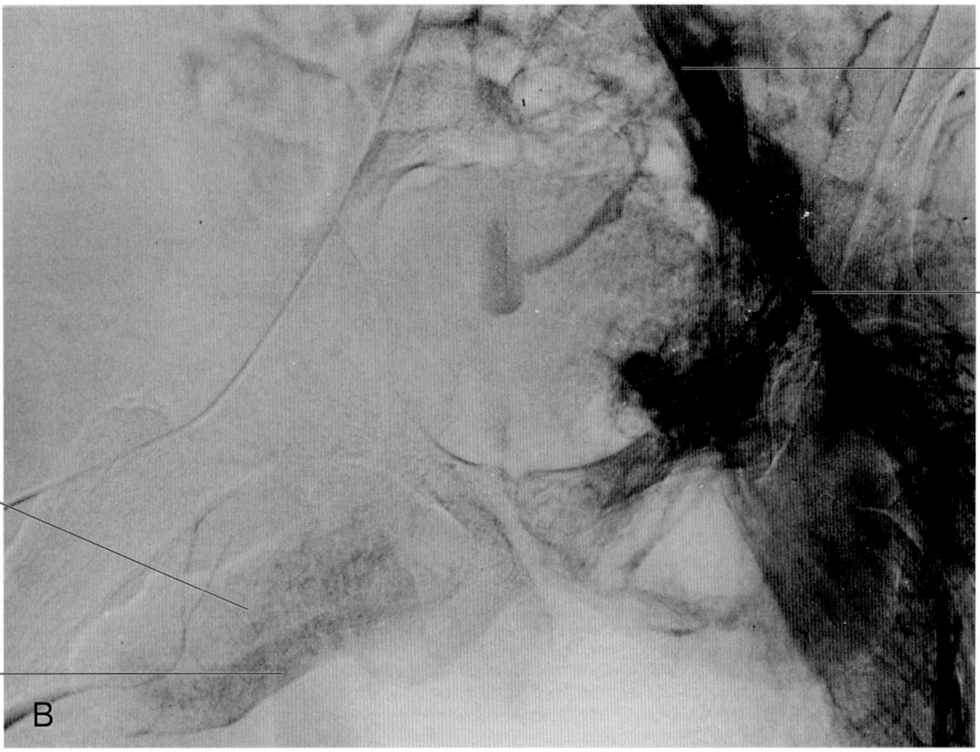

Figure 19.10. *Continued*

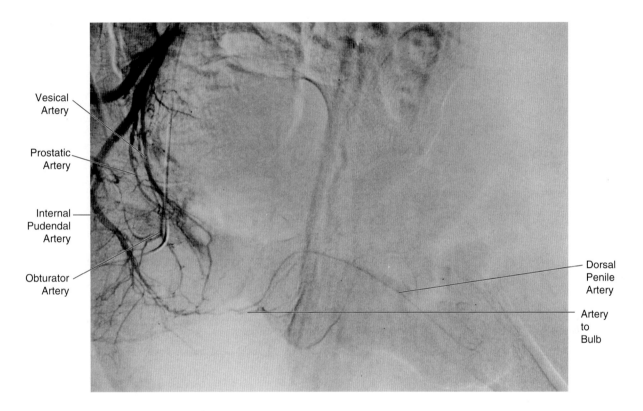

Vesical
Artery

Prostatic
Artery

Internal
Pudendal
Artery

Obturator
Artery

Dorsal
Penile
Artery

Artery
to
Bulb

Figure 19.11. Selective angiography of the right internal iliac artery showing only the dorsal penile artery. The cavernosal artery either may be occluded or originate from the left side.

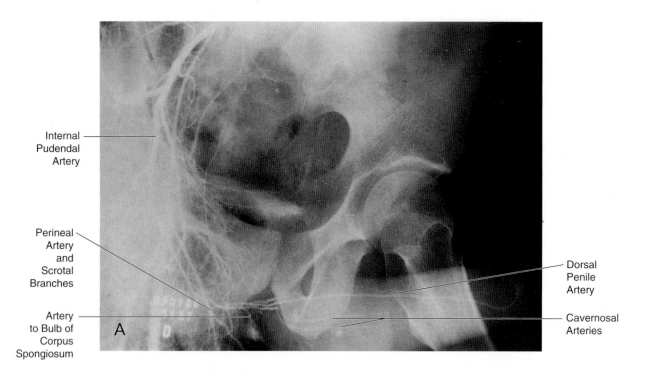

Internal
Pudendal
Artery

Perineal
Artery
and
Scrotal
Branches

Artery
to Bulb of
Corpus
Spongiosum

Dorsal
Penile
Artery

Cavernosal
Arteries

Figure 19.12. A. Selective angiography of the right internal iliac artery shows the right dorsal penile artery and right and left cavernosal artery filling from the right hand side injection. The bulbar artery is very small. **B.** Right internal iliac angiography shows the dorsal penile artery and the cavernosal artery. The bulbar artery is small. **C.** Right internal iliac artery shows a small dorsal penile artery, a even smaller cavernosal artery and a long and relatively large spongiosal artery.

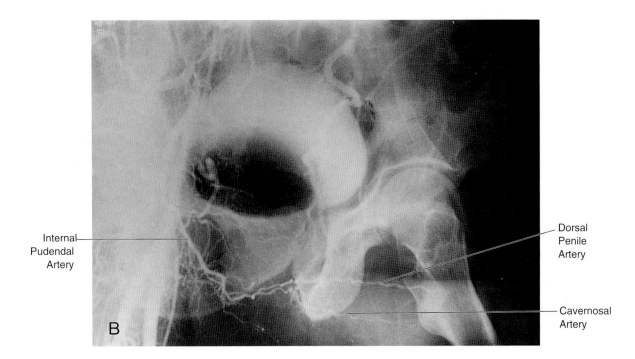

Internal
Pudendal
Artery

Dorsal
Penile
Artery

Cavernosal
Artery

B

Figure 19.12. *Continued*

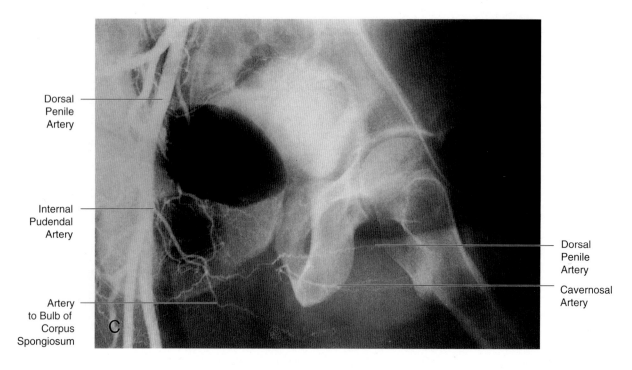

Dorsal
Penile
Artery

Internal
Pudendal
Artery

Artery
to Bulb of
Corpus
Spongiosum

C

Dorsal
Penile
Artery

Cavernosal
Artery

Figure 19.12. *Continued*

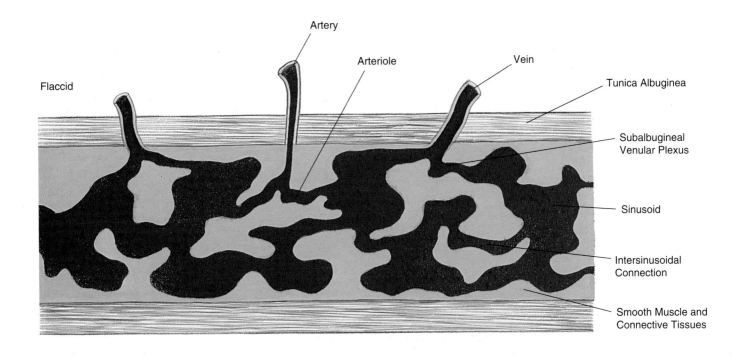

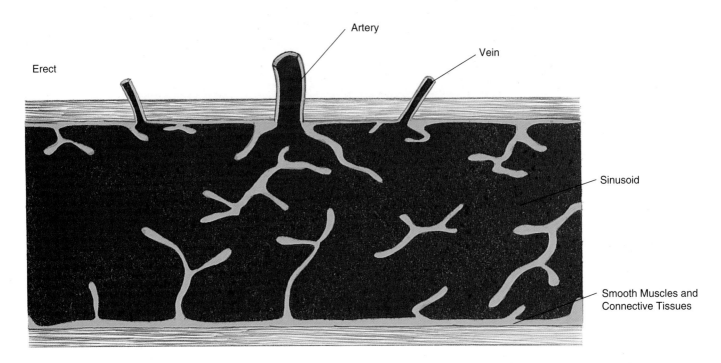

Figure 19.13. Schematic diagram of the cavernosal smooth muscle and sinusoids. When flaccid the sinusoids are smaller in capacity and the muscle has a high tonus, limiting arterial inflow. Venous outflow in free. After stimulation the sinusoidal smooth muscle relaxes and the sinusoids distend, reducing resistance to arterial flow, and obstructing the venous outflow by compressing the peripheral venules against the tunica albuginea, rising the cavernosal pressure close to systolic pressure.

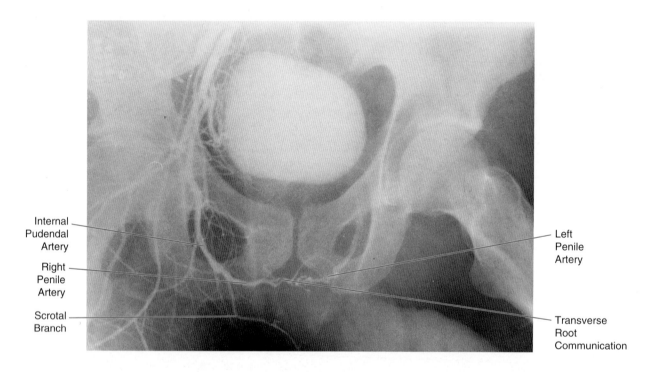

Internal
Pudendal
Artery

Right
Penile
Artery

Scrotal
Branch

Left
Penile
Artery

Transverse
Root
Communication

Figure 19.14. Right internal iliac angiography showing the transverse root communication between the right and left arterial systems.

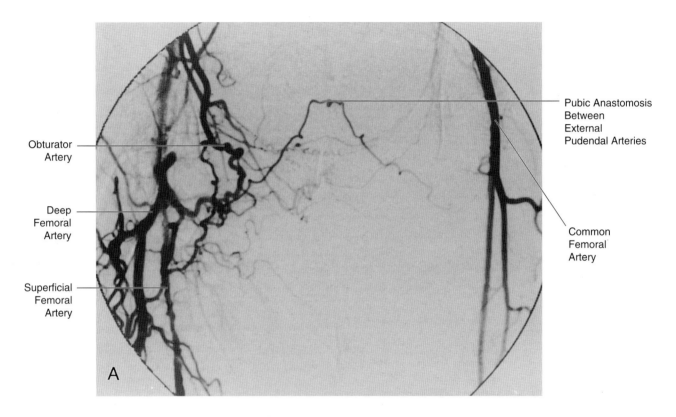

Figure 19.15. Pelvic angiography showing the communications between the right and left arterial systems through the transverse root communication **(A)** and between medial femoral circumflex arteries or external pudendal arteries **(B)** in a patient with vascular disease.

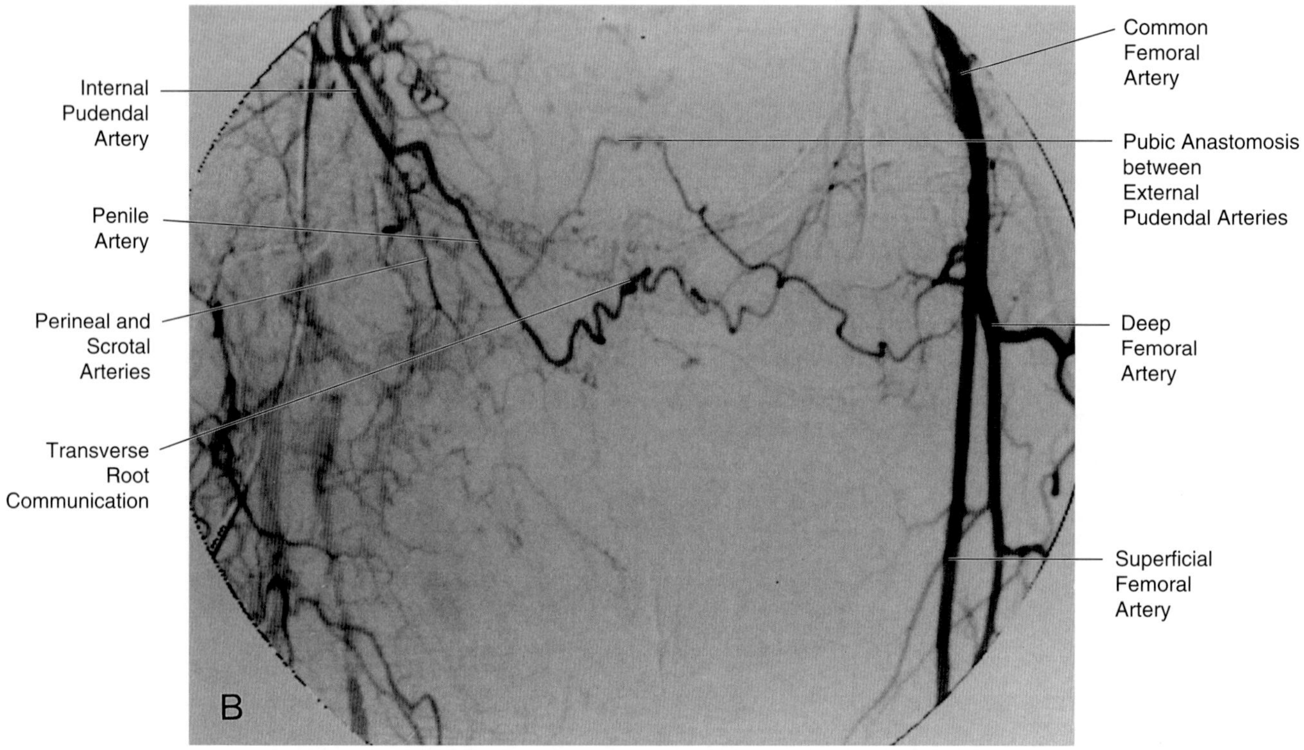

Figure 19.15. *Continued*

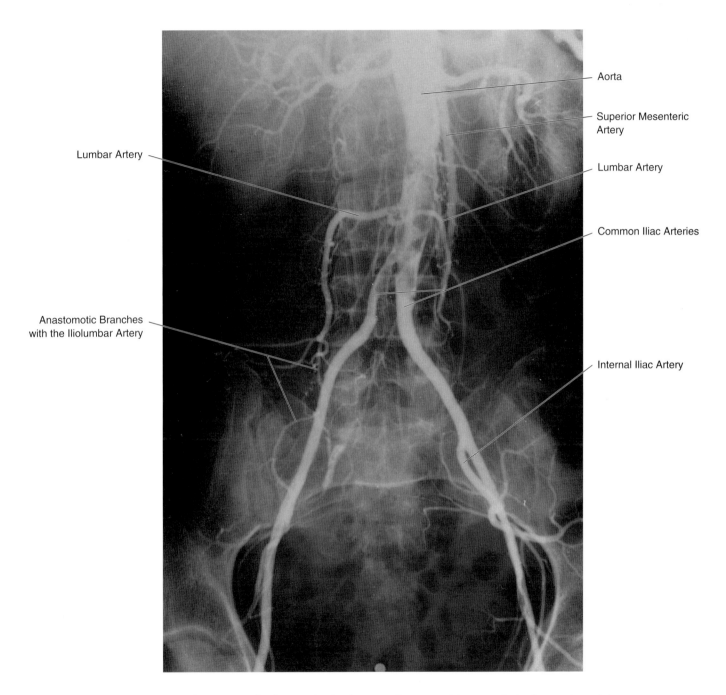

Figure 19.16. Pelvic angiography showing the development of anastomosis between the lumbar arteries and the internal iliac branches, due to an occlusion at the aortic bifurcation.

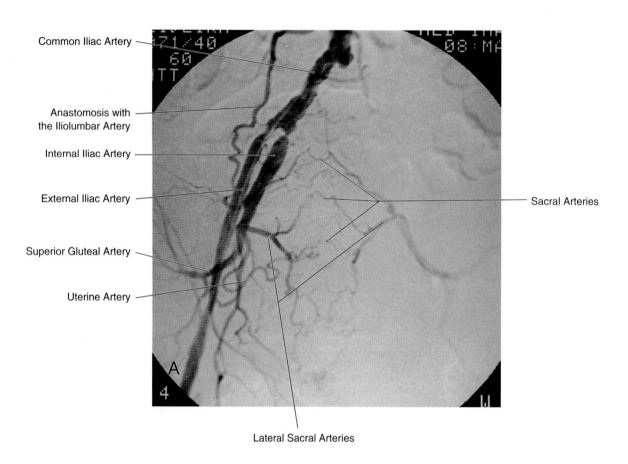

Figure 19.17. Pelvic angiography in a patient with arterial occlusion showing the development of the lateral sacral arteries and the gluteal arteries.

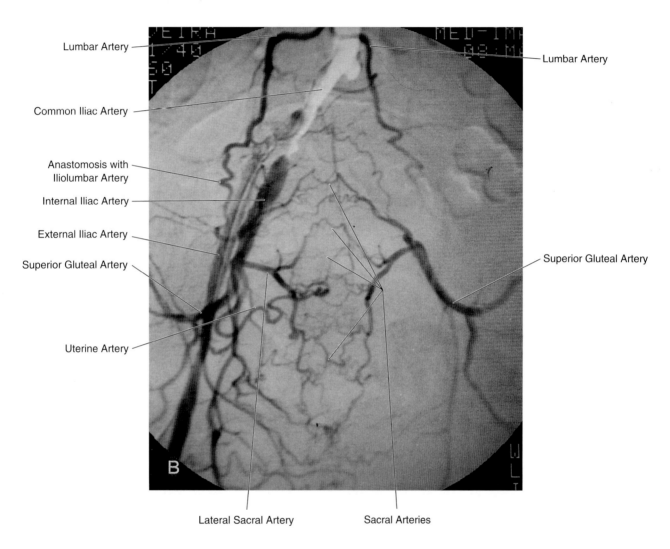

Figure 19.17. *Continued*

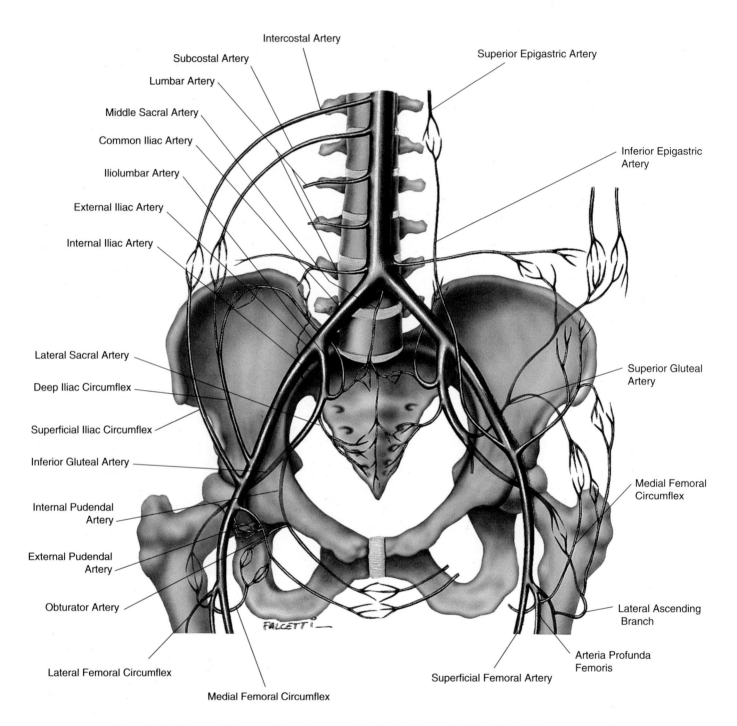

Intercostal Artery

Subcostal Artery

Lumbar Artery

Middle Sacral Artery

Common Iliac Artery

Iliolumbar Artery

External Iliac Artery

Internal Iliac Artery

Superior Epigastric Artery

Inferior Epigastric Artery

Lateral Sacral Artery

Deep Iliac Circumflex

Superficial Iliac Circumflex

Inferior Gluteal Artery

Internal Pudendal Artery

External Pudendal Artery

Obturator Artery

Superior Gluteal Artery

Medial Femoral Circumflex

Lateral Ascending Branch

Lateral Femoral Circumflex

Medial Femoral Circumflex

Superficial Femoral Artery

Arteria Profunda Femoris

FALCETT

Figure 19.18. Schematic diagram of the major potential parietal pathways of collateral circulation encountered in chronic obstructive vascular disease at the abdominal and pelvic levels.

20

VEINS OF THE ABDOMEN AND PELVIS

VEINS OF THE PELVIS (FIGS. 20.1, 20.2)

External Iliac Vein

The external iliac vein is the continuation of the femoral vein, begins at the inguinal ligament, and joins the internal iliac vein, thus forming the common iliac vein. The external iliac vein is medial to the iliac artery. This vein is usually valveless.

Tributaries
    Inferior epigastric vein
    Deep circumflex iliac vein
    Pubic vein

Internal Iliac Vein (Fig. 20.3)

Several veins converge superiorly in the great sciatic foramen to form the internal iliac vein, to join the external iliac vein, forming the common iliac vein, anteriorly to the sacroiliac joint.

Tributaries
    Origin outside the pelvis
        Superior gluteal veins
        Inferior gluteal veins
        Internal pudendal veins
        Obturator vein
    Anterior to the sacrum
        Lateral sacral veins
    Origin in visceral venous plexus
        Middle rectal veins
        Rectal venous plexus
        Prostatic venous plexus
        Vesical plexus
        Dorsal veins of the penis and penile venous plexus
        Uterine plexuses
        Vaginal plexuses

Superior Gluteal Veins (Fig. 20.4)

Vena comitans of the superior gluteal artery. They enter the pelvis through the greater sciatic foramen, above the muscle piriformis and join the internal iliac vein as a single trunk.

Inferior Gluteal Veins

Vena comitans of the inferior gluteal artery. They arise proximal and posteriorly in the thigh, anastomose with the medial circumflex femoral and 1st perforating veins. They enter low in the greater sciatic foramen, joining the internal iliac vein and connect with the superficial gluteal veins through the gluteal perforating veins.

Internal Pudendal Veins (Fig. 20.5)

Vena comitans of the internal pudendal artery, commencing in the prostatic venous plexus and ending in the internal iliac vein. They receive veins from the penile bulb and the scrotal (or labial) and inferior rectal veins. The deep dorsal vein of the penis ends in the prostatic plexus, but is connected through that plexus to the internal pudendal veins.

Obturator Vein

This vein commences in the proximal adductor region and enters the pelvis through the obturator foramen, coursing a retroperitoneal path, passing between the ureter and the internal iliac artery to join the internal iliac vein.

Lateral Sacral Veins (Figs. 20.1, 20.3, 20.4)

These veins are interconnected by the sacral venous plexus and follow the lateral sacral arteries.

Middle Rectal Vein

This vein arises from the rectal venous plexus, receiving tributaries from the bladder, prostate and seminal vesicle.

Rectal Venous Plexus (Figs. 18.102, 18.106, 18.107)

The rectal venous plexus surrounds the rectum and is connected anteriorly to the vesical plexus in males and to the uterovaginal plexus in females. It has an internal rectal plexus, under the rectal and anal epithelium and an external rectal plexus outside the muscular layer. In the anal canal, the internal plexus has longitudinal dilatations, most prominent in the left lateral, right anterolateral, and right posterolateral sectors. These veins are apt to become varicose and will be known as internal hemorrhoids. The internal plexus drains mostly to the superior rectal vein, but connects extensively with the external rectal plexus. The external rectal plexus drains inferiorly by the inferior rectal veins, tributary of the internal pudendal vein. The external rectal plexus drains in the middle to a middle rectal vein, tributary of the internal iliac vein. The superior rectal vein is the beginning of the inferior mesenteric vein and drains the superior part of the external rectal plexus. The veins in the subcutaneous part of the external rectal plexus, may thrombose and form the so-called external hemorrhoids.

The wide anastomoses between the rectal venous plexus and the internal iliac vein, as well as with the inferior mesenteric vein, establish communication between the portal and systemic venous systems.

Prostatic Venous Plexus

The periprostatic venous plexus is composed of a superficial and a deep plexus. The deep plexus is popularly known as Santorini's plexus. The periprostatic plexus is originated from the deep dorsal vein of the penis, when this vessel leaves the penis under the Buck's fascia and penetrates the pelvis passing under the symphysis of the pubis. After penetrating the pelvis, the vein divides into three major branches: the superficial branch and the right and left deep lateral venous plexuses, (Figs. 20.6, 20.7). The superficial branch is centrally located and emerges in the retropubic adipose tissue between the pubic-prostatic ligaments, overlying the bladder neck and the prostate (Figs. 20.8, 20.9). This vein often has communicating branches over the bladder and into the endopelvic fascia (Fig. 20.8). Mostly (80% of cases), this vein is really a single midline vessel, presenting early or late bifurcation in 20% of the cases. In 10% of the cases this superficial vein may be double or may have other anatomical variations. In 10% of cases, the superficial vein is absent.

The lateral venous plexuses (deep plexus, Santorini's) pass posterolaterally, beneath the visceral or preprostatic fascia (Figs. 20.10, 20.11, 20.12) and communicate freely with the internal iliac vein (hypogastric vein) through the pudendal, obturator, and vesical venous plexuses. The deep venous plexus (Santorini's plexus) can be visualized in dissected specimens only after opening the endopelvic fascia and its right and left condensations, which unite the prostate to the dorsal surface of the pubis (the so-called "pubic-prostatic ligaments") (Figs. 20.10, 20.11, 20.12).

Because the lateral plexuses (deep plexus) anastomose freely with other pelvic plexuses, any laceration of this structure can lead to considerable blood loss during any kind of retropubic surgery. Also, since the periprostatic plexus communicates with the paravertebral venous network (Batsons's plexus), osseous metastases constitute the most common form of hematogenous metastasis of prostatic carcinoma, which occurs through this paravertebral plexus (Fig. 20.33). The most frequent sites involved are the pelvic bone, lumbar spine, femora, thoracic spine, and ribs.

Vesical Plexus

The vesical plexus covers the lower bladder and the prostatic base in males and is connected to the prostatic venous plexus in males and to the vaginal venous plexus in females. It is drained by several vesical veins, tributaries of the internal iliac vein.

Dorsal Veins of the Penis and Penile Venous Anatomy (Fig. 20.13, 20.14, 20.15, 20.16, 20.17)

There is a superficial and a deep dorsal vein of the penis. The superficial dorsal vein of the penis drains the prepuce and skin, and is positioned longitudinally along the penis, draining to the external pudendal veins. The superficial dorsal vein of the penis receives, along its course, flow from the corpora cavernosa penis through circumflex veins. The deep dorsal vein of the penis runs backward in the midline, under the fibrous penile sheath. It receives blood flow from the glans penis and corpora cavernosa penis, through the circumflex veins. It reaches the prostatic venous plexus after dividing into right and left branches, but has also communications with the internal pudendal veins (Figs. 20.18, 20.19, 20.20, 20.21, 20.22, 20.23, 20.44). The deep dorsal vein of the penis has a venous valve beneath the symphysis pubis.

The superficial venous system of the penis including the superficial dorsal vein drains into the superficial femoral vein through the external pudendal vein and the saphenous vein (Figs. 20.25, 20.25, 20.27, 20.28).

The corpora cavernosa penis are formed by sinusoids surrounded by smooth muscle and connective tissues with high wall tonus. The sinusoidal vascular space and arterial inflow are limited in flaccid state. The venous outflow is unimpeded. During erection, after neurostimulation or intracavernosal papaverine injection, the sinusoidal smooth muscle relaxes, and distended sinusoids compress and obstruct peripheral venules against tunica albuginea. Simultaneously, resistance to arterial flow decreases until cavernosal pressure approaches systolic pressure (Fig. 19.13).

The crura of the corpora cavernosa penis are drained by crural perforating veins, which are tributaries of the internal pudendal veins (Fig. 20.13).

Uterine Plexuses

The uterine venous plexus extends laterally in the broad ligaments, communicating with the ovarian and vaginal plexuses. The uterine plexus is drained by the uterine vein, which is a tributary of the internal iliac vein (Figs. 20.29, 20.30a).

Vaginal Plexuses

The vaginal plexuses connect with the uterine, vesical, and rectal plexuses and are drained by vaginal veins to the internal iliac veins.

Common Iliac Veins

The common iliac vein arises from the junction of the external and the internal iliac veins at the level of the sacroiliac joint. The common iliac vein follows an oblique direction ending at the level of the 5th lumbar vertebra, joining the contralateral common iliac vein to form the inferior vena cava. The right common iliac vein is almost vertical while the left is oblique and longer. The left common iliac vein crosses behind the right common iliac artery and is sometimes compressed by this vessel. The common iliac vein is joined by the iliolumbar and lateral sacral veins (Figs. 20.1, 20.2).

Variations

The left common iliac vein may ascend left of the aorta to the level of the left renal vein, where it crosses anterior to the aorta to join the inferior vena cava.

Median Sacral Veins

The median sacral veins are companions of the median sacral artery, anteriorly to the sacrum, joining into a single vein, ending in the left common iliac vein or at the junction of the common iliac veins (Figs. 20.1, 20.4).

ABDOMINAL VEINS

Inferior Vena Cava

Tributaries
    Lumbar veins
    Ascending lumbar veins
    Gonadal veins
    Renal veins
    Suprarenal veins
    Inferior phrenic veins

Inferior Vena Cava (Figs. 20.1, 20.2, 20.31, 20.32)

The inferior vena cava carries blood from all the structures and abdominal organs, below the diaphragm, being formed by the confluence of the common iliac veins. It follows an upward direction in front of the lumbar spine, to the right of the abdominal aorta. The IVC reaches the liver and has an intrahepatic segment, which may be totally encircled by hepatic parenchyma. It reaches the right atrium of

the heart, through the tendinous part of the diaphragm. At the entrance of the inferoposterior part of the right atrium, there is a semilunar valve of the inferior vena cava.

Variations

A number of anomalies may occur during the development phase of the inferior vena cava in fetal life. It may be totally replaced by two or more vessels, with failure of interconnection between the common iliac veins, and persistence of a longitudinal channel on the left, supracardinal, or subcardinal veins. It may also suffer a complete transposition to the left of the aorta.

Collateral Circulation

There is a rich collateral venous network bypassing the inferior vena cava in cases of thrombosis or occlusion, either through a superficial or deep venous network. The superficial system includes the epigastric veins, the circumflex iliac, the lateral thoracic veins, the thoracoepigastric, the internal thoracic, the posterior intercostal, the external pudendal and lumbovertebral anastomotic veins. The deep system includes the azygos vein, the hemiazygos and the lumbar veins. The vertebral venous plexus, including the Batson's venous plexus, are also in the collateral venous circuit (Figs. 20.33, 20.34).

Tributaries

Lumbar Veins

There are four pairs of lumbar veins, draining the lumbar muscles and skin from the abdominal wall. The lumbar veins also drain the vertebral venous plexuses and are connected by the ascending lumbar veins. The left side lumbar veins are longer and cross behind the abdominal aorta. The 1st and 2nd lumbar veins may connect to the inferior vena cava, the ascending lumbar veins or the lumbar azygos vein (Figs. 20.1, 20.33, 20.35).

Ascending Lumbar Veins

The ascending lumbar veins originate from the common iliac veins and make connections between the common iliac veins to the iliolumbar and lumbar veins. They ascend behind the psoas major muscles and in front of the vertebral transverse processes. Cranially they join the subcostal veins and turn medially forming the azygos vein in the right side and the hemiazygos vein on the left (Fig. 20.35).

Gonadal Veins (Figs. 20.36, 20.37)

Testicular Veins

These veins arise from the posterior aspect of the testis and drain the epididymis to form the pampiniform plexus. They follow the spermatic cord, anteriorly to the ductus deferens, crossing the inguinal ring and the inguinal canal, ascending retroperitoneally close to the ureter, anterior to the psoas major, as two or more veins, with abundant collaterals and anastomoses, in both sides of the testicular artery. The left testicular vein joins in a single vessel and opens into the left renal vein to form a right angle. The right testicular vein joins in a single vessel and opens in the inferior vena cava, just below the right renal vein, forming an acute angle. The testicular veins have several valves that may be nonfunctioning and cause varicoceles on the testis, mainly on the left side.

Ovarian Veins

There is a venous plexus in the broad ligament of the uterus, which communicates with the uterine plexus, from which originate the two ovarian veins in each side, following the path of the ovarian artery, and coursing together in each side of the artery, opening at the inferior vena cava on the right and on the left renal vein on the left. They have valves and the valvular incompetence may lead to pelvic varices (Figs. 20.30, 20.36, 20.37).

Renal Veins

Intrarenal Veins

In contrast to the arteries, there is free circulation throughout the venous system and, therefore, the veins do not have a segmental model. Nevertheless, the renal venous system presents some anatomic characteristics that are reasonably constant, and should be known during angiographic examinations.

Material of Investigation

Fifty-two three-dimensional endocasts of the kidney-collecting system together with the intrarenal veins were obtained from 26 fresh cadavers of both sexes, who died of causes not related to the urinary tract.

A blue polyester resin (volume approximately 15.0 ml) was injected into the main trunk of the renal vein to fill in the kidney venous tree and a yellow resin into the ureter (about 5.0 ml) to fill in the collecting system, according to the proportions and technique described previously.

Findings

The intrarenal venous arrangement demonstrates free anastomosis between the veins. The small veins of the cortex, called Stellate Veins, drain into the Interlobular Veins, which form a series of arches (Figs. 20.38, 20.39). Within the kidney substance, these arches are arranged in arcades, which lie mainly in the longitudinal axis. There are usually three systems of longitudinal anastomotic arcades and the anastomoses occur at different levels; between the

stellate veins (more peripherally), between the arcuate veins (at the base of the pyramids), and between the interlobar (infundibular) veins (close to the renal sinus) (Figs. 20.38, 20.39). These anastomoses are named as first order, second order, and third order, from periphery to the center (Fig. 20.40).

Around the caliceal necks, there were large venous anastomoses (collar's like), formed mainly when the veins draining the posterior half of the kidney cross over at the necks of the minor calices to join the anterior main trunks (Fig. 20.41). There were also horizontal arches, crossing over the calices to link the anterior and posterior veins, as well as the longitudinal systems at different levels (Fig. 20.42). The venous arcades join one another in both the longitudinal and horizontal planes to produce larger veins that unite to form large trunks. The main renal vein was formed by these trunks, which course toward the hilum where they unite, prior to emptying into the vena cava.

In one series, three trunks (28 of 52 casts: 53.8%) and two trunks (15 of 52 casts: 28.8%) joining each other to form the main renal vein were found (Fig. 20.43). Less frequently, four trunks (8 of 52 casts: 15.4%) or five trunks (1 of 52 casts: 1.9%) were found.

Dorsal Kidney

In 36 of 52 casts (69.2%), there was a posterior (retropelvic) vein that coursed on the back of the kidney collecting system either to drain into the renal vein or empty directly into the vena cava. In 25 of 52 casts (48.1%), the retropelvic vein had a close relationship to the upper infundibulum or to the junction of the pelvis with the upper calix (Fig. 20.44a). In the other 11 of 52 casts (21.1%), the retropelvic vein crossed and was related to the middle posterior surface of the renal pelvis (Fig. 20.44b). In 16 of 52 casts (30.8%), there were no veins on the posterior aspect of the renal pelvis because the veins draining the posterior region crossed anteriorly to join the main anterior trunks of the renal vein (Fig. 20.44c).

Relationship to Ureteropelvic Junction

In 40.4% of the cases (21 of 52 casts), we found a close relationship between an important tributary of the renal vein and the anterior aspect of the UPJ (Fig. 20.45a). Among these cases, there was one vein anterior and another vein posterior to the UPJ, simultaneously (Fig. 20.46 a,b). In the other 59.6% of cases (31 of 52 casts), the UPJ was not related to veins, either anteriorly or posteriorly (Fig. 20.45 b).

Extrarenal Veins

Mostly, the renal vein is formed by the union of two (53.8% of the cases) or three intrarenal trunks (28.8%). Less frequently, there were four trunks (15.4%) or five trunks (1.9%), joining to form the main renal vein. After leaving the renal hilus on each side, both renal veins drain into the inferior vena cava. The left renal vein is longer than the right vein and usually has a higher penetration into the vena cava. The left renal vein has a ventral course in relation to the abdominal aorta and is caudally located in relation to the origin of the superior mesenteric artery.

The right renal vein does not have tributaries. In contrast, the left renal vein drains an extensive body area and usually receives the left inferior suprarenal vein, the left inferior diaphragmatic vein, the left gonadal vein, and the left second lumbar vein.

Anatomic variations of the renal veins are less common than the arterial variations. Also, when exist anatomic variations, they are more frequent in the right side (Fig. 20.47). The left renal vein almost always is single.

Material of Investigation

The extrarenal veins in 88 "in situ" kidneys, dissected from 44 formalin-fixed cadavers of adult patients, of both sexes, who died of causes unrelated to the urinary tract, were analyzed.

Findings

The left renal vein was single in all of the 44 left kidneys that were analyzed.

Considering the right side, in three cases, two renal veins draining to the inferior vena cava were present (7.0% of right kidneys or 3.5% of the total kidneys). Among these, in one case the two veins had similar calibers, being the inferior vein slightly greater in diameter. In the other two cases, the caliber of the inferior vein was less than a half of the superior vein caliber.

Capsular and Perirenal Veins

There is a rich venous network around the kidneys, draining the renal capsule and with anastomoses between the intrarenal venous system and the capsular veins. The perirenal veins drain into the gonadal vein, inferior phrenic vein, and suprarenal veins. There are direct anastomoses directly with the main renal vein and with the ureteric veins (Figs. 20.1, 20.47).

Suprarenal Veins (See Fig. 18.116)

There is only one draining adrenal vein for each adrenal hilum. The right adrenal vein is short, small opening directly and horizontally into the lateroposterior aspect of the inferior vena cava, far above the right renal vein (Figs. 20.48, 20.49, 20.50).

The left adrenal vein is longer, larger and descends from the adrenal gland posteriorly to the body of the pancreas to open in the left renal vein, joined by a branch of the left inferior phrenic vein, about 1 cm from the inferior vena cava (Figs. 20.50, 20.51, 20.52).

Angiographically the hepatic veins of the lower group may be mistakenly identified as the right adrenal vein (Fig. 20.53). Occasionally the right adrenal vein drains into one of the small hepatic veins of the lower group.

Inferior Phrenic Veins

The inferior phrenic veins follow the same distribution of the companion inferior phrenic arteries on the lower diaphragmatic surface. The right ends in the inferior vena cava, above or together with the right hepatic vein. The left is frequently double and one branch opens in the inferior vena cava or together with the left hepatic vein, while the other may join the left adrenal vein or the left renal vein (Figs. 20.54, 18.114, 18.115).

HEPATIC VEINS AND PORTAL VENOUS SYSTEM

Hepatic Veins

Distribution of the Hepatic Veins

The hepatic veins drain the liver parenchyma and start as intralobular veins, draining the sinusoids of the hepatic lobules. According to the classical description, these end at the sublobular veins, which will drain into the hepatic veins. The hepatic veins are valveless and are contiguous with the hepatic tissue.

There are three main hepatic veins emerging from the upper, posterior surface of the liver, opening at the inferior vena cava and an individual vein from the caudate lobe (Figs. 20.55, 20.56). These are called the upper group, consisting of the large, right, middle, and left hepatic veins, and the smaller caudate lobe vein which delineates four well-defined territories of drainage (Figs. 20.55, 20.56, 20.57).

The right hepatic veins run at the right hepatic fissure, which divides the right hepatic lobe in the anterior and the posterior sector. The right hepatic vein drains both the anterior (segments VIII and V) and the posterior (segments VI and VII) sectors of the right hepatic lobe (Fig. 20.55).

In 16 of 25 casts of liver specimens, there was only one right hepatic vein of large diameter receiving several tributaries from the several segments of the right lobe (Figs. 20.58, 20.59, 20.60, 20.61, 20.62). In two cases, the tributaries from segment VIII were large and reached the right hepatic vein near the IVC. One cast showed two RHV, parallel to each other and with similar sizes. In two cases, the right hepatic vein had a single short trunk of about 1 cm, but was bifid with two parallel veins peripherally. Six livers showed an accessory right hepatic vein, caudal and distal, but parallel to the main vein and posterior to the portal vein bifurcation. In two casts the right hepatic vein was extremely underdeveloped. In 1.6 % of the cases (out of a series of 60 cases) three right hepatic veins were identified, and the most anterior one was located anteriorly to the portal vein bifurcation and to the anterior branch of the right portal trunk (Fig. 20.65).

The distance from the anterior aspect of the right hepatic vein, at 1 cm from the IVC and the posterior aspect of the portal bifurcation, was measured in a straight line. This distance ranged from 2.7 to 5.4 cm, with a mean distance of 4.41 cm. In the cases in which there were two right hepatic veins, the distance was 1.8 cm from the medial branch and 4.2 cm from the lateral branch. The accessory right hepatic veins and the portal bifurcation were very close. The distance between the anterior aspect of the accessory right hepatic veins measured at 1 cm from the IVC and the portal bifurcation was 2.2 to 4.3 cm with a mean distance of 3.1 cm.

The middle hepatic vein runs at the middle hepatic fissure, dividing the right hepatic lobe from the left hepatic lobe and drains most of the medial aspect of the left liver lobe (segment IV), but in general receives a large tributary from the right hepatic lobe (segment V), crossing from the right to the left hepatic lobes. The middle hepatic vein joins the left hepatic vein to form a single venous trunk ending in the anterolateral aspect of the inferior vena cava.

There was only one middle hepatic vein in all 25 cases of the series analyzed; they joined the IVC directly in about 20% of the cases and formed a common trunk with the left hepatic vein in 80% of the cases.

The distance between the inferior aspect of the middle hepatic vein, at 1 cm from the IVC and the superior posterior aspect of the portal bifurcation and left portal trunk, was measured in a straight line. This distance ranged from 2.4 to 4.5 cm, with a mean distance of 3.9 cm.

The left hepatic vein runs partially at the fissure for the ligamentum teres and at the left hepatic fissure, between the segments II and III, and drains preferentially the lateral sector (segments II and III) of the left hepatic lobe, but also receives tributaries from the segment IV (Fig. 20.66). The left hepatic vein is always anterior to the left portal vein

The caudate lobe vein is an independent tributary of the inferior vena cava and opens in the cava in a much lower position, in relation with the three main hepatic veins.

The lower group of hepatic veins are smaller in size and numerous and drain liver parenchyma directly to the inferior vena cava, from the right liver lobe and the caudate lobe.

Variations of the Hepatic Veins

There may be several large accessory hepatic veins draining the upper (diaphragmatic) part of the right and left liver lobes, joining the main hepatic veins, close to the outlet ring at the inferior vena cava. Several additional draining veins, from territories not usually drained by the three main veins, may be tributaries of the right, middle and left hepatic veins (Fig. 20.59).

Accessory hepatic veins may also be encountered in the lower group, draining a variable amount of parenchyma from the right liver lobe, with an incidence of up to 15% of the population.

Venous Collateral Channels

When obstruction of the hepatic veins or the suprahepatic segment of the inferior vena cava happens, several collateral pathways develop and may be divided into three types:

1. Extrahepatic
   Collaterals developed through the liver capsule toward retroperitoneal and intercostal veins
2. Intrahepatic-Interlobar
   Collaterals developed from the hepatic segment with venous obstruction to adjacent patent hepatic veins (Fig. 20.67)
3. Indeterminate Type ("Spiderweb" appearance)
   Fine and/or coarse collateral networks emanating from the occluded vein (at phlebography), without certain flow direction

Portal Vein

The portal vein is about 7 to 8 cm in length and carries the visceral blood to the liver, where it ramifies following the segmental pattern, like the hepatic artery, reaching the sinusoids, from which the blood again converges to drain into the inferior vena cava through the hepatic veins. There are no valves at the portal vein during the adult life. The portal vein results from the confluence of the splenic vein and the superior mesenteric vein, and follows a path, posteriorly to the pancreatic head and anteriorly to the inferior vena cava, reaching the liver through the lesser omentum, and anterior to the epiploic foramen (Figs. 20.55, 20.68, 20.69, 20.70, 20.71, 20.72). Inside the lesser omentum and at the porta hepatis, it is posterior to the bile duct and the hepatic artery. The bile duct is parallel, but lateral, whereas the hepatic artery is parallel, but medial.

At the porta hepatis, the portal vein divides in the right and left branches. The right portal branch enters the right hepatic lobe, after receiving the cystic vein. It branches into the four segments of the right hepatic lobe (V, VI, VII, and VIII hepatic segments), and in some cases also branches to the caudate lobe (segment I). The left portal branch enters the right hepatic lobe, it is longer and with smaller diameter, and branches into the four segments of the left lobe (I, IV, II and III hepatic segments) (Figs. 20.55, 20.73, 20.74). At the left lobe of the liver, it is joined by the paraumbilical veins and the ligamentum teres (residum of the obliterated left umbilical vein). There is also a connection with the inferior vena cava by the ligamentum venosum (remnant of the occluded ductus venosus).

Anatomy of the Portal Bifurcation

In 24 livers, the portal vein presented a very short and thin right trunk and a long left trunk. In almost every specimen, branches to the caudate lobe were seen, arising from the bifurcation of the portal vein or from the first 1 cm of the left trunk. One liver presented an anomalous variation at the portal bifurcation. The portal vein bifurcated in a larger left trunk and a smaller right trunk. The left trunk further divided into a real left trunk and branches to segments V and VIII of the right lobe.

In one liver, the artery crossed posteriorly to the origin of the portal trunk to the segment V and segment VIII and followed a joint path close to the posterosuperior aspect of the portal branch to the segments VI and VII. In another liver the hepatic artery bifurcated proximally and to the left of the portal bifurcation, giving off one large anterior branch and a smaller branch which crossed posterior to the portal bifurcation and followed a path on the posterosuperior aspect of the right trunk for the portal vein. In one case there was a posterior arterial branch in the first 2 cm of the left portal trunk. In 9 specimens there were arterial and/or biliary structures in the way between the first 1 cm of the right hepatic vein and

the portal bifurcation (Figs. 20.58, 20.59, 20.60). These biliary and arterial branches were oriented towards the segment VII or segments VI and VII. In these cases there was an intimate relationship between these two bilio-arterial structures, but overall the biliary branches were posterior. In general the biliary and arterial structures are close to the superior aspect of the portal trunks and more frequently are anterosuperior.

Tributaries

Besides the splenic and the superior mesenteric veins, other tributaries are the left gastric, right gastric, the paraumbilical, and cystic veins.

Right Gastric Vein

The right gastric vein runs to the right along the lesser curvature of the stomach, draining both faces of the stomach, eventually reaching the portal vein. It forms a loop with the left gastric vein (Fig. 20.75).

Left Gastric Vein (Coronary Vein)

The left gastric vein drains both gastric walls, upward in the lesser curvature of the stomach, and through the lesser omentum reaches the portal vein. It is connected to the lower esophageal veins through plentiful anastomoses (Figs. 20.76, 20.77, 20.78, 20.79).

Paraumbilical Veins

These are small veins, in variable number, extending along the ligamentum teres and median umbilical ligament, connecting veins of the anterior abdominal wall to the left branch of the portal vein. Since the paraumbilical veins connect the portal venous system to the systemic venous system, they form a direct potential portosystemic shunt. The umbilical vein remnant (Baumgarten recess) shows no visible lumen in normal patients. The ligamentum teres shows no lumen even in cirrhotic patients with portal hypertension.

Cystic Veins

There are two types of cystic veins. The first type comprehend veins originated at the superior surface of the gallbladder, entering the liver parenchyma directly or joining the bile duct veins system. The second, and more rare type, is a single or a double cystic vein joining the right portal branch.

Variations and Anomalies of the Portal Vein

The variations of the portal vein are mostly related to the different arrangement of the tributaries. The left gastric vein may enter at the junction of the splenic and the portal vein. The left gastric vein may join the splenic vein. The inferior mesenteric vein may enter the superior mesenteric vein and high intestinal veins may enter directly at the portal vein. The anomalies of the portal vein are mostly related to anomalies of position: portal vein anterior to the head of the pancreas and first part of the duodenum; portal vein entering the inferior vena cava; pulmonary vein entering portal vein; congenital stricture of the portal vein.

Splenic Vein

The splenic vein is one of the two larger tributaries of the portal vein, and its confluence with the superior mesenteric vein actually forms the portal vein. It is a large vein, about 1 cm in diameter, enlarging as reaches the portal vein. Normally it is a relatively straight vein, but may get very tortuous due to portal hypertension. The main splenic vein is formed by the union of two veins in 76% of the cases, by three branches in 20% of the cases, and by four branches in 4% of the 50 specimens studied. The spleen has a venous segmentation which varies in number, but make totally independent compartments, as visualized in the corrosion endocasts obtained of the intrasplenic venous vasculature (Figs. 20.80, 20.81). It is originated from the splenic hilum, and follows a path from left to right, behind the tail and body of the pancreas, receiving several pancreatic venous branches. There is a close correspondence concerning number and path between the hilar splenic veins and the hilar splenic arteries in 80.6% of the cases. There is no correspondence in 19.4% of the cases. The analysis of 25 casts injected with polyester resin showed 2 venous segments in 85.0% of the cases and 3 venous segments in 11.0% of the cases. There is also a correspondence between splenic venous segments and splenic arterial segments, where each trabecular artery corresponds to a trabecular vein. The splenic venous segments are entirely independent at the venous or arterial circulation (Figs. 20.80, 20.81)

Tributaries

Short Gastric Veins

There are 4 or 5 short gastric veins, draining the gastric fundus and part of the greater gastric curvature, reaching the splenic vein or one of its large tributaries. These veins are also in communication with the lower esophageal veins, and may enlarge markedly when submitted to portal hypertension, reverting the blood flow (Figs. 20.76, 20.82, 20.83).

Left Gastroepiploic Vein

This vein runs along the greater gastric curvature, from right to left, draining the walls of the stomach and the greater omentum, reaching the initial part of the splenic vein (Figs. 20.82, 20.83).

Pancreatic Veins

There is a variable number of pancreatic veins draining the body and tail of the pancreas. They may be small, draining directly into the splenic vein, or larger and few resulting from the confluence of smaller tributaries, eventually draining into the splenic vein. The full description of the pancreatic vein drainage follows.

Inferior Mesenteric Vein (Fig. 20.84)

The inferior mesenteric vein drains the rectum, the sigmoid colon and the left colon, joining the splenic vein distally, close to the confluence with the inferior mesenteric vein, posterior to the body of the pancreas. Occasionally it ends at the union of the splenic and superior mesenteric vein, and sometimes at the superior mesenteric vein itself.

Tributaries

Superior Rectal Vein

Sigmoid Veins

Left Colic Vein

The inferior mesenteric vein begins as the superior rectal vein, arising from the rectal plexus, having connections with the middle and inferior rectal veins. It ascends posterior to the peritoneum, and receives the sigmoid veins and the left colic vein. The left colic vein continues with the middle colic vein at the splenic flexure of the colon.

Superior Mesenteric Vein

The superior mesenteric vein is the largest tributary to the portal vein. It drains the small intestine, cecum, ascending and transverse parts of the colon carrying the blood to enter the portal circulation. It passes behind the pancreatic head and horizontal part of the duodenum and is anterior to the inferior vena cava and joins the splenic vein forming the portal vein. The superior mesenteric vein is formed by the union of the tributaries from the terminal ileum, the cecum and the appendix, receiving several other tributaries along its length (Figs. 20.85, 20.86, 20.87).

Tributaries

Jejunal and Ileal Veins

These are the most numerous tributaries of the superior mesenteric vein. They are named after the respective arteries and conform with the arcade distribution, placed, as a rule on the left side of the superior mesenteric veins, from the duodenojejunal junction to the vicinity of the ileocecal junction where ends the ileocolic vein. The 1st and sometimes the 1st and 2nd jejunal veins are joined by the inferior pancreaticoduodenal vein, either as a trunk or as separate vessels (Figs. 20.88, 20.89, 20.90).

Ileocolic Vein

The ileocolic vein is formed by the union of the anterior and posterior cecal veins, plus the appendicular veins, the last ileal vein and a colic vein, eventually joining the superior mesenteric vein on its right aspect. Anastomoses freely with the ileal veins and the right colic vein (Fig. 20.88).

Right Colic Vein

This vein drains the right colon and results from the junction of the several venous arcades of the right colon wall and from the marginal vein. It anastomoses freely with the ileocolic vein and the middle colic vein. It is retroperitoneal and joins the superior mesenteric vein at the level where it crosses over the 3rd part of the duodenum (Fig. 20.85).

Middle Colic Vein

The middle colic vein drains the transverse colon and has a right and left branch. The right middle colic vein anastomoses with the right colic vein, while the left anastomoses with the left colic vein (tributary of the inferior mesenteric vein) at the splenic flexure of the colon. The middle colic vein joins the superior mesenteric vein through the gastrocolic trunk in the majority of the cases, but may end directly into the superior mesenteric vein itself.

Right Gastroepiploic Vein

This vein drains the greater omentum and the distal part of the body and the antrum of the stomach. It is a long vein and runs along the greater gastric curvature, from left to right. It anastomoses freely with the left gastroepiploic vein and is a major collateral path to drain the spleen when the splenic vein is occluded. The right gastroepiploic vein ends at the gastrocolic trunk, tributary of the superior mesenteric vein, joining the middle colic and anterior pancreaticoduodenal vein. It may occasionally end directly at the superior mesenteric vein (Figs. 20.91, 20.92).

Pancreaticoduodenal Veins

The pancreaticoduodenal veins drain the head of the pancreas and the duodenal wall, and follow similar anatomical architecture to its arterial structure. There is a posterior pancreaticoduodenal venous arcade and an anterior pancreaticoduodenal venous arcade between the superior and inferior pancreaticoduodenal veins. The posterior superior ends at the portal vein, the anterior superior ends at the gastrocolic trunk, while both posterior and anterior inferior end at the superior mesenteric vein, through the 1st jejunal vein (Fig. 20.93).

Anastomoses Between the Portal and Systemic Circulation

In portal vein obstruction or portal vein hypertension due to liver disease, anastomosis between the portal vein and systemic veins may develop, carrying portal blood into the systemic circulation (Fig. 20.94).

There are four main groups of portal systemic collaterals.

Group I

Where protective mucosal epithelium adjoins absorptive mucosal epithelium

Group I (A)

At the cardia of the stomach, where the left gastric vein and short gastric veins of the portal system anastomoses with the intercostal, diaphragm-esophageal and azygos tributaries, veins of the caval system, creating esophageal and gastric fundus varices

Group I (B)

At the anal canal the superior rectal (hemorrhoidal) vein, tributary of the inferior mesenteric vein (portal system), anastomoses with the middle and inferior rectal (hemorrhoidal) veins of the inferior vena cava system, creating hemorrhoids.

Group II

In the falciform ligament through the paraumbilical veins, vestiges of the umbilical circulation of the fetal life. Enlargement of these connections, in presence of portal hypertension, may produce varices of veins radiating from the umbilicus, the Caput Medusae (part of the Cruveilhier-Baumgarten syndrome). The umbilical vein remnant does not recanalize, within the ligamentum teres.

Group III

Where the abdominal organs are in contact with retroperitoneal tissues or adherent to the abdominal wall (Intercostal Veins, Lumbar Veins). Includes veins from the liver to the diaphragm (Veins of Sappey), veins in the lienorenal ligament and omentum, lumbar veins (veins of Retzius), and veins developed in adhesions and scars of previous surgeries.

Group IV

Connections between the portal system and the left renal vein. This may be through communications directly from the splenic vein or via diaphragmatic, pancreatic, left adrenal, gonadal, or gastric veins.

Other Collaterals

The communications from the gastroesophageal collaterals, retroperitoneal and venous systems of the abdomen eventually reach the superior vena cava via the azygos or hemiazygos systems. Very rarely a patent ductus venosus connects the left branch of the portal vein to the inferior vena cava. In cases of extra-hepatic portal venous obstructions additional collaterals develop towards the liver, entering the liver through the portal vein in the porta hepatis. These collaterals include the veins at the hilum, venae comitantes of the portal vein and hepatic arteries, veins in the suspensory ligaments of the liver, unnamed veins around the gallbladder, and diaphragmatic and omental veins.

Pancreatic Venous System

The anatomy of the pancreatic veins corresponds roughly to the distribution of the pancreatic arteries (Fig. 20.95).

The head of the pancreas has the venous drainage related to the main stem of the portal vein and to the superior mesenteric vein. The venous drainage of the head of the pancreas is constituted by four main veins, forming two arcades, one posterior and one anterior. The posterior aspect of the pancreas head is drained by one or several posterior superior pancreaticoduodenal (PSPD) veins directly connected to the dorsal aspect of the portal vein, usually about 2 cm from the point of confluence of the splenic, the superior mesenteric and the portal veins. The posterior arcade also empties into the first jejunal vein or directly into the superior mesenteric vein via the posterior inferior pancreaticoduodenal vein (PIPD). This arcade runs posteriorly to the pancreatic head in the pancreaticoduodenal sulcus, receiving tributaries from the pancreas and duodenum. The anterior aspect of the pancreas head is drained by the anterior superior pancreaticoduodenal vein (ASPD) emptying directly into the gastrocolic trunk (GT) beside several smaller veins. The GT receives the right gastroepiploic (RGE) vein and the middle colic vein (MCV) and empties itself into the right aspect of the superior mesenteric vein (SMV), from 1 to 3 cm from the junction of the superior mesenteric, splenic (SV), and portal (PV) veins.

The lower ventral aspect of the head of the pancreas is drained by the anterior inferior pancreaticoduodenal vein (AIPD) which drains into the 1st jejunal vein or, in some cases, into the SMV. The AIPD is usually joined by the PIPD vein in the last few centimeters before emptying into the 1st jejunal vein.

The ventral aspect of the pancreas head may be occasionally drained by a vein emptying in the ventral surface of the PV, near the confluence or up to 3 or 4 cm from that point. The larger pancreatic veins draining the pancreas head run on the surface of the organ and not within the parenchyma itself (Figs. 20.96, 20.97, 20.98, 20.99, 20.100, 20.101, 20.102).

The venous drainage of the pancreas head is usually connected through collaterals to the dorsal pancreatic vein (DP) which drains part of the mediodorsal part of the head and empties in the dorsal aspect of the portal confluence wall (Figs. 20.103, 20.104, 20.105, 20.106).

The body of the pancreas is drained by the transverse pancreatic (TP) vein, which empties either into the inferior mesenteric vein, SMV, or SV (Figs. 20.107, 20.108). The TP vein runs along the inferior border of the pancreatic body, parallel to the SV and receives a large number of small branches from the pancreas body and may be connected to the left gastric vein (LGV) (Fig. 20.109). Several of the smaller veins draining the body of the pancreas empty into the PSPD, the LGV, or directly into the large venous trunks near the confluence (Fig. 20.107, 20.108).

The tail of the pancreas is drained by a large number of small and short veins that are usually connected to the caudal aspect of the splenic vein. These are mainly intrapancreatic veins that are part of a rich anastomotic venous bed connecting the TP vein and the SV. Some of the lower polar veins of the spleen may also participate in the distal caudal pancreatic venous drainage (Figs. 20.110, 20.111, 20.112 and 20.113).

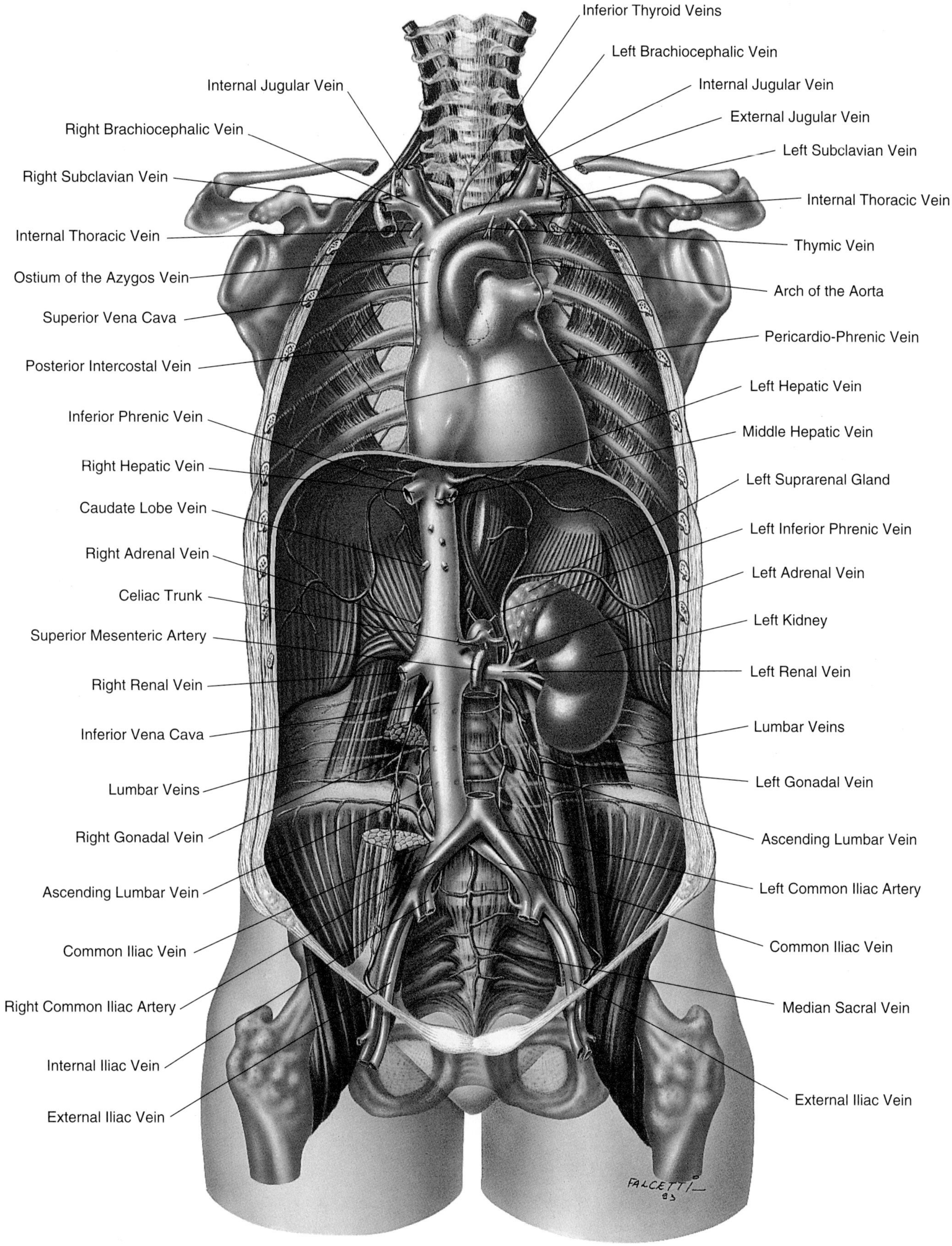

Inferior Thyroid Veins

Left Brachiocephalic Vein

Internal Jugular Vein

External Jugular Vein

Left Subclavian Vein

Internal Thoracic Vein

Thymic Vein

Arch of the Aorta

Pericardio-Phrenic Vein

Left Hepatic Vein

Middle Hepatic Vein

Left Suprarenal Gland

Left Inferior Phrenic Vein

Left Adrenal Vein

Left Kidney

Left Renal Vein

Lumbar Veins

Left Gonadal Vein

Ascending Lumbar Vein

Left Common Iliac Artery

Common Iliac Vein

Median Sacral Vein

External Iliac Vein

Internal Jugular Vein

Right Brachiocephalic Vein

Right Subclavian Vein

Internal Thoracic Vein

Ostium of the Azygos Vein

Superior Vena Cava

Posterior Intercostal Vein

Inferior Phrenic Vein

Right Hepatic Vein

Caudate Lobe Vein

Right Adrenal Vein

Celiac Trunk

Superior Mesenteric Artery

Right Renal Vein

Inferior Vena Cava

Lumbar Veins

Right Gonadal Vein

Ascending Lumbar Vein

Common Iliac Vein

Right Common Iliac Artery

Internal Iliac Vein

External Iliac Vein

Figure 20.1. Schematic diagram of the inferior vena cava, tributaries veins of the abdomen and pelvis, as well as the superior vena cava and main venous tributaries of the chest.

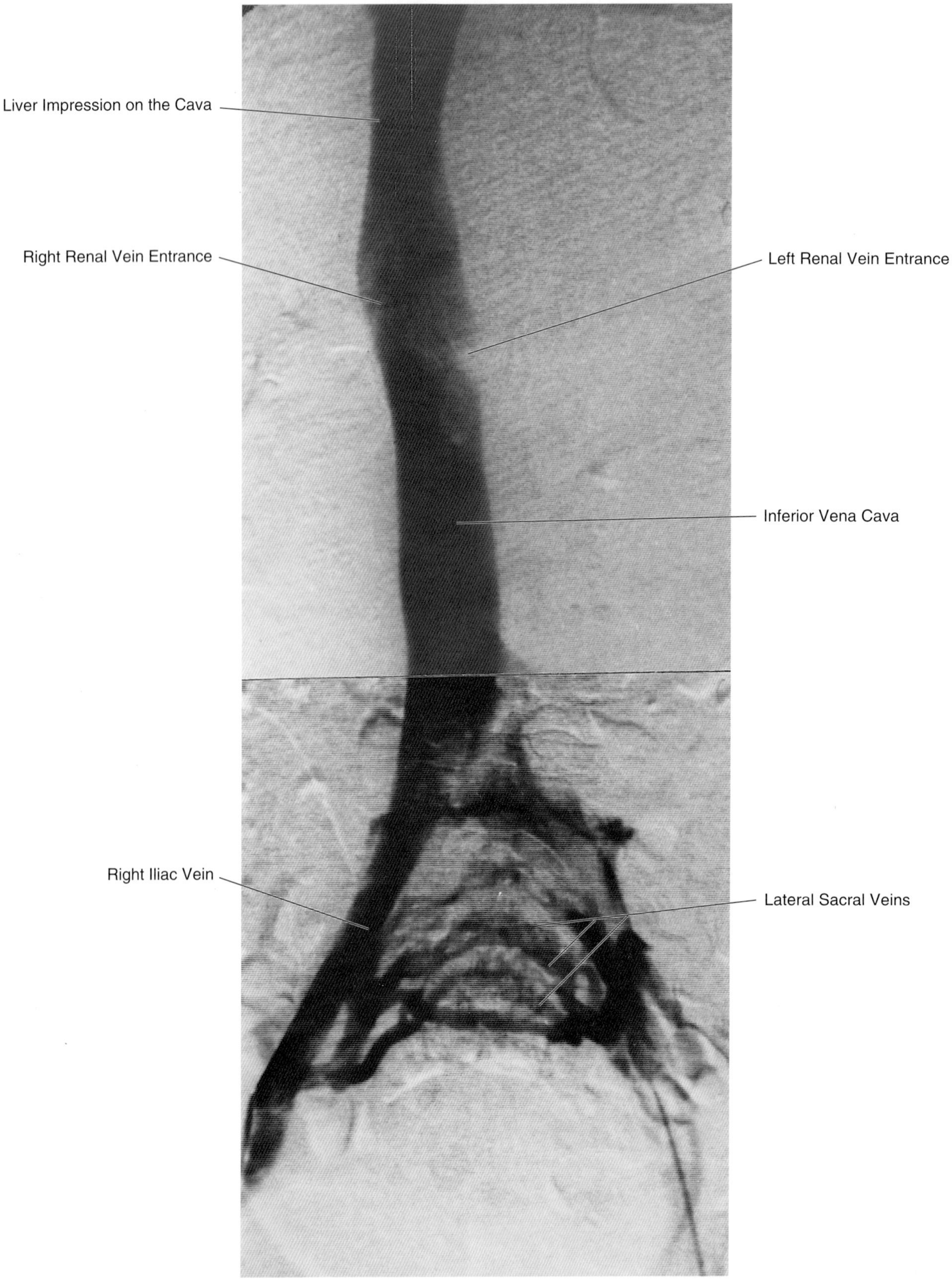

Liver Impression on the Cava

Right Renal Vein Entrance

Left Renal Vein Entrance

Inferior Vena Cava

Right Iliac Vein

Lateral Sacral Veins

Figure 20.2. Venography of the iliac veins and inferior vena cava. Due to occlusion of the left iliac, there is filling of the lateral sacral veins and internal iliac veins. Note the filling defects at the confluence of the renal veins with the inferior vena cava. The liver causes some constriction of the cava.

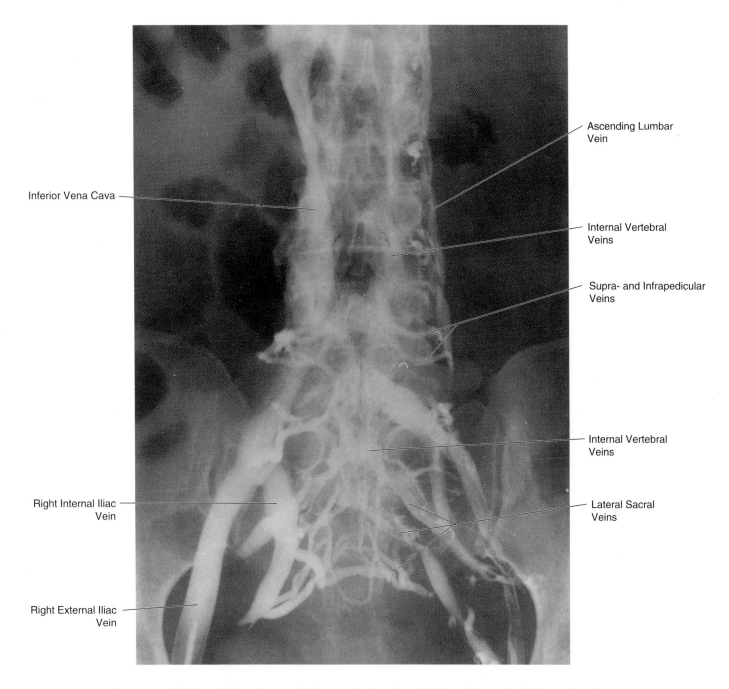

Inferior Vena Cava —

Right Internal Iliac
Vein

Right External Iliac
Vein

Ascending Lumbar
Vein

Internal Vertebral
Veins

Supra- and Infrapedicular
Veins

Internal Vertebral
Veins

Lateral Sacral
Veins

Figure 20.3. The internal iliac veins are filled. Note the lateral sacral veins and the epidural plexus. The inferior vena cava is constricted and there is occlusion of the left iliac vein. The ascending lumbar vein is also visible on the left.

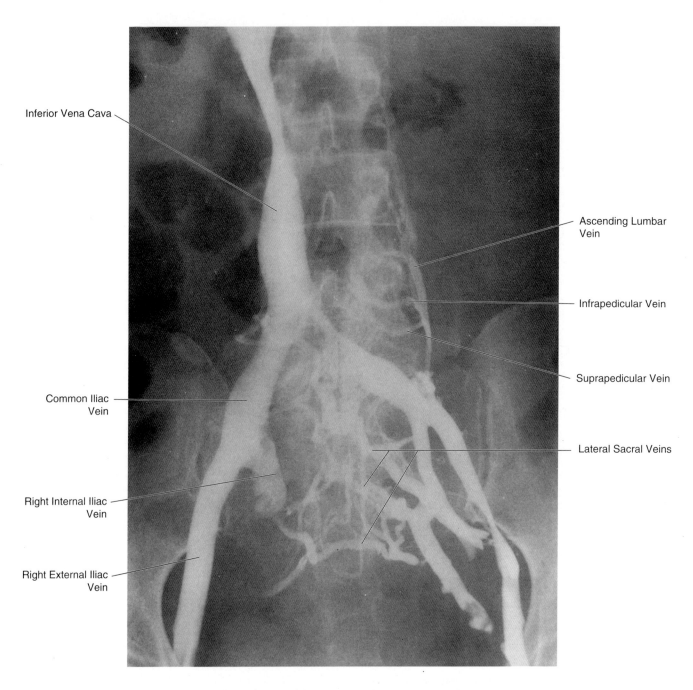

Inferior Vena Cava

Ascending Lumbar
Vein

Infrapedicular Vein

Suprapedicular Vein

Common Iliac
Vein

Lateral Sacral Veins

Right Internal Iliac
Vein

Right External Iliac
Vein

Figure 20.4. Angiographic demonstration of the lateral sacral veins and internal iliac veins. The inferior vena
cava is stenotic. The left ascending lumbar vein is visible.

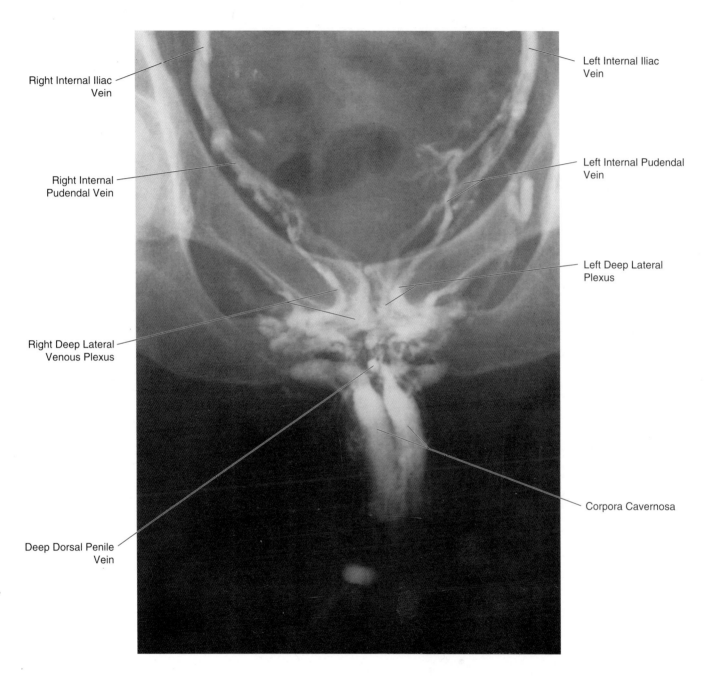

Right Internal Iliac
Vein

Right Internal
Pudendal Vein

Right Deep Lateral
Venous Plexus

Deep Dorsal Penile
Vein

Left Internal Iliac
Vein

Left Internal Pudendal
Vein

Left Deep Lateral
Plexus

Corpora Cavernosa

Figure 20.5. Percutaneous cavernosogram showing the corpora cavernosa, the prostatic venous plexus, the internal pudendal veins and the internal iliac veins.

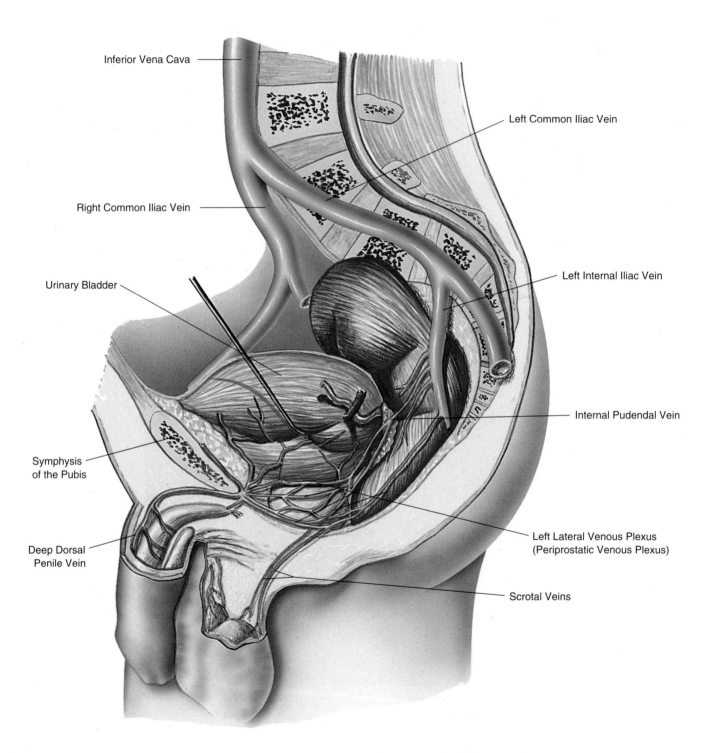

Inferior Vena Cava

Right Common Iliac Vein

Urinary Bladder

Symphysis
of the Pubis

Deep Dorsal
Penile Vein

Left Common Iliac Vein

Left Internal Iliac Vein

Internal Pudendal Vein

Left Lateral Venous Plexus
(Periprostatic Venous Plexus)

Scrotal Veins

Figure 20.6. Schematic diagram of the male pelvis on a lateral view. It reveals the deep dorsal vein of the penis
penetrating the pelvis under the symphysis of the pubis. The left lateral plexus is also seen.

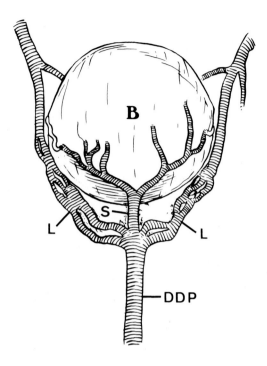

Figure 20.7. Schematic drawing from a superior view of the deep dorsal vein of the penis (DDV) dividing into three major branches; the superficial branch (S) and the right and left deep lateral plexuses (L). B = urinary bladder.

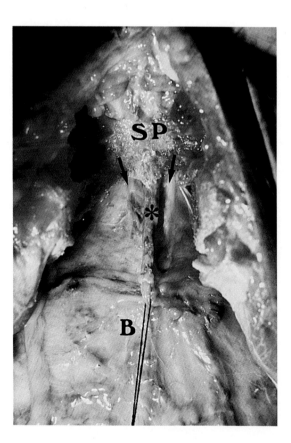

Figure 20.8. Specimen injected with blue latex through the deep dorsal vein of the penis. Superior view of the retropubic space reveals the right and left puboprostatic ligaments (arrows) and the superficial branch of the periprostatic plexus (superficial plexus) cen-trally located (asterisk) and emerging above the endopelvic fascia, between the puboprostatic ligaments. Note the communication venous branches over the bladder. SP = symphysis pubis; B = urinary bladder.

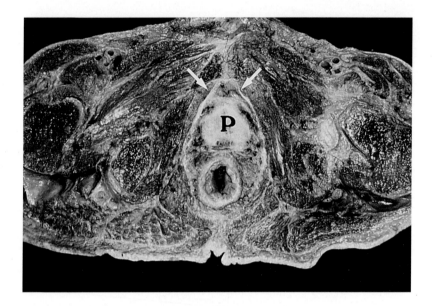

Figure 20.9. Transverse section through the pelvis of a male specimen, reveals the prostate (P) involved by the lateral deep venous plexuses. The whitish band embracing the prostate, the plexuses, and the rectum, is the endopelvic fascia. The arrows point out the anterior condensa-tions of the endopelvic fascia, attached to the posterior surface of the symphysis pubis (puboprostatic ligaments). Note the superficial branch (superficial plexus) in the retropubic adipose tissue, between the pubo-prostatic ligaments.

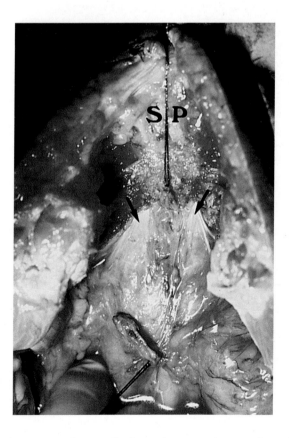

Figure 20.10. Same specimen shown in Figure 20.8. The superficial branch of the deep dorsal vein (superficial plexus) was divided. Note the endopelvic fascia and the puboprostatic ligaments (arrows). The lat-eral venous plexuses (deep plexus) are located on the right and left sides, beneath the endopelvic fascia (preprostatic fascia). SP = Symphysis pubis.

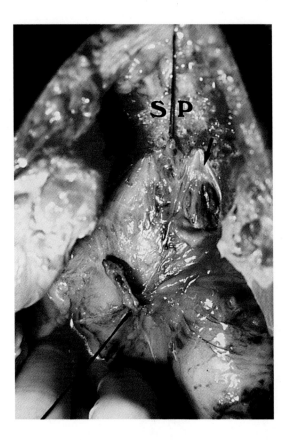

Figure 20.11. Same specimen shown in Figure 20.10. The right puboprostatic ligament was divided (arrow) and the endopelvic fascia was opened in the right side. Note the right deep lateral plexus injected with blue latex.
SP = Symphysis pubis.

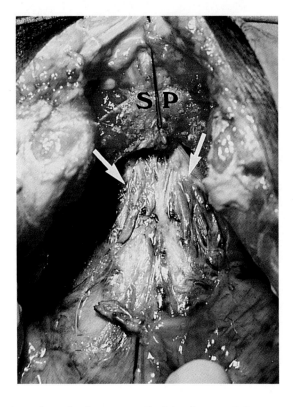

Figure 20.12. Same specimen shown in Figure 20.11. The left puboprostatic ligament was also divided and the endopelvic fascia was completely opened, exposing the right and left deep venous plexuses (deep plexus, Santorini's) (arrows). SP = Symphysis pubis.

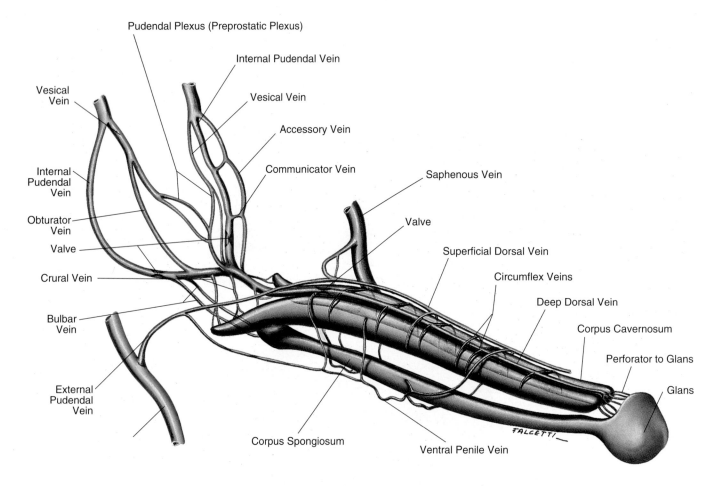

Figure 20.13. Diagrammatic demonstration of the penile venous anatomy draining the corpora cavernosa, as observed on an oblique view. It is noteworthy to observe crural drainage into internal pudendal veins, bulbar drainage via several veins into the internal pudendal vein. There are few communications or none at all, between the deep and superficial dorsal veins. The drainage of the glans is predominantly into the deep dorsal penile vein, there are, however, direct communications between the glans and corpus cavernosum. The circumflex veins from corpora cavernosa drain into the deep dorsal penile vein but also into superficial dorsal penile vein. The drainage of the deep dorsal penile vein is into the preprostatic plexus and internal pudendal veins. The drainage of the superficial dorsal penile vein is into the external pudendal and then into the saphenous veins.

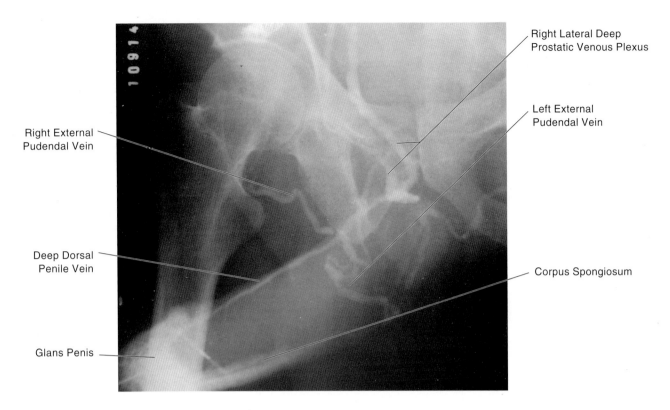

Figure 20.14. Direct contrast medium injection into glans show opacification of glans, corpus spongiosum and deep dorsal vein. Note communications of the deep dorsal penile vein with the pudendal plexus (preprostatic) and the external pudendal veins.

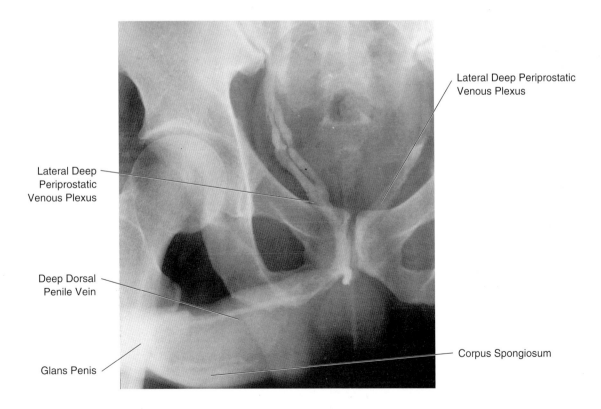

Figure 20.15. Direct contrast injection into glans show opacification of glans, corpus spongiosum and deep dorsal vein. The deep dorsal vein drains into the preprostatic plexus.

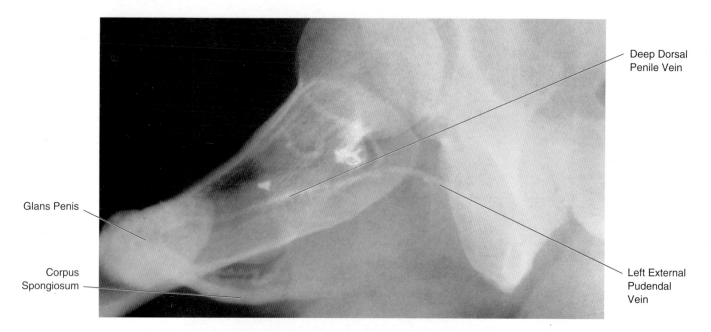

Deep Dorsal
Penile Vein

Glans Penis

Corpus
Spongiosum

Left External
Pudendal
Vein

Figure 20.16. Contrast injection into glans show opacification of glans, corpus spongiosum and deep dorsal vein. There is a communication with the right external pudendal. No communication with the preprostatic plexus is observed.

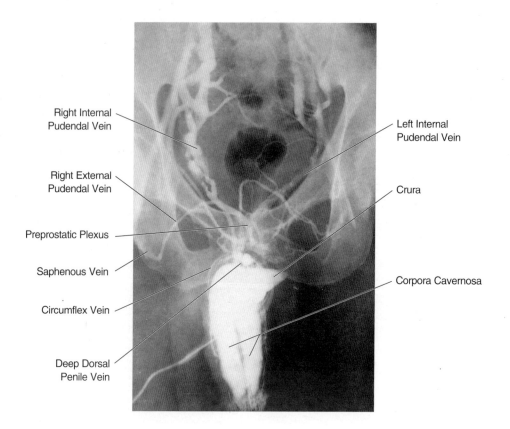

Right Internal
Pudendal Vein

Left Internal
Pudendal Vein

Right External
Pudendal Vein

Crura

Preprostatic Plexus

Saphenous Vein

Circumflex Vein

Corpora Cavernosa

Deep Dorsal
Penile Vein

Figure 20.17. Cavernosogram showing opacification of the corpora cavernosa, the deep dorsal vein, the circumflex veins and the communications with the pudendal plexus and the external pudendal veins, with subsequent opacification of the femoral veins.

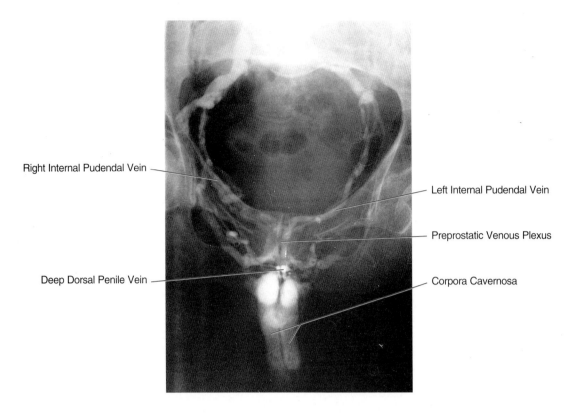

Right Internal Pudendal Vein

Left Internal Pudendal Vein

Preprostatic Venous Plexus

Deep Dorsal Penile Vein

Corpora Cavernosa

Figure 20.18. Cavernosogram showing opacification of the corpora cavernosa, the deep dorsal vein, and the communication with the preprostatic plexus and the internal pudendal and internal iliac veins.

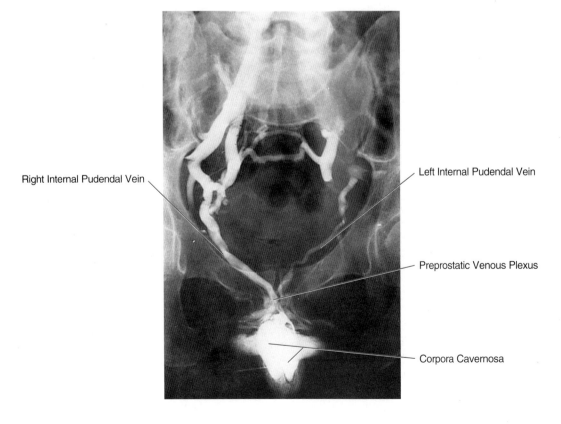

Right Internal Pudendal Vein

Left Internal Pudendal Vein

Preprostatic Venous Plexus

Corpora Cavernosa

Figure 20.19. Cavernosogram showing opacification of the corpora cavernosa, the deep dorsal vein and the crura of the corpora cavernosa, and the drainage of the penis to the prostatic venous plexus with right and left branches. Note the direct communication with the internal pudendal veins and the internal iliac veins.

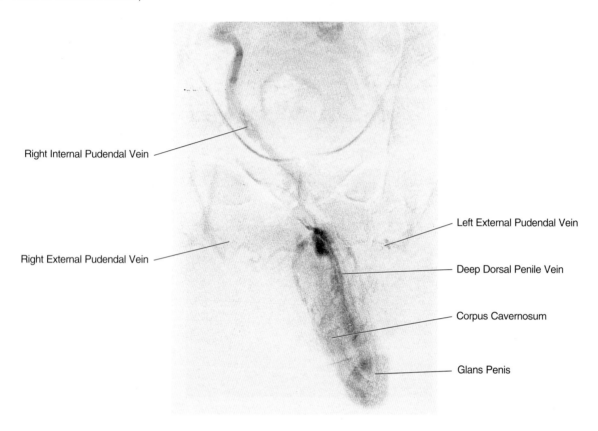

Right Internal Pudendal Vein

Left External Pudendal Vein

Right External Pudendal Vein

Deep Dorsal Penile Vein

Corpus Cavernosum

Glans Penis

Figure 20.20. Photographic subtraction of the cavernosogram showing opacification of the corpora cavernosa of the penis and the deep and superficial dorsal penile veins. The drainage to the internal pudendal vein on the right is noted.

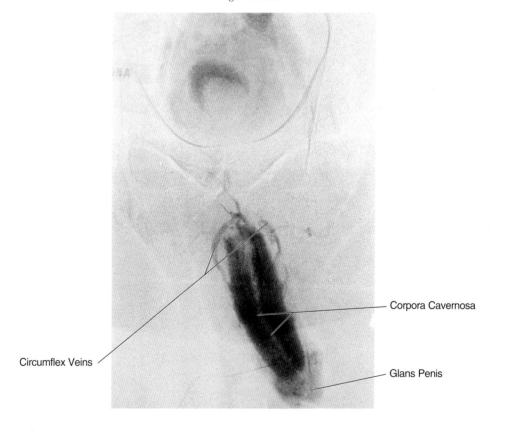

Corpora Cavernosa

Circumflex Veins

Glans Penis

Figure 20.21. Cavernosogram showing opacification of the corpora cavernosa and the drainage through the circumflex veins into the deep dorsal penile vein. Note very faint opacification of the external pudendal vein on the left.

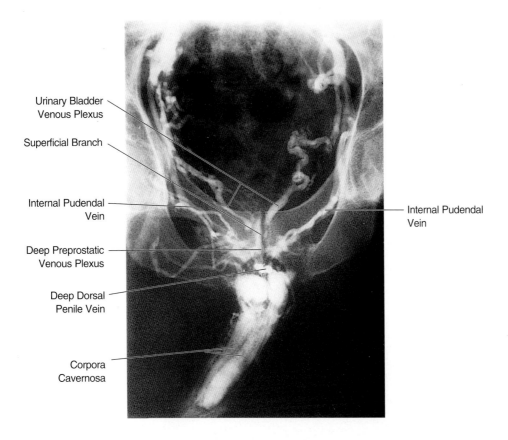

Urinary Bladder
Venous Plexus

Superficial Branch

Internal Pudendal
Vein

Deep Preprostatic
Venous Plexus

Deep Dorsal
Penile Vein

Corpora
Cavernosa

Internal Pudendal
Vein

Figure 20.22. Cavernosogram showing opacification of the corpora cavernosa and the drainage through the deep dorsal penile vein and preprostatic venous lexus. The prostatic venous plexus drains into the internal pudendal veins and internal iliac veins.

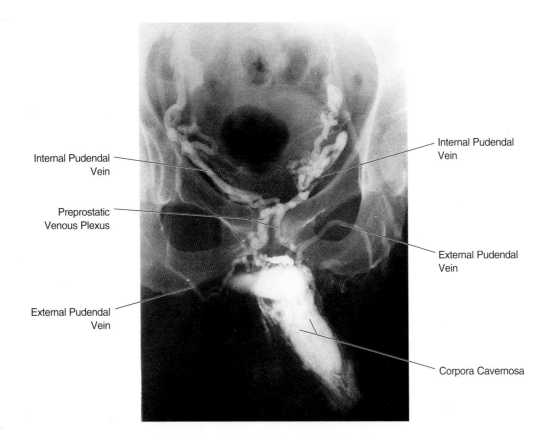

Internal Pudendal
Vein

Preprostatic
Venous Plexus

External Pudendal
Vein

Internal Pudendal
Vein

External Pudendal
Vein

Corpora Cavernosa

Figure 20.23. Cavernosogram showing opacification of the corpora cavernosa and the drainage through the deep dorsal penile vein and the preprostatic venous plexus. There is a deep venous plexus divided in left and right plexuses. Note the opacification of the external pudendal veins.

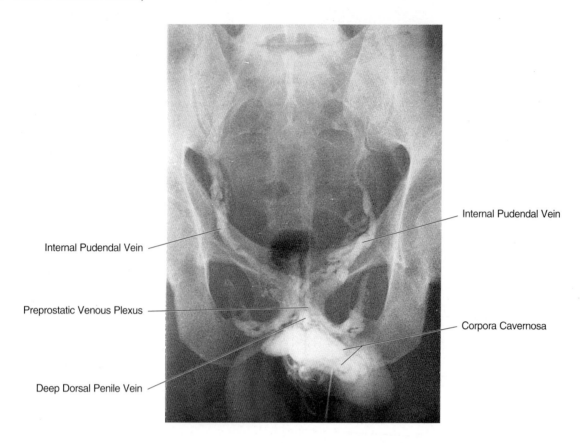

Internal Pudendal Vein

Internal Pudendal Vein

Preprostatic Venous Plexus

Corpora Cavernosa

Deep Dorsal Penile Vein

Figure 20.24. Cavernosogram showing the lateral venous plexuses (Santorini's deep venous plexus) and the free communications with other pelvic venous plexuses. Note the drainage through the internal pudendal veins. The deep dorsal penile vein is seem.

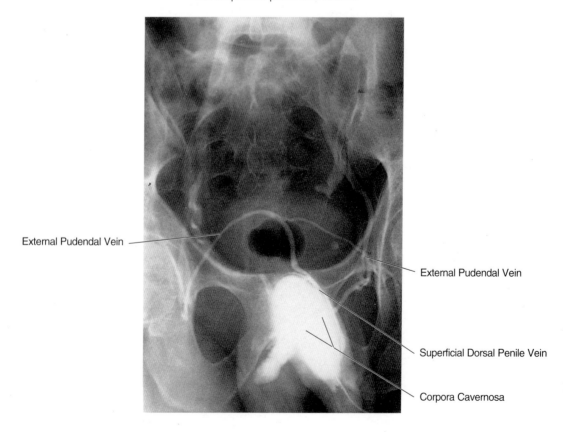

External Pudendal Vein

External Pudendal Vein

Superficial Dorsal Penile Vein

Corpora Cavernosa

Figure 20.25. Cavernosogram showing the corpora cavernosa and filling of the superficial dorsal penile vein, draining into the external pudendal veins and with partial opacification of the saphenous veins.

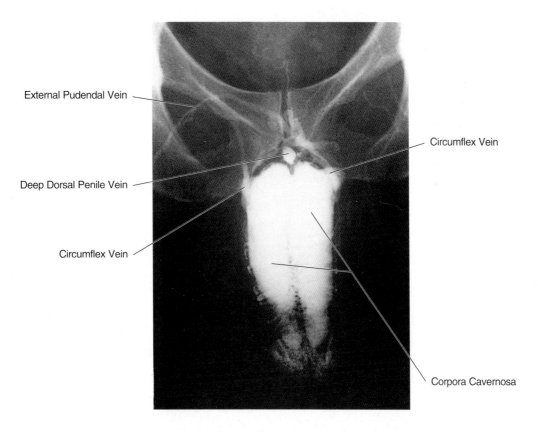

Figure 20.26. Cavernosogram showing the corpora cavernosa and filling of the deep dorsal penile vein, draining partially into the preprostatic venous plexus and into superficial veins. Note the circumflex veins.

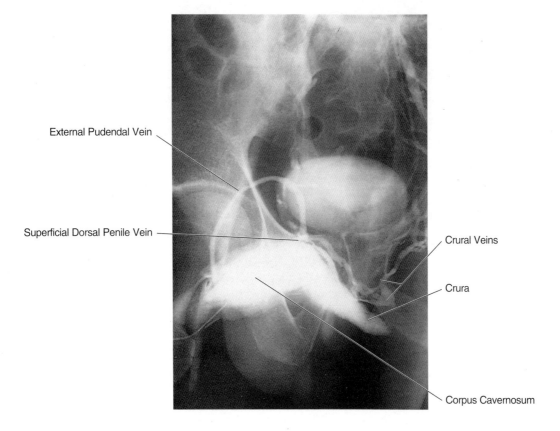

Figure 20.27. Oblique view of a cavernosogram showing the corpora cavernosa and the drainage through the preprostatic venous plexus and vesical plexus. A right external pudendal vein is observed.

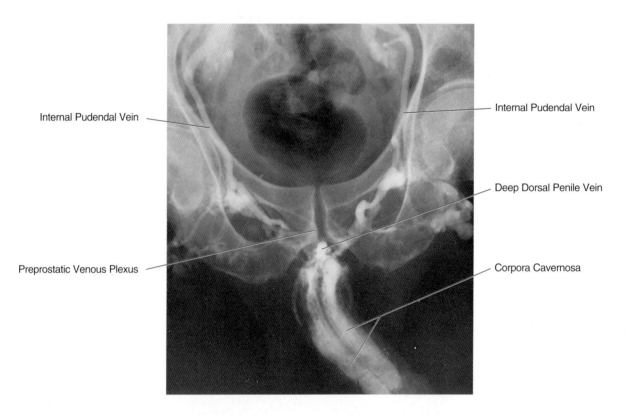

Internal Pudendal Vein

Internal Pudendal Vein

Deep Dorsal Penile Vein

Preprostatic Venous Plexus

Corpora Cavernosa

Figure 20.28. Cavernosogram showing the corpora cavernosa and the drainage through the deep venous plexus (preprostatic plexus) and the external pudendal veins.

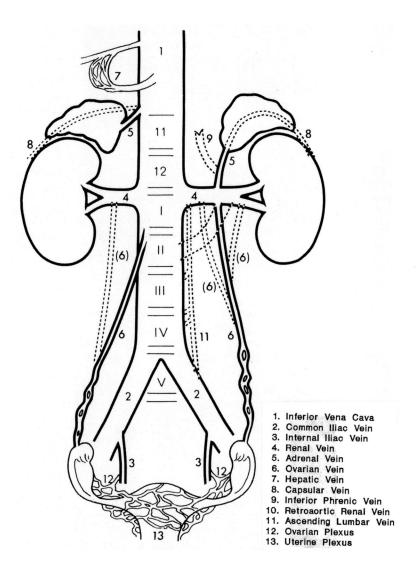

Figure 20.29. Schematic diagram of the uterine venous plexuses, ovarian and vaginal venous plexuses, showing also the ovarian veins. Note the possible variations in position of the ovarian veins, renal veins, adrenal veins and the multiple possible anastomosis and relationships.

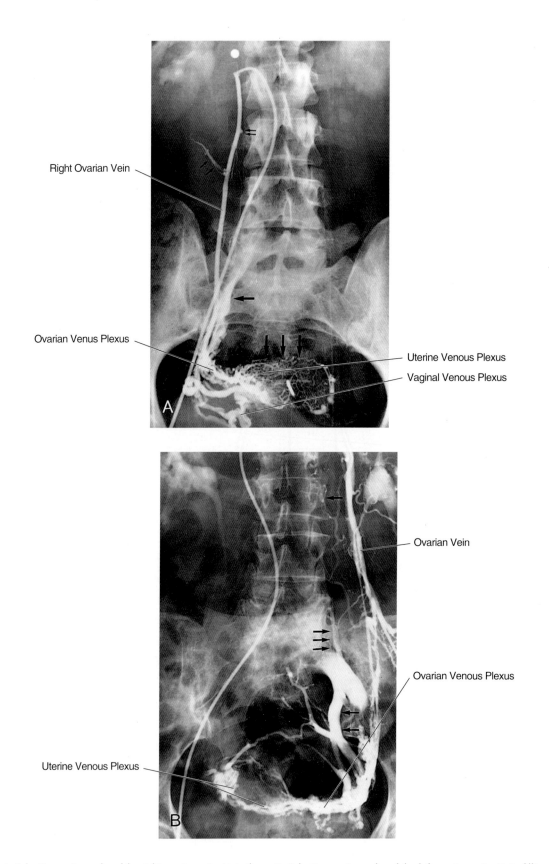

Figure 20.30. A. Selective angiography of the right ovarian vein. Note the filling of the uterine venous plexus (three arrows). The ovarian plexus and partial filling of the vaginal plexus is seen. The right internal and common iliac veins are visualized (single arrow). Note the multiple anastomosis of the right ovarian vein with retroperitoneal veins (small arrows). **B.** Selective angiography of the left ovarian vein. Note filling of the uterine venous plexus. This system has wide anastomosis with the internal iliac vein (two arrows) and with the common iliac vein. Note filling of the ascending lumbar vein on the left (three arrows). Note also the multiple anastomosis of the left ovarian vein with the retroperitoneal veins.

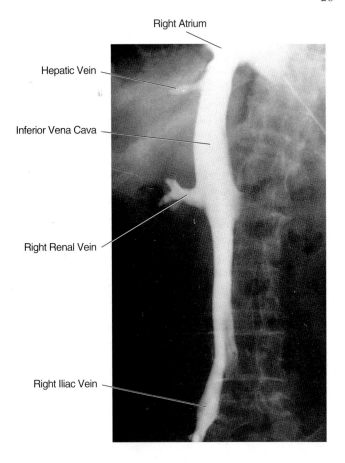

Right Atrium

Hepatic Vein

Inferior Vena Cava

Right Renal Vein

Right Iliac Vein

Figure 20.31. Angiography of the iliac veins and inferior vena cava. Note reflux of the contrast medium into the right renal vein and into a hepatic vein. The right atrium is filled with contrast medium.

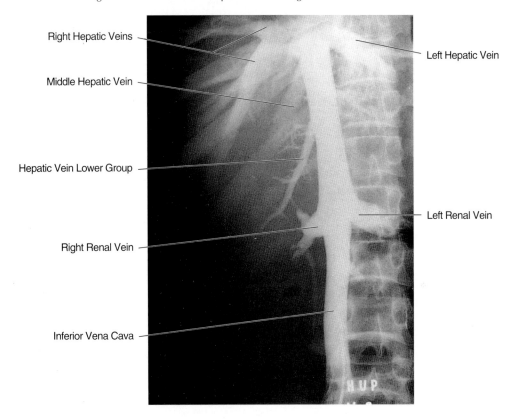

Right Hepatic Veins

Middle Hepatic Vein

Hepatic Vein Lower Group

Right Renal Vein

Inferior Vena Cava

Left Hepatic Vein

Left Renal Vein

Figure 20.32. Angiography of the inferior vena cava. Note the reflux of contrast medium into the renal veins and into the hepatic veins. The hepatic veins are large and the inferior one is well visualized.

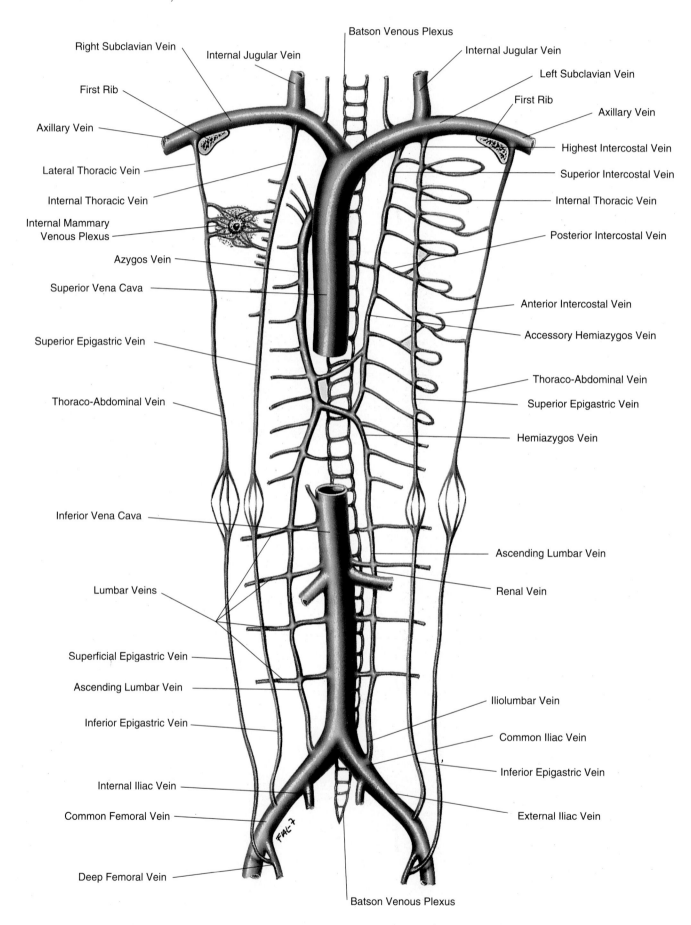

Figure 20.33. Diagram depicting the venous collateral pathways available between the thorax and the abdomen.

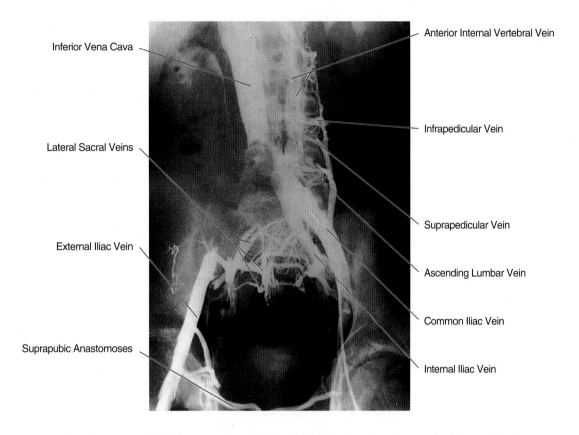

Figure 20.34. Angiogram of the iliac veins and inferior vena cava showing the collateralization into the pelvis and perilumbar veins. Due to the occlusion of the right common iliac and inferior vena cava there is development of the collaterals. Note the anastomosis between the two iliac veins through the lateral sacral veins. The left ascending lumbar vein is clearly seen and the anastomosis with the epidural plexus is observed through the suprapedicular and infrapedicular veins. The lateral and medial anterior internal vertebral veins are also seem as a plexus along the medullar canal.

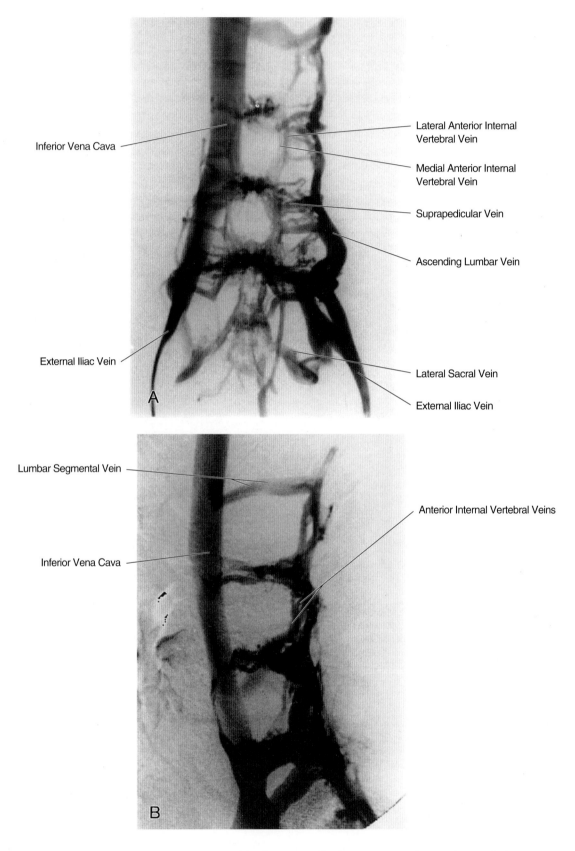

Figure 20.35. A. Anterior view of an angiogram of the iliac veins and inferior vena cava showing the vertebral venous plexus. **B.** Lateral view of the angiogram showing the inferior vena cava and the communications through the lumbar segmental veins. Posteriorly the epidural venous plexus is observed as a dense venous plexus.

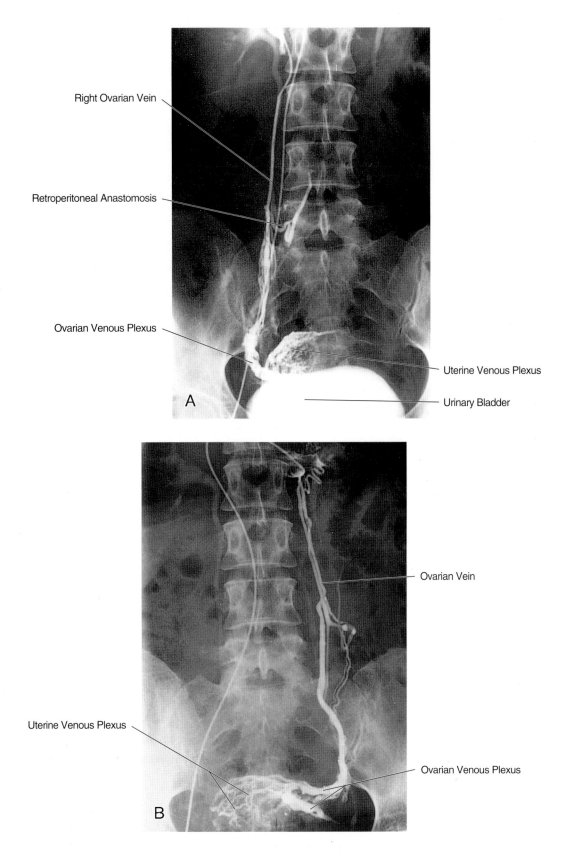

Right Ovarian Vein

Retroperitoneal Anastomosis

Ovarian Venous Plexus

Uterine Venous Plexus

Urinary Bladder

A

Ovarian Vein

Uterine Venous Plexus

Ovarian Venous Plexus

B

Figure 20.36. A. Selective angiography of the right ovarian vein. Note the filling of the ovarian plexus and part of the uterine plexus. Anastomosis with retroperitoneal veins is observed. **B.** Selective angiography of the left ovarian vein. Note the duplication of the vein and the anastomosis with retroperitoneal veins. The uterine venous plexus is also seem.

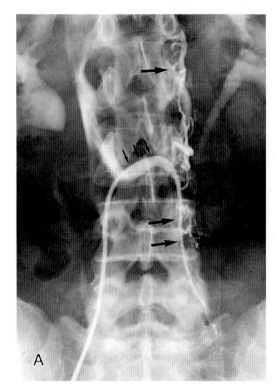

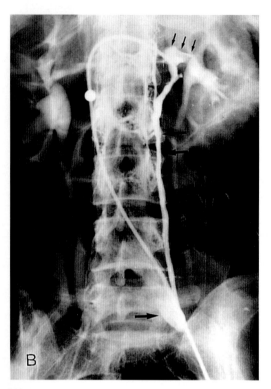

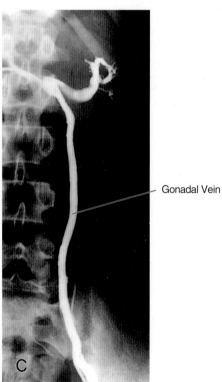

Gonadal Vein

Figure 20.37. A. Injection into a segmental lumbar vein (three small arrows). Note opacification of part of the left ovarian vein (one large arrow) and partial opacification of the ascending lumbar vein (two large arrows). **B.** Selective injection into the left ovarian vein (two large arrows). The left renal vein is partially opacified (three arrows). The left common iliac vein is also opacified (one arrow). **C.** Selective injection into the left ovarian vein. There is partial filling of the left renal vein.

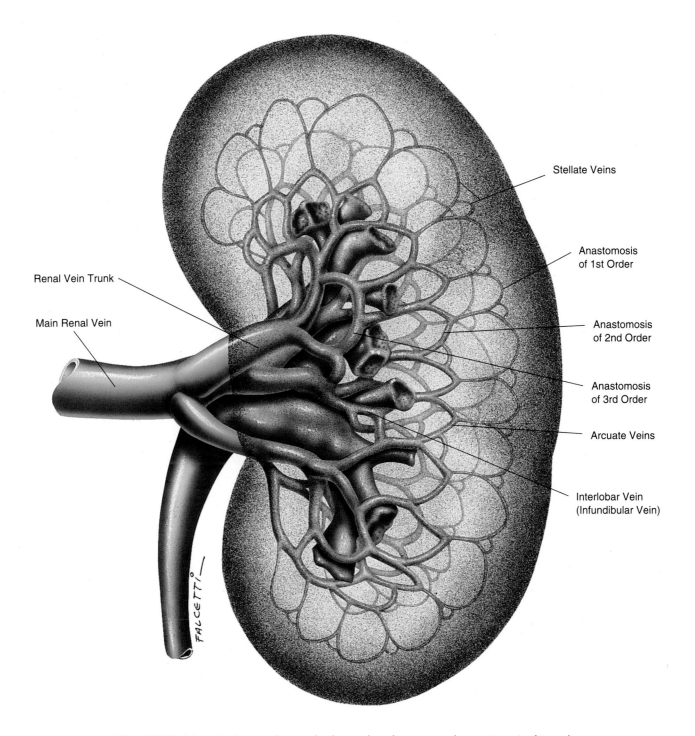

Stellate Veins

Anastomosis
of 1st Order

Anastomosis
of 2nd Order

Anastomosis
of 3rd Order

Arcuate Veins

Interlobar Vein
(Infundibular Vein)

Renal Vein Trunk

Main Renal Vein

Figure 20.38. Schematic drawing showing the three orders of venous arcades; anastomosis of 1st order, anastomosis of 2nd order, and anastomosis of 3rd order.

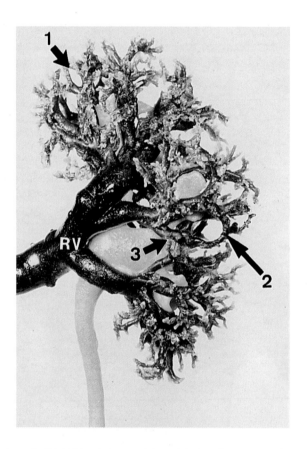

Figure 20.39. Anterior view of a left kidney endocast of the pelvicaliceal system together with the venous vascular tree shows the three systems or longitudinal anastomotic arcades; from lateral (periphery) to medial (hilar): stellate veins (1), arcuate veins (2) and interlobar veins (3). RV= renal vein.

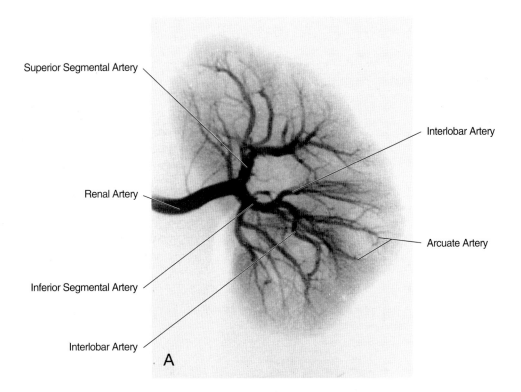

Superior Segmental Artery

Interlobar Artery

Renal Artery

Arcuate Artery

Inferior Segmental Artery

Interlobar Artery

A

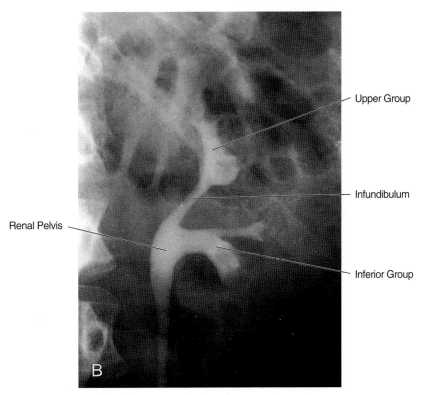

Upper Group

Infundibulum

Renal Pelvis

Inferior Group

B

Figure 20.40. A. Renal angiogram showing the arterial phase. **B.** Intravenous pyelogram showing the caliceal system in the same subject. **C.** Renal venogram showing the intra and extrarenal veins. **D.** More peripheral venogram showing the medial, stellate and arcuate veins.

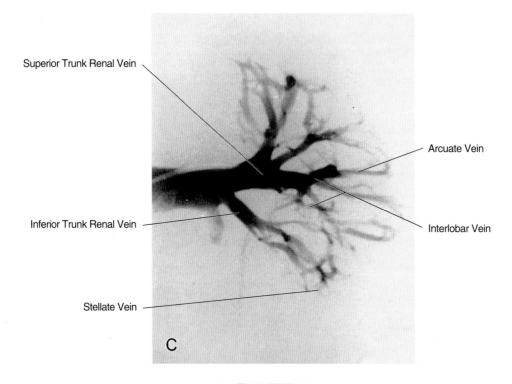

Superior Trunk Renal Vein

Arcuate Vein

Inferior Trunk Renal Vein

Interlobar Vein

Stellate Vein

C

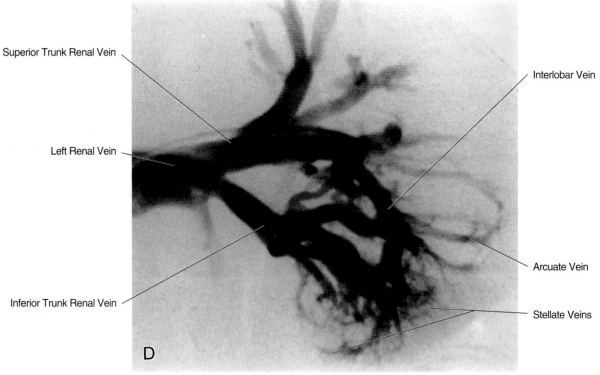

Superior Trunk Renal Vein

Interlobar Vein

Left Renal Vein

Inferior Trunk Renal Vein

Arcuate Vein

Stellate Veins

D

Figure 20.40. *Continued*

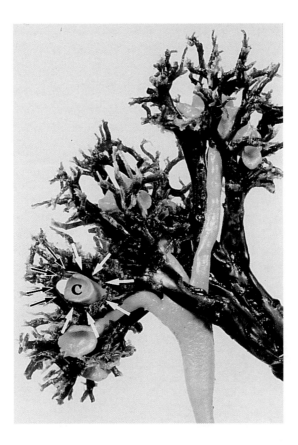

Figure 20.41. Posterior view of an endocast from left kidney shows large venous anastomosis like a collar (arrows) around the neck of a calix (C).

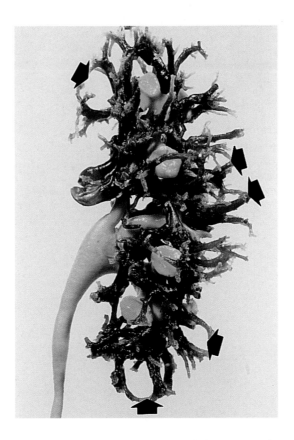

Figure 20.42. Posterior oblique view of an endocast from a right kidney shows horizontal arches linking the anterior and posterior veins, as well as the longitudinal system (arrows).

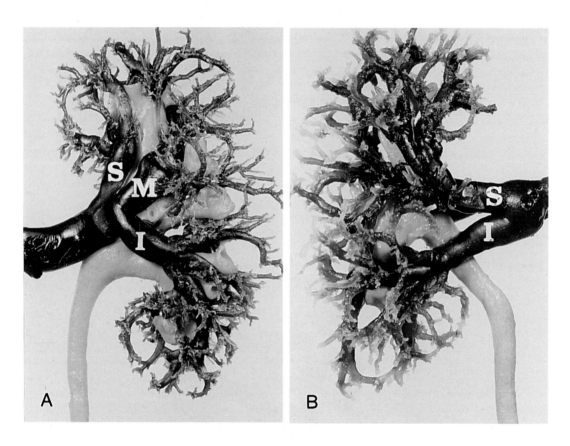

Figure 20.43. A. Anterior view of an endocast from a left kidney shows the main renal vein formed by three trunks. S: superior; M: middle; I: inferior. **B.** Anterior view of endocast from a right kidney shows the main renal vein formed by two trunks. S: superior; I: inferior.

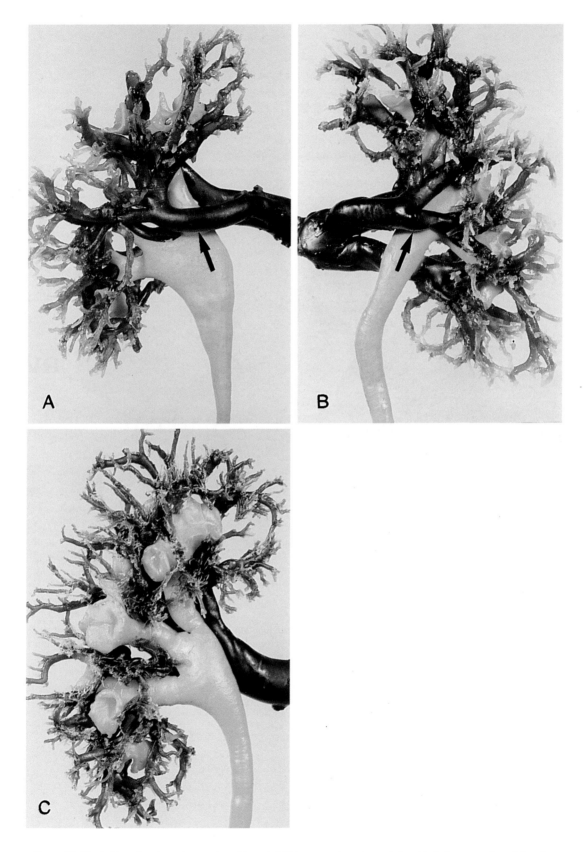

Figure 20.44. A. Posterior view of an endocast from left kidney reveals a close relationship between a retropelvic vein (arrow) and the junction of renal pelvis with upper calix. **B.** Posterior view of an endocast from right kidney shows a prominent retropelvic vein (arrow) crossing the middle posterior aspect of the renal pelvis. **C.** Posterior view of an endocast from the left kidney reveals that there are no veins on the posterior aspect of the renal pelvis.

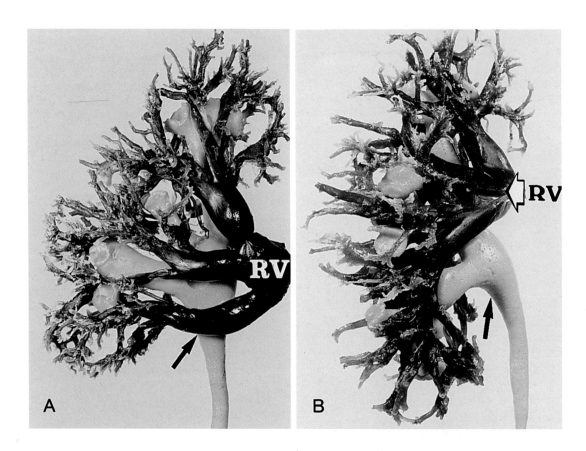

Figure 20.45. Anatomic relationship between ureteropelvic junction (UPJ) and renal veins. **A.** Anterior view of an endocast from a right kidney shows a close relationship between a prominent inferior tributary of the renal vein and the anterior aspect of the UPJ (arrow). **B.** Anterior view of an endocast from a right kidney shows the UPJ free from veins (nonvascular area), arrow. RV= renal vein.

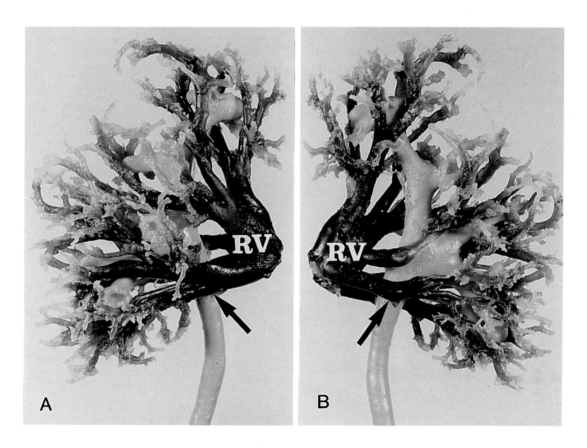

Figure 20.46. Anatomic relationships between the ureteropelvic junction (UPJ) and the renal vein. A. Anterior view of an endocast of a right kidney shows a close relationship between an anterior tributary of the renal vein and the UPJ (arrow). **B.** Posterior view of the endocast shown in A reveals the UPJ in close relationship to a retropelvic vein (arrow). RV = renal vein.

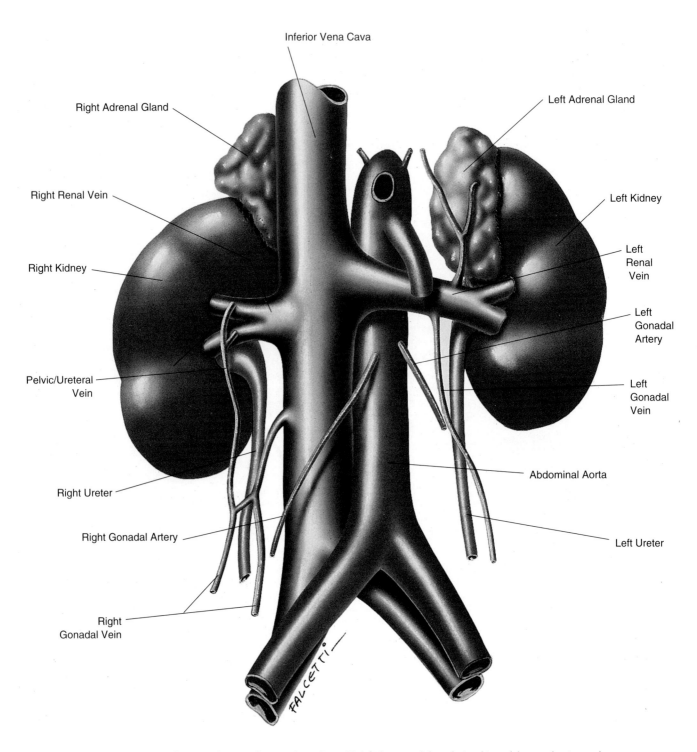

Figure 20.47. Schematic diagram showing the right and left kidneys and the relationships of the renal veins and the gonadal veins and variations. The renal veins may be partially or totally duplicated.

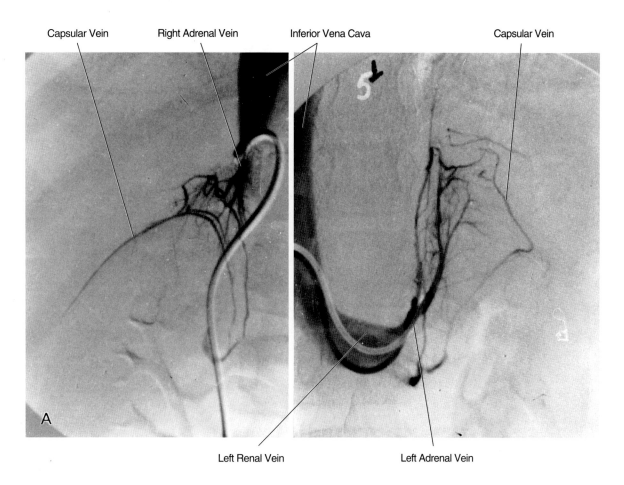

Capsular Vein   Right Adrenal Vein   Inferior Vena Cava   Capsular Vein

Left Renal Vein   Left Adrenal Vein

Figure 20.48. Selective venography of the right and left adrenal veins. The right adrenal vein ends in the posterolateral aspect of the inferior vena cava. Note the anastomosis with the renal capsular veins. The gland is triangular and small. On the left the adrenal vein is longer and ends in the superior aspect of the left renal vein. Note anastomosis with renal capsular veins and with inferior phrenic veins. The gland is longer and located medially to the kidney.

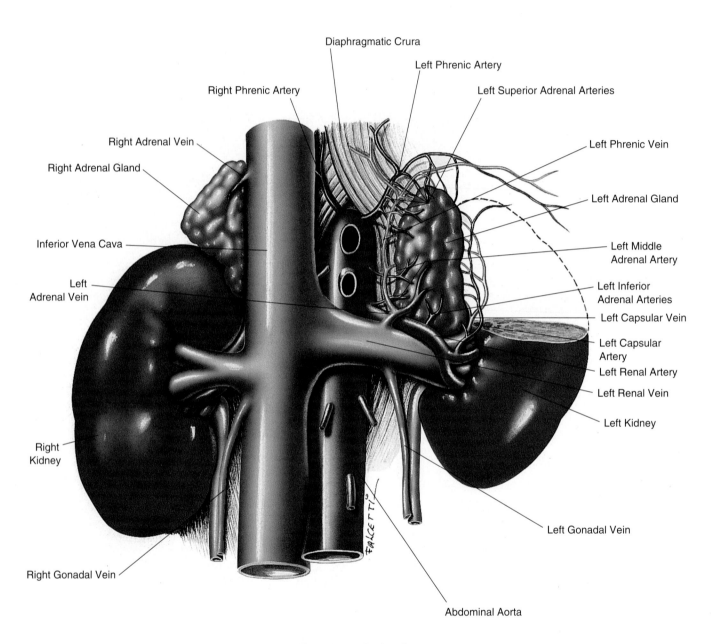

Figure 20.48. *Continued*

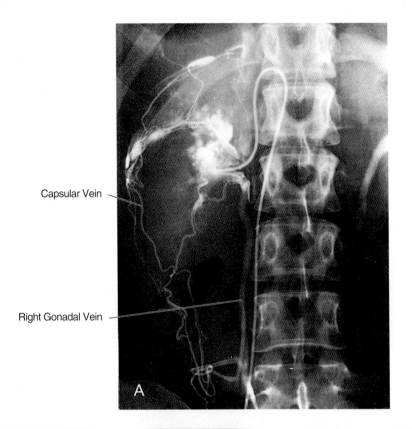

Capsular Vein

Right Gonadal Vein

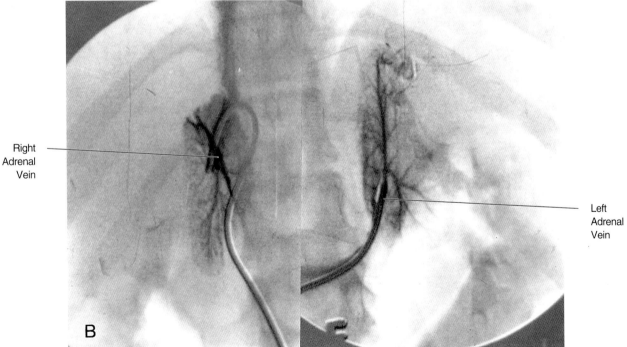

Right
Adrenal
Vein

Left
Adrenal
Vein

Figure 20.49. A. Selective injection into a renal capsular vein, showing retrograde stain of soft tissues and filling of retroperitoneal veins and gonadal vein. **B.** Selective injection at the right and left adrenal veins showing the enlarged right and left adrenal glands. Again the right adrenal vein ends in the inferior vena cava and the left adrenal vein ends in the left renal vein.

Right Adrenal Vein

Capsular Vein

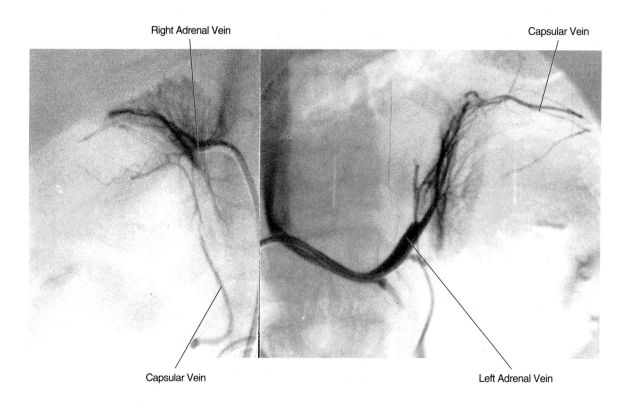

Capsular Vein

Left Adrenal Vein

Figure 20.50. Selective injection into the right and left adrenal veins showing the small triangular right adrenal gland riding the upper pole of the kidney and the left longer adrenal gland draining into the left renal vein, located medially to the left kidney.

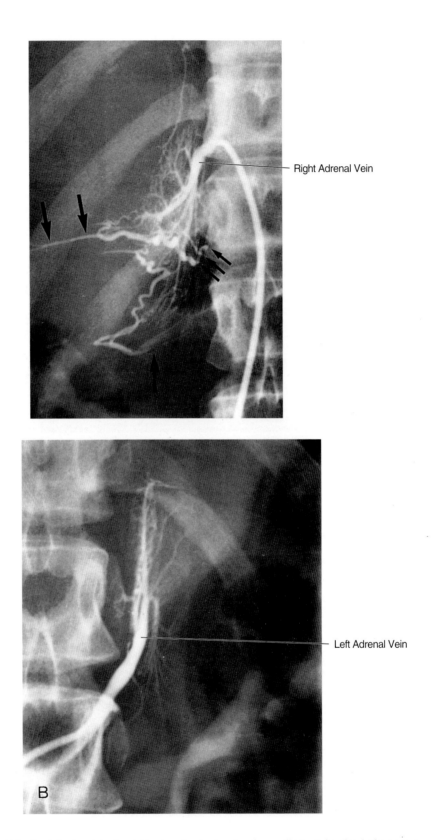

Right Adrenal Vein

Left Adrenal Vein

Figure 20.51. A. Selective injection into the right adrenal vein showing the small triangular gland. The arrows point to collaterals and anastomosis with the capsular veins. **B.** Selective injection into the left adrenal vein showing the long vein and gland. The left adrenal vein drains into the left renal vein.

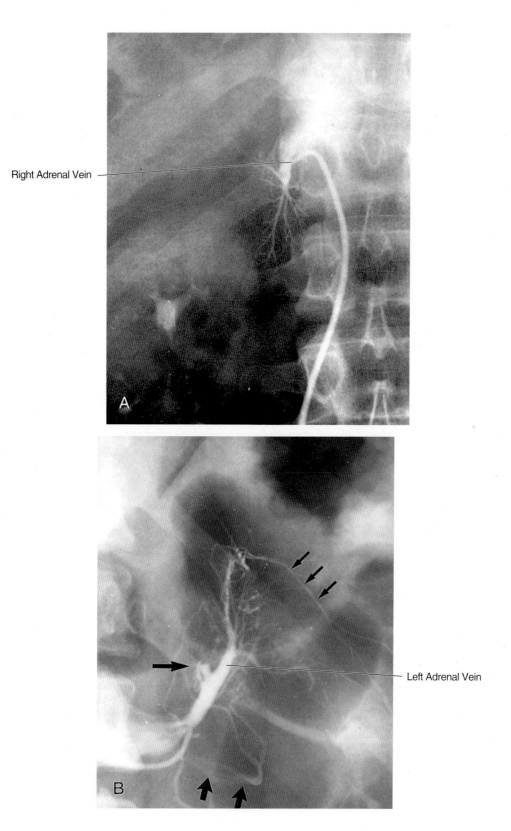

Figure 20.52. A. Selective injection into the right adrenal vein showing the small triangular gland. The right adrenal vein end into the posterolateral aspect of the inferior vena cava. **B.** Selective injection into the left adrenal vein. The large arrow shows the stump of the left inferior phrenic vein. The three small arrows show a capsular vein anastomosed with the adrenal vein circulation. The two small arrows show anastomosis with the intrarenal veins.

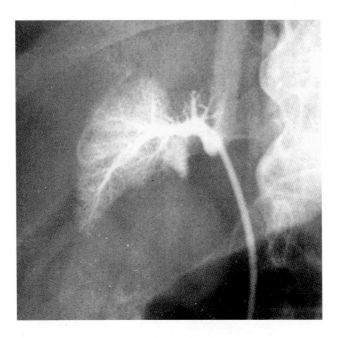

Figure 20.53. Selective injection into one hepatic vein of the inferior group. This vein may mimic the right adrenal vein when an angiographic search is performed.

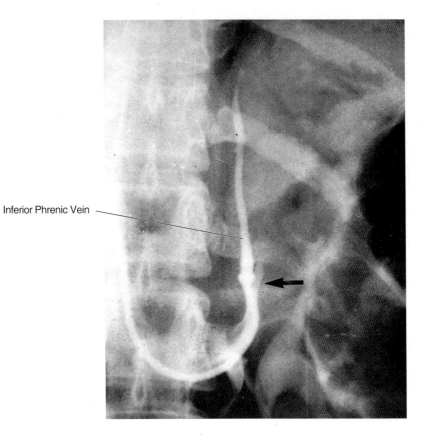

Inferior Phrenic Vein

Figure 20.54. Selective injection into a left adrenal vein showing only the left inferior phrenic vein. The arrow shows the real left adrenal vein.

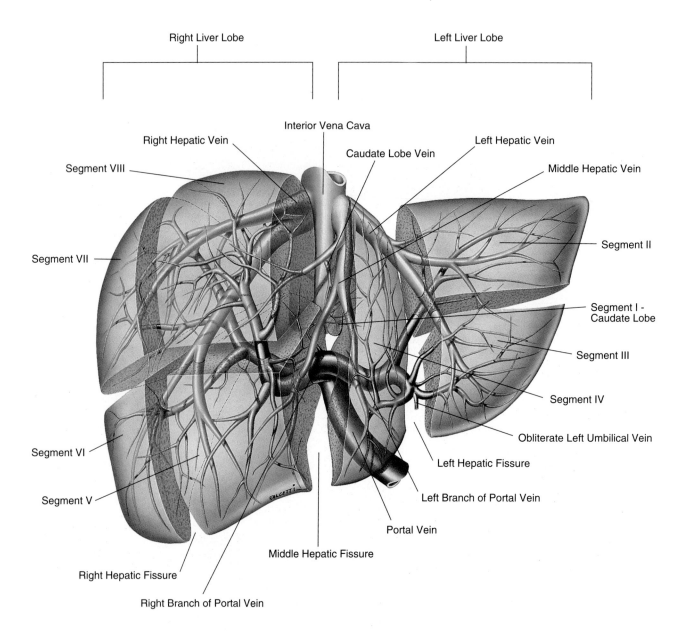

Figure 20.55. Schematic drawing showing the anatomy of the hepatic veins, the portal vein and the Couinaud segments. The right hepatic vein runs into the right hepatic fissure, while the middle hepatic vein runs into the middle hepatic fissure. The right branch of the middle hepatic vein drain part of the right liver lobe.

Right Hepatic Vein   Accessory Right Hepatic Vein   Middle Hepatic Vein   Left Hepatic Vein (Duplicated)

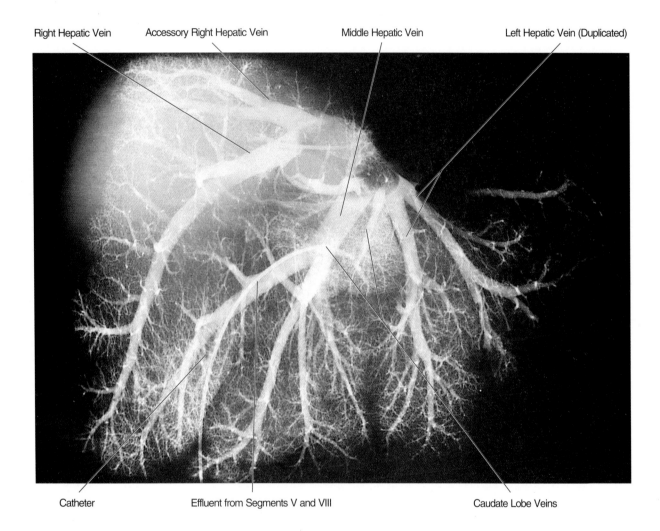

Catheter   Effluent from Segments V and VIII   Caudate Lobe Veins

Figure 20.56. Angiography in a liver specimen showing the classic distribution of the hepatic veins. Note the
catheter into the caudate lobe vein.

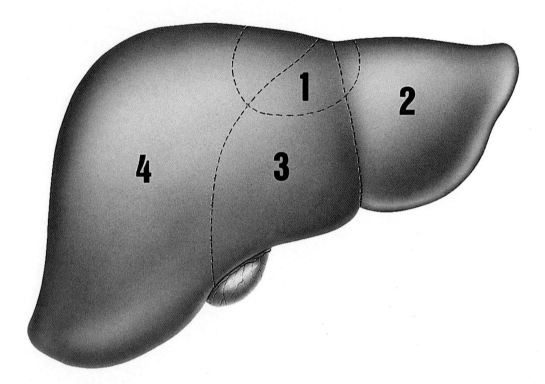

Figure 20.57. Territories of drainage of the four main hepatic veins. The distribution of the territories follows a clockwise direction when seem from above.

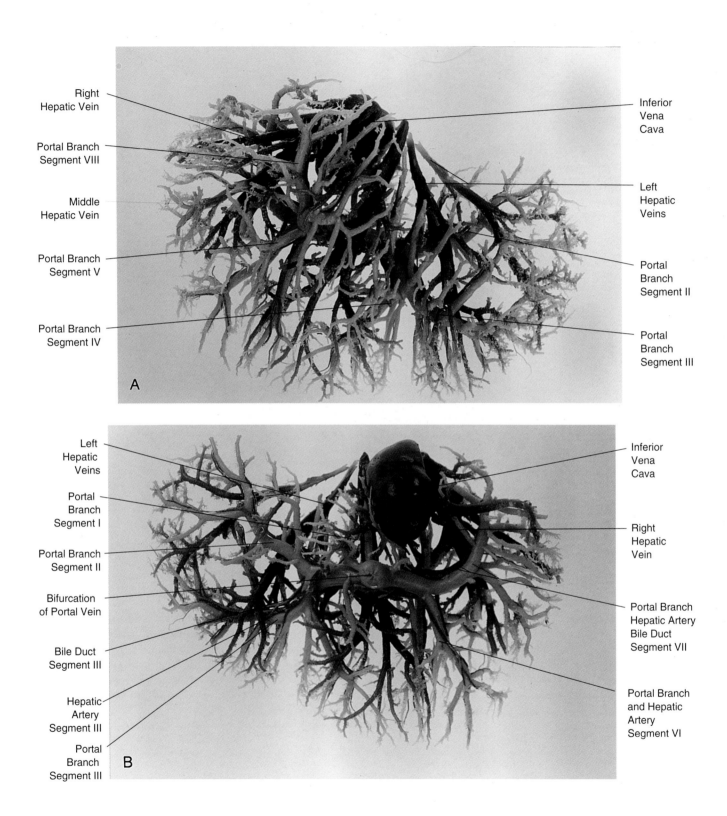

Right
Hepatic Vein

Portal Branch
Segment VIII

Middle
Hepatic Vein

Portal Branch
Segment V

Portal Branch
Segment IV

Inferior
Vena
Cava

Left
Hepatic
Veins

Portal
Branch
Segment II

Portal
Branch
Segment III

A

Left
Hepatic
Veins

Portal
Branch
Segment I

Portal Branch
Segment II

Bifurcation
of Portal Vein

Bile Duct
Segment III

Hepatic
Artery
Segment III

Portal
Branch
Segment III

Inferior
Vena
Cava

Right
Hepatic
Vein

Portal Branch
Hepatic Artery
Bile Duct
Segment VII

Portal Branch
and Hepatic
Artery
Segment VI

B

Figure 20.58. A. Anterior view of a plastic endocast of a liver specimen. The hepatic veins and inferior vena cava are blue. The portal vein is yellow. The hepatic artery is red and the bile duct is green. **B.** Posterior view of the endocast shows the relationship of the right hepatic artery and right bile duct with the right portal vein.

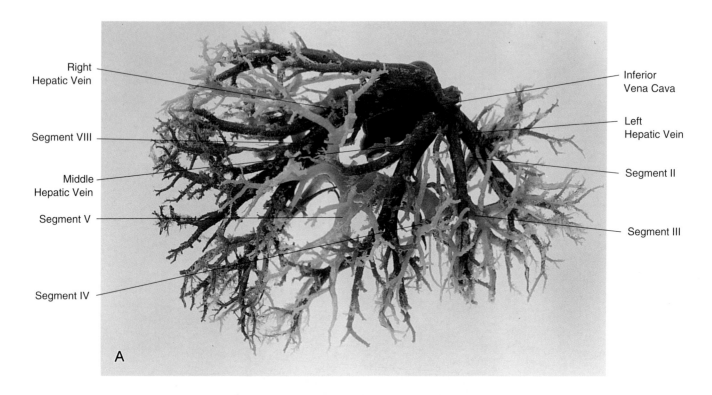

Right
Hepatic Vein

Segment VIII

Middle
Hepatic Vein

Segment V

Segment IV

Inferior
Vena Cava

Left
Hepatic Vein

Segment II

Segment III

A

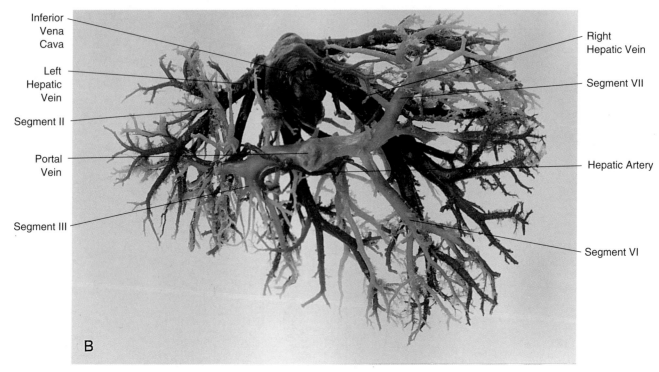

Inferior
Vena
Cava

Left
Hepatic
Vein

Segment II

Portal
Vein

Segment III

Right
Hepatic Vein

Segment VII

Hepatic Artery

Segment VI

B

Figure 20.59.   A. Anterior view of a plastic endocast of a liver specimen. The hepatic veins and inferior vena cava are blue. The portal vein is yellow. The hepatic artery is red and the bile duct is green. In the periphery of the right lobe, the portal vein is red due to mixture of the plastic mate-rial from the portal vein with the arterial injection, due to occlusion of the peripheral portal vein. **B.** Posterior view of the plastic endocast of the liver. Note the position of the hepatic artery in relation to the portal vein. The bile duct is less visible.

Segment VIII

Right Hepatic Vein

Inferior Vena Cava

Left Hepatic Vein

Segment II

Bile Duct
Segment VIII

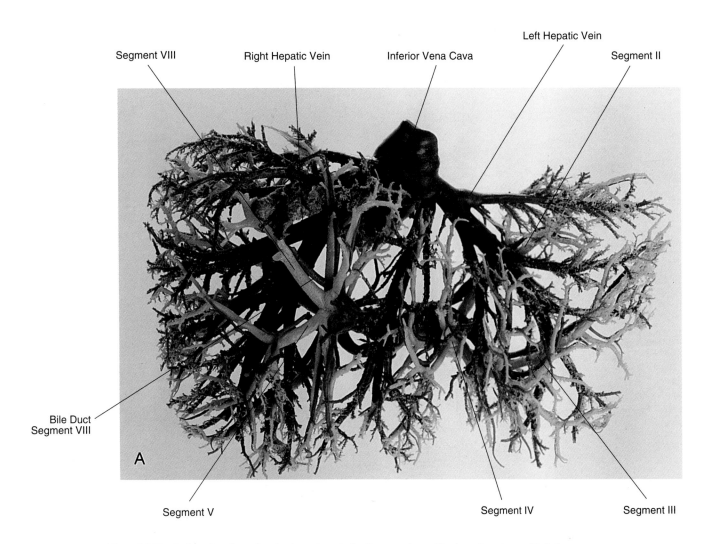

A

Segment V

Segment IV

Segment III

Figure 20.60. A. Anterior view of a plastic endocast of a liver specimen. The hepatic veins and inferior vena cava are blue. The portal vein is yellow. The bile duct is green. Note the relationship of the bile duct with the right portal vein. **B.** Posterior view of the endocast. Note the relationship of the bile duct with the portal vein.

Segment II — Left Hepatic Vein — Inferior Vena Cava — Right Hepatic Vein

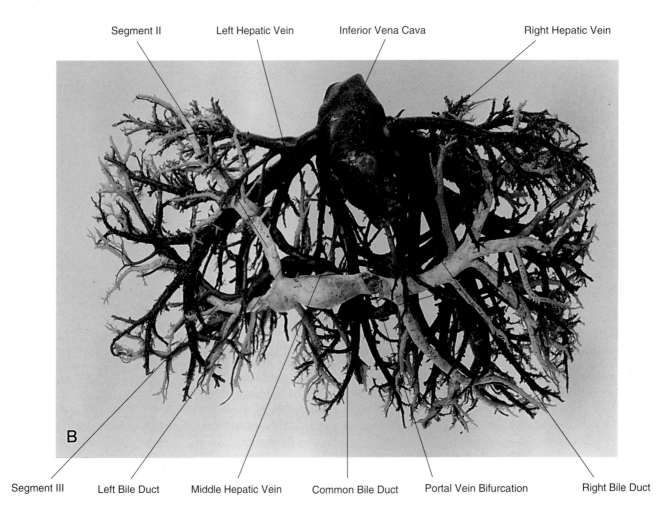

Segment III — Left Bile Duct — Middle Hepatic Vein — Common Bile Duct — Portal Vein Bifurcation — Right Bile Duct

Figure 20.60. *Continued*

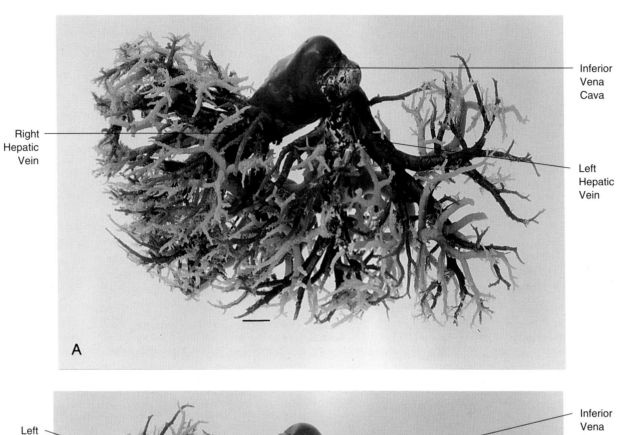

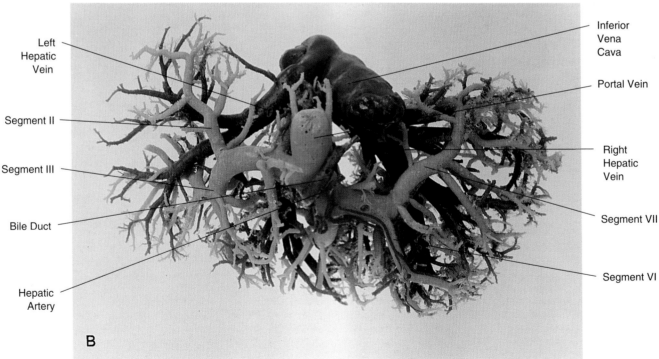

Figure 20.61. A. Anterior view of a plastic endocast of a liver specimen. The hepatic veins and inferior vena cava are blue. The portal vein is yellow. The bile duct is green. The hepatic artery is red. Note the relationship of the hepatic artery and bile duct with the portal vein. **B.** Posterior view of the endocast. Note the relationship of the hepatic artery and the bile duct with the portal vein.

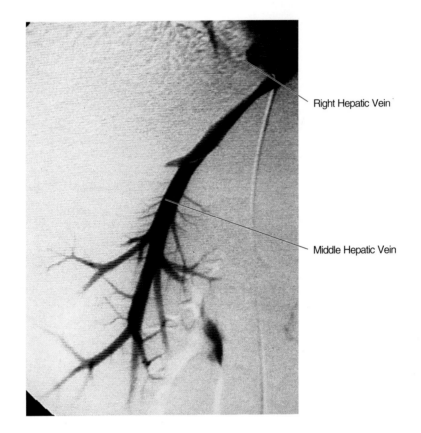

Figure 20.62. Angiogram of the middle hepatic vein.

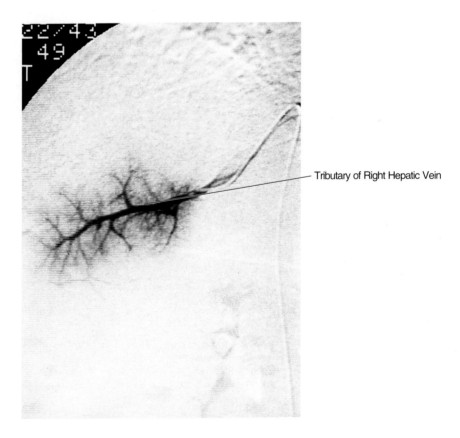

Figure 20.63. Angiogram of the right hepatic vein.

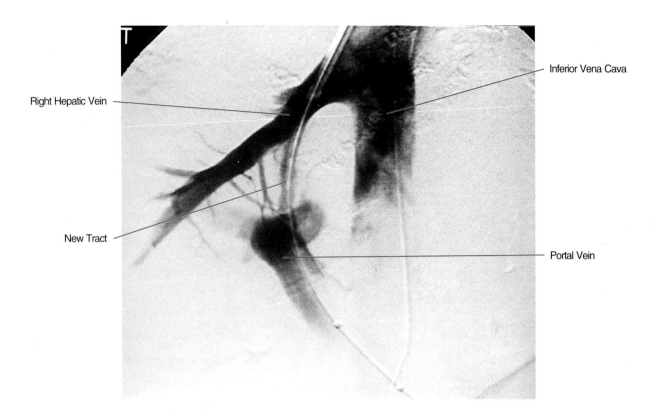

Figure 20.64. Angiogram during a TIPS procedure showing the relationships of the right hepatic vein, the portal vein, and the inferior vena cava. There is a tract created by the puncture.

Right Hepatic Veins   Inferior Vena Cava   Left Hepatic Vein

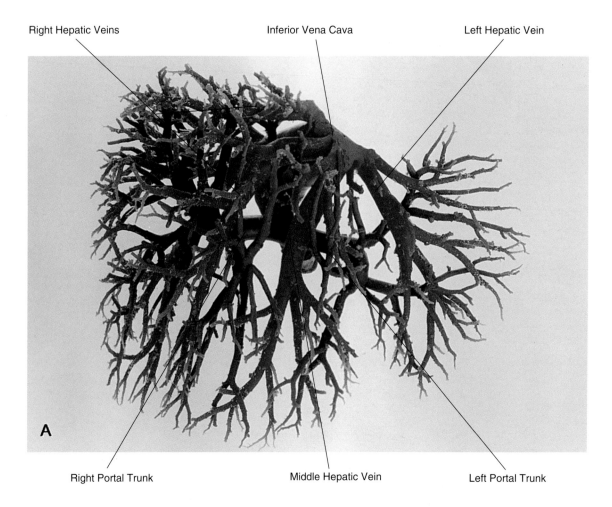

A

Right Portal Trunk   Middle Hepatic Vein   Left Portal Trunk

Figure 20.65. A. Anterior view of a plastic endocast of a liver specimen. The hepatic veins and inferior vena cava are red. The portal vein is green. There are three right hepatic veins, as an anatomical variation. The most anterior hepatic vein is anterior to the right portal vein. **B.** Posterior view of the plastic endocast. Note the relationship of the hepatic veins with the portal vein.

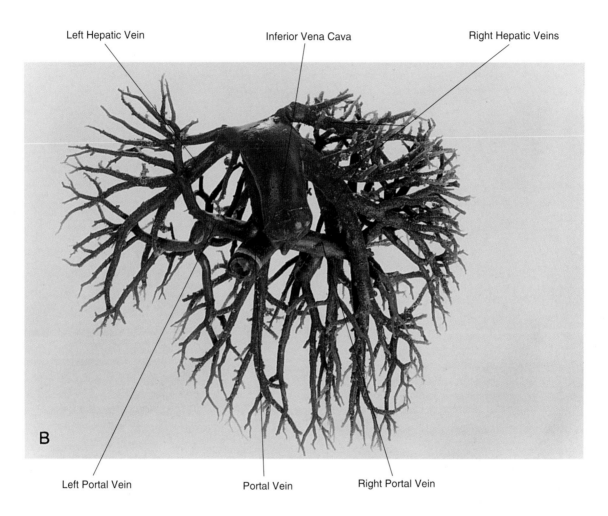

Left Hepatic Vein

Inferior Vena Cava

Right Hepatic Veins

Left Portal Vein

Portal Vein

Right Portal Vein

B

Figure 20.65. *Continued*

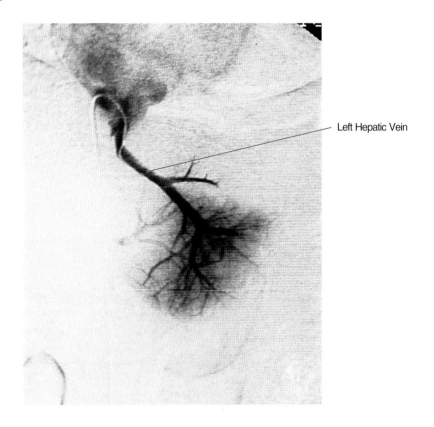

Left Hepatic Vein

Figure 20.66. Angiogram of the left hepatic vein.

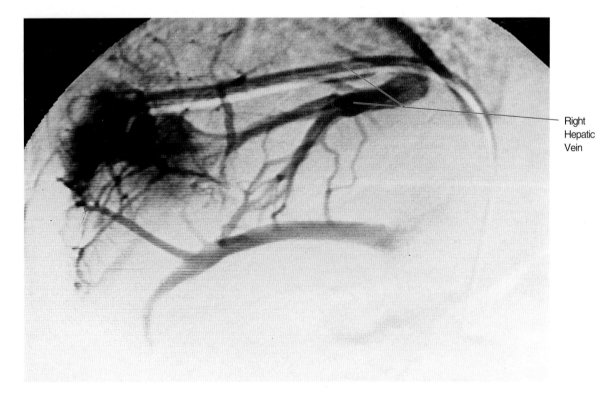

Right
Hepatic
Vein

Figure 20.67. Wedged angiogram of the right hepatic vein. Note the reflux of contrast medium into other branches of the right hepatic vein.

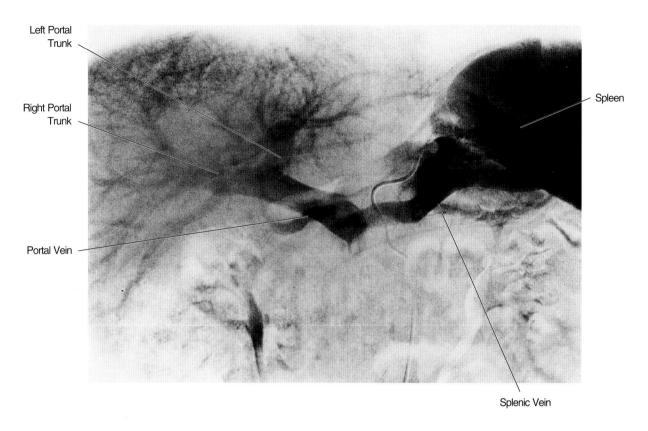

Left Portal Trunk

Right Portal Trunk

Portal Vein

Spleen

Splenic Vein

Figure 20.68. Arterial portography showing the opacification of the splenic vein and the portal vein as well as the intrahepatic radicles.

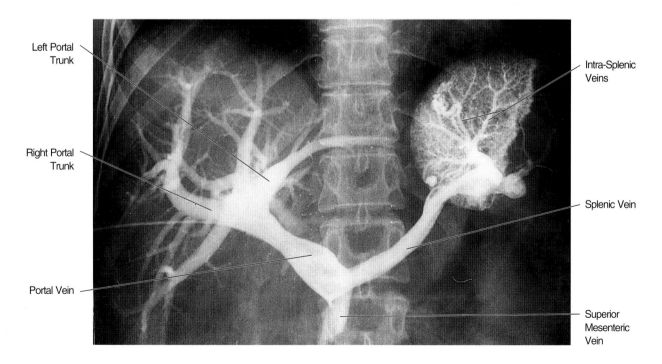

Left Portal Trunk

Right Portal Trunk

Portal Vein

Intra-Splenic Veins

Splenic Vein

Superior Mesenteric Vein

Figure 20.69. Transhepatic portography shows the opacification of the splenic vein, intrasplenic venous branches and filling of the portal vein and intrahepatic radicles.

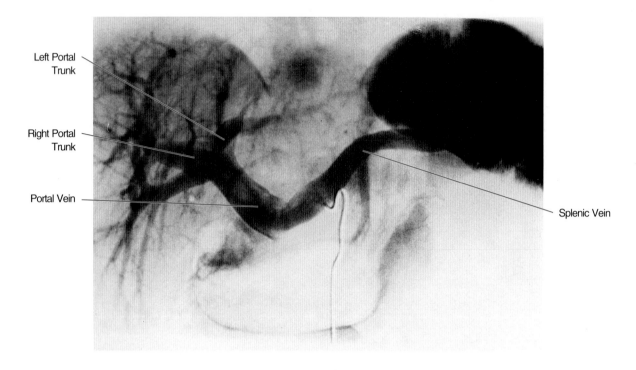

Figure 20.70. Arterial portography shows the splenic blush, the splenic vein opacification and the portal vein filling.

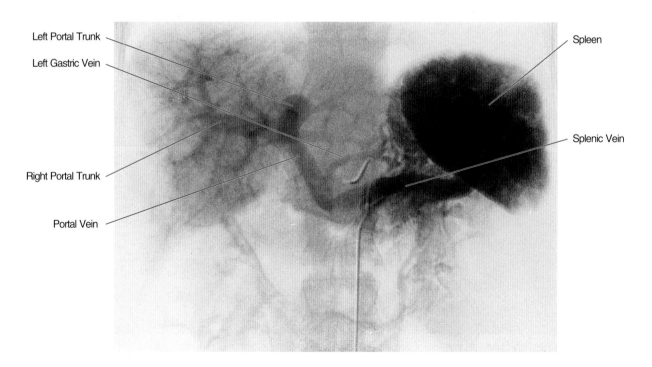

Figure 20.71. Arterial portography shows the splenic blush, the splenic vein opacification and the portal vein filling.

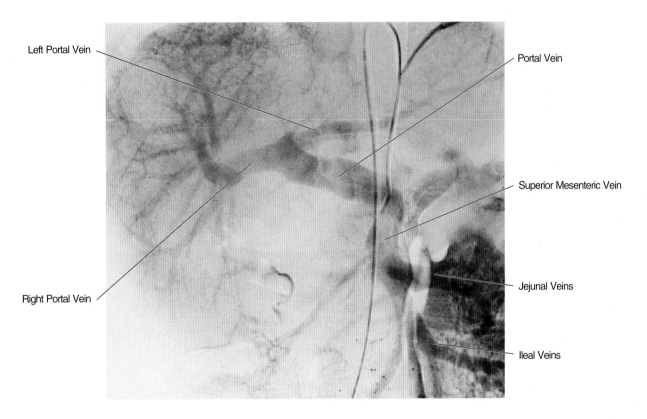

Figure 20.72. Arterial portography with injection into the superior mesenteric artery, shows the superior mesenteric artery, and the portal vein.

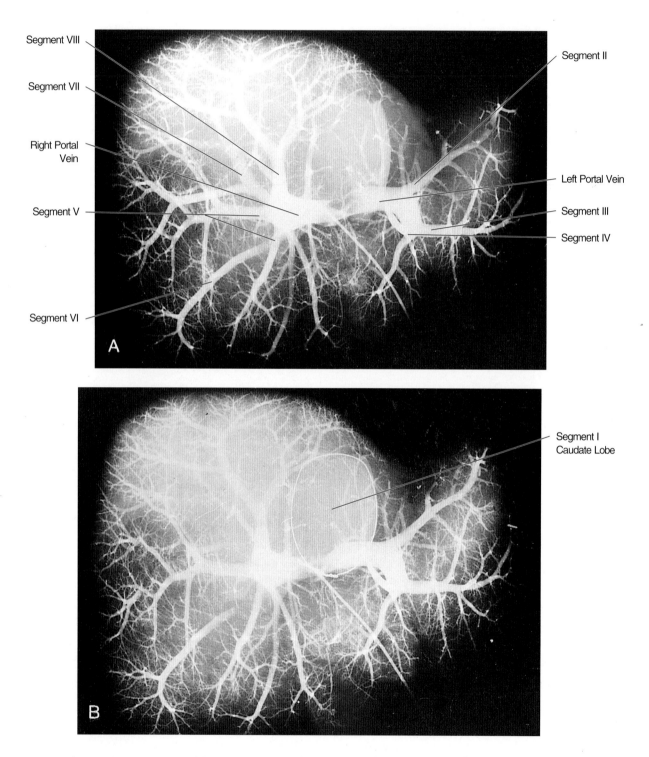

Segment VIII

Segment VII

Right Portal
Vein

Segment V

Segment VI

Segment II

Left Portal Vein

Segment III

Segment IV

A

B

Segment I
Caudate Lobe

Figure 20.73. A. Specimen of the liver injected into the portal vein. Note the segmental distribution of the portal vein. **B.** Note the radiopaque mark around the caudate lobe.

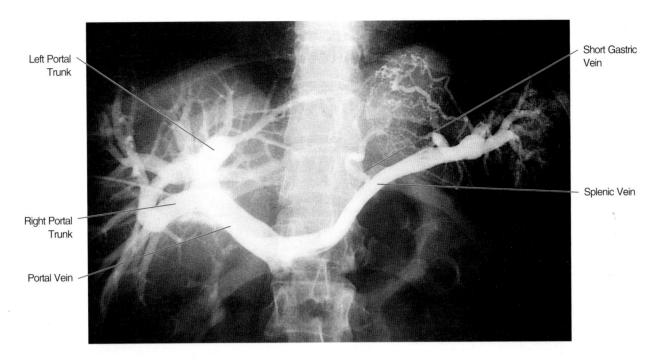

Figure 20.74. Transhepatic portography shows the splenic vein and portal vein densely opacified.

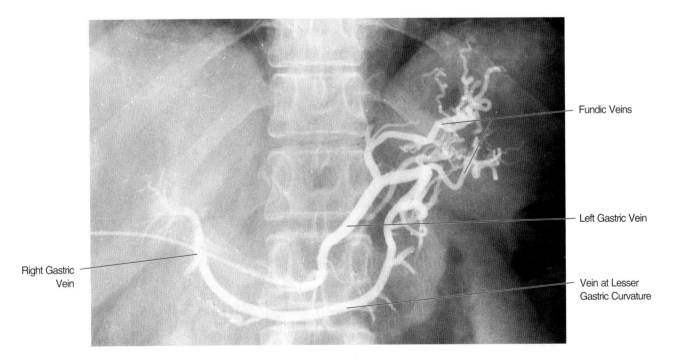

Figure 20.75. Selective injection angiography, by transhepatic approach, into the left gastric vein (coronary vein), showing the retrograde filling of the gastric wall veins and filling of the vein along the lesser curvature of the stomach. Note filling of the right gastric vein anastomosed with the intrahepatic portal vein.

Left Portal Trunk   Left Gastric Vein   Fundic Veins

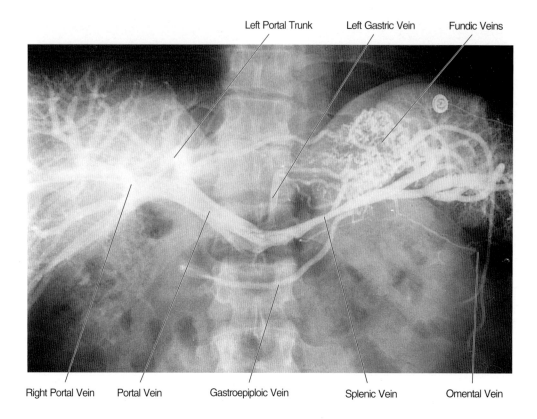

Right Portal Vein   Portal Vein   Gastroepiploic Vein   Splenic Vein   Omental Vein

Figure 20.76. Transhepatic portography shows the retrograde filling of the left gastric vein and filling of the short gastric veins and filling of the left gastroepiploic vein.

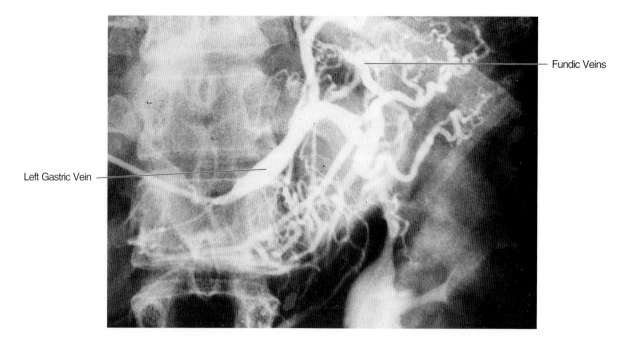

Fundic Veins

Left Gastric Vein

Figure 20.77. Selective injection into the left gastric vein showing the retrograde filling of the short gastric veins in the stomach fundus.

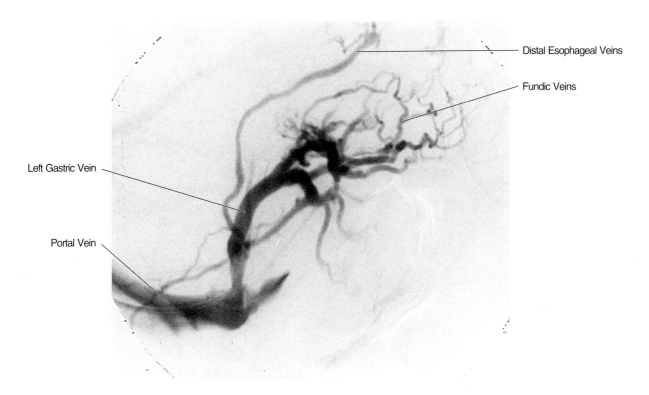

Distal Esophageal Veins

Fundic Veins

Left Gastric Vein

Portal Vein

Figure 20.78. Selective injection into the left gastric vein shows filling of the fundic gastric veins and distal esophageal veins.

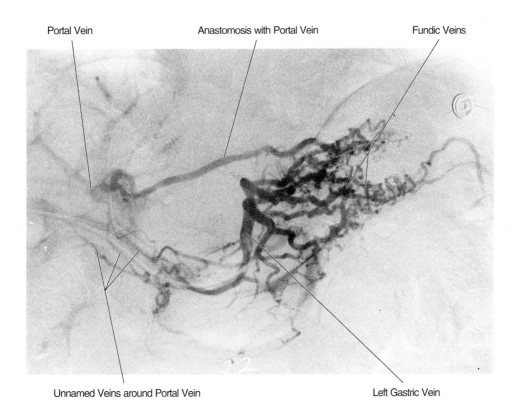

Portal Vein

Anastomosis with Portal Vein

Fundic Veins

Unnamed Veins around Portal Vein

Left Gastric Vein

Figure 20.79. Selective injection into the left gastric vein shows filling of the fundic gastric veins and multiple collaterals and anastomoses in the gastric wall. Note the unnamed veins around the portal vein. There is also an anastomosis between the left gastric vein and the intrahepatic portal vein.

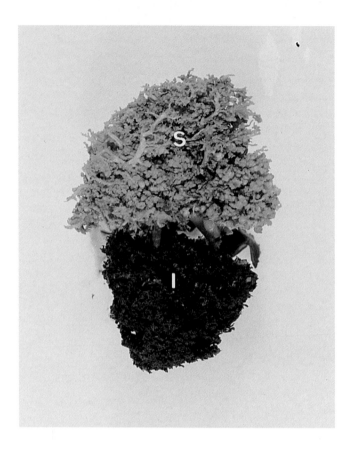

Figure 20.80. Vinilite resin corrosion endocast of the intrasplenic venous vasculature. View of the parietal surface shows two venous segments injected with different colors. S = superior venous segment, I = inferior venous segment.

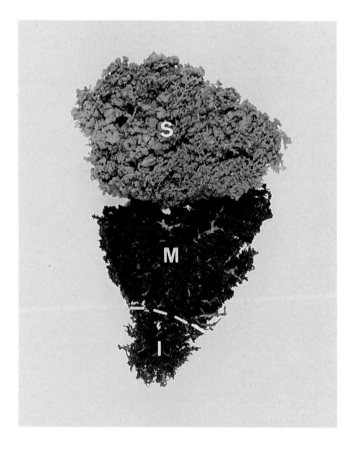

Figure 20.81. Vinilite resin corrosion endocast of the intrasplenic venous vasculature. View of the parietal surface shows three venous segments injected with different colors. S = superior venous segment, M = middle venous segment, I = inferior venous segment.

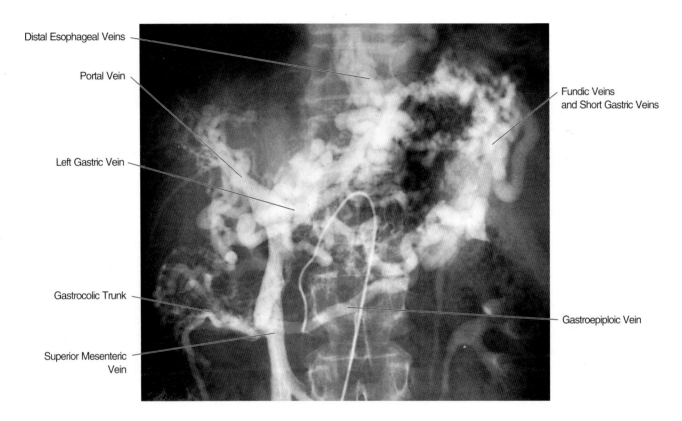

Distal Esophageal Veins

Portal Vein

Left Gastric Vein

Gastrocolic Trunk

Superior Mesenteric
Vein

Fundic Veins
and Short Gastric Veins

Gastroepiploic Vein

Figure 20.82. Late phase of a superior mesenteric arteriogram showing the opacification of the superior mesenteric vein, portal vein and short gastric veins, left and right gastroepiploic veins.

Right Portal Trunk   Left Portal Trunk   Left Gastric Vein   Fundic Veins   Spleen

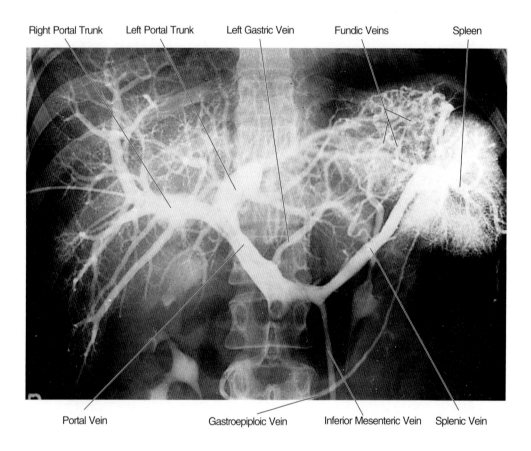

Portal Vein   Gastroepiploic Vein   Inferior Mesenteric Vein   Splenic Vein

Figure 20.83. Direct transhepatic portography showing the splenic vein, left gastric vein and short gastric veins and the fundic veins in the stomach. The portal vein is well filled.

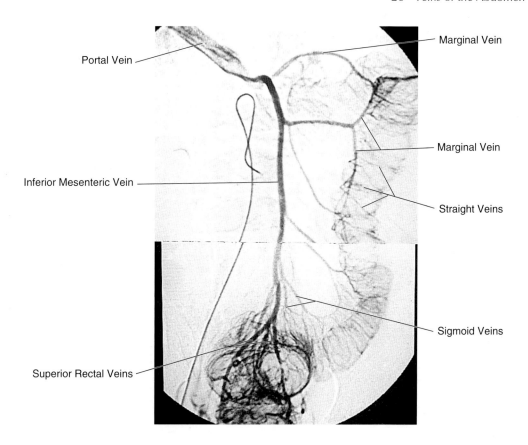

Portal Vein

Marginal Vein

Inferior Mesenteric Vein

Marginal Vein

Straight Veins

Sigmoid Veins

Superior Rectal Veins

Figure 20.84. Late phase of inferior mesenteric angiogram showing the inferior mesenteric vein and tributaries. Note portal vein filling.

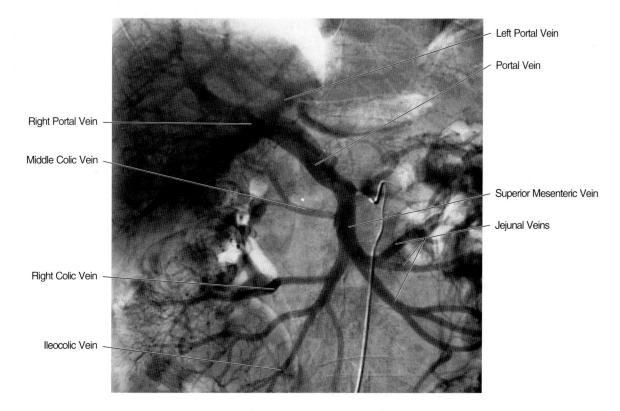

Left Portal Vein

Portal Vein

Right Portal Vein

Middle Colic Vein

Superior Mesenteric Vein

Jejunal Veins

Right Colic Vein

Ileocolic Vein

Figure 20.85. Arterial portography obtained through superior mesenteric artery injection. Excellent filling of the superior mesenteric vein and tributaries. The portal vein is also opacified.

Left Portal
Trunk

Right Portal
Trunk

Portal Vein

Superior Mesenteric
Vein

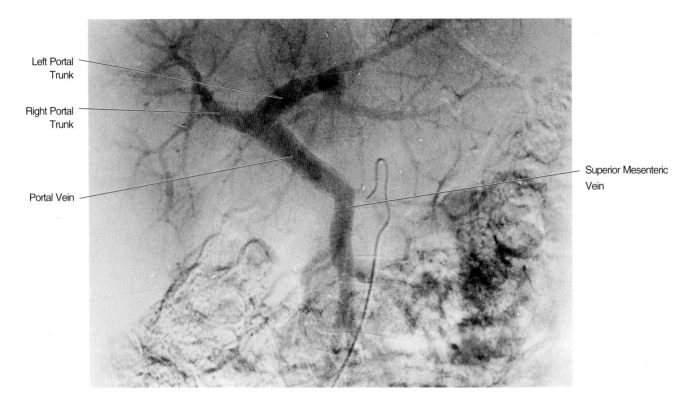

Figure 20.86.   Arterial portography obtained by superior mesenteric artery injection. Filling of the superior
mesenteric vein and tributaries. The portal vein is also opacified.

Portal Vein

Superior Mesenteric Vein

Jejunal Veins

Right Colic Vein

Ileal Veins

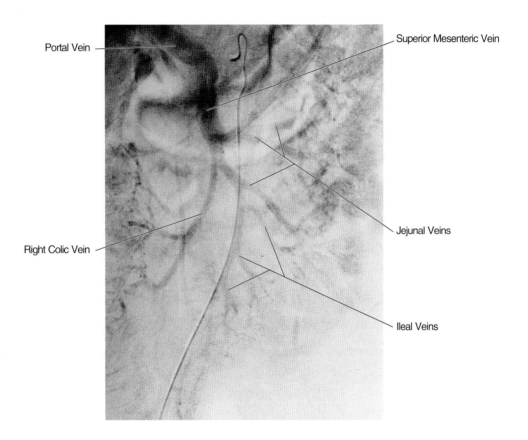

Figure 20.87. Arterial portography showing the superior mesenteric vein.

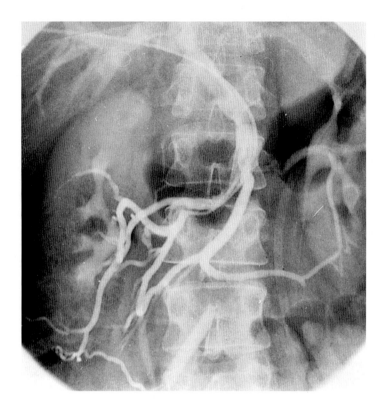

Figure 20.88.   Selective injection at the right colic vein. Some of the ileal veins are also opacified.

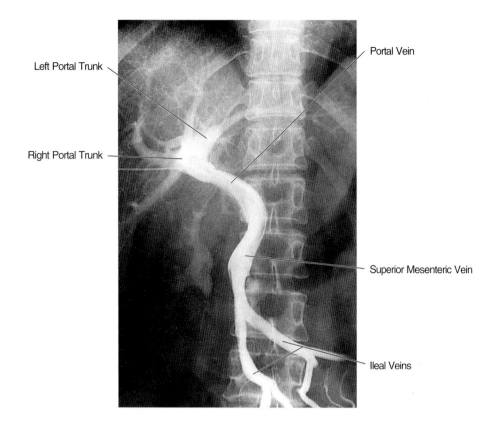

Figure 20.89. Selective injection at ileal veins.

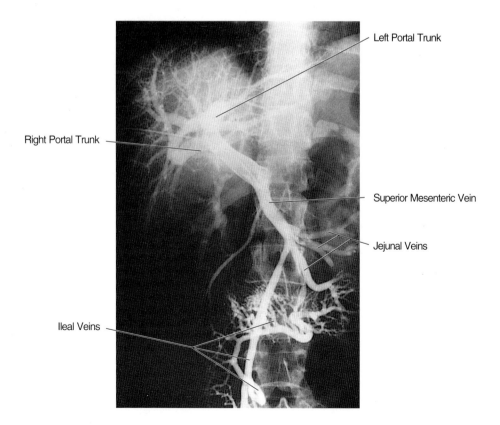

Figure 20.90. Selective injection at jejunal and ileal veins.

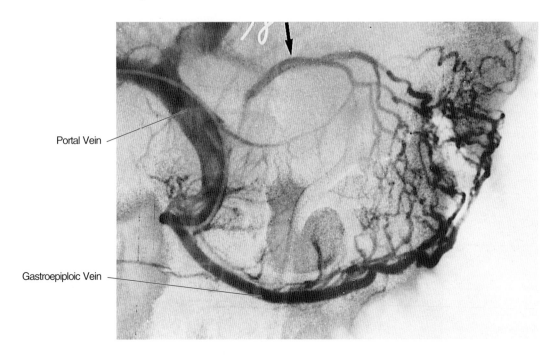

Portal Vein

Gastroepiploic Vein

Figure 20.91. Selective injection into the right gastroepiploic vein, shows filling of the gastric wall veins and opacification of the left gastric vein (arrow). The portal vein is opacified.

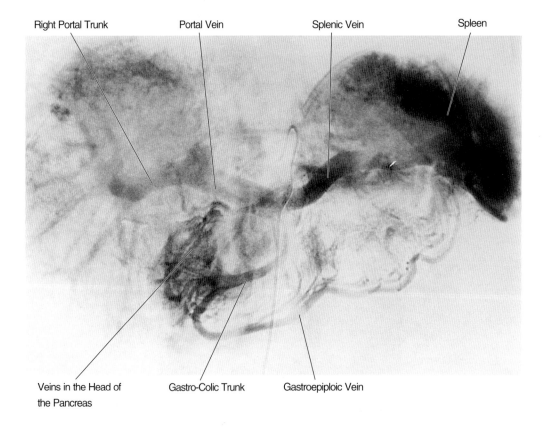

Right Portal Trunk   Portal Vein   Splenic Vein   Spleen

Veins in the Head of   Gastro-Colic Trunk   Gastroepiploic Vein
the Pancreas

Figure 20.92. Late phase of a selective injection in the celiac trunk. Note filling of the right and left gastroepiploic veins. Note visualization of the gastrocolic trunk with opacification of the pancreatic head veins. The portal vein and splenic vein are well opacified.

Portal Vein

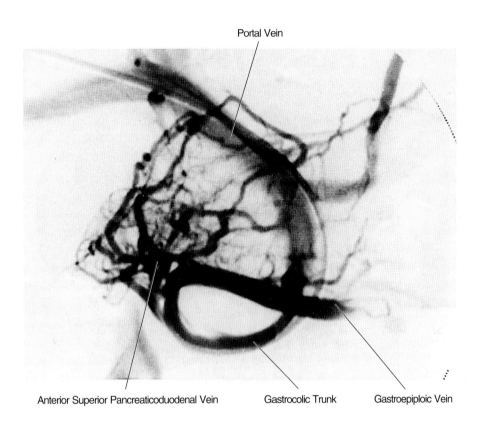

Anterior Superior Pancreaticoduodenal Vein   Gastrocolic Trunk   Gastroepiploic Vein

Figure 20.93. Selective injection at the gastrocolic trunk with filling of the pancreatic head veins and the right gastroepiploic vein.

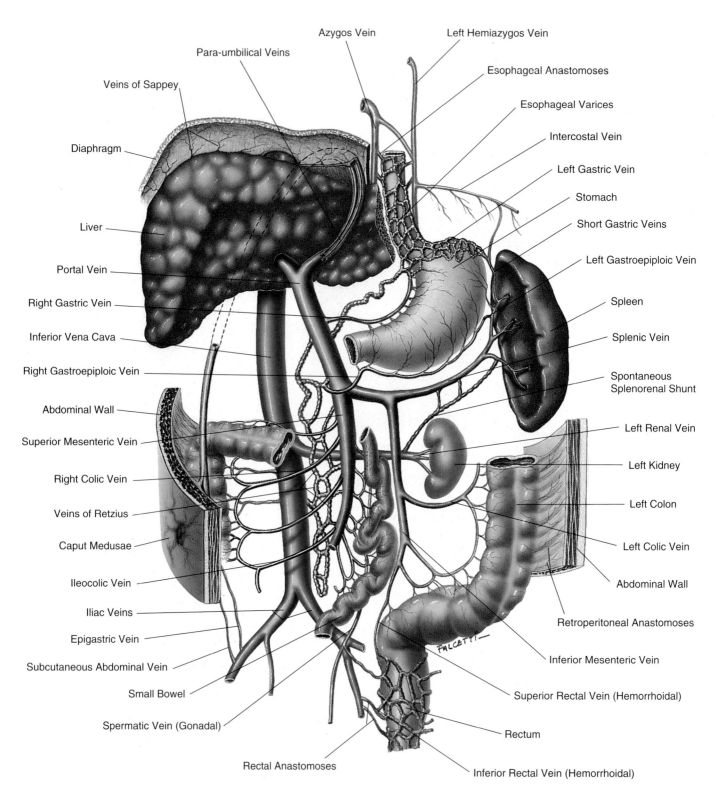

Veins of Sappey

Para-umbilical Veins

Azygos Vein

Left Hemiazygos Vein

Esophageal Anastomoses

Esophageal Varices

Intercostal Vein

Left Gastric Vein

Stomach

Short Gastric Veins

Left Gastroepiploic Vein

Spleen

Splenic Vein

Spontaneous Splenorenal Shunt

Left Renal Vein

Left Kidney

Left Colon

Left Colic Vein

Abdominal Wall

Retroperitoneal Anastomoses

Inferior Mesenteric Vein

Superior Rectal Vein (Hemorrhoidal)

Rectum

Inferior Rectal Vein (Hemorrhoidal)

Diaphragm

Liver

Portal Vein

Right Gastric Vein

Inferior Vena Cava

Right Gastroepiploic Vein

Abdominal Wall

Superior Mesenteric Vein

Right Colic Vein

Veins of Retzius

Caput Medusae

Ileocolic Vein

Iliac Veins

Epigastric Vein

Subcutaneous Abdominal Vein

Small Bowel

Spermatic Vein (Gonadal)

Rectal Anastomoses

Figure 20.94. Sites of portosystemic collaterals and communications.

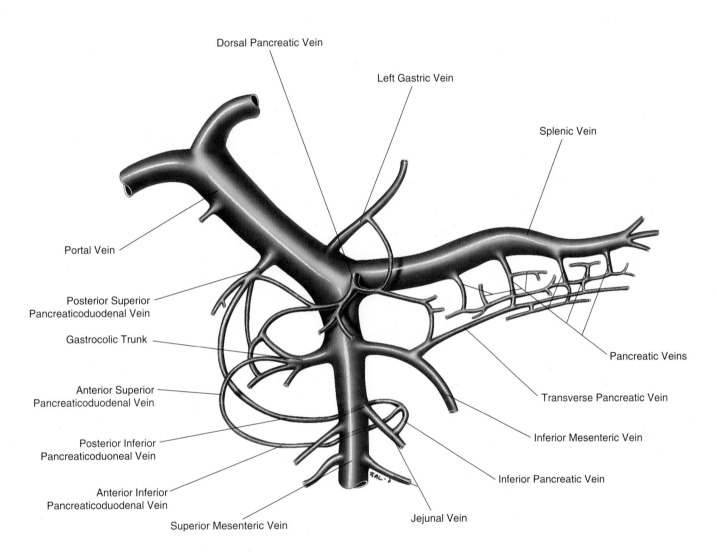

Figure 20.95. Schematic drawing showing the pancreatic venous drainage.

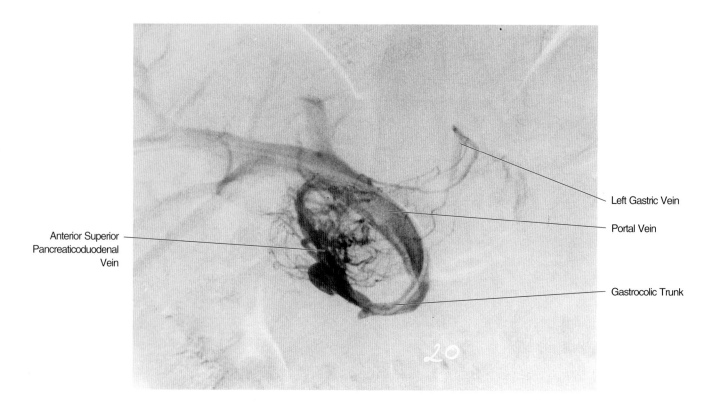

Figure 20.96. Selective injection into the gastrocolic trunk.

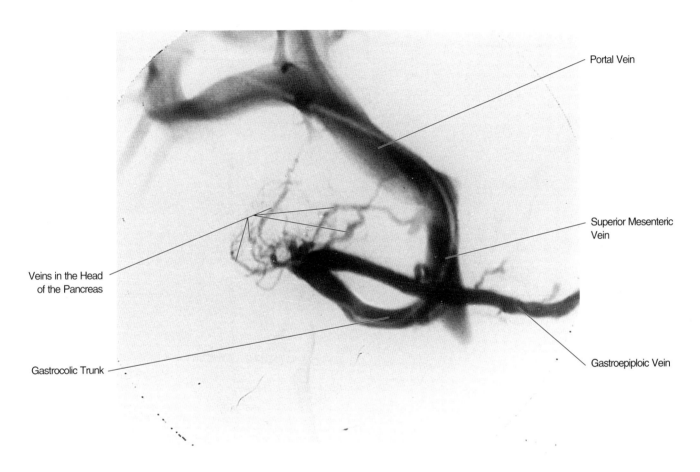

Portal Vein

Superior Mesenteric
Vein

Veins in the Head
of the Pancreas

Gastroepiploic Vein

Gastrocolic Trunk

Figure 20.97. Selective injection into the gastrocolic trunk.

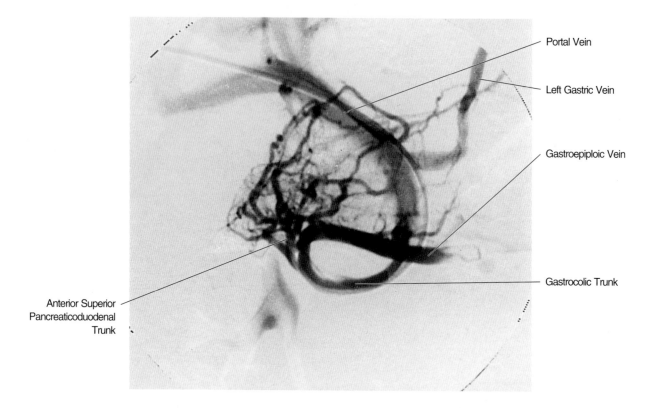

Portal Vein

Left Gastric Vein

Gastroepiploic Vein

Gastrocolic Trunk

Anterior Superior Pancreaticoduodenal Trunk

Figure 20.98. Selective injection into the gastrocolic trunk.

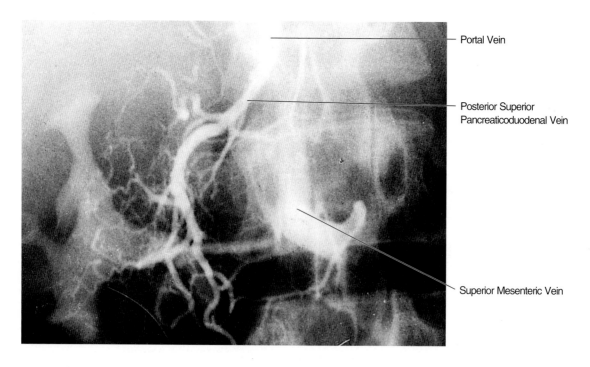

Portal Vein

Posterior Superior Pancreaticoduodenal Vein

Superior Mesenteric Vein

Figure 20.99. Selective injection into the posterior superior pancreaticoduodenal vein.

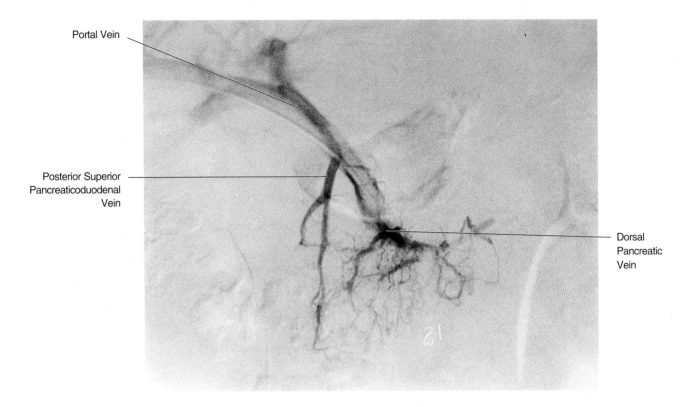

Figure 20.100. Selective injection into the dorsal pancreatic vein with simultaneous opacification of the posterior superior pancreaticoduodenal vein.

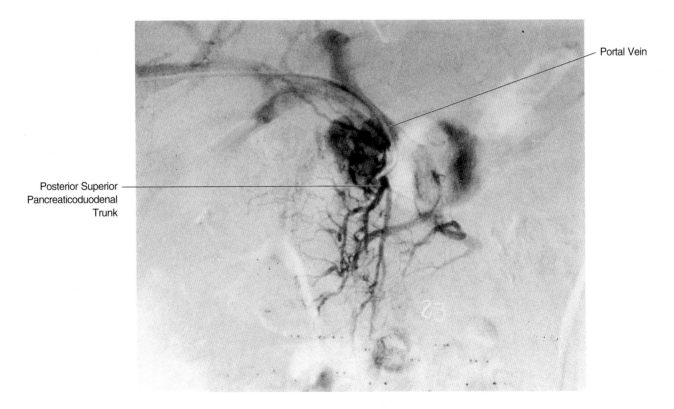

Figure 20.101. Selective injection into the posterior superior pancreaticoduodenal vein.

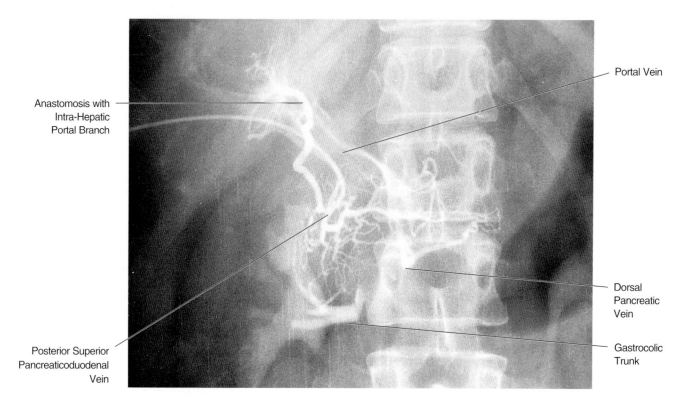

Portal Vein

Anastomosis with
Intra-Hepatic
Portal Branch

Dorsal
Pancreatic
Vein

Gastrocolic
Trunk

Posterior Superior
Pancreaticoduodenal
Vein

Figure 20.102. Selective venogram at the posterior superior pancreaticoduodenal vein.

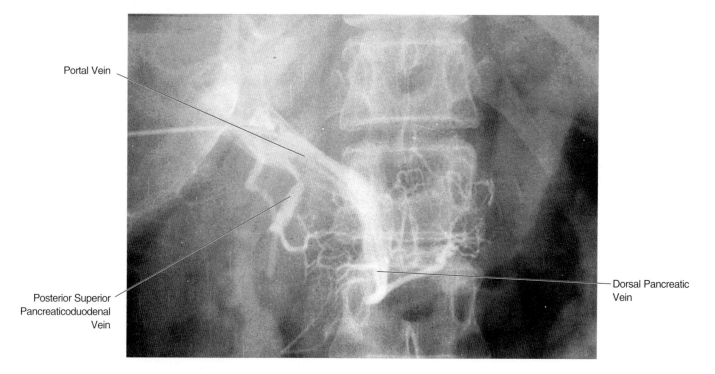

Portal Vein

Dorsal Pancreatic
Vein

Posterior Superior
Pancreaticoduodenal
Vein

Figure 20.103. Selective venogram of the dorsal pancreatic vein.

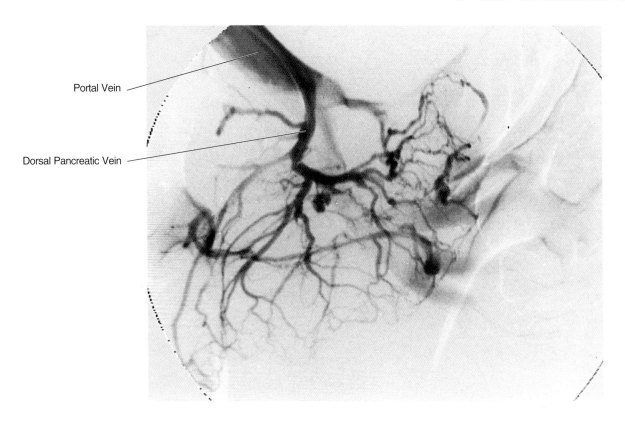

Portal Vein

Dorsal Pancreatic Vein

Figure 20.104. Selective venogram of the dorsal pancreatic vein. Note the large size of this vein and the wide anastomotic network with opacification of veins from the head to the pancreatic body. A few venous aneurysms are also seem.

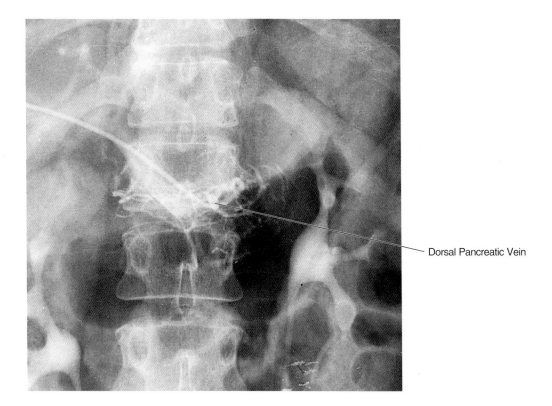

Dorsal Pancreatic Vein

Figure 20.105. Selective venogram of the dorsal pancreatic vein. Note the small size of this vein.

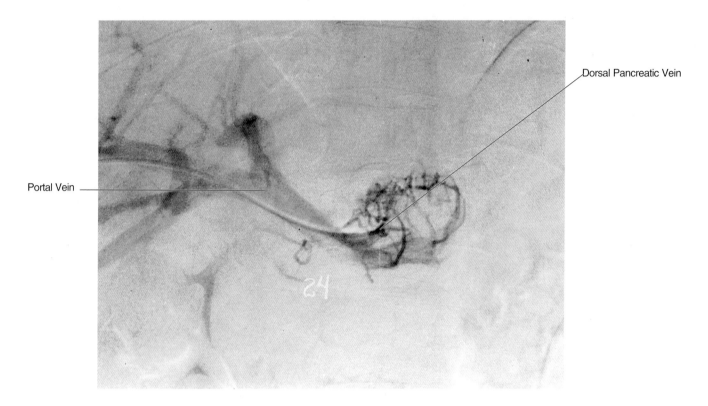

Figure 20.106. Selective venogram of the dorsal pancreatic vein, in an unusual position.

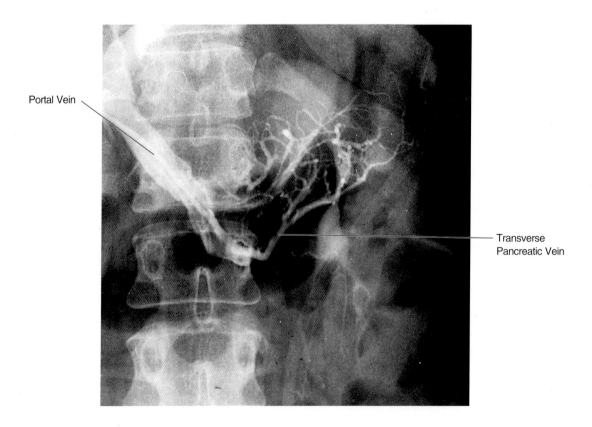

Figure 20.107. Selective venogram of the transverse pancreatic vein.

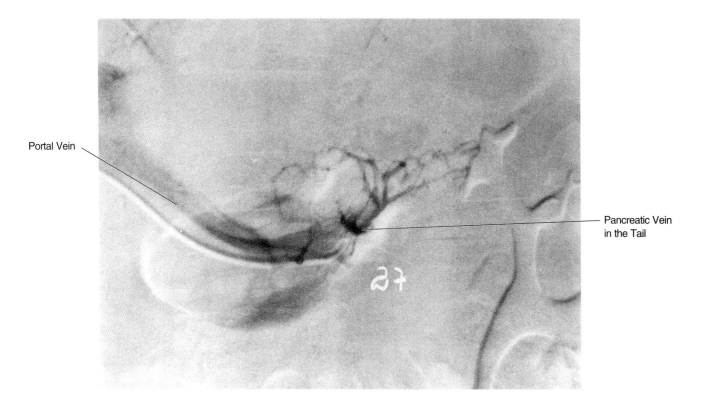

Figure 20.108. Selective venogram of the transverse pancreatic vein.

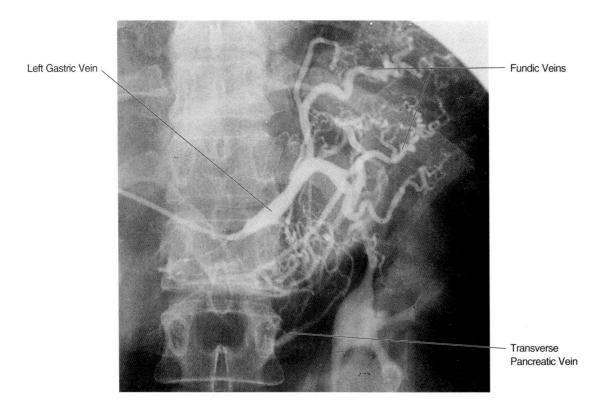

Figure 20.109. Selective venogram of the left gastric vein. Note the anastomosis with the gastric veins and pancreatic veins.

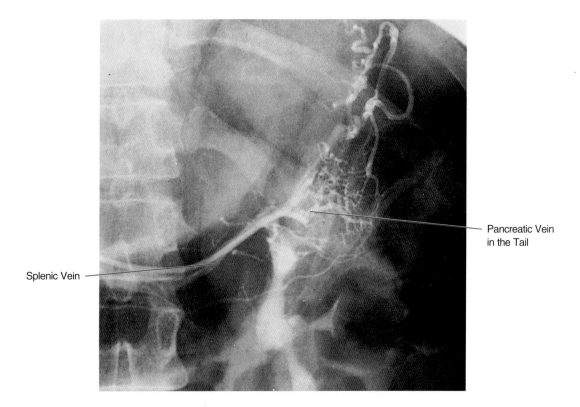

Figure 20.110. Selective venogram of pancreatic veins of the tail.

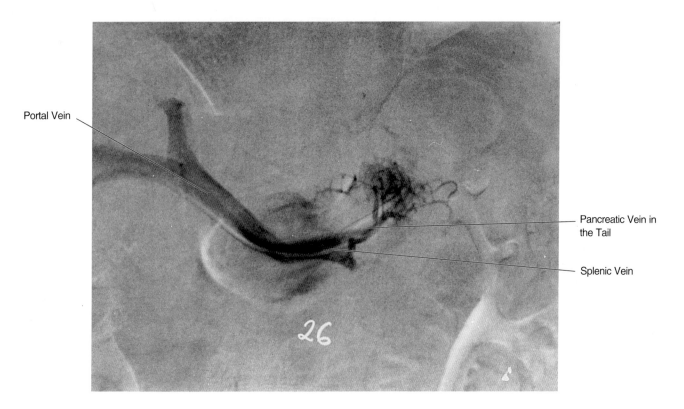

Figure 20.111. Selective venogram of pancreatic veins of the tail.

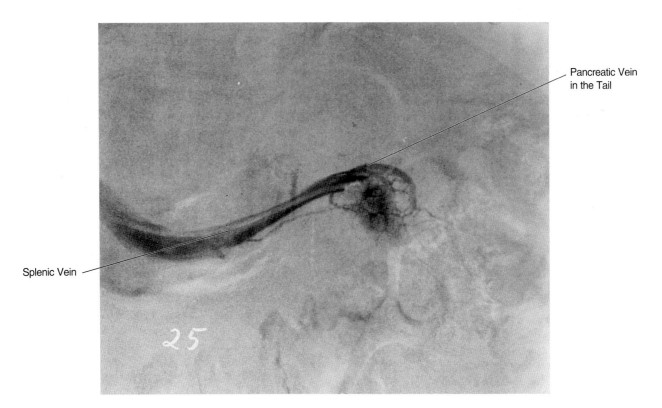

Pancreatic Vein
in the Tail

Splenic Vein

Figure 20.112. Selective venogram of the pancreatic veins of the tail.

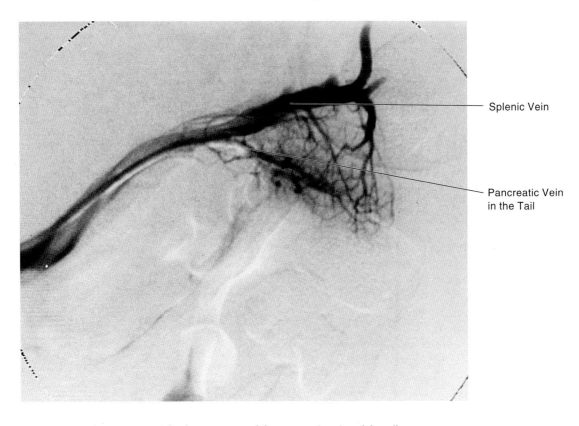

Splenic Vein

Pancreatic Vein
in the Tail

Figure 20.113. Selective venogram of the pancreatic veins of the tail.

21

LYMPHATIC SYSTEM OF THE ABDOMEN AND PELVIS

LUMBAR LYMPH NODES

There are three main groups of lumbar lymph nodes, the preaortic, lateral aortic (right and left), and retroaortic. The preaortic receives drainage from the ventral splanchnic; the lateral aortic drains the viscera supplied by the lateral splanchnic and dorsolateral somatic vessels. The retroaortic lymph nodes drain no specific territory, but are mainly an interconnection of the other groups (Figs. 21.1, 21.2)

Preaortic Lymph Nodes

The preaortic lymph nodes comprise the group located anteriorly to the abdominal aorta and receive the intestinal trunks, named after the arteries with which they are companions. Celiac lymph nodes, superior mesenteric lymph nodes, and inferior mesenteric lymph nodes.

Celiac Lymph Nodes

There are three main groups of lymph nodes sending afferents to the celiac lymph nodes, from gastric lymphatic vessels and nodes (from left gastric nodes, right gastroepiploic nodes, pyloric nodes) (Fig. 21.3), from hepatic lymphatic vessels and nodes (Fig. 21.4) (from the stomach, duodenum, liver, gallbladder, bile ducts, and head of the pancreas), and from splenopancreatic lymphatic vessels and nodes (from stomach, spleen, and pancreas) (Fig. 21.3).

Superior and Inferior Mesenteric Lymph Nodes

The superior and inferior mesenteric lymph nodes are located close to the origin of the corresponding arteries. They collect lymphatic drainage from the duodenojejunal flexure to the upper anal canal, including the mesenteric, ileocolic, colonic, and pararectal lymph nodes, discharging into the celiac lymph nodes. There are hundreds of lymph nodes in the territory comprised by the mesentery. The lymphatic drainage of the rectum and anal canal has a double path. The upper half of the rectum drains to

the pararectal nodes and subsequently to the superior mesenteric lymph nodes, while the lower half of the rectum and the anal canal drains to the internal iliac lymph nodes. Lymphatic vessels of the mucocutaneous junction reaches the medial superficial inguinal nodes (Fig. 21.5).

Lateral Aortic Lymph Nodes

Comprise the group of lymph nodes flanking the abdominal aorta and the inferior vena cava. Several afferents reach those nodes, from the kidney, suprarenal gland, abdominal ureter, posterior abdominal wall, testis and ovary. The pelvic organs lymph reaches the lateral aortic lymph nodes, after passing through regional groups as the internal iliac nodes, external iliac nodes, and common iliac nodes (Fig. 21.6). The internal iliac group receives deep gluteal lymph, and the external iliac group receives the efferents from the inguinal lymph nodes, whereas the common iliac nodes are grouped around the common iliac artery, draining the external and internal iliac nodes and sending efferents to the lateral aortic nodes.

Lymphatic Drainage of the Urinary and Reproductive Organs

From the Kidney

The intrarenal lymphatics of the kidney are divided into a superficial plexus and a deep plexus. The superficial plexus is located immediately below the renal capsule and is connected with cortical lymphatics. In pathologic conditions (pyelonephritis, for example), this plexus may communicate with an extrarenal plexus located in the perirenal fat, which drains, in its turn, into the lumbo-aortic lymph nodes.

The deep plexus is subcortical and also pyramidal (more deeply located). These deep plexuses are perivascular and drain together, along the arcuate and interlobar vessels, converging to the renal hilus. The collecting channels emerge from the renal hilus and, if a polar artery is present, usually a lymphatic channel follows the polar vessel. There are one to four lymphatic channels which emerge from the renal hilus, either anteriorly or posteriorly to the renal vein. These lymphatics may be anastomosed, giving a plexiform aspect. The lymphatics usually are periarterial, forming an anterior plexus when they come from the kidney ventral surface or a posterior plexus when they come from the kidney dorsal surface. In some cases, the lymphatic channels may connect their lymph nodes directly, without following the arterial branches. The drainage of the lymphatic vessels differs in some aspects, between right and left sides:

Right Side. The lymphatic channels of the right kidney may be divided into posterior, anterior, and middle. The posterior lymphatic vessels follow the renal artery, posteriorly to the vena cava. These lymphatics reach the lumbo-aortic lymph nodes, which are located just bellow the renal artery origin. Afterward, they end up in the retrocaval nodes, inter-aorto-caval nodes (L-1 to L-3), lateral caval nodes, and surrounding the deep surface of the renal artery, they follow the right diaphragmatic crus to reach the right abdominal lymphatic channel. The anterior lymphatic channels, running above the vessels, drain into the posterior lymphatics or, when running medially, end in the precaval nodes. Sometimes, they can cross the vena cava to reach the superior inter-aorto-caval nodes. The middle lymphatics run between the renal vein and the renal artery to reach the anterior and posterior lymphatic groups (Figs. 21.7, 21.8).

Left Side. The lymphatic vessels of the left kidney may be divided into posterior and anterior. The posterior channels leave the renal hilum and run behind the renal vessels to reach the lymphatic nodes of the diaphragmatic crus. The anterior channels run ventrally to the renal vein; they reach the lymph nodes located above or bellow the renal artery origin, when draining the superior pole or the inferior pole, respectively. There are also lymphatics that come from the inferior pole to reach the lymph nodes that are located in the spermatic artery origin, on the lateral surface of the aorta (Figs. 21.7, 21.9).

On both sides, the lymphatic drainage of the kidney posterior region (dorsal surface), reaches directly the lymph nodes of the diaphragmatic crus, in contact with the hiatus of the splanchnic nerve. From this point, through the diaphragm, these lymphatics drain into the retroaortic nodes, from T-11 to L-1 (mediastinal lymphatics) (Fig. 21.7). This detail is very important to be remembered when assessing the spread of renal cell carcinoma metastases.

From the Ureter

The draining lymphatic vessels of the ureter begin in the submucous, intramuscular, and adventitial plexuses with intercommunications. The lymphatic vessels from the pelvic part of the ureter drain to the common, internal, and external iliac nodes. The lower abdominal part of the ureter drains directly to the common iliac nodes, while the proximal ureter drains

to the renal collecting vessels or pass directly to the lateral aortic nodes.

From the Bladder

Lymphatic drainage originates at the mucous, intramuscular, and extramuscular plexuses. The collecting vessels end in the external iliac lymph nodes (Fig. 21.10).

From the Urethra

The lymphatic vessels from the prostatic and membranous urethra in the male and the female urethra drain to the internal iliac nodes. The lymphatic vessels of the anterior male urethra drain to the deep inguinal nodes.

From the Testis

There is a superficial (under the tunica vaginalis) and a deep (in the substance of the testis and epididymis) plexuses. Four to eight collecting lymphatic trunks ascend at the spermatic cord following the testicular vessels, draining to the lateral and preaortic lymph nodes. The drainage of the ovary is, like the testicular, made by lymphatic trunks, which ascend with the ovarian vessels to the lateral and preaortic lymph nodes.

From the Ductus Deferens, Seminal Vesicle, and Prostate Gland

The lymphatic vessels from the ductus drain to the external iliac nodes, those from the seminal vesicle drain to the internal and external iliac nodes, while the prostatic vessels drain to the internal iliac and sacral nodes.

From the Scrotum and Penis

The skin drainage of these organs drain to the superficial inguinal nodes.

From the Uterus and Uterine Tubes

Lymphatic from the cervix pass laterally to the parametrium and the external iliac nodes, to the internal iliac nodes and to the rectal and sacral nodes. Lymphatic vessels from the lower part of the uterine body drain mostly to the external iliac nodes, following those from the cervix. The lymphatic vessels from the upper part of the uterine body, the fundus and the tubes, accompany the ovarian lymphatics with the ovarian vessels (Fig. 21.10).

From the Vagina

The lymphatic vessels from the vagina join the lymphatics of the cervix, rectum, and vulva (Fig. 21.10).

Retroaortic Lymph Nodes

The retroaortic lymph nodes have no special area of drainage; they are mostly regarded with the drainage of the posterior abdominal wall, to comprise the periphery of the lateral aortic groups and to participate in the interconnection of the surrounding groups.

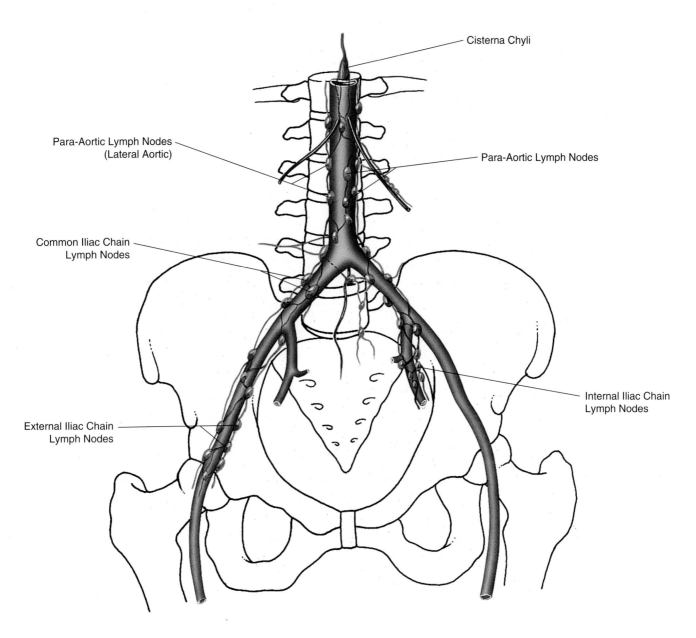

Figure 21.1. Schematic drawing showing the lymphatic drainage of the pelvis and abdomen through the internal iliac, external iliac, and para-aortic lymphatics and lymph nodes. Note the cisterna chyli behind the aorta.

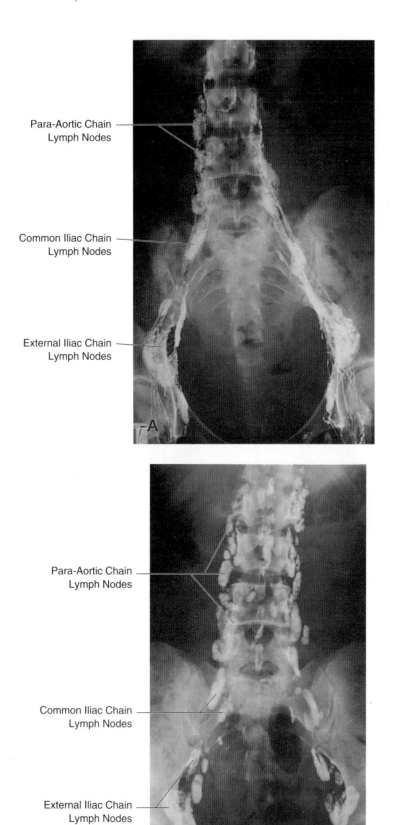

Para-Aortic Chain
Lymph Nodes

Common Iliac Chain
Lymph Nodes

External Iliac Chain
Lymph Nodes

A

Para-Aortic Chain
Lymph Nodes

Common Iliac Chain
Lymph Nodes

External Iliac Chain
Lymph Nodes

B

Figure 21.2. A. Early phase of a bilateral lymphangiogram showing the external iliac lymph nodes and the para-aortic lymphatics. **B.** Late phase of the lymphangiogram showing the lymph nodes of the external iliac and para-aortic groups.

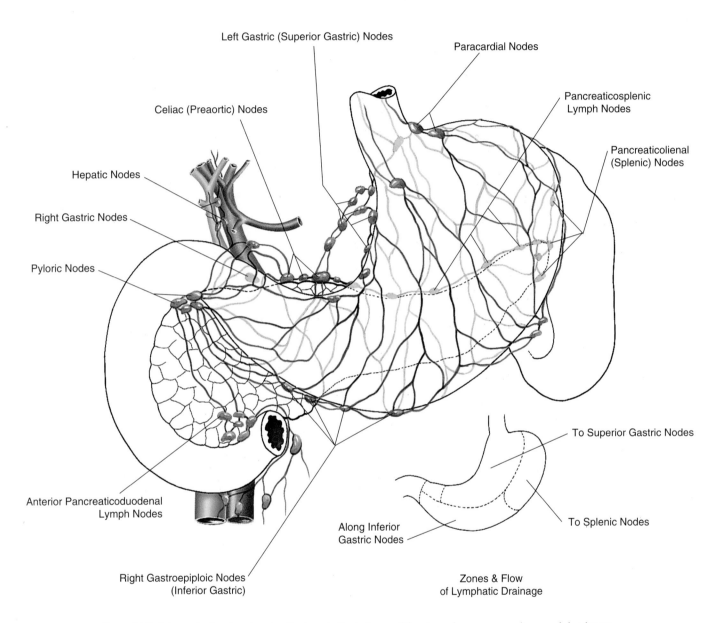

Left Gastric (Superior Gastric) Nodes

Paracardial Nodes

Pancreaticosplenic Lymph Nodes

Celiac (Preaortic) Nodes

Pancreaticolienal (Splenic) Nodes

Hepatic Nodes

Right Gastric Nodes

Pyloric Nodes

To Superior Gastric Nodes

Anterior Pancreaticoduodenal Lymph Nodes

Along Inferior Gastric Nodes

To Splenic Nodes

Right Gastroepiploic Nodes (Inferior Gastric)

Zones & Flow of Lymphatic Drainage

Figure 21.3. Schematic drawing showing the lymphatic drainage of the stomach, pancreas, spleen, and duodenum. Note in the insert the zones & flow of lymphatic drainage of the stomach.

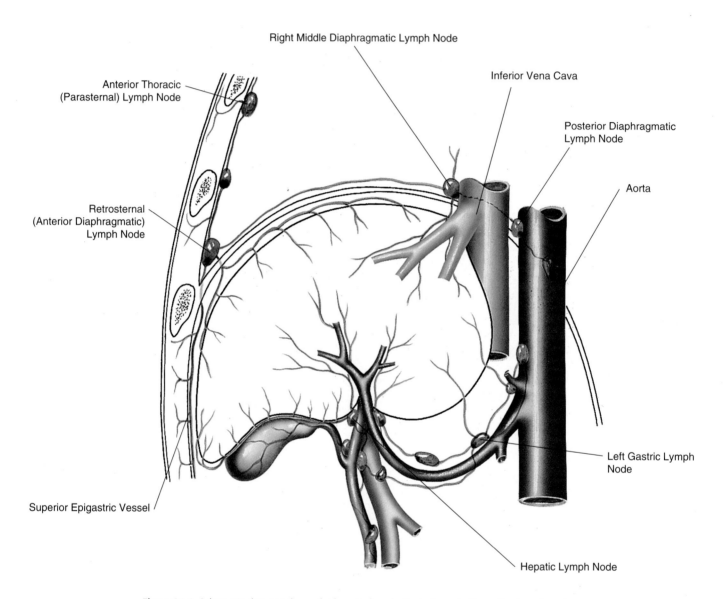

Figure 21.4. Schematic drawing shows the hepatic lymphatic drainage to the celiac lymph nodes.

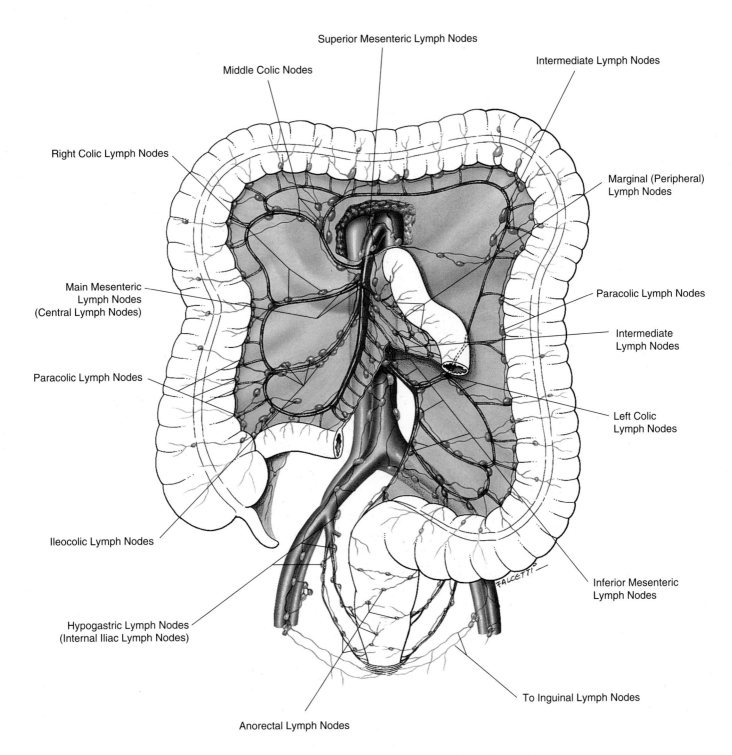

Figure 21.5. Schematic drawing showing the superior and inferior mesenteric lymphatic drainage. Note also the rectal lymphatic drainage demonstrated.

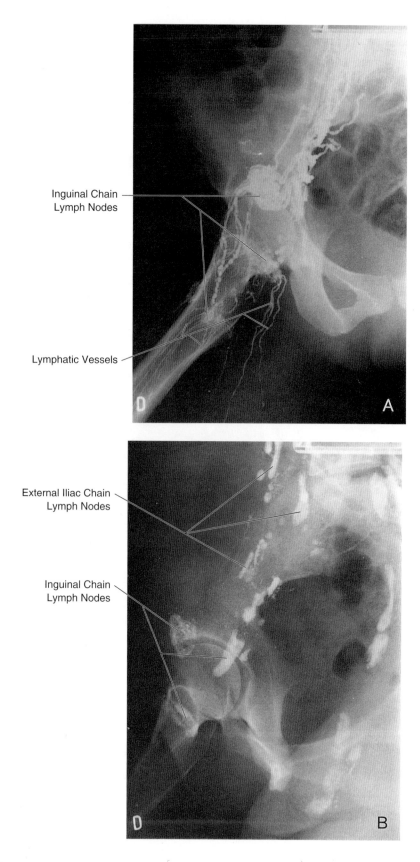

Figure 21.6. A. Lymphangiogram of the inguinal group of lymphatics and nodes draining into the external iliac group. **B.** Late phase of a lymphangiogram showing both sides of the external iliac lymph nodes in right oblique. **C.** Late phase of a lymphangiogram showing both sides of the external iliac lymph nodes in left oblique.

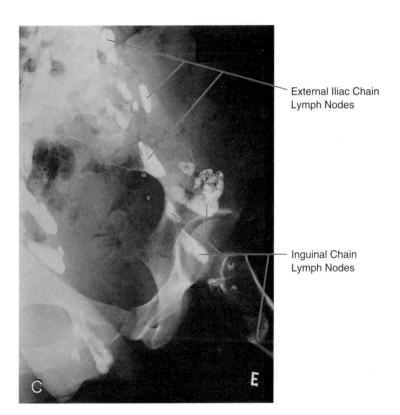

External Iliac Chain
Lymph Nodes

Inguinal Chain
Lymph Nodes

Figure 21.6. *Continued*

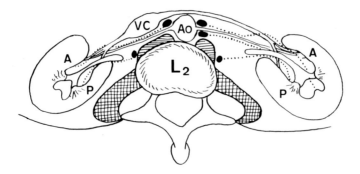

Figure 21.7. Inferior view of a schematic drawing from a transverse section in the retroperitoneal region. The collecting lymphatics are demonstrated with dotted lines. They run to the lateral aortic lymph nodes, in the renal artery origin. Note the lymphatics of the posterior region running to the diaphragmatic crux, from there they can reach the mediastinal lymphatics. Ao = abdominal aorta; VC = inferior vena cava; A = anterior region of the kidney (ventral surface); P = posterior region of the kidney (dorsal surface); L2 = second lumbar vertebra.

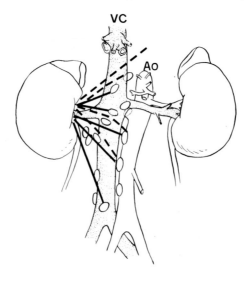

Figure 21.8. Lymphatic drainage of the right kidney. The anterior lymphatic channels are shown with the continuous lines; the posterior channels are shown with the dashed lines. VC = inferior vena cava; Ao = abdominal aorta.

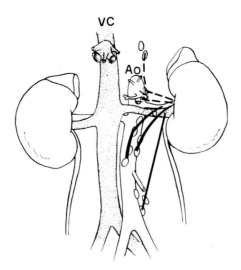

Figure 21.9. Lymphatic drainage of the left kidney. The anterior lymphatic channels are shown with the continuous line; the posterior channels are shown with the dashed line. VC= inferior vena cava; AO = abdominal aorta.

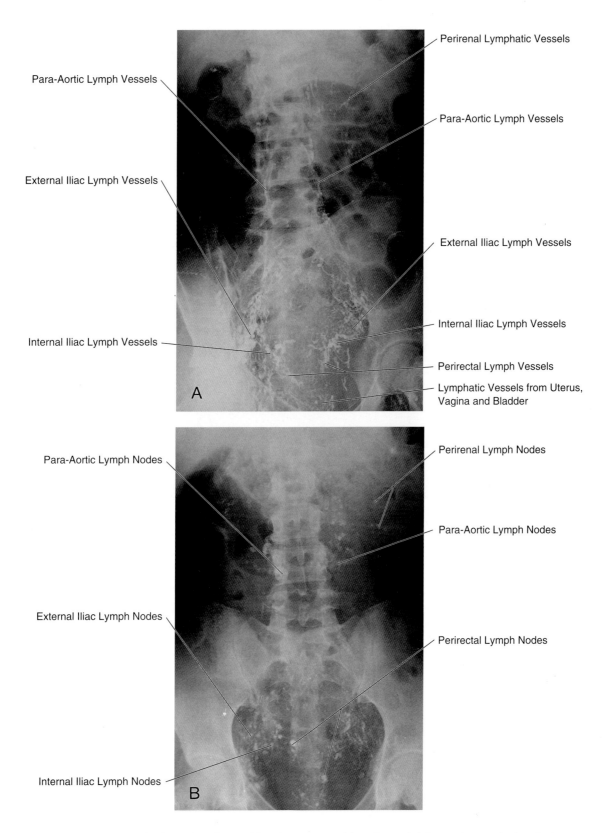

Figure 21.10. **A.** Early phase of an abnormal lymphangiogram of the pelvis and abdomen showing the lymphatics of the pelvic organs and the different anastomosis. **B.** Late phase of the lymphangiogram showing the pelvic Lymph Nodes. **C.** Close up view of the pelvis showing the lymphatic drainage of the internal iliac, external iliac, anorectal lymphatics and lymphatic vessels around the uterus and vagina.

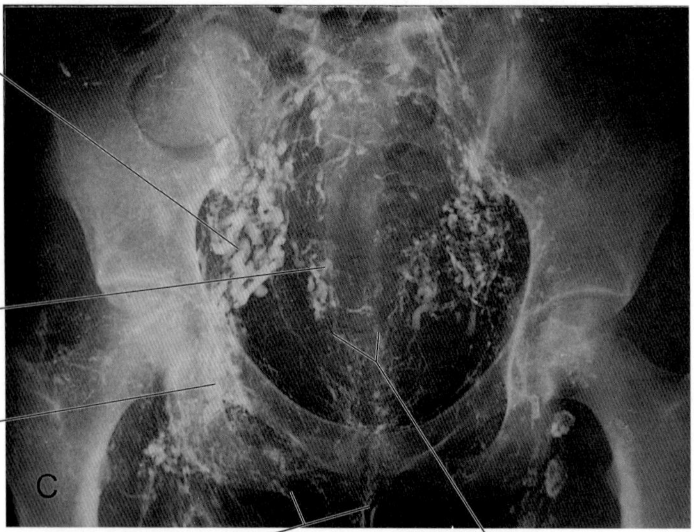

External Iliac Lymphatic Vessels

Internal Iliac Lymphatic Vessels

Inguinal Lymphatic Vessels

C

Perineal Lymphatic Vessels

Peri-Rectal Lymphatic Vessels
Vaginal, Uterine and Bladder
Vessels

Figure 21.10. *Continued*

22

ARTERIES OF THE LOWER EXTREMITY

FEMORAL ARTERY

The femoral artery is the continuation of the external iliac artery. It begins behind the inguinal ligament, and ends when it passes through the adductor canal (Figs. 22.1, 22.2).

Branches

Superficial epigastric artery
Superficial circumflex iliac artery
Superficial external pudendal artery
Deep external pudendal artery
Muscular branches
Arteria profunda femoris
Descending genicular arteries

Superficial Epigastric Artery

This artery arises about 1 cm below the inguinal ligament and anastomoses with branches of the inferior epigastric artery and the opposite vessels (See Fig. 19.1).

Superficial Circumflex Iliac Artery (Fig. 22.3)

Superficial External Pudendal Artery (Fig. 22.3)

Deep External Pudendal Artery (Fig. 22.3)

Muscular Branches

Arteria Profunda Femoris (Fig. 22.4)

It is the largest branch of the femoral artery and has the origin about 3.5 cm from the inguinal ligament. It arises laterally and posteriorly from the femoral artery (Figs. 22.5, 22.6, 22.7).

Branches

Lateral circumflex femoral artery
   Ascending branch
   Descending branch
Medial circumflex femoral artery
Perforating arteries. Usually three (Fig. 22.4)
   1st Perforating artery
   2nd Perforating artery
     Femoral nutrient artery
   3rd Perforating artery

The end of arteria profunda femoris is called 4th perforating. Numerous muscular branches are present at that level
Anastomoses
   Gluteal arteries - with terminal branches of the medial circumflex femoral artery
   Circumflex femoral arteries - with 1st perforating artery
   Perforating arteries - with each other
   4th Perforating artery - with superior muscular branches of popliteal arteries

Descending Genicular Artery (Figs. 22.1 and 22.8)

This artery branches from the superficial femoral artery before the adductor's canal and anastomoses with medial superior genicular artery.

Branches

Saphenous branch. Anastomoses with medial inferior genicular artery
Muscular branches. Articular branches

POPLITEAL ARTERY

The popliteal artery is the continuation of the superficial femoral artery passing the adductor's canal, continuing until branching into anterior and posterior tibial arteries (Figs. 22.8, 22.9).

Branches

Cutaneous branches
Superior muscular branches
Sural arteries
Superior genicular arteries
Middle genicular artery
Inferior genicular arteries

Cutaneous Branches

Superior Muscular Branches (Figs. 22.10 and 22.11)

Two or three branches

Sural Arteries (Figs. 22.9 and 22.12)

Two arteries as a rule

Superior Genicular Arteries
(Figs. 22.8, 22.9, 22.10 and 22.13)

Branches

Medial superior genicular artery
    Anastomoses with descending genicular artery and
    medial inferior genicular artery
Lateral superior genicular artery
    Anastomoses with the descending lateral circum-
    flex, with the lateral inferior genicular artery,
    descending genicular artery, medial superior
    genicular artery

Middle Genicular Artery
(Figs. 22.8, 22,9, 22.10 and 22.13)

This artery is small and not always recognizable.

Inferior Genicular Arteries
(Figs. 22.8, 22.9, 22.10, 22.13 and 22.14)

Branches

Medial inferior genicular artery
    Anastomoses with the lateral inferior genicular
    artery, the medial superior genicular artery,
    anterior tibial recurrent artery and the saphe-
    nous branch and the descending genicular
    artery.
Lateral inferior genicular artery
    Anastomosis with the medial inferior genicular
    artery, the lateral superior genicular artery, ante-
    rior and posterior tibial recurrent circumflex
    peroneal artery.

Genicular Anastomosis (Figs. 22.8 and 22.14)

Superficial Network

    Fascia
    Skin
    Fat

Deep Network

    Articular surface
    Bone
    Marrow
    Capsule
    Synovial membrane

Participating Vessels

    Medial genicular artery
    Lateral genicular artery
    Descending genicular artery
    Descending branch of lateral circumflex femoral
    Circumflex peroneal
    Anterior tibial recurrent arteries
    Posterior tibial recurrent arteries

The popliteal artery branches into the anterior and
posterior tibial arteries. It is also called trifurcation of
the popliteal artery. The initial portion of the posteri-
or tibial artery is commonly called tibial peroneal
trunk (Figs. 22.15, 22.16). Some variations in the
popliteal trifurcation are encountered (Fig. 22.17).

ANTERIOR TIBIAL ARTERY

This artery is one of the terminal branches of the
popliteal artery. It originates in the back of the leg
and passes forward between the two heads of tibialis
posterior muscle and through the upper part of the
interosseous membrane to the front of the leg, medial to the neck of the fibula, descending to the ankle
and continuing to the dorsum of the foot where it is
named arteria dorsalis pedis (dorsal artery of the
foot). Sometimes the anterior tibial artery originates
high in the middle of the popliteal artery.

Branches (Figs. 22.18, 22.19)

Posterior tibial recurrent artery
Anterior tibial recurrent artery
Muscular branches
Anterior medial malleolar artery
Anterior lateral malleolar artery

Posterior Tibial Recurrent Artery (Fig. 22.15)

This inconstant branch arises before crossing the
interosseous membrane.

Anterior Tibial Recurrent Artery (Figs. 22.15, 22.16)

This artery arises from the frontal part of the anterior tibial artery, after crossing the interosseous membrane.

Muscular Branches (Figs. 22.16)

Muscular branches are numerous and anastomose
with the posterior tibial and peroneal artery.

Anterior Medial Malleolar Artery (Figs. 22.20, 22.21)

This artery anastomoses with the posterior tibial
artery and medial plantar artery.

Anterior Lateral Malleolar Artery (Fig. 22.21)

The anterior lateral malleolar artery anastomoses
with the perforating branch of the peroneal artery and
ascending twigs from lateral tarsal artery.

Anastomosis at the Ankle Level (Fig. 22.18)

Medial malleolar network
    Anterior medial malleolar branch of anterior tibial
        artery
    Medial tarsal branch of dorsalis pedis

Malleolar - Calcanean branches of posterior tibial arteries
Branches from the medial plantar artery
Lateral malleolar network
Anterior lateral malleolar branch of anterior tibial artery
Lateral tarsal branch of dorsalis pedis
Perforating and calcanean branch of peroneal and twigs from the lateral plantar artery

ARTERIES OF THE FOOT

The anterior arteries of the foot are distal branches of the anterior tibial artery.

Anterior Tibial Branches in the Foot
(Figs. 22.22, 22.23, 22.24, 22.25, 22.26)

Arteria Dorsalis Pedis (Dorsal Artery of the Foot)

Extension of the anterior tibial artery on the dorsal aspect of the foot.

Branches

Tarsal arteries
Laterals
Medials - join the medial malleolar network
Arcuate artery
Anastomoses with the lateral tarsal and lateral plantar arteries; gives off the 2nd, 3rd, and 4th dorsal metatarsal arteries
Dorsal metatarsal arteries

Joined by the proximal and distal perforating arteries from the plantar arch, and plantar metatarsal arteries respectively. The dorsal metatarsal arteries divide distally into two dorsal digital branches for the sides of adjoining toes. The 4th dorsal metatarsal artery gives off a lateral branch to the 5th toe.

The 1st dorsal metatarsal artery arises from the dorsal artery of the foot before it passes into the sole branching distally to the great toe and to the adjoining sides of the first and 2nd toes.

POSTERIOR TIBIAL ARTERY

This artery arises from the popliteal artery after the bifurcation with the anterior tibial artery. The segment before giving off the peroneal artery is commonly called the tibial-peroneal trunk positioned in between the tibia and fibula. The posterior tibial artery passes downwards on the back of the leg reaching the foot and passing in the back of the medial malleolus. It divides into the medial and lateral plantar arteries (Figs. 22.16, 22.18, 22.19, 22.20, 22.22, 22.23).

Branches

Circumflex fibular artery
Peroneal artery (fibular artery)

Nutrient artery
Muscular branches
Communicating branch
Medial malleolar branches

Circumflex Fibular Artery

The circumflex fibular artery may arise from the anterior tibial artery.

Peroneal Artery (Fibular Artery)
(Figs. 22.15–22.20, 22.27–22.30)

This artery originates from the first centimeter of the posterior tibial artery and may arise directly from the popliteal artery. It is the largest branch of the posterior tibial artery.

Branches

Muscular branches
Nutrient artery of the fibula
Perforating branch (through interosseous membrane)
Arises 5 cm above the lateral malleolus. Anastomoses with the anterior lateral malleolar artery. May take the place of the arteria dorsalis pedis.
Communicating branch (anastomoses with the communicating branch of the posterior tibial artery) (Figs. 22.27–22.30).
Calcanean (terminal) branches (communicates with the calcanean branches of the posterior tibial artery, and anterior lateral malleolar artery)

Nutrient Artery of the Tibia

The nutrient artery of the tibia is one of the largest nutrient arteries in the body and arises from the proximal posterior tibial artery.

Muscular Branches

These branches provide nutrition to the muscles in the back of the leg.

Communicating Branch

The communication branch is the transverse artery in the back of the tibia and anastomoses with the communicating branch of the peroneal artery.

Medial Malleolar Branches

The medial malleolar branches are part of the malleolar network.

ARTERIES OF THE FOOT

The arteries of the foot are distal branches of the posterior tibial artery.

Posterior Tibial Branches in the Foot
(Figs. 22.20, 22.22, 22.31 – 22.34)

Calcaneal Branches

These branches anastomose with the medial malle olar arteries and calcanean branches of the peroneal artery.

Medial Plantar Artery

It is the smaller terminal plantar branch of the posterior artery. It passes along the base of the first metatarsal bone and the medial border of the first toe, anastomosing with a branch of the 1st metatarsal artery. This artery supplies three small superficial digital branches, joining the 1st, 2nd, and 3rd plantar arteries.

Lateral Plantar Artery

This artery is the largest terminal plantar branch of the posterior tibial artery. It runs lateral and distal to the base of the 5th metatarsal bone and turns medially to the area between the base of the 1st and 2nd metatarsal bone, connecting with the distal aspect of the dorsal artery of the foot, completing the plantar arch.

Branches

Muscular branches
Superficial branches
Anastomotic branches—to the lateral tarsal and arcuate arteries
Calcanean branch—occasionally present

Plantar Arch

Branches

Three perforating branches
Anastomoses with the dorsal metacarpal arteries
Four plantar metatarsal arteries
Each divides into two plantar digital arteries. Distal perforating branch joining the dorsal metatarsal artery; 1st plantar metatarsal artery springs from the junction of the lateral plantar and dorsal artery of the foot. The digital branch for the lateral side of the 5th toe arises from the lateral plantar artery.

Variations in the Arteries of the Foot

There are about six variations described for the plantar arteries of the foot (Fig. 22.35): Type Ia, Ib, Type IIa, IIb, IIc and Type III.

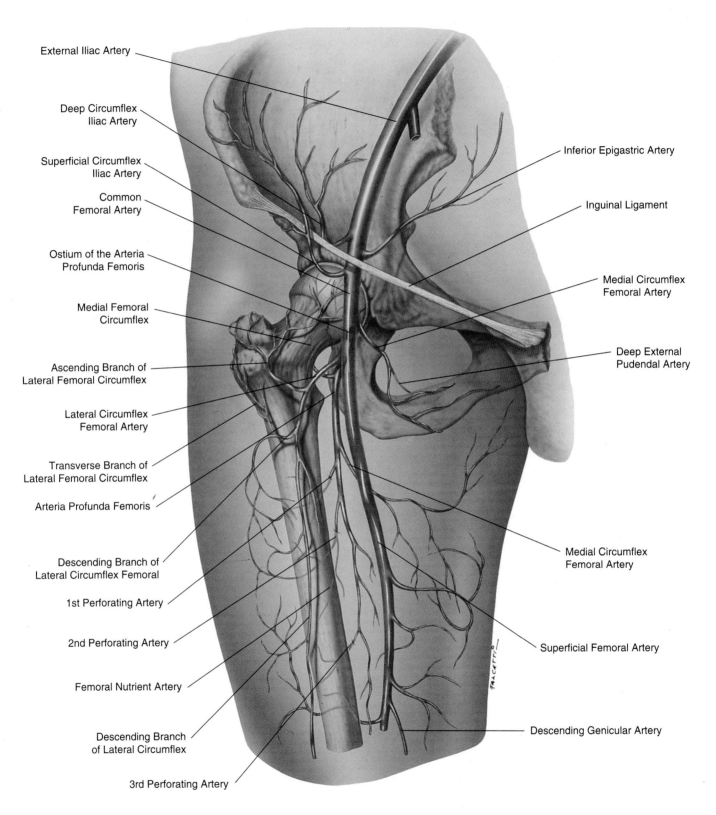

External Iliac Artery

Deep Circumflex
Iliac Artery

Superficial Circumflex
Iliac Artery

Common
Femoral Artery

Ostium of the Arteria
Profunda Femoris

Medial Femoral
Circumflex

Ascending Branch of
Lateral Femoral Circumflex

Lateral Circumflex
Femoral Artery

Transverse Branch of
Lateral Femoral Circumflex

Arteria Profunda Femoris

Descending Branch of
Lateral Circumflex Femoral

1st Perforating Artery

2nd Perforating Artery

Femoral Nutrient Artery

Descending Branch
of Lateral Circumflex

3rd Perforating Artery

Inferior Epigastric Artery

Inguinal Ligament

Medial Circumflex
Femoral Artery

Deep External
Pudendal Artery

Medial Circumflex
Femoral Artery

Superficial Femoral Artery

Descending Genicular Artery

Figure 22.1. Schematic drawing demonstrating the femoral artery and main branches. Note the perforating arteries,
branches of the arteria profunda femoris.

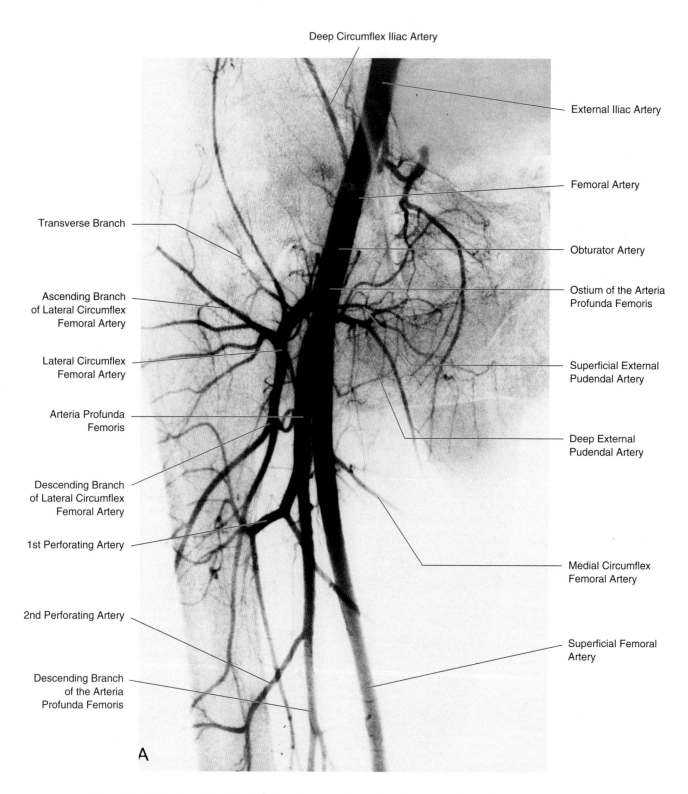

Deep Circumflex Iliac Artery

External Iliac Artery

Femoral Artery

Transverse Branch

Obturator Artery

Ascending Branch
of Lateral Circumflex
Femoral Artery

Ostium of the Arteria
Profunda Femoris

Lateral Circumflex
Femoral Artery

Superficial External
Pudendal Artery

Arteria Profunda
Femoris

Deep External
Pudendal Artery

Descending Branch
of Lateral Circumflex
Femoral Artery

1st Perforating Artery

Medial Circumflex
Femoral Artery

2nd Perforating Artery

Superficial Femoral
Artery

Descending Branch
of the Arteria
Profunda Femoris

A

Figure 22.2. A. Angiography of the right femoral artery and main branches. **B.** Late phase of the femoral arteriography showing the companion veins of the femoral artery and branches.

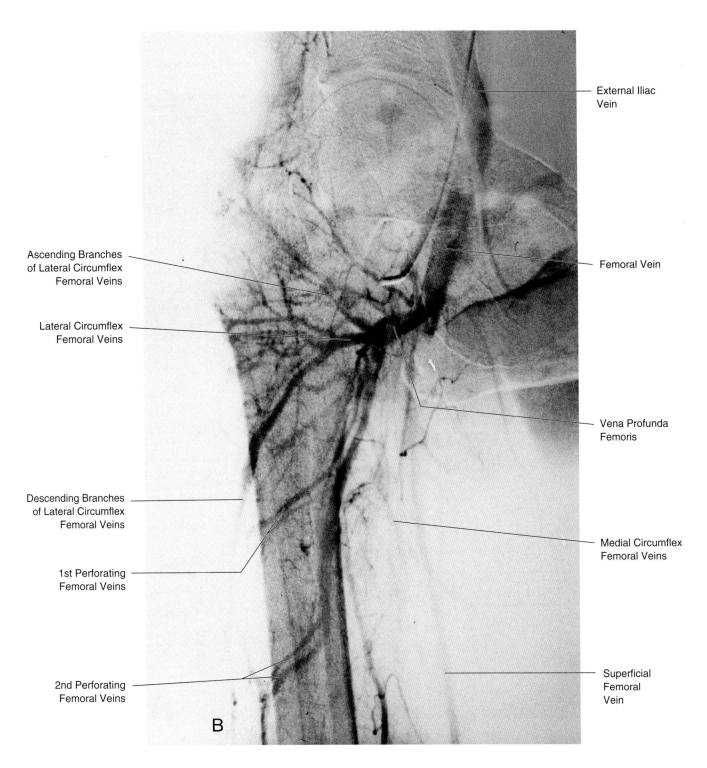

Ascending Branches
of Lateral Circumflex
Femoral Veins

Lateral Circumflex
Femoral Veins

Descending Branches
of Lateral Circumflex
Femoral Veins

1st Perforating
Femoral Veins

2nd Perforating
Femoral Veins

B

External Iliac
Vein

Femoral Vein

Vena Profunda
Femoris

Medial Circumflex
Femoral Veins

Superficial
Femoral
Vein

Figure 22.2. *Continued*

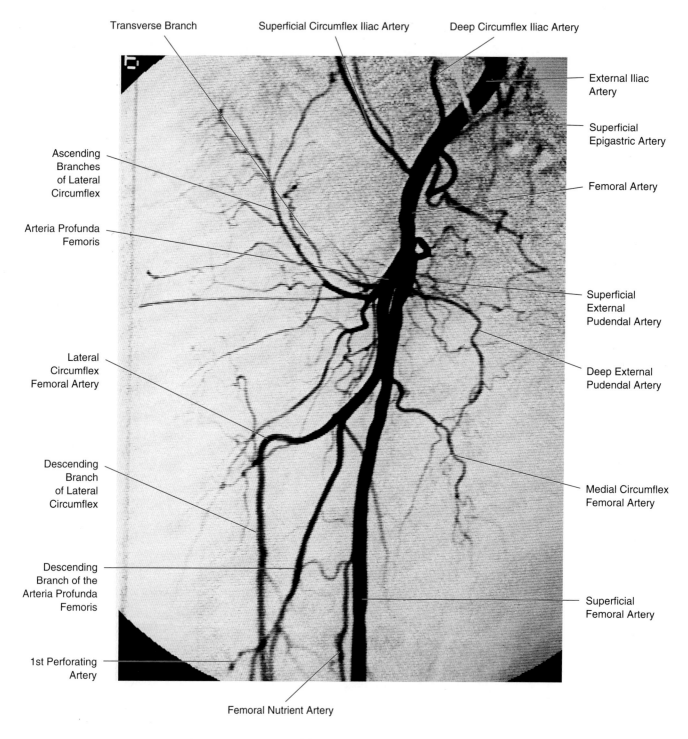

Transverse Branch

Superficial Circumflex Iliac Artery

Deep Circumflex Iliac Artery

External Iliac Artery

Superficial Epigastric Artery

Ascending Branches of Lateral Circumflex

Femoral Artery

Arteria Profunda Femoris

Superficial External Pudendal Artery

Lateral Circumflex Femoral Artery

Deep External Pudendal Artery

Descending Branch of Lateral Circumflex

Medial Circumflex Femoral Artery

Descending Branch of the Arteria Profunda Femoris

Superficial Femoral Artery

1st Perforating Artery

Femoral Nutrient Artery

Figure 22.3. Angiogram of the right femoral artery and main branches.

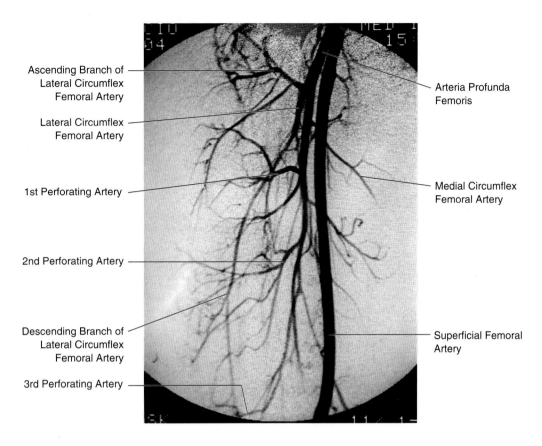

Figure 22.4. Angiogram of the right femoral artery and main branches.

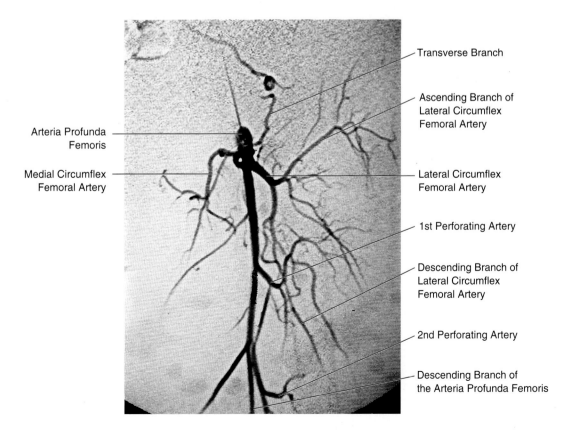

Figure 22.5. Angiogram of the left arteria profunda femoris.

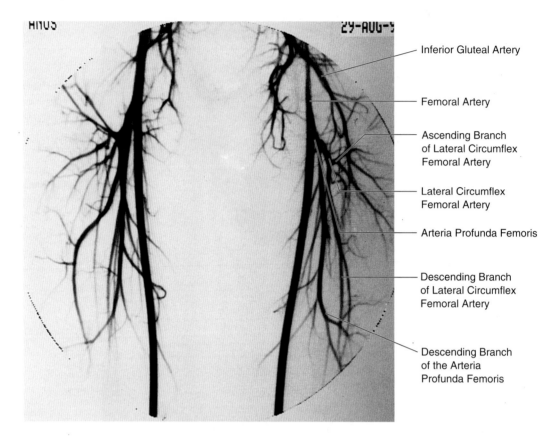

Figure 22.6. Angiogram of both femoral arteries.

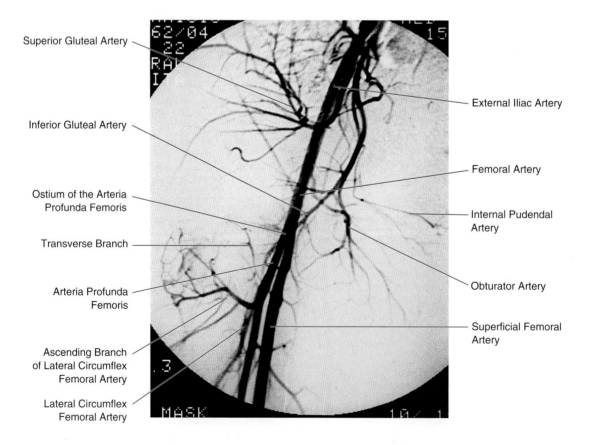

Figure 22.7. Angiogram of the right femoral artery and branches.

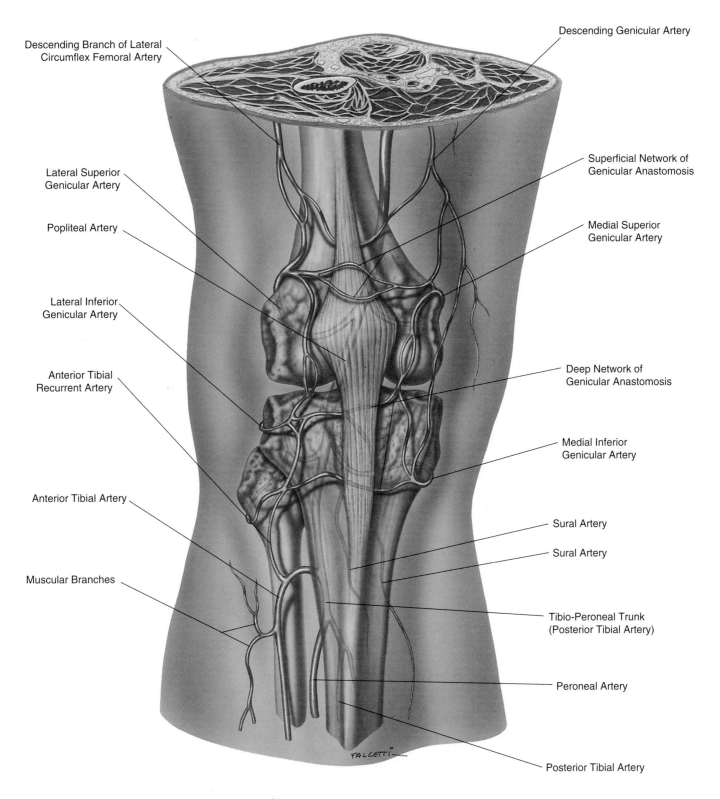

Descending Branch of Lateral Circumflex Femoral Artery

Descending Genicular Artery

Lateral Superior Genicular Artery

Superficial Network of Genicular Anastomosis

Popliteal Artery

Medial Superior Genicular Artery

Lateral Inferior Genicular Artery

Anterior Tibial Recurrent Artery

Deep Network of Genicular Anastomosis

Medial Inferior Genicular Artery

Anterior Tibial Artery

Sural Artery

Sural Artery

Muscular Branches

Tibio-Peroneal Trunk (Posterior Tibial Artery)

Peroneal Artery

Posterior Tibial Artery

Figure 22.8. Schematic drawing of the popliteal artery and knee branches, including the genicular anastomotic network.

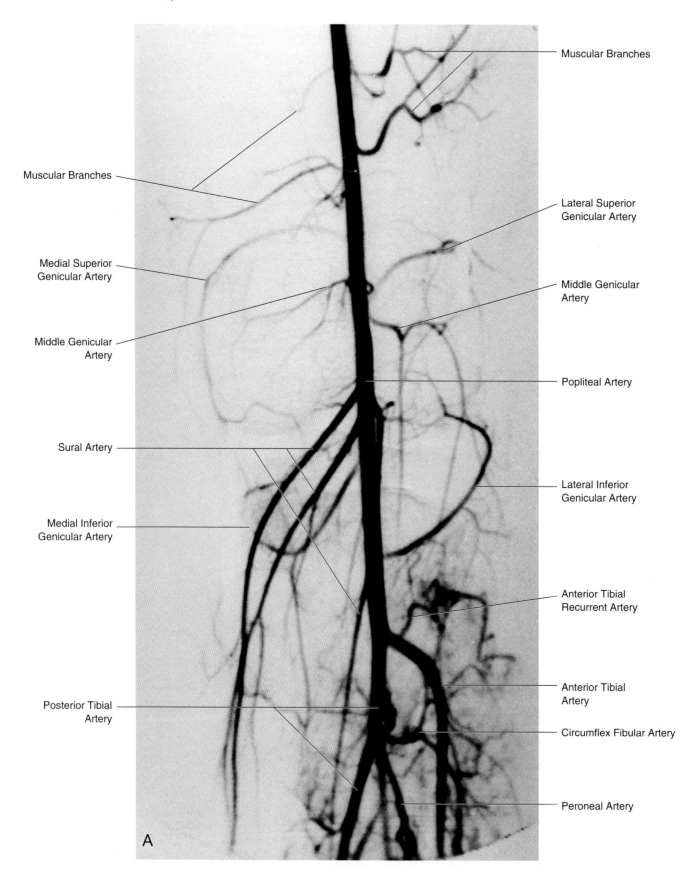

Muscular Branches

Muscular Branches

Medial Superior
Genicular Artery

Middle Genicular
Artery

Sural Artery

Medial Inferior
Genicular Artery

Posterior Tibial
Artery

Lateral Superior
Genicular Artery

Middle Genicular
Artery

Popliteal Artery

Lateral Inferior
Genicular Artery

Anterior Tibial
Recurrent Artery

Anterior Tibial
Artery

Circumflex Fibular Artery

Peroneal Artery

A

Figure 22.9. A. Anterior view of an angiogram of the popliteal artery and branches. **B.** Lateral view of the popliteal artery, showing the main branches. Note that the circumflex fibular artery supplies a hypervascular lesion in the popliteal fossa.

Middle
Genicular Artery

Muscular
Branches

Popliteal
Artery

Muscular
Branches

Lateral Superior
Genicular Artery

Medial Superior
Genicular Artery

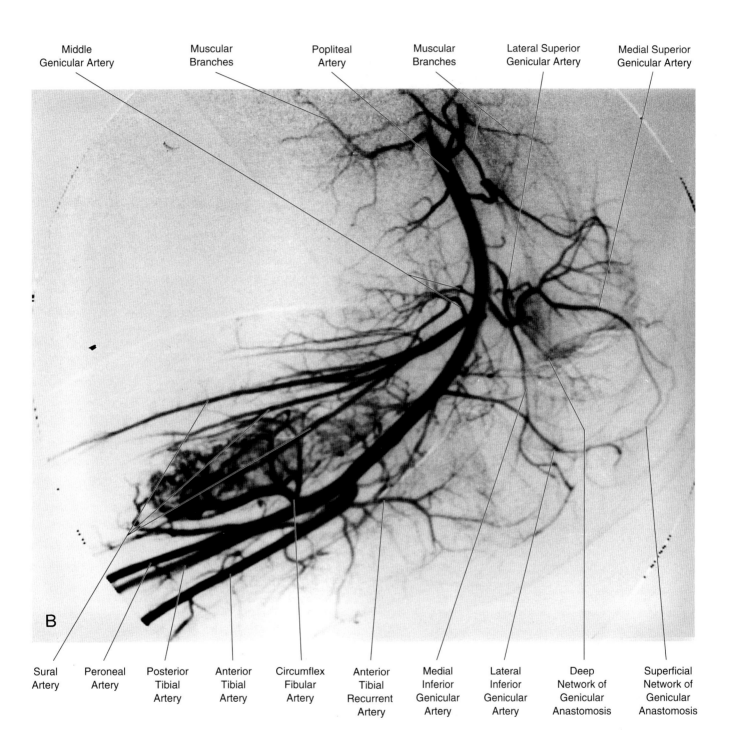

B

Sural
Artery

Peroneal
Artery

Posterior
Tibial
Artery

Anterior
Tibial
Artery

Circumflex
Fibular
Artery

Anterior
Tibial
Recurrent
Artery

Medial
Inferior
Genicular
Artery

Lateral
Inferior
Genicular
Artery

Deep
Network of
Genicular
Anastomosis

Superficial
Network of
Genicular
Anastomosis

Figure 22.9. *Continued*

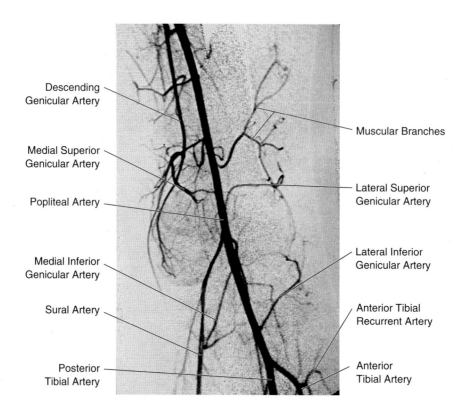

Descending Genicular Artery

Medial Superior Genicular Artery

Popliteal Artery

Medial Inferior Genicular Artery

Sural Artery

Posterior Tibial Artery

Muscular Branches

Lateral Superior Genicular Artery

Lateral Inferior Genicular Artery

Anterior Tibial Recurrent Artery

Anterior Tibial Artery

Figure 22.10. Anterior view of an angiogram of the popliteal artery and main branches.

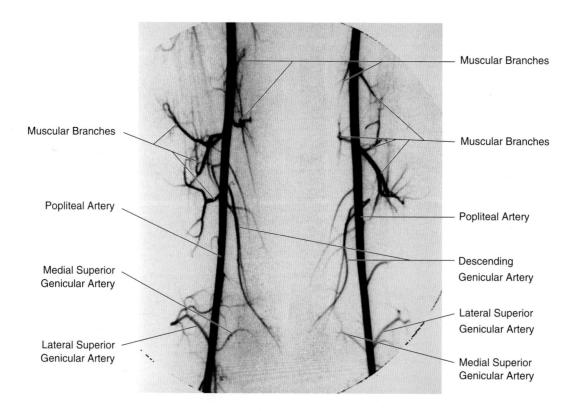

Muscular Branches

Popliteal Artery

Medial Superior Genicular Artery

Lateral Superior Genicular Artery

Muscular Branches

Muscular Branches

Popliteal Artery

Descending Genicular Artery

Lateral Superior Genicular Artery

Medial Superior Genicular Artery

Figure 22.11. Anterior view of a bilateral angiogram of the popliteal arteries and main branches.

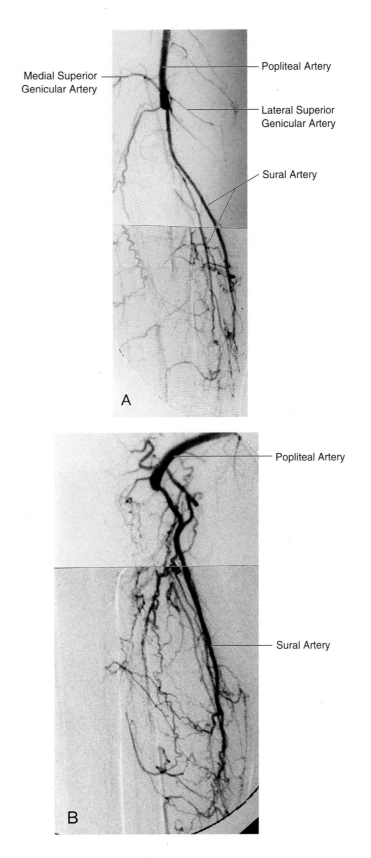

Figure 22.12. A. Anterior view of an occluded popliteal artery with the prominent sural arteries. **B.** Lateral view of the occluded popliteal artery showing the prominent sural arteries.

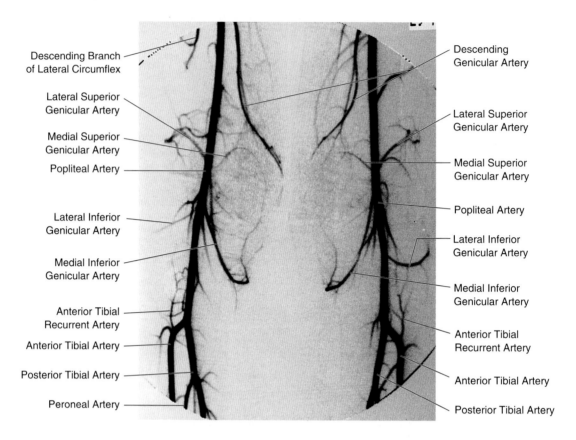

Descending Branch
of Lateral Circumflex

Lateral Superior
Genicular Artery

Medial Superior
Genicular Artery

Popliteal Artery

Lateral Inferior
Genicular Artery

Medial Inferior
Genicular Artery

Anterior Tibial
Recurrent Artery

Anterior Tibial Artery

Posterior Tibial Artery

Peroneal Artery

Descending
Genicular Artery

Lateral Superior
Genicular Artery

Medial Superior
Genicular Artery

Popliteal Artery

Lateral Inferior
Genicular Artery

Medial Inferior
Genicular Artery

Anterior Tibial
Recurrent Artery

Anterior Tibial Artery

Posterior Tibial Artery

Figure 22.13. Anterior view of an angiogram of both popliteal arteries showing the main branches.

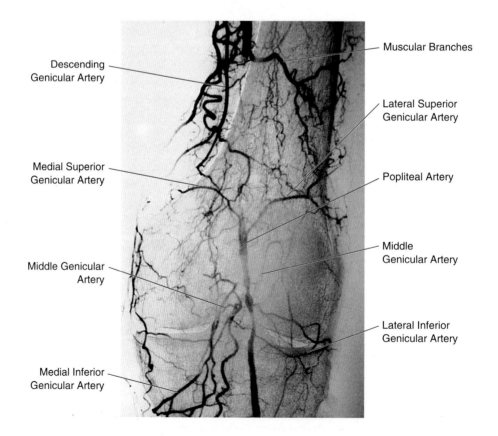

Descending
Genicular Artery

Medial Superior
Genicular Artery

Middle Genicular
Artery

Medial Inferior
Genicular Artery

Muscular Branches

Lateral Superior
Genicular Artery

Popliteal Artery

Middle
Genicular Artery

Lateral Inferior
Genicular Artery

Figure 22.14. Anterior view of an angiogram of an occluded left popliteal artery showing the prominent genicular
arteries and anastomotic branches.

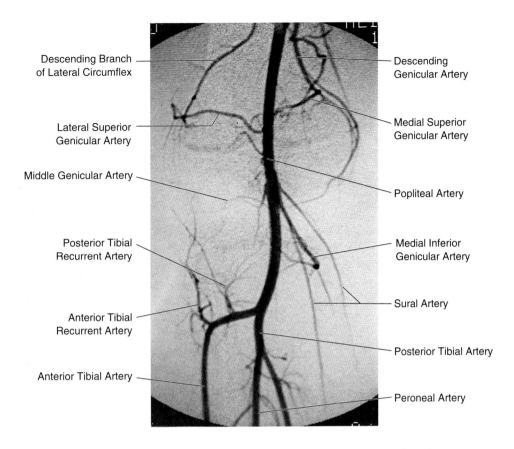

Descending Branch of Lateral Circumflex

Descending Genicular Artery

Lateral Superior Genicular Artery

Medial Superior Genicular Artery

Middle Genicular Artery

Popliteal Artery

Posterior Tibial Recurrent Artery

Medial Inferior Genicular Artery

Sural Artery

Anterior Tibial Recurrent Artery

Posterior Tibial Artery

Anterior Tibial Artery

Peroneal Artery

Figure 22.15. Anterior view of an popliteal angiogram showing the main branches.

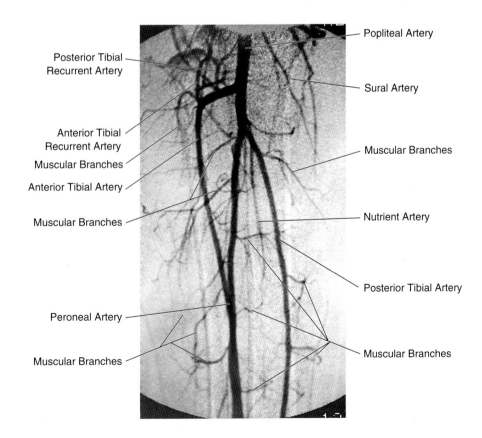

Popliteal Artery

Posterior Tibial Recurrent Artery

Sural Artery

Anterior Tibial Recurrent Artery

Muscular Branches

Muscular Branches

Anterior Tibial Artery

Nutrient Artery

Muscular Branches

Posterior Tibial Artery

Peroneal Artery

Muscular Branches

Muscular Branches

Figure 22.16. Anterior view of the popliteal artery trifurcation showing the origins of the anterior tibial artery, posterior tibial artery, and peroneal artery.

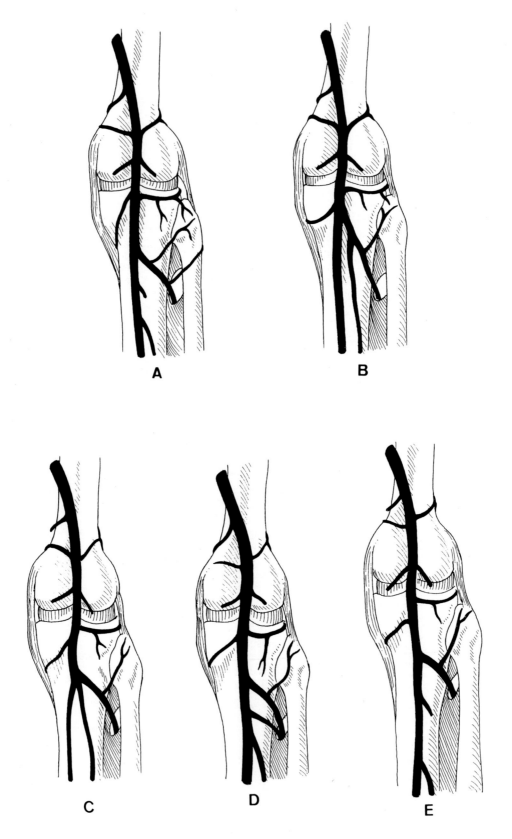

Figure 22.17. Variations of the popliteal bifurcation. A. Regular most frequent trifurcation. **B.** Tibioperoneal trunk with the anterior tibial artery. **C.** Trifurcation of the three main arteries at the same level. **D.** Anastomosis of the anterior tibial artery and tibioperoneal trunk. **E.** Long tibioperoneal trunk.

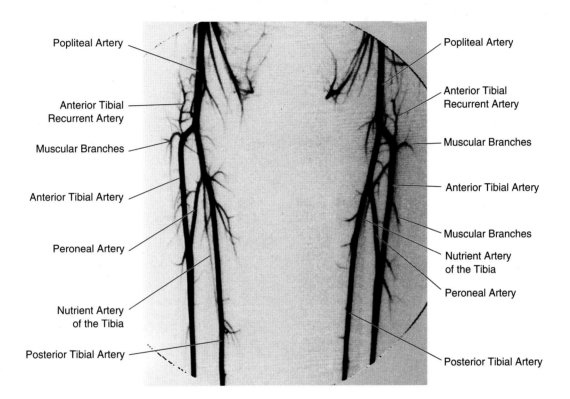

Popliteal Artery

Anterior Tibial
Recurrent Artery

Muscular Branches

Anterior Tibial Artery

Peroneal Artery

Nutrient Artery
of the Tibia

Posterior Tibial Artery

Popliteal Artery

Anterior Tibial
Recurrent Artery

Muscular Branches

Anterior Tibial Artery

Muscular Branches

Nutrient Artery
of the Tibia

Peroneal Artery

Posterior Tibial Artery

Figure 22.18. Bilateral angiogram of the trifurcation of the popliteal arteries.

Anterior Tibial Artery ——————

Posterior Tibial Artery ——————

Peroneal Artery ——————

—— Anterior Tibial Artery

—— Posterior Tibial Artery

—— Peroneal Artery

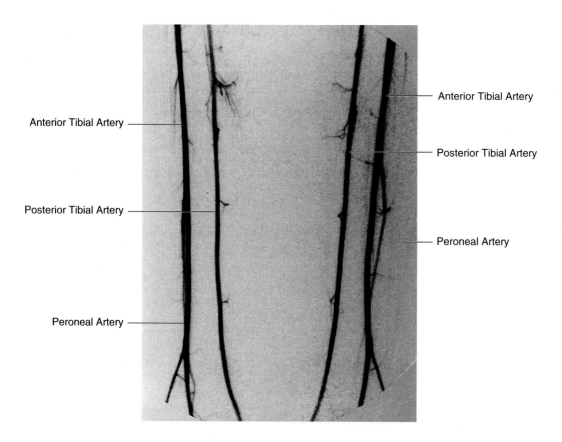

Figure 22.19. Bilateral angiogram of the distal segment of the tibial and peroneal arteries.

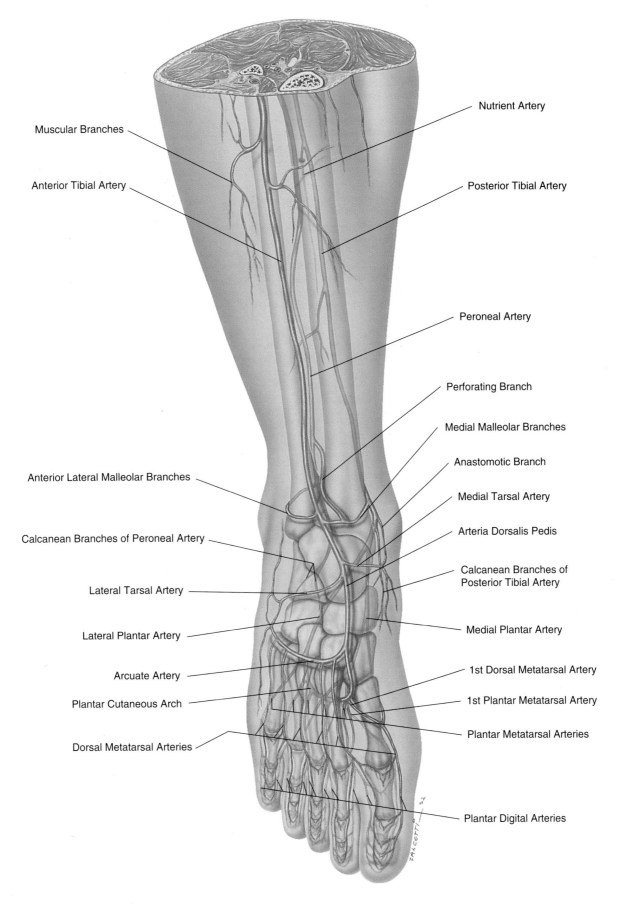

Muscular Branches

Anterior Tibial Artery

Nutrient Artery

Posterior Tibial Artery

Peroneal Artery

Perforating Branch

Medial Malleolar Branches

Anastomotic Branch

Anterior Lateral Malleolar Branches

Medial Tarsal Artery

Arteria Dorsalis Pedis

Calcanean Branches of Peroneal Artery

Calcanean Branches of Posterior Tibial Artery

Lateral Tarsal Artery

Lateral Plantar Artery

Medial Plantar Artery

Arcuate Artery

1st Dorsal Metatarsal Artery

Plantar Cutaneous Arch

1st Plantar Metatarsal Artery

Plantar Metatarsal Arteries

Dorsal Metatarsal Arteries

Plantar Digital Arteries

Figure 22.20. Schematic drawing of the arterial circulation of the ankle and foot in an anterior view.

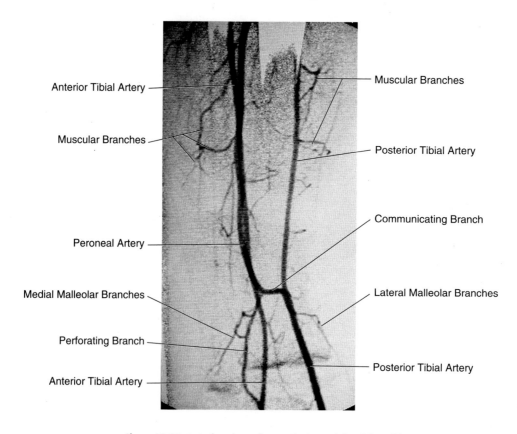

Anterior Tibial Artery

Muscular Branches

Muscular Branches

Posterior Tibial Artery

Peroneal Artery

Communicating Branch

Medial Malleolar Branches

Lateral Malleolar Branches

Perforating Branch

Anterior Tibial Artery

Posterior Tibial Artery

Figure 22.21. Anterior view of an angiogram of the right ankle.

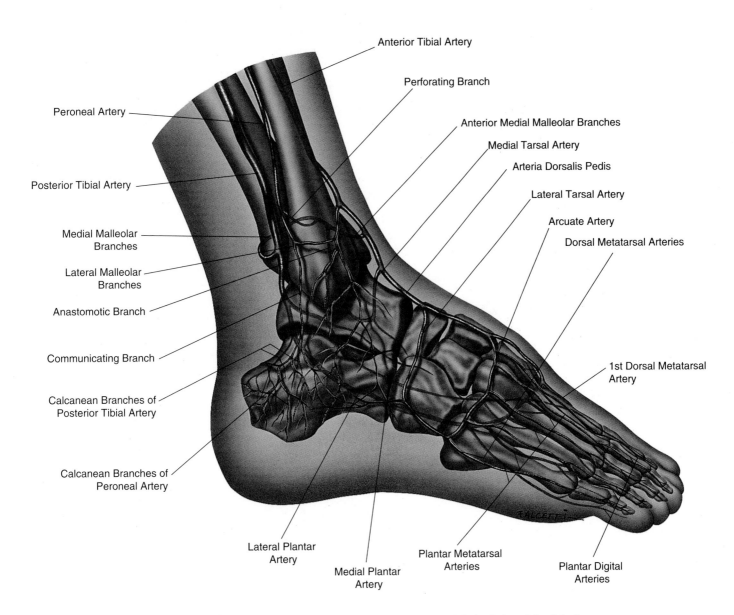

Figure 22.22. Lateral view of a schematic drawing showing the arterial circulation of the right foot.

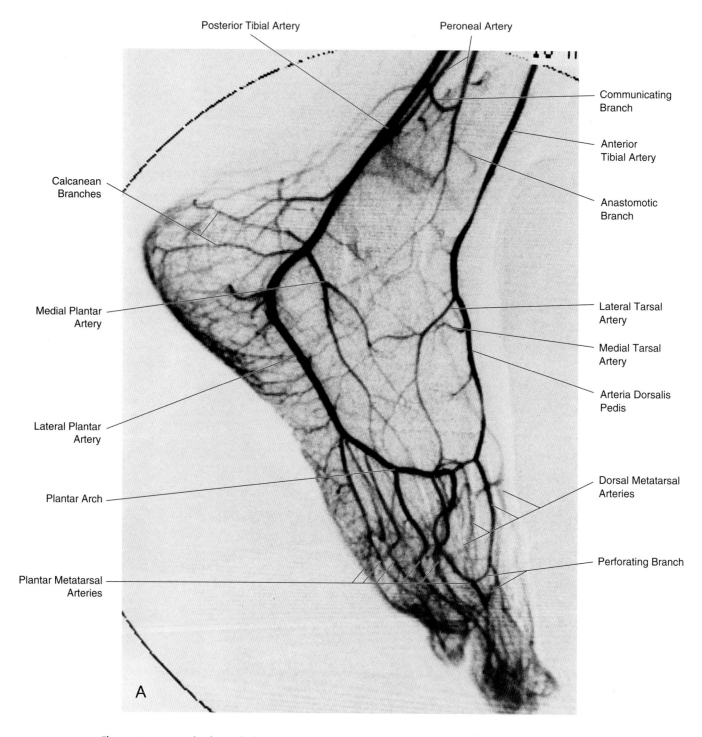

Posterior Tibial Artery

Peroneal Artery

Communicating Branch

Anterior Tibial Artery

Anastomotic Branch

Calcanean Branches

Medial Plantar Artery

Lateral Tarsal Artery

Medial Tarsal Artery

Arteria Dorsalis Pedis

Lateral Plantar Artery

Plantar Arch

Dorsal Metatarsal Arteries

Plantar Metatarsal Arteries

Perforating Branch

A

Figure 22.23. A. Early phase of a lateral view of an angiogram of the foot. **B.** Late phase of the foot angiogram showing the venous drainage of the foot.

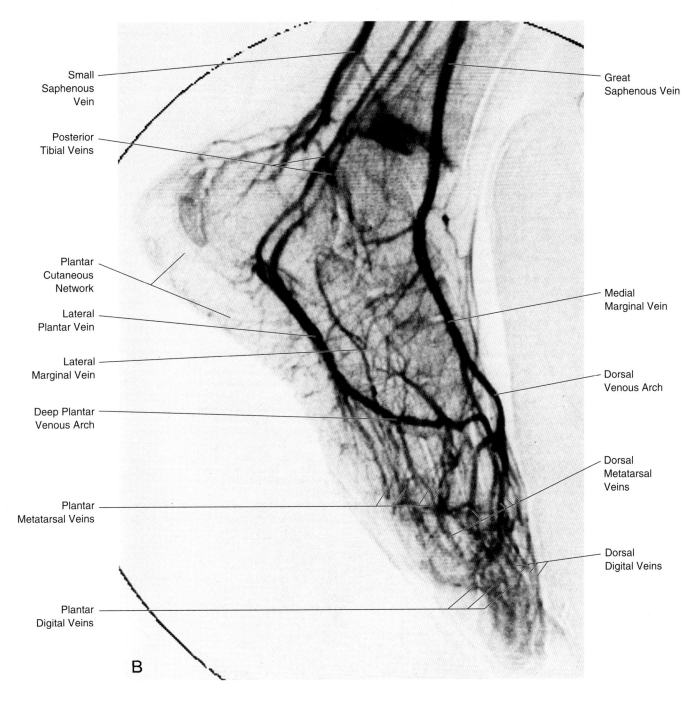

Small Saphenous Vein

Posterior Tibial Veins

Plantar Cutaneous Network

Lateral Plantar Vein

Lateral Marginal Vein

Deep Plantar Venous Arch

Plantar Metatarsal Veins

Plantar Digital Veins

Great Saphenous Vein

Medial Marginal Vein

Dorsal Venous Arch

Dorsal Metatarsal Veins

Dorsal Digital Veins

B

Figure 22.23. *Continued*

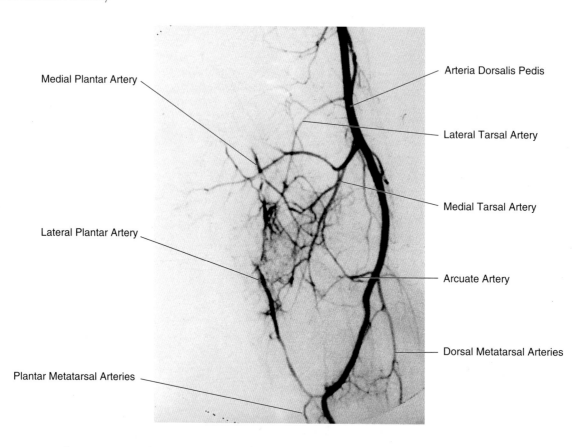

Figure 22.24. Lateral view of a superselective angiogram of the arteria dorsalis pedis and branches.

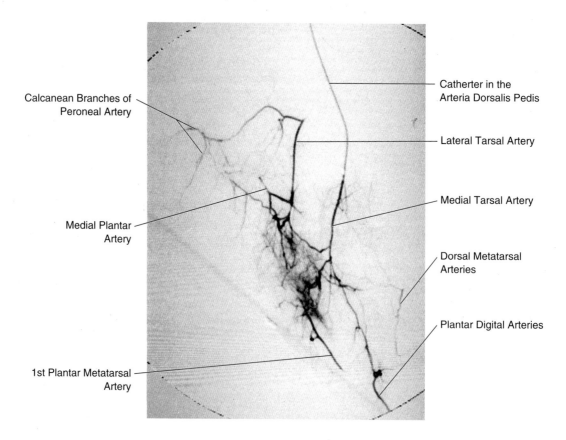

Figure 22.25. Lateral view of a superselective angiogram of the medial tarsal artery, branch of the arteria dorsalis pedis.

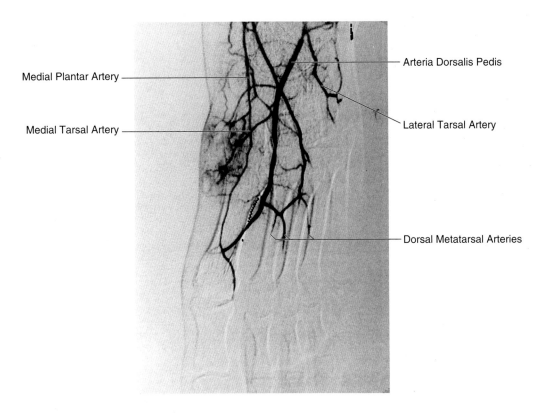

Medial Plantar Artery

Medial Tarsal Artery

Arteria Dorsalis Pedis

Lateral Tarsal Artery

Dorsal Metatarsal Arteries

Figure 22.26. Anterior view of the left foot showing the superselective injection into the arteria dorsalis pedis and main branches.

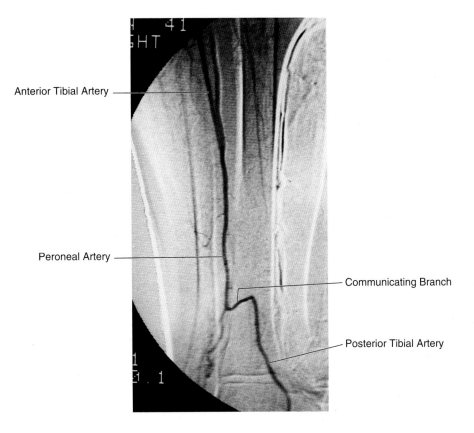

Anterior Tibial Artery

Peroneal Artery

Communicating Branch

Posterior Tibial Artery

Figure 22.27. Anterior view of an angiogram of the arterial circulation of the right ankle.

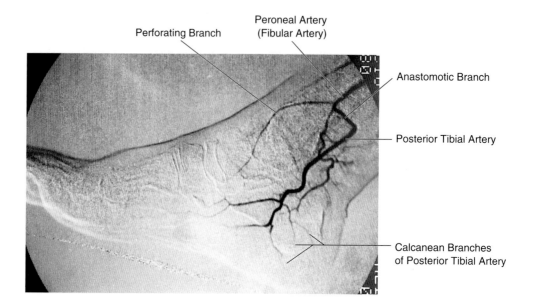

Figure 22.28. Lateral view of the angiogram of the arterial circulation of the peroneal artery and anastomotic branches with the posterior tibial artery.

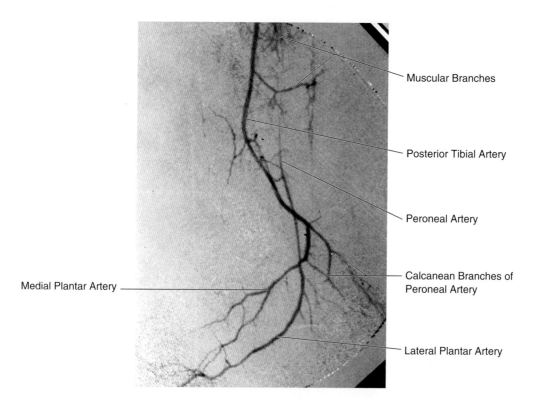

Figure 22.29. Lateral view of the angiogram of the arterial circulation of the posterior tibial artery and the calcanean branches and plantar arteries.

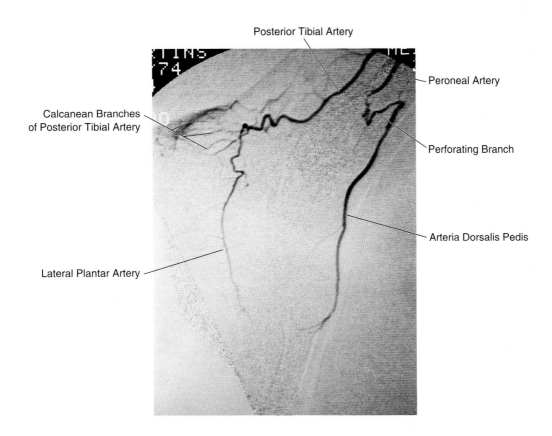

Figure 22.30. Lateral view of the angiogram of the arterial circulation of the posterior tibial artery and anastomotic branches with the anterior tibial artery and arteria dorsalis pedis.

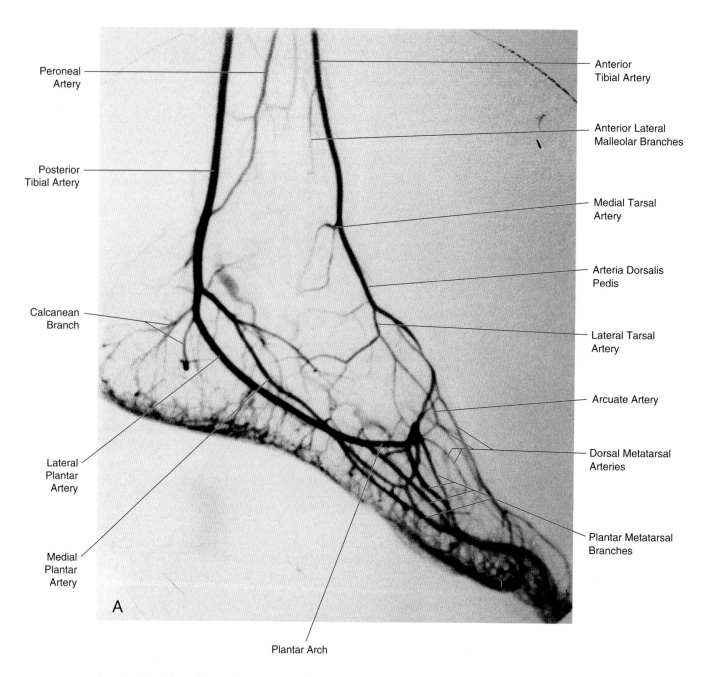

Peroneal Artery

Posterior Tibial Artery

Calcanean Branch

Lateral Plantar Artery

Medial Plantar Artery

A

Anterior Tibial Artery

Anterior Lateral Malleolar Branches

Medial Tarsal Artery

Arteria Dorsalis Pedis

Lateral Tarsal Artery

Arcuate Artery

Dorsal Metatarsal Arteries

Plantar Metatarsal Branches

Plantar Arch

Figure 22.31. A. Lateral view of an angiogram of the arterial circulation of the foot. **B.** Late phase of the angiogram of the left foot showing the venous drainage. Note that there is a venous malformation in the plantar veins of the foot.

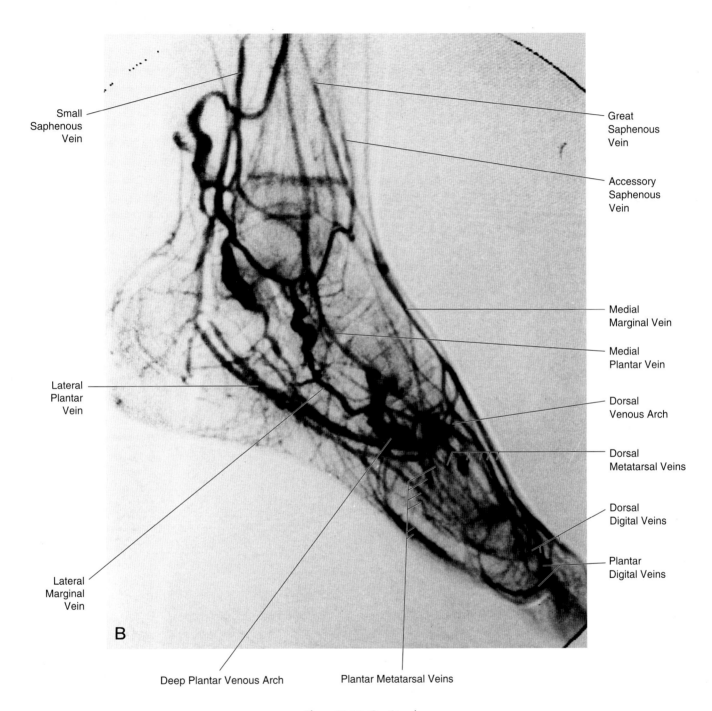

Small Saphenous Vein

Great Saphenous Vein

Accessory Saphenous Vein

Medial Marginal Vein

Medial Plantar Vein

Lateral Plantar Vein

Dorsal Venous Arch

Dorsal Metatarsal Veins

Dorsal Digital Veins

Plantar Digital Veins

Lateral Marginal Vein

B

Deep Plantar Venous Arch

Plantar Metatarsal Veins

Figure 22.31. *Continued*

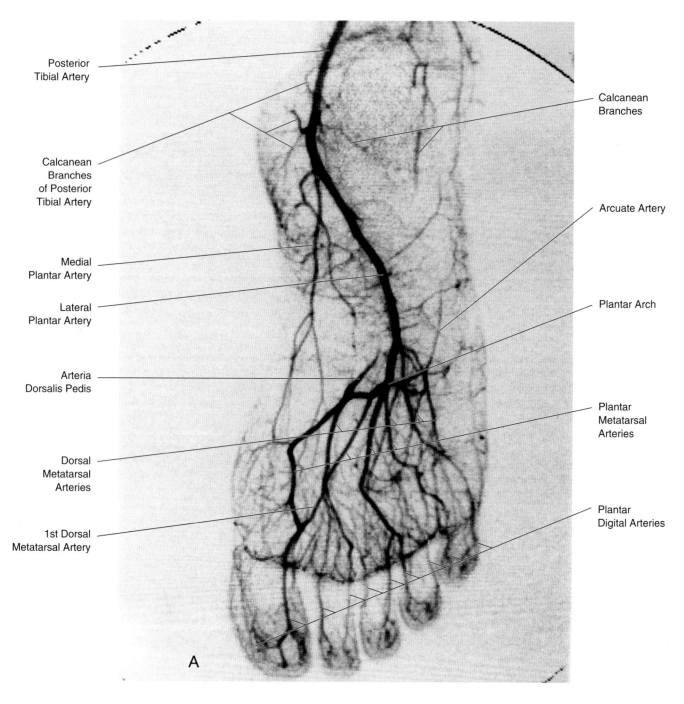

Posterior
Tibial Artery

Calcanean
Branches
of Posterior
Tibial Artery

Medial
Plantar Artery

Lateral
Plantar Artery

Arteria
Dorsalis Pedis

Dorsal
Metatarsal
Arteries

1st Dorsal
Metatarsal Artery

Calcanean
Branches

Arcuate Artery

Plantar Arch

Plantar
Metatarsal
Arteries

Plantar
Digital Arteries

A

Figure 22.32. A. Anterior view of the angiogram of the left foot with a selective injection in the posterior tibial artery, showing the plantar and metatarsal arteries as well as the plantar arch. **B.** Late phase of the angiogram of the foot showing the venous drainage and the deep plantar venous arch. **C.** Late phase of the angiogram showing the plantar cutaneous arch.

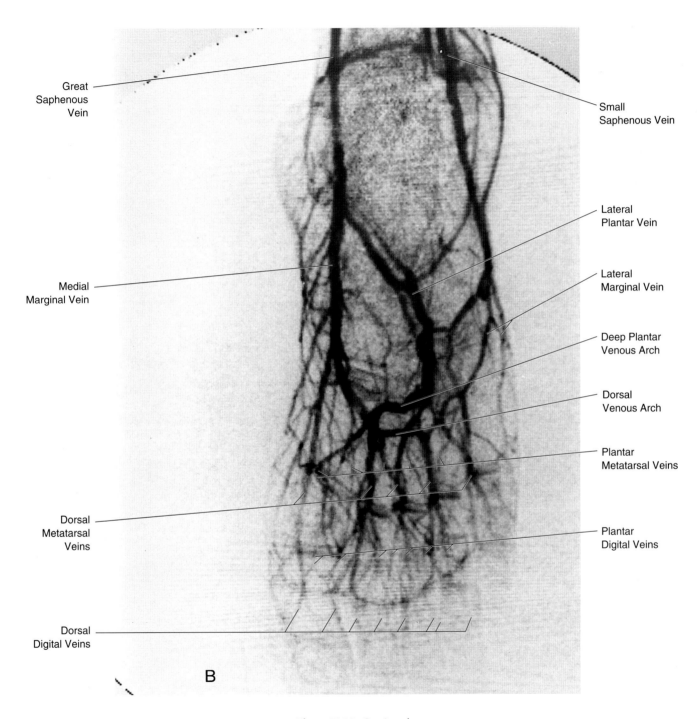

Great Saphenous Vein

Small Saphenous Vein

Lateral Plantar Vein

Medial Marginal Vein

Lateral Marginal Vein

Deep Plantar Venous Arch

Dorsal Venous Arch

Plantar Metatarsal Veins

Dorsal Metatarsal Veins

Plantar Digital Veins

Dorsal Digital Veins

B

Figure 22.32. *Continued*

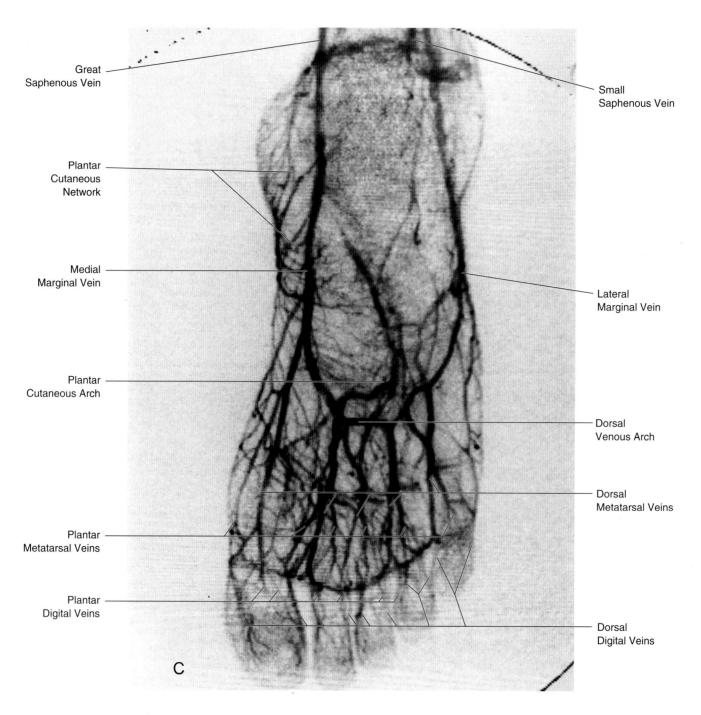

Great Saphenous Vein

Small Saphenous Vein

Plantar Cutaneous Network

Medial Marginal Vein

Lateral Marginal Vein

Plantar Cutaneous Arch

Dorsal Venous Arch

Dorsal Metatarsal Veins

Plantar Metatarsal Veins

Plantar Digital Veins

Dorsal Digital Veins

C

Figure 22.32. *Continued*

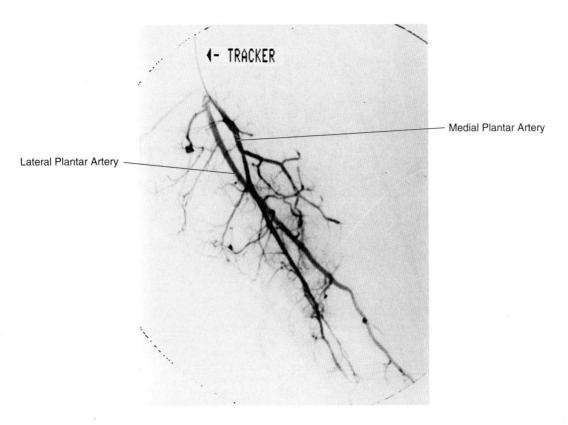

Figure 22.33. Superselective angiography of the lateral and medial plantar arteries.

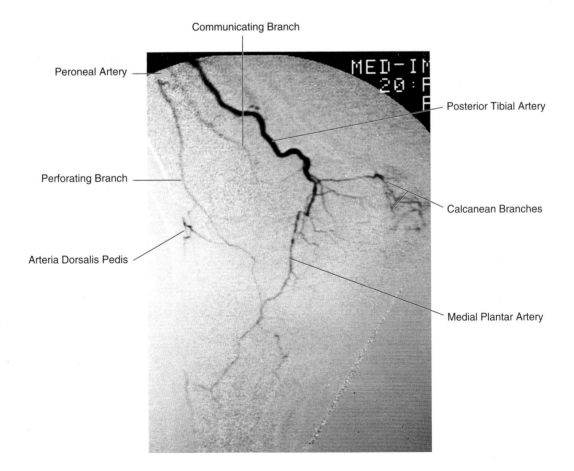

Figure 22.34. Lateral view of the foot with occlusion of the anterior tibial artery, showing the anastomosis between the anterior and posterior systems.

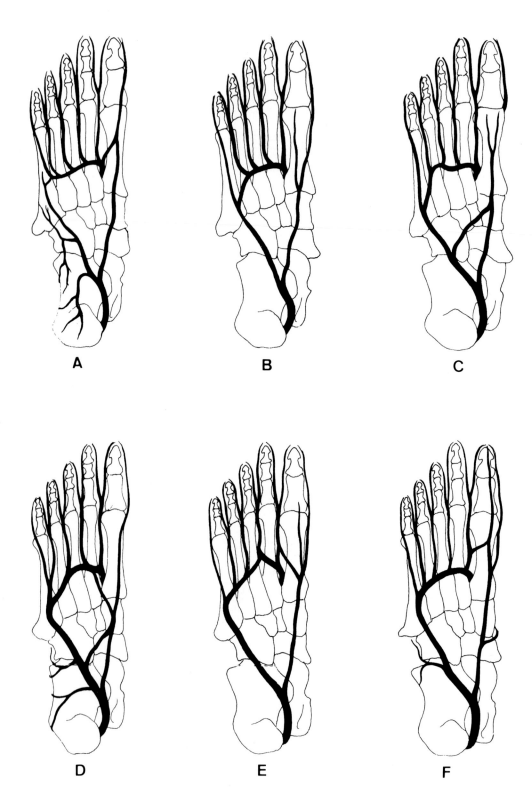

Figure 22.35. Variations of the plantar arteries. A. Type Ia - deep plantar artery originated from the anterior dorsalis pedis, which gives origin to all the metatarsal arteries. **B.** Type Ib - deep plantar artery originated from the arteria dorsalis pedis and partially from the lateral plantar artery. **C.** Type IIa - lateral plantar artery originates the 4th space metatarsal artery.

D. Type IIb - lateral plantar artery originates the 4th, 3th metatarsal arteries. **E.** Type IIc - lateral plantar artery originates the 4th, 3th, and 2nd metatarsal arteries. **F.** Type III - lateral plantar artery after originating the metatarsal arteries goes to the dorsal aspect of the foot and communicates with the arteria dorsalis pedis.

23

VEINS OF THE LOWER EXTREMITY

The veins of the lower extremities may be divided in two main groups, deep and superficial. The superficial veins are found under the skin in the superficial fascia. The deep venous system accompany the arteries. Valves are present in both systems, but are more numerous in the deep veins.

SUPERFICIAL VEINS OF THE LOWER LIMB

The main named superficial veins are the great (long, magna) and small (lesser, parva) saphenous veins. Most of the tributaries to this system are unnamed (Fig. 23.1).

Great (Long, Magna, Internal) Saphenous Vein

This vein begins in the medial marginal vein of the foot and end in the femoral vein below the inguinal ligament. It is often duplicated below the knee (Fig. 23.2).

Tributaries

At the ankle - medial marginal vein
In the leg - free communications with the small saphenous vein and deep veins, perforating veins, frontal vein, tibial malleolus vein and from the calf
In the thigh - from the medial and posterior aspect, may form the accessory saphenous vein

Tributaries

Superficial epigastric
Superficial circumflex iliac
Superficial external pudendal vein
Thoraco epigastric vein

Small (Short, Parva, External, Lesser) Saphenous Vein

This vein is a continuation of the lateral marginal vein of the foot, at the back of the leg, ending in the popliteal vein. It receives numerous cutaneous tributaries and communicates with the great saphenous vein (Fig. 23.3).

Perforating Veins

The great and lesser saphenous veins are connected with the deep veins through the perforating veins. The perforating veins have valves arranged so that normally they prevent the flow of blood from the deep to the superficial veins.

The perforating veins are found in the foot, leg, and thigh.

In the Foot

There are four perforating veins.

One 2.5 cm below the medial malleolus
One 3.5 cm below and anterior to the medial malleolus
Two 3.0 cm below and anterior to the lateral malleolus

In the Leg

There are 16 constant perforating veins.

8 drain into the posterior tibial veins (Cockett's and Boyd's veins)
4 drain into the peroneal veins
4 drain into the soleal and gemelar veins

In the Thigh

There are two constant perforating veins (Dodd's Group or perforating veins of Hunter)

DEEP VEINS OF THE LOWER LIMB

These veins are companions of the arteries and their branches.

In the Foot (Figs. 23.1, 23.5, 23.6)

The plantar digital veins arise from plexuses on the surface of the digits and communicate with the dorsal digital veins and join to form four plantar metatarsal veins.

The plantar metatarsal veins communicate through perforating veins with the veins of the dorsum of the foot forming the deep plantar venous arch, accompanying the plantar arterial arch.

The medial and lateral plantar veins run backwards, arising from the deep plantar venous arch, following the corresponding tract of the arteries. After communicating with the great and small saphenous veins, they join behind the medial malleolus to form the posterior tibial veins.

In the Leg (Fig. 23.6, 23.7)

Posterior Tibial Veins (Fig. 23.8)

These veins are companions of the posterior tibial artery. Major effluents are peroneal veins (companions of the peroneal artery) and perforating veins from the superficial system.

Anterior Tibial Veins (Fig. 23.8)

The anterior tibial veins are companions of the anterior tibial artery and dorsal artery of the foot. They cross the interosseous membrane and join the posterior tibial veins to form the popliteal veins.

Popliteal Vein (Figs. 23.9, 23.10)

This vein follows an upward direction through the popliteal fossa and the adductor's canal, where it is named femoral vein. Tributaries are the small saphenous vein, gastrocnemius veins, and other muscular veins.

In the Thigh

Femoral Vein (Superficial Femoral Vein) (Fig. 23.11)

This vein follows the tract of the femoral artery as the continuation of the popliteal vein, ending about the level of the inguinal ligament, becoming the external iliac vein. At this level, it is sometimes called common femoral vein. At the inguinal ligament, the vein is medial to the corresponding artery, occupying the middle compartment of the femoral sheath.

Tributaries are muscular veins, vena profunda femoris (deep femoral vein), and the great saphenous vein. The lateral and medial circumflex femoral veins are also usual tributaries.

The vena profunda femoris is anterior to the arteria profunda femoris and receives muscular tributaries and perforating branches, establishing anastomoses with the popliteal vein (below it) and inferior gluteal vein.

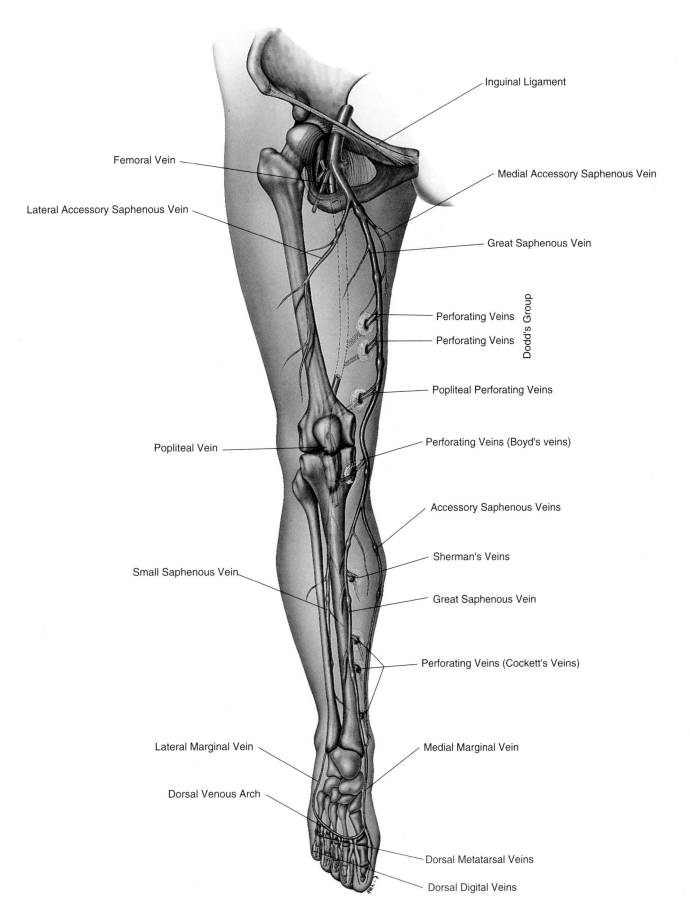

Figure 23.1. Schematic drawing showing the superficial venous system of the lower extremity.

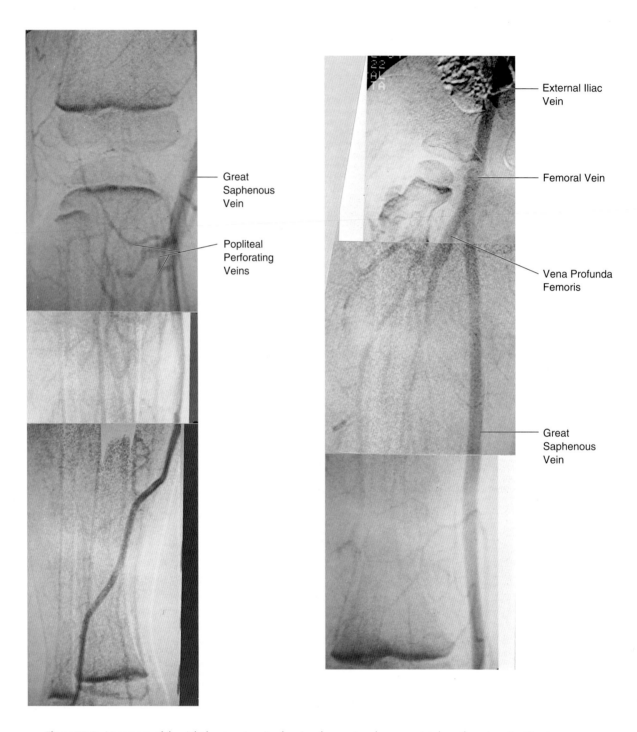

Figure 23.2.   Venogram of the right lower extremity showing the great saphenous vein along the extremity. Due to hypoplasia of the deep venous system, the superficial venous system is prominent.

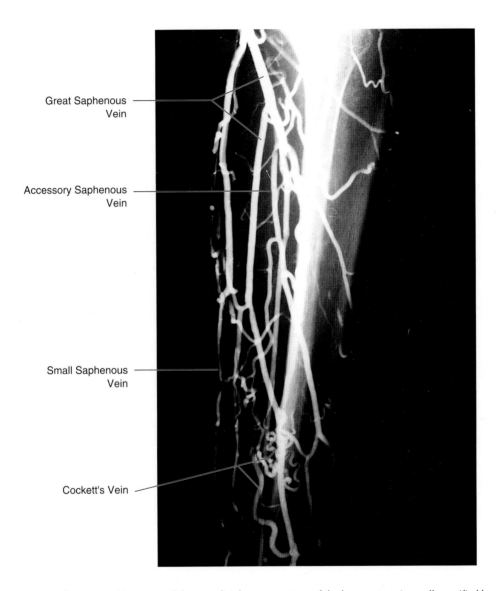

Great Saphenous Vein

Accessory Saphenous Vein

Small Saphenous Vein

Cockett's Vein

Figure 23.3. Venogram of the superficial venous system of the lower extremity, well opacified because of obstruction of the deep venous system.

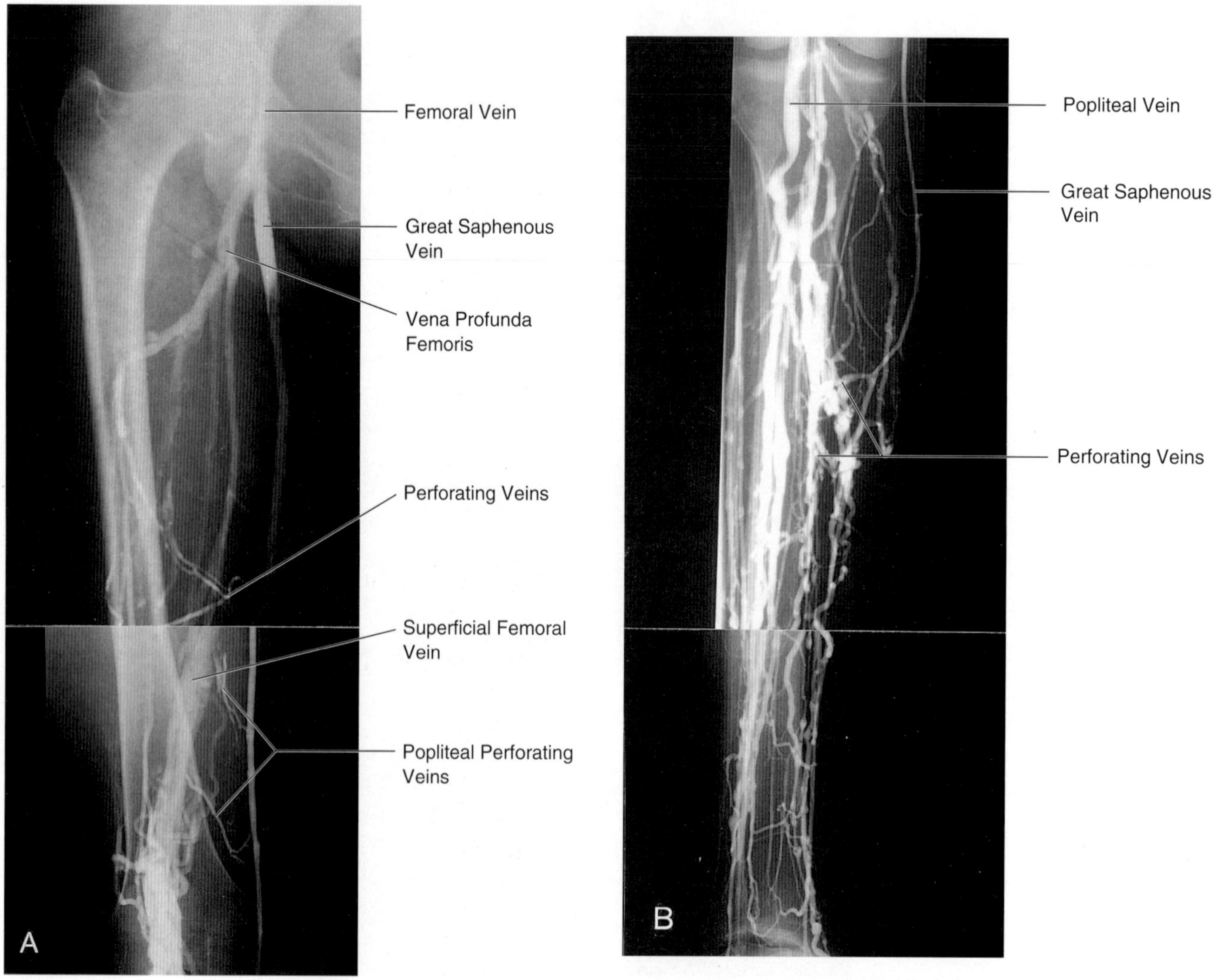

Figure 23.4. A, B. Venogram of the superficial and deep venous system of the right lower extremity.

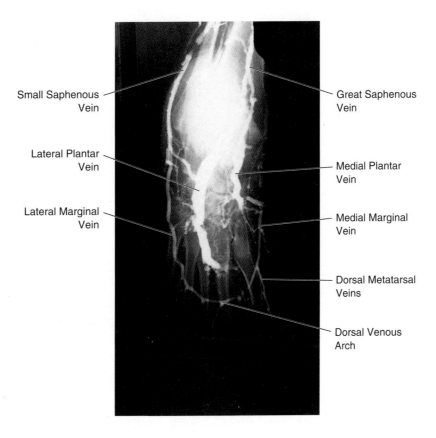

Small Saphenous
Vein

Great Saphenous
Vein

Lateral Plantar
Vein

Medial Plantar
Vein

Lateral Marginal
Vein

Medial Marginal
Vein

Dorsal Metatarsal
Veins

Dorsal Venous
Arch

Figure 23.5. Venogram of the right foot.

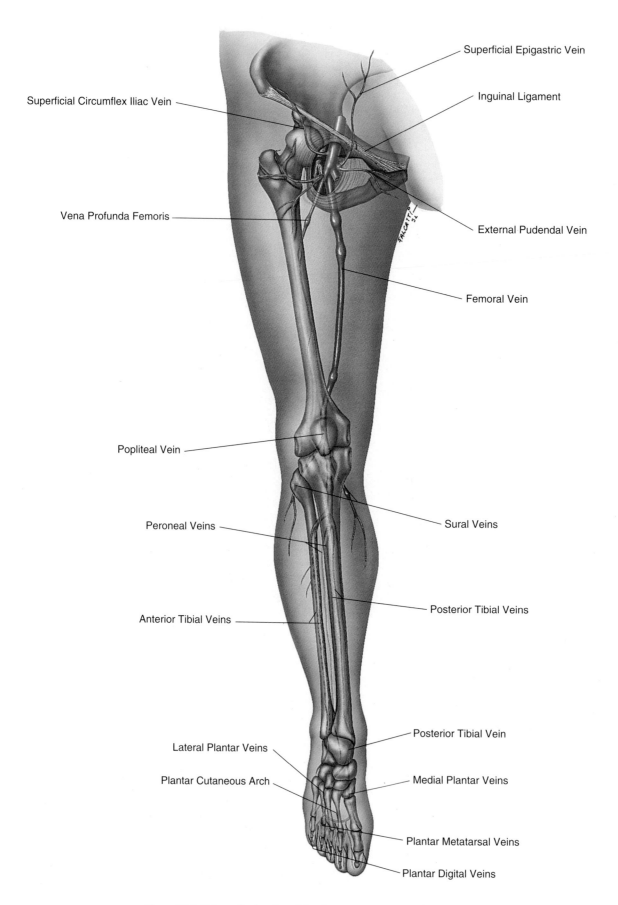

Superficial Epigastric Vein

Inguinal Ligament

Superficial Circumflex Iliac Vein

External Pudendal Vein

Vena Profunda Femoris

Femoral Vein

Popliteal Vein

Sural Veins

Peroneal Veins

Posterior Tibial Veins

Anterior Tibial Veins

Posterior Tibial Vein

Lateral Plantar Veins

Medial Plantar Veins

Plantar Cutaneous Arch

Plantar Metatarsal Veins

Plantar Digital Veins

Figure 23.6. Schematic drawing of the deep venous system of the lower extremity.

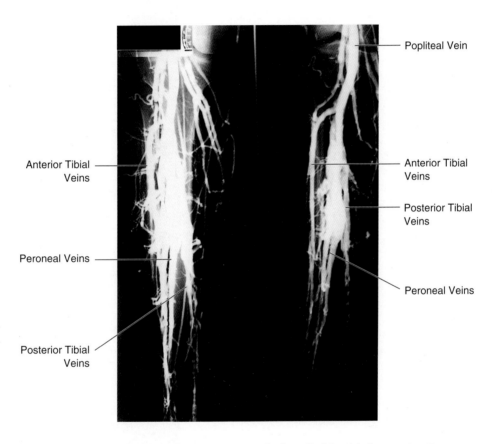

Figure 23.7. Venogram of the deep venous system in the calf of the right lower extremity.

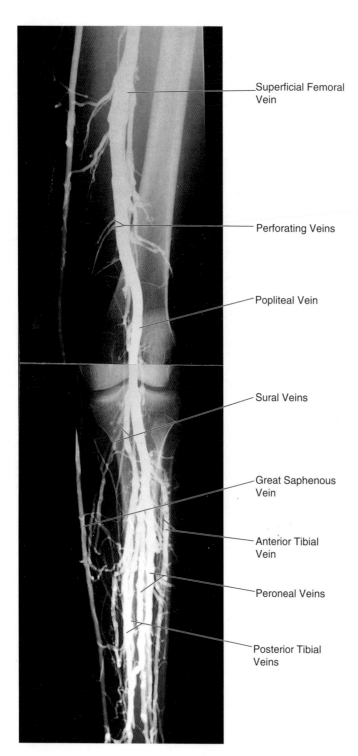

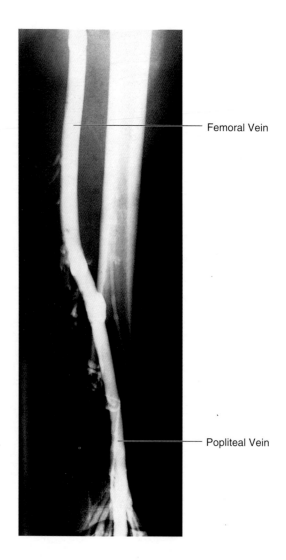

Superficial Femoral
Vein

Perforating Veins

Popliteal Vein

Sural Veins

Great Saphenous
Vein

Anterior Tibial
Vein

Peroneal Veins

Posterior Tibial
Veins

Femoral Vein

Popliteal Vein

Figure 23.9. Venogram of the deep venous system of the left lower extremity showing the popliteal and femoral vein.

Figure 23.8. Venogram of the deep venous system of the left lower extremity.

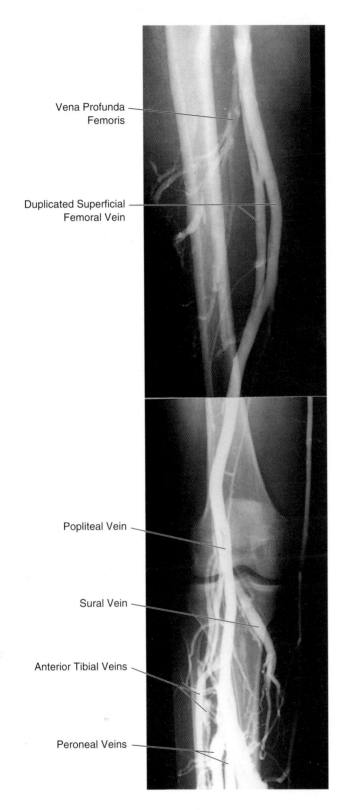

Vena Profunda Femoris

Duplicated Superficial Femoral Vein

Popliteal Vein

Sural Vein

Anterior Tibial Veins

Peroneal Veins

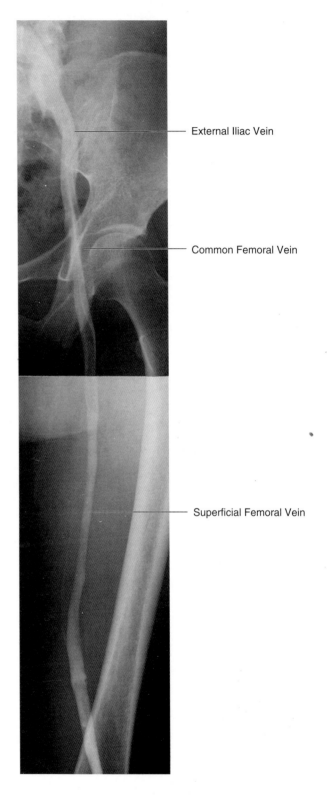

External Iliac Vein

Common Femoral Vein

Superficial Femoral Vein

Figure 23.10. Venogram of the deep venous system of the left lower extremity showing the popliteal and femoral vein. Note that there is a partial duplication of the superficial femoral vein.

Figure 23.11. Venogram of the left lower extremity showing the superficial femoral vein, the common femoral vein, and the left iliac vein.

24

LYMPHATIC SYSTEM OF THE LOWER EXTREMITY

SUPERFICIAL LYMPHATIC DRAINAGE

The superficial lymphatic vessels drain the superficial tissues, beginning in lymphatic plexuses beneath the skin. The foot is drained by a group of larger medial vessels following the path of the great saphenous vein and a lateral group of smaller vessels that follows the small saphenous vein (Fig. 24.1).

The lymphatics of the medial group follow the great saphenous vein up to the groin ending in the lower group of the superficial inguinal lymph nodes. The lateral group of lymphatic vessels follows the small saphenous vein ending in the popliteal lymph nodes. Some of these lymphatic vessels, however, will cross to the front of the leg joining the medial group. The buttock lymphatic drainage is oriented to the upper group of the superficial inguinal lymph nodes.

DEEP LYMPHATIC DRAINAGE

The lymphatic vessels of the deep group follow the main blood vessels and are divided in several groups, named after the related artery and veins, such as: anterior tibial, posterior tibial, peroneal, popliteal, and femoral. The deep lymphatic vessels of the foot and leg reach the popliteal lymph nodes, while the drainage of the thigh reaches the deep inguinal lymph nodes. The deep lymphatic drainage of the gluteal and ischial regions follows the blood vessels and are named after them. The superior gluteal lymphatics drain to a lymph node at the greater sciatic foramen and the inferior gluteal lymphatics drain to the internal iliac lymph nodes after passing through a couple of small lymph nodes close to the piriformis muscle.

POPLITEAL LYMPH NODES

The popliteal lymph nodes lie at the popliteal fossa, are small, and are six or seven in number. They receive lymphatic drainage from the small saphenous vein territory, knee joint, and genicular arteries territory and the trunks from the tibial vessels (Fig. 24.1).

DEEP INGUINAL LYMPH NODES

The deep inguinal lymph nodes are two or three nodes in number, medial to the femoral vein. They receive the deep lymphatic afferents from the femoral vessels group and from the penis or clitoris. They may receive also the superficial lymphatics from the superficial inguinal lymph nodes. The efferents drain to the external iliac lymph nodes.

SUPERFICIAL INGUINAL LYMPH NODES

There are two groups of superficial inguinal lymph nodes: upper and lower groups. The upper group forms a chain below the inguinal ligament. Laterally they receive afferents draining the gluteal tissues and abdominal wall. Medially, they receive the superficial lymphatics from the external genitalia, anal canal and perineal region, uterine vessels, and abdominal wall. The lower group forms a chain along the terminal great saphenous vein. They receive the superficial lymphatic vessels of the lower extremity except from the back and lateral side of the calf (Fig. 24.1). The drainage of the superficial inguinal lymph nodes is directly to the external iliac lymph nodes.

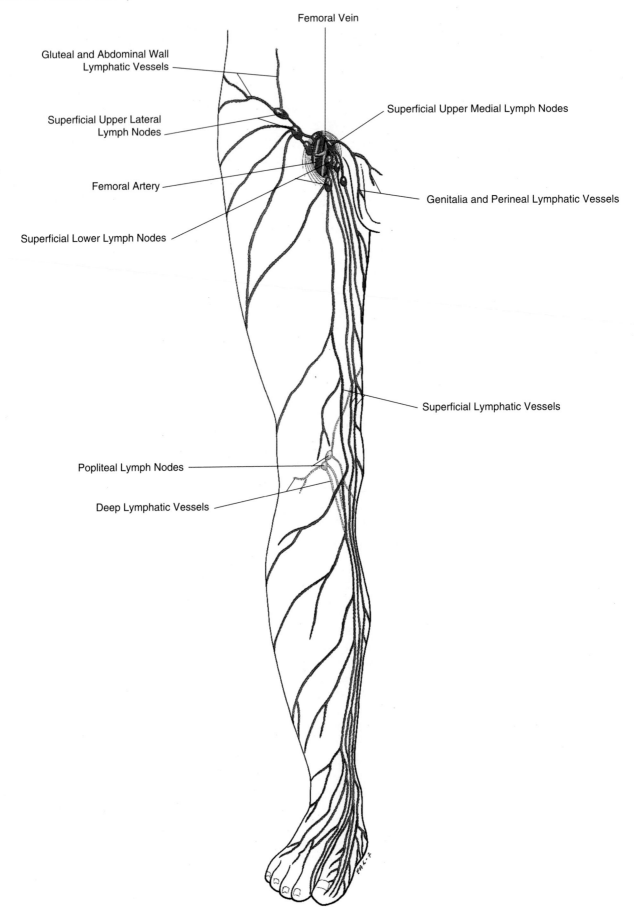

Femoral Vein

Gluteal and Abdominal Wall
Lymphatic Vessels

Superficial Upper Medial Lymph Nodes

Superficial Upper Lateral
Lymph Nodes

Femoral Artery

Genitalia and Perineal Lymphatic Vessels

Superficial Lower Lymph Nodes

Superficial Lymphatic Vessels

Popliteal Lymph Nodes

Deep Lymphatic Vessels

Figure 24.1. Schematic diagram of the lymphatic drainage of the lower extremity.

25

SUGGESTED READINGS

FETAL CIRCULATION

Carlson BM. The cardiovascular system. In Human embryology and developmental biology. Mosby, St. Louis 1994;372-406.

Corliss CE. The circulatory system. In Patten's Human Embryology. Elements of clinical development. McGraw-Hill. New York. 1976;389-452.

Rudolph AM. Hepatic and ductus venous blood flows during fetal life. Hepatology 1983;3:254-258.

Obel W. The umbilical vein in different periods of life in man. Folia Morphol 1976;35:173-179.

ARTERIES OF THE HEAD AND NECK

Djindjian R, Merland JJ. Super-selective arteriography of the external carotid artery. 1st edition. Berlin: Springer-Verlag. 1978;1-550.

Lasjaunias P, Berenstein A. Functional anatomy of craniofacial arteries. Volume 1 Surgical Neuroangiography. New York: Springer-Verlag New York. 1987;1-426.

Lasjaunias P, Berenstein A. Functional vascular anatomy of brain, spinal cord and spine. Volume 3. Surgical Neuroangiography. New York: Springer-Verlag New York. 1990;1-337.

Newton TH, Potts DG. Radiology of the skull and brain. Vol 2, Book 2; Angiography. St. Louis, CV Mosby, 1974.

VEINS OF THE HEAD AND NECK

Lasjaunias P, Berenstein A. Functional vascular anatomy of brain, spinal cord and spine. Volume 3. Surgical Neuroangiography. New York: Springer-Verlag New York. 1990;1-337.

Newton TH, Potts DG. Radiology of the skull and brain. Vol 2, Book 3; Angiography. St. Louis, CV Mosby, 1974.

Schild HH, Strack TR. Selective simultaneous bilateral sampling from the inferior petrosal sinuses. In Uflacker R, Sörensen R (eds) Percutaneous venous blood sampling in endocrine diseases. Springer Verlag, New York, 1992, pp 48-74.

Williams PL, Warwick R, Dyson M, Bannister LH. Angiology, Chapter 6. Gray's Anatomy. 37th edition. Edinburgh: Churchill Livingstone. 1989;661-858.

LYMPHATIC SYSTEM OF THE HEAD AND NECK

Fischer HW, Lawrence MS, Thornbury JR. Lymphography of the normal adult male: observations and their relation to the diagnosis of metastatic neoplasm. Radiology 1962;78:399-406.

Fischer HW, Zimmerman GR. Roentgenographic visualization of lymph nodes and lymphatic channels. AJR 1959;81:517-534.

Willians PL, Warwick R, Dyson M, Bannister LH. Angiology, Chapter 6. Gray's Anatomy. 37th edition. Edinburgh: Churchill Livingstone. 1989;661-858.

ARTERIES OF THE SPINAL CORD AND SPINE

Doppman JL, Di Chiro G, Ommaya AK. Selective arteriography of the spinal cord. 1st ed. St. Louis: Warren H. Green, Inc. 1969;3-16.

Lasjaunias P, Berenstein A. Functional vascular anatomy of brain, spinal cord and spine. Volume 3. Surgical Neuroangiography. New York: Springer-Verlag New York. 1990;1-337.

Rodesch G, Lasjaunias P, Berenstein A. Functional vascular anatomy of the spine and spinal cord. Rivista Neuroradiologia (Suppl 2) 1992;5:63-66.

Tveten L. Spinal cord vascularity. I. Extraspinal sources of spinal cord arteries in man. Acta Radiol (Diagn) 1976;17:1-16.

Tveten L. Spinal cord vascularity. III. The spinal cord arteries in man. Acta Radiol (Diagn) 1976;17:257-273.

VEINS OF THE SPINAL CORD AND SPINE

Batson OV. The function of the vertebral veins and their role in the spread of metastases. Ann Surg 1940;112:138-148.

Drasin GF, Daffner RH, Sexton RF, Cheatham WC. Epidural venography: Diagnosis of herniated lumbar intervertebral disc and other disease of the epidural space. AJR 1976;126:1010-1016.

Gershater R, St. Louis EL. Lumbar Epidural Venography. Review of 1,200 cases. Radiology 1979;131:409-421.

Gershater R, Holgate RC. Lumbar epidural venography in the diagnosis of disc herniations. AJR 1976;126:992-1002.

Tveten L. Spinal cord vascularity. I. Extraspinal sources of spinal cord arteries in man. Acta Radiol (Diagn) 1976;17:1-16.

Tveten L. Spinal cord vascularity. III. The spinal cord arteries in man. Acta Radiol (Diagn) 1976;17:257-273.

THORACIC AORTA AND ARTERIES OF THE TRUNK

Blake HA, Manion WC. Thoracic arterial arch anomalies. Circulation 1962;26:251-265.

Botenga ASJ. Selective bronchial and intercostal arteriography. Baltimore: The Williams and Wilkins Co. 1970;1-159.

Caix M, Descottes B, Rousseay DG, Rousseau D. The arterial vascularization of the middle thoracic and lower esophagus. Anat Clin 1982;3:95-106.

Cauldwell EW, Siekert RG, Lininger RE, Anson BJ. The bronchial arteries: An anatomic study of 150 cadavers. Surg Gynecol Obst 1948;86:395-412.

Hellekant C. Bronchial angiography and intra-arterial chemotherapy in lung carcinoma. Thesis. University of Lund. Malmo, Sweden, 1978; 1-100.

Hollinshead WH. Anatomy for surgeons, vol 2: The thorax, abdomen, and pelvis. New York, Harper & Row, 1971.

Jardin M, Remy J. Control of hemoptysis: Systemic angiography and anastomoses of the internal mammary artery. Radiology 1988;168:377-383.

Jonsson K, Karlsson S. Angiography of the internal mammary artery. Acta Radiol 1985;26:113-120.

Netter FH. Anatomy of the esophagus. In Netter FH (ed) Digestive System. Part I. Upper Digestive Tract. Vol 3. New York: The Ciba Collection of Medical Illustrations, 1966; 34-46.

Pisco JBM. Angioplastia Transluminal Percutânea. Thesis. Universidade Nova de Lisboa. Lisboa, Portugal 1990; 1-334.

Tan RT, McGahan JP, Link DP, Lantz BMT. Bronchial artery embolization in management of haemoptysis. J Interv Radiol 1991;6:67-76.

Uflacker R, Kaemmerer A. Picon PD, Rizzon CFC, Neves CMC, Oliveira ESB, Oliveira MEM, Azevedo SNB, Ossanai R. Bronchial artery embolization in the management of hemoptysis: Technical aspects and long-term results.

VEINS OF THE THORAX

Abrams HL. The vertebral and azygos venous systems and some variations in systemic venous return. Radiology 1957;69:508-525.

Drane WE, Watt AC, Marks DS. Obstruction of the superior vena cava or its major tributaries demonstrated by bolus-injection excretory urography. Radiology 1982;144:499-504.

Fritzsche P, Andersen C, Smith DC. Collateral circulation secondary to upper extremity venous thrombosis visualized during excretory urography. Radiology 1982;144:495-498.

Hollinshead WH. Anatomy for surgeons, vol 2: The thorax, abdomen, and pelvis. New York, Harper & Row, 1971.

Sörensen R. Selective venous sampling for parathyroid hormone excess. In Uflacker R, Sörensen R (eds) Percutaneous venous blood sampling in endocrine diseases. Springer Verlag, New York, 1992, pp 125-150.

Thomas ML. Phlebography. Arch Surg 1972;104:145-151.

Yune HY, Klatte EC. Mediastinal venography. AJR 1986;147:674-684.

Willians PL, Warwick R, Dyson M, Bannister LH. Angiology, Chapter 6. Gray's Anatomy. 37th edition. Edinburgh: Churchill Livingstone. 1989;661-858.

LYMPHATIC SYSTEM OF THE THORAX

Fischer HW, Lawrence MS, Thornbury JR. Lymphography of the normal adult male: observations and their relation to the diagnosis of metastatic neoplasm. Radiology 1962;78:399-406.

Fischer HW, Zimmerman GR. Roentgenographic visualization of lymph nodes and lymphatic channels. AJR 1959;81:517-534.

Fraser RG, Paré JAP, Paré PD, Fraser RS, Genereux GP. The normal chest. In: Fraser RG, Paré JAP, Paré PD, Fraser RS, Genereux GP. eds 3rd ed. Philadelphia: W.B. Saunders Co. 1988:1-314.

Hollinshead WH. Anatomy for surgeons, vol 2: The thorax, abdomen, and pelvis. New York, Harper & Row, 1971.

PULMONARY ARTERIAL CIRCULATION

Boyden EA. Segmental anatomy of the lungs. New York, McGraw-Hill, 1955.

Dotter CT. The Normal Pulmonary Arteriogram. In: Abrams HL, ed. Abrams Angiography. Vascular and Interventional Radiology. 3rd ed. Boston: Little, Brown and Co., 1983; 715-722.

Elliott FM, Reid L. Some new facts about the pulmonary artery and its branching pattern. Clin Radiol 1965;16:193-198.

Fraser RG, Paré JAP, Paré PD, Fraser RS, Genereux GP. The normal chest. In: Fraser RG, Paré JAP, Paré PD, Fraser RS, Genereux GP. eds 3rd ed. Philadelphia: W.B. Saunders Co. 1988:1-314.

Murata K, Itoh H, Todo G, Itoh T, Kanaoka M, Furuta M, Torizuka K. Bronchial venous plexus and its communication with pulmonary circulation. Invest Radiol 1986;21:24-30.

Nagaishi C. Functional anatomy and histology of the lung. Baltimore, University Park Press, 1972.

Rigatto M. Funçoes da Circulaçao Pulmonar. In Rigatto M (ed) Fisiopatologia da Circulaçao Pulmonar. 1st ed. Sao Paulo: Fundo Editorial Byk-Procienx, 1973; 13-41.

PULMONARY VENOUS CIRCULATION

Dotter CT. The Normal Pulmonary Arteriogram. In: Abrams HL, ed. Abrams Angiography. Vascular and Interventional Radiology. 3rd ed. Boston: Little, Brown and Co., 1983; 715-722.

Fraser RG, Paré JAP, Paré PD, Fraser RS, Genereux GP. The normal chest. In: Fraser RG, Paré JAP, Paré PD, Fraser RS, Genereux GP. eds 3rd ed. Philadelphia: W.B. Saunders Co. 1988:1-314.

Murata K, Itoh H, Todo G, Itoh T, Kanaoka M, Furuta M, Torizuka K. Bronchial venous plexus and its communication with pulmonary circulation. Invest Radiol 1986;21:24-30.

Nagaishi C. Functional anatomy and histology of the lung. Baltimore, University Park Press, 1972.

Rigatto M. Funçoes da Circulaçao Pulmonar. In Rigatto M (ed) Fisiopatologia da Circulaçao Pulmonar. 1st ed. Sao Paulo: Fundo Editorial Byk-Procienx, 1973; 13-41.

PULMONARY AND THORACIC LYMPHATIC SYSTEM

Nagaishi C. Functional anatomy and histology of the lung. Baltimore, University Park Press, 1972.

Fraser RG, Paré JAP, Paré PD, Fraser RS, Genereux GP. The normal chest. In: Fraser RG, Paré JAP, Paré PD, Fraser RS, Genereux GP. eds 3rd ed. Philadelphia: W.B. Saunders Co. 1988:1-314.

HEART AND CORONARY ARTERIES

Netter FH. Heart. In Netter FH (ed) Vol 5. 1st ed. New York: The Ciba Collection of Medical Illustrations, 1969; 1-293.

Netter FH. Atlas of Human Anatomy. Summit, New Jersey. Ciba-Geigy Corporation, 1989.

Pansky B, House EL. Review of Gross Anatomy. 2nd ed. London: The Macmillan Co. 1971;1-493.

Willians PL, Warwick R, Dyson M, Bannister LH. Angiology, Chapter 6. Gray's Anatomy. 37th edition. Edinburgh: Churchill Livingstone. 1989;661-858.

CARDIAC VEINS

Netter FH. Heart. In Netter FH (ed) Vol 5. 1st ed. New York: The Ciba Collection of Medical Illustrations, 1969; 1-293.

Willians PL, Warwick R, Dyson M, Bannister LH. Angiology, Chapter 6. Gray's Anatomy. 37th edition. Edinburgh: Churchill Livingstone. 1989;661-858.

ARTERIES OF THE UPPER EXTREMITIES

Coleman SS, Anson BJ. Arterial patterns in the hand. Based upon a study of 650 specimens. Surg Gyn Obst 1961;113:409-424.

Daseler EH, Anson BJ. Surgical anatomy of the subclavian artery and its branches. Surg Gynecol Obstet 1959;108:149-174.

Ikeda A, Ugawa A, Kazihara Y, Hamada N. Arterial patterns in the hand based on a three dimensional analysis of 220 cadaver hands. J Hand Surg 1988;13A:501-509.

Janevski BK. Angiography of the upper extremity. The Hague, Martinus Nijhoff Publishers, 1982, pp 37-122.

Netter FH. Anatomy. Upper Limb. In Netter FH. (ed) Musculoskeletal System. Part I. Anatomy, Physiology and Metabolic Disorders. Vol 8. New York: The Ciba Collection of Medical Illustrations, 1987; 20-74.

VEINS OF THE UPPER EXTREMITY

Janevski BK. Angiography of the upper extremity. The Hague, Martinus Nijhoff Publishers, 1982, pp 37-122.

Netter FH. Anatomy. Upper Limb. In Netter FH (ed) Musculoskeletal System. Part I. Anatomy, Physiology and Metabolic Disorders. Vol 8. New York: The Ciba Collection of Medical Illustrations, 1987; 20-74.

Netter FH. Atlas of Human Anatomy. Summit, New Jersey. Ciba-Geigy Corporation, 1989.

Thomas ML. Phlebography. Arch Surg 1972;104:145-151.

LYMPHATIC SYSTEM OF THE UPPER EXTREMITY

Fischer HW, Lawrence MS, Thornbury JR. Lymphography of the normal adult male: observations and their relation to the diagnosis of metastatic neoplasm. Radiology 1962;78:399-406.

Fischer HW, Zimmerman GR. Roentgenographic visualization of lymph nodes and lymphatic channels. AJR 1959;81:517-534.

Netter FH. Anatomy. Upper Limb. In Netter FH (ed) Musculoskeletal System. Part I. Anatomy, Physiology and Metabolic Disorders. Vol 8. New York: The Ciba Collection of Medical Illustrations, 1987; 20-74.

ABDOMINAL AORTA AND BRANCHES

Adams DB. The importance of extrahepatic biliary anatomy in preventing complications at laparoscopic cholecystectomy. Surg Clin North Am 1993;73:861-871.

Anson BJ, Cauldwell EW, Pick JW, Beaton LE. The blood supply of the kidney, suprarenal gland, and associated structures. Surg Gynecol Obstet 1947;84:313.

Baum S. Normal anatomy and collateral pathways of the mesenteric circulation. In Boley SJ. ed. Vascular disorders of the intestine. 1st edition. New York: Apple-Century-Crofts. 1971;1-18.

Bismuth H. Surgical anatomy and anatomical surgery of the liver. World J Surg 1982;6:3-9.

Boijsen E. Angiographic studies of the anatomy of single and multiple renal arteries. Acta Radiol (Suppl 183) 1959;1-135.

Charnsangavej C, Chuang VP, Wallace S, Soo C-S, Bowers T. Angiographic classification of hepatic arterial collaterals. Radiology 1982;144:485-494.

Cho KJ, Lunderquist A. The peribiliary plexus: The microvascular architecture of the bile duct in the rabbit and in clinical cases. Radiology 1983;147:357-364.

Couinaud C. Le foie: Etudes anatomiques et chirurgicales. 1st edition. Paris: Masson & Cie. 1957;1-530.

Daseler EH, Anson BJ, Hambley WC, Reiman AF. The cystic artery and constituents of the hepatic pedicle: A study of 500 specimens. Surg Gynecol Obstet 1947;85:47-63.

da Silva Filho, AR. Vascularização arterial do baço: Estudo da independência e análise proporcional dos seus segmentos. Thesis. Escola Paulista de Medicina, Sao Paulo, Brazil. 1991; 1-63.

Demachi H, Matsui O, Takashima T. Scanning electron microscopy of intrahepatic microvasculature casts following experimental hepatic artery embolization. Cardiovasc Intervent Radiol 1991;14:158-162.

Ekataksin W, Zou Z, Wake K. A new look at the "hepatic" artery: Intrahepatic arterial compartmentation in mammalian livers. Hepatology 1995;22:159A.

Ekataksin W, Wake K. Liver units in three dimensions. I. Organization of argyrophilic connective tissue skeleton in porcine liver with particular reference to the "compound hepatic lobule." Am J Anat 1991;191:113-153.

Fine H, Keen EN. The arteries of the human kidney. J Anat 1966;100:881-894.

Flint ER. Abnormalities of the right hepatic, cystic and gastroduodenal arteries, and of the bile ducts. Brit J Surg 1923;10:509-512.

Garti I, Meiraz D. Ectopic origin of main renal artery. Urology 1980;15:627-629.

Gazelle GS, Haaga JR. Hepatic neoplasms: Surgically relevant segmental anatomy and imaging techniques. AJR 1992; 158:1015-1018.

Healey JE Jr. Vascular anatomy of the liver. Ann NY Acad Sci. 1970;170:8-17.

Kan Z, Ivancev K, Lunderquist A, McCuskey PA, Wright KC, Wallace S, McCuskey RS. In vivo microscopy of hepatic tumors in animal models: A dynamic investigation of blood supply to hepatic metastases. Radiology 1993;187:621-626.

Kardon RH, Kessel RG. Three-dimensional organization of the hepatic microcirculation in the rodent as observed by scanning electron microscopy of corrosion casts. Gastroenterology 1980;79:72-81.

Kinnunem J, Totterman S, Tervahartiala P. Ten renal arteries. Eur J Radiol 1985; 5: 300-301.

Lafortune M, Madore F, Patriquin H, Breton G. Segmental anatomy of the liver: A sonographic approach to the Couinaud nomenclature. Radiology 1991;181:443-448.

Le Bail B, Balaubaud C, Bioulac-Sage P. Anatomy and Structure of the liver and biliary Tree. In Prieto J, Rodés J, Shafritz DA (ed). Hepatobiliary diseases. Springer-Verlag. Berlin 1992. pg 1-38.

Lunderquist A. Angiography in carcinoma of the pancreas. Acta Radiol (Suppl 235) 1965;1-143.

Lunderquist A. Arterial segmental supply of the liver. Acta Radiol (Suppl 272) 1967;1-86.

MacSween RNM, Scothorne RJ. Developmental anatomy and normal structure. In MacSween RNM, Anthony PP, Scheuer PJ (ed). Pathology of the Liver. 2nd ed. Churchill Livingstone. Edinburgh, 1987, pg 1-45.

Marston A. Intestinal ischaemia. 1st edition. London: Edward Arnold Publisher Ltd. 1977;1-190.

Merklin RJ. Arterial supply of the suprarenal gland. Anat Rec 1962;144:359.

Merklin RJ, Michels NA. The variant renal and suprarenal blood supply with data on inferior phrenic, ureteral and gonadal arteries. A statistical analysis based on 185 dissections and review of the literature. J Int Coll Surg 1958;29:41.

Michels NA. The hepatic, cystic and retroduodenal arteries and their relations to the biliary ducts. Ann Surg 1951;133:503-524.

Michels NA. The variational anatomy of the spleen and splenic artery. Am J Anat 1942;70:21-26.

Michels NA. Blood supply and anatomy of the upper abdominal organs with a descriptive atlas. Philadelphia, J.B. Lippincott Co, 1955.

Millward-Sadler GH, Jezequel A-M. Normal histology and ultrastructure. In Millward-Sadler GH, Wright R, Arthur MJP (ed), Wright's - Liver and biliary disease. 3rd ed. Vol. 1. WB Saunders, London, 1992; pg 3-11.

Mizumoto R, Suzuki H. Surgical Anatomy of the hepatic hilum with special reference to the caudate lobe. World J Surg 1988;12: 2-10.

Moar JJ, Tobias PV. Multiple renal arteries. (Letter) S Afr Med J 1958;67:399.

Motta PM. Scanning electron microscopy of the liver. In. Popper H, Schaffner F (ed) Progress in liver diseases. Vol VII. Grune & Stratton, New York, 1982, pg 1-16.

Myers MA. Normal anatomic relationships and variants. In Myers MA, ed. Dynamic radiology of the abdomen. New York, NY. Springer-Verlag 1992.

Netter FH. Anatomy of the Abdomen. In Netter FH (ed) Digestive System. Part II. Lower Digestive Tract. Vol 3. 1st ed. New York: The Ciba Collection of Medical Illustrations, 1969; 10-44.

Netter FH. Anatomy of the lower digestive tract. In Netter FH (ed) Digestive System. Part II. Lower Digestive Tract. Vol 3. New York: The Ciba Collection of Medical Illustrations, 1969; 47-81.

Netter FH. Anatomy of the stomach and duodenum. In Netter FH (ed) Digestive System. Part I. Upper Digestive Tract. Vol 3. New York: The Ciba Collection of Medical Illustrations, 1966; 49-65.

Netter FH. Normal anatomy of the liver, biliary tract and pancreas. In Netter FH (ed) Digestive System. Part III. Liver, Biliary Tract and Pancreas. Vol 3. New York: The Ciba Collection of Medical Illustrations, 1967; 2-31.

Nordmark L. Angiography of the testicular artery. Acta Radiol [Diagn] 1977;18:25-32.

Northover JMA, Terblanche J. A new look at the arterial supply of the bile duct in man and its surgical implications. Br J Surg 1979;66:379-384.

Notkovich H. Variations of the testicular and ovarian arteries in relation to the renal pedicle. Surg Gynecol Obstet 1956;103:487-495.

Pierson JM. The arterial blood supply of the pancreas. Surg Gynec Obst 1943;77:426-430.

Pick JW, Anson BJ. The inferior phrenic artery: Origin and suprarenal branches. Anat Rec 1940;78:413.

Sampaio FJB, Passos MARF. Renal arteries: anatomic study for surgical and radiologic practice. Surg Radiol Anat 1992;14:113-117.

Sampaio FJB. Renal arterial pedicle: anatomic analysis applied to urologic and radiologic procedures. In: Sampaio FJB, Uflacker R, eds. Renal Anatomy Applied to Urology, Endourology and Interventional Radiology. 1st ed. New York: Thieme Medical Publishers, 1993: 47-53.

Sampaio FJB. Anatomic study and proportional analysis of the kidney arterial segments. In: Sampaio FJB, Uflacker R, eds. Renal Anatomy Applied to Urology, Endourology and Interventional Radiology. 1st ed. New York: Thieme Medical Publishers, 1993: 39-46.

Sampaio FJB. Relationships of intrarenal arteries and the kidney collecting system. In: Sampaio FJB, Uflacker R, eds. Renal Anatomy Applied to Urology, Endourology and Interventional Radiology. 1st ed. New York: Thieme Medical Publishers, 1993:23-32.

Sampaio FJB, Aragao AHM. Anatomical relationship between the intrarenal arteries and the kidney collecting system. J Urol 1990;143:679-681.

Sampaio FJB, Mandarin-de-Lacerda CA. 3-Dimensional and radiological pelvicaliceal anatomy for endourology. J Urol 1988;140:1352-1355.

Sampaio FJB. Anatomical background for nephron-sparing surgery in renal cell carcinoma. J Urol 1992;147:999-1005.

Sampaio FJB, Mandarin-de-Lacerda CA. Anatomical classification of the kidney collecting system for endourologic procedures. J Endourol 1988;2:247-251.

Sampaio FJB, Favorito LA. Endopyélotomie. Etude anatomique des rapports vasculaires de la jonction pyélo-urétérale (JPU). J d'Urol 1991;97:73-77.

Sampaio FJB. Arterial and venous anatomic relationships to the ureteropelvic junction. In: Sampaio FJB, Uflacker R (eds) Renal Anatomy Applied to Urology, Endourology and Interventional Radiology. 1st ed. New York: Thieme Medical Publishers 1993;77-81.

Sherlock S. Diseases of the liver and biliary system. 8th edition. Oxford: Blackwell Scientific Publications. 1992;1-578.

Soyer P, Roche A. Three-dimensional imaging of the liver. Acta Radiol 1991;32:432-435.

Sugarbaker PH, Nelson RC, Murray DR, Chezmar JL, Bernardino ME. A segmental approach to computerized tomographic portography for hepatic resection. Surg Gynecol Obstet 1990;171:189-195.

Sundgren R. Selective angiography of the left gastric artery. Acta Radiol (Suppl 299) 1970;1-100.

Terblanche J, Allison HF, Northover JMA. An ischemic basis for biliary strictures. Surgery 1983;94:52-57.

Uflacker R, Reichert P, D'Albuquerque LC, Oliveira e Silva A. Liver anatomy applied to the placement of transjugular intrahepatic portosystemic shunt (TIPS). Radiology 1994;191:705-712.

VanDamme J-P, Bonte J. Vascular Anatomy in Abdominal Surgery. 1st edition. New York: Thieme Medical Publishers, Inc. 1990;1-142.

Yamauchi T, Furui S, Ohtomo K, Itai Y. Stereoscopic digital subtraction angiography of hepatic artery and vein. AJR 1987;148:825-826.

Yule E. The arterial supply of the duodenum. J Anat 1927;61:344-348.

Zanier JFC. Acesso percutâneo ao rim em endourologia. Thesis. Universidade Federal do Rio de Janeiro. Rio de Janeiro, Brazil, 1990;1-109.

ARTERIES OF THE PELVIS

Bookstein JJ, Lang EV. Penile magnification pharmacoarteriography: Details of intrapenile arterial anatomy. AJR 1987;148:883-888.

Bookstein JJ. Penile angiography: The last angiographic frontier. AJR 1988;150:47-54.

Borell U, Fernström I. The ovarian artery. An arteriographic study in human subjects. Acta Radiol 1954;42:253-265.

Delcour C, Vandenbosch G, Delatte, et al. Penile arteriography: Technical advances. AJR 1988;150:803-804.

Fernstrom I. Arteriography of the uterine artery. Acta Radiol (Stock) (Suppl) 1955.

Hassen-Khodja R, Batt M, Michetti C, et al. Radiologic anatomy of the anastomotic systems of the internal iliac artery. Surg Radiol Anat 1987;9:135-140.

VanDamme J-P, Bonte J. Vascular Anatomy in Abdominal Surgery. 1st edition. New York: Thieme Medical Publishers, Inc. 1990;1-142.

Walsh PC. Radical retropubic prostatectomy. In Campbell's Urology. WB Saunders, Philadelphia, vol 3, 1986, pp 2754-2775.

Willians PL, Warwick R, Dyson M, Bannister LH. Angiology, Chapter 6. Gray's Anatomy. 37th edition. Edinburgh: Churchill Livingstone. 1989;661-858.

Willians PL, Warwick R, Dyson M, Bannister LH. Splanchnology, Chapter 7. Gray's Anatomy. 37th edition. Edinburgh: Churchill Livingstone. 1989;1245-1475.

VEINS OF THE ABDOMEN AND PELVIS

Anderson RC, Adams P, Burke B. Anomalous inferior vena cava with azygos continuation (infrahepatic interruption of the inferior vena cava). Report of 15 new cases. J Pediatr 1961;59:370-383.

Bergstrand I, Eckman CA. Portal circulation in portal hypertension. Acta Radiol [Diagn] (Stock) 1957;47:1-22.

Bookstein JJ. Cavernosal venoocclusive insufficiency in male impotence: evaluation of degree and location. Radiology 1987;164:175-178.

Bookstein JJ. Penile angiography: The last angiographic frontier. AJR 1988;150:47-54.

Bookstein JJ, Lurie AL. Selective penile venography: Anatomical and hemodynamic observations. J Urol 1988;140:55-60.

Chermet J, Bigot JM. Venography of the inferior vena cava and its branches. New York: Springer-Verlag. 1980;1-232.

Cho KJ, Geisinger KR, Shields JJ, Forrest ME. Collateral channels and histopathology in hepatic vein occlusion. AJR 1982;139:703-709.

Coolsaet BLRA. The varicocele syndrome: Venography determining the optimal level for surgical management. J Urol 1980;124:833-839.

Couinaud C. The parabiliary venous system. Surg Radiol Ana 1988;10:311-316.

da Silva Filho, AR. Vascularizaçao venosa do baço: Estudo morfológico da formaçao da veia esplênica e análise segmentar intraparenquimatosa. Thesis. Universidade Federal do Ceará, Fortaleza, Brazil. 1992;1-46

Delcour C, Wespes E, Schulman CC, et al. Investigation of the venous system in impotence of vascular origin. Urol Radiol 1984;6:190-193.

Doehner GA. The hepatic venous system. Its pathologic roentgen anatomy. Radiology 1968;90:1124-1131.

Doehner GA. The hepatic venous system. Its normal roentgen anatomy. Radiology 1968;90:1119-1123.

Doehner GA, Ruzicka FF, Hoffman G, Rousselot LM. The portal venous system: Its roentgen anatomy. Radiology 1955;64:675-687.

Göthlin J, Lunderquist A, Tylén U. Selective phlebography of the pancreas. Acta Radiol 1974;15:474-480.

Healey JE Jr. Vascular anatomy of the liver. Ann NY Acad Sci. 1970;170:8-17.

Helander CG, Lindblon A. retrograde pelvic venography. Acta Radiol (Diagn) 1959;51:401-414.

Johnstone FRC. The suprarenal veins. Am J Surg 1957;94:615.

Juttner HU, Jenney JM, Ralls PW, Goldstein LI, Reynolds TB. Ultrasound demonstration of portosystemic collaterals in cirrhosis and portal hypertension. Radiology 1982;142:459-463.

Kardon RH, Kessel RG. Three-dimensional organization of the hepatic microcirculation in the rodent as observed by scanning electron microscopy of corrosion casts. Gastroenterology 1980;79:72-81.

Keller FS, Niles NR, Rösch J, et al. Retrograde pancreatic venography: Autopsy study. Radiology 1980;135;285-293.

Lafortune M, Constantin A, Breton G, Légaré AG, Lavoie. The recanalized umbilical vein in portal hypertension: A myth. AJR 1985;144:549-553.

Lavoie P. Légaré AG, Viallet A. Portal catheterization via the round ligament of the liver. Am J Surg 19967;144:822-830.

Leger L, Lenriot JP, Lemaigre G. Physiopathology of portal hypertension. Circulatory neophysiology after portacaval shunt. In Child CG (ed). Portal Hypertension. Major Problems in Clinical Surgery. Philadelphia: W.B. Saunders Co. 1974;165-195.

Le Bail B, Balaubaud C, Bioulac-Sage P. Anatomy and Structure of the liver and biliary Tree. In Prieto J, Rodés J, Shafritz DA (ed). Hepatobiliary diseases. Springer-Verlag. Berlin 1992. pg 1-38.

MacSween RNM, Scothorne RJ. Developmental anatomy and normal structure. In MacSween RNM, Anthony PP, Scheuer PJ (ed). Pathology of the Liver. 2nd ed. Churchill Livingstone. Edinburgh, 1987, pg 1-45.

Madrazo B, Jafri SZ, Shirkhoda A, Roberts JL, Ellwood RA. Portosystemic collaterals: Evaluation with color Doppler imaging and correlation with CT and MRI. Seminars Interv Radiol 1990;7:169-184.

Merklin RJ, Eger SA. The adrenal venous system in man. J Int Coll Surg 1961;35:572.

Michels NA. Blood supply and anatomy of the upper abdominal organs with a descriptive atlas. Philadelphia, J.B. Lippincott Co, 1955.

Mikaelsson CG. Venous communications of the adrenal glands. Acta Radiol (Stock) 1970;10:369.

Millward-Sadler GH, Jezequel A-M. Normal histology and ultrastructure. In Millward-Sadler GH, Wright R, Arthur MJP (ed), Wright's - Liver and biliary disease. 3rd ed. Vol. 1. WB Saunders, London, 1992. pg 3-11.

Moltz L, Sörensen R. Selective venous sampling for the differential diagnosis of female hyperandrogenemia. In Uflacker R, Sörensen R (eds) Percutaneous venous blood sampling in endocrine diseases. Springer Verlag, New York, 1992, pp 1-27.

Morin C, Lafortune M, Pomier G, Robin M, Breton G. Patent paraumbilical vein: Anatomic and hemodynamic variants and their clinical importance. Radiology 1992;185:253-256.

Motta PM. Scanning electron microscopy of the liver. In. Popper H, Schaffner F (ed) Progress in liver diseases. Vol VII. Grune & Stratton, New York, 1982, pg 1-16.

Myers MA. Normal anatomic relationships and variants. In Myers MA, ed. Dynamic radiology of the abdomen. New York, NY. Springer-Verlag 1992.

Myers RP. Anatomical variation of the superficial preprostatic veins in respect to radical retropubic prostatectomy. J Urol 1991;145:992-993.

Netter FH. Anatomy of the Abdomen. In Netter FH (ed) Digestive System. Part II. Lower Digestive Tract. Vol 3. 1st ed. New York: The Ciba Collection of Medical Illustrations, 1969; 10-44.

Netter FH. Anatomy of the lower digestive tract. In Netter FH (ed) Digestive System. Part II. Lower Digestive Tract. Vol 3. New York: The Ciba Collection of Medical Illustrations, 1969; 47-81.

Netter FH. Anatomy of the stomach and duodenum. In Netter FH (ed) Digestive System. Part I. Upper Digestive Tract. Vol 3. New York: The Ciba Collection of Medical Illustrations, 1966; 49-65.

Netter FH. Normal anatomy of the liver, biliary tract and pancreas. In Netter FH (ed) Digestive System. Part III. Liver, Biliary Tract and Pancreas. Vol 3. New York: The Ciba Collection of Medical Illustrations, 1967; 2-31.

Obel W. The umbilical vein in different periods of life in man. Folia Morphol 1976;35:173-179

Reiner WG, Walsh PC. An anatomical approach to the surgical management of the dorsal vein and Santorini's plexus during radical retropubic surgery. J Urol 1979;121:198-200.

Sampaio FJB, Aragao AHM. Anatomical relationship between the renal venous arrangement and the kidney collecting system. J Urol 1990; 144:1089-1093.

Sampaio FJB. Arterial and venous anatomic relationships to the ureteropelvic junction. In Sampaio FJB, Uflacker R (eds) Renal Anatomy Applied to Urology, Endourology and Interventional Radiology. 1st. ed. New York: Thieme Medical Publishers 1993;77-81.

Sano A, Kuroda Y, Moriyasu F, Takahashi Y, Koizumi S, Kimura S, Okuda K. Portopulmonary venous anastomosis in portal hypertension demonstrated by percutaneous transhepatic cine-portography. Radiology 1982;144:479-484.

Sherlock S. Diseases of the liver and biliary system. 8th edition. Oxford: Blackwell Scientific Publications. 1992;1-578.

Soyer P, Roche A. Three-dimensional imaging of the liver. Acta Radiol 1991;32:432-435.

Sugarbaker PH, Nelson RC, Murray DR, Chezmar JL, Bernardino ME. A segmental approach to computerized tomographic portography for hepatic resection. Surg Gynecol Obstet 1990;171:189-195.

Uflacker R. Pancreatic venous sampling. In Uflacker R, Sörensen R (eds) Percutaneous venous blood sampling in endocrine diseases. Springer Verlag, New York, 1992, pp 75-118.

Uflacker R, Reichert P, D'Albuquerque LC, Oliveira e Silva A. Liver anatomy applied to the placement of transjugular intrahepatic portosystemic shunt (TIPS). Radiology 1994;191:705-712.

VanDamme J-P, Bonte J. Vascular Anatomy in Abdominal Surgery. 1st edition. New York: Thieme Medical Publishers, Inc. 1990;1-142.

van Leeuwen MS, Fernandez MA, van Es HW, Stokking R, Dillon EH, Feldberg MAM. Variations in venous and segmental anatomy of the liver: Two- and three-dimensional MR imaging in healthy volunteers. AJR 1994;162:1337-1345.

Yamauchi T, Furui S, Ohtomo K, Itai Y. Stereoscopic digital subtraction angiography of hepatic artery and vein. AJR 1987;148:825-826.

Walsh PC. Radical retropubic prostatectomy. In Campbell's Urology. WB Saunders, Philadelphia, vol 3, 1986, pp 2754-2775.

Willians PL, Warwick R, Dyson M, Bannister LH. Angiology, Chapter 6. Gray's Anatomy. 37th edition. Edinburgh: Churchill Livingstone. 1989;661-858.

Zanier JFC. Acesso percutâneo ao rim em endourologia. Thesis. Universidade Federal do Rio de Janeiro. Rio de Janeiro, Brazil, 1990;1-109.

LYMPHATIC SYSTEM OF THE ABDOMEN

Delmas V, Hidden G, Dauge MCL. Remarques sur les lymphatiques du rein: le premier relais nodal. Bull Soc Anat Paris. 1989;13:105-109.

Delmas V, Hidden G, Dauge MCL. Organisation du drainage lymphatique au niveau de l'appareil urinaire et genital de l'homme. Bull Soc Anat Paris 1989;13:95-103.

Fischer HW, Lawrence MS, Thornbury JR. Lymphography of the normal adult male: observations and their relation to the diagnosis of metastatic neoplasm. Radiology 1962;78:399-406.

Fischer HW, Zimmerman GR. Roentgenographic visualization of lymph nodes and lymphatic channels. AJR 1959;81:517-534.

Giuliani L, Gilberti C, Martorana G. Lymphadenectomy. Lymphatic drainage of the kidney. In Giuliaini L, Gilberti C, Martorana G eds. Atlas of Surgery for Renal Cancer. 2nd ed. Milan: Grafiche Mazzucchelli. 1989; 43-45.

VanDamme J-P, Bonte J. Vascular Anatomy in Abdominal Surgery. 1st edition. New York: Thieme Medical Publishers, Inc. 1990;1-142.

ARTERIES OF THE LOWER EXTREMITY

Golan JF, Garrett WV. Smith BL, et al. Persistent sciatic artery and vein: An unusual case. J Vasc Surg 1986;3:162-165.

Mussbichler H. Arteriographic investigation of the normal hip in adults. Evaluation of methods and vascular findings. Acta Radiol 1971;11:195-215.

Netter FH. Anatomy. Lower Limb. In Netter FH (ed) Musculoskeletal System. Part I. Anatomy, Physiology and Metabolic Disorders. Vol 8. New York: The Ciba Collection of Medical Illustrations, 1987; 75- 121.

VEINS OF THE LOWER EXTREMITY

Greitz T. Phlebography of the normal leg. Acta Radiol (Diagn) 1955;44:1-20.

Jacobsen BH. The venous drainage of the foot. Surg Gynecol Obstet 1970;131:22-24.

Netter FH. Anatomy. Lower Limb. In Netter FH (ed) Musculoskeletal System. Part I. Anatomy, Physiology and Metabolic Disorders. Vol 8. New York: The Ciba Collection of Medical Illustrations, 1987; 75- 121.

Thomas ML. Phlebography. Arch Surg 1972;104:145-151.

LYMPHATIC SYSTEM OF THE LOWER EXTREMITY

Heman PG, Benninghoff DL, Nelson JH. Mellins HZ. Roentgen anatomy of the ilio-pelvic-aortic lymphatic system. Radiology 1963;80:182-193.

Larson DL, Lewis SR. Deep lymphatic system of the lower extremity. Am J Surg 1967;113:217-220.

Netter FH. Anatomy. Lower Limb. In Netter FH (ed) Musculoskeletal System. Part I. Anatomy, Physiology and Metabolic Disorders. Vol 8. New York: The Ciba Collection of Medical Illustrations, 1987; 75- 121.

Vitek J, Kaspar Z. The radiology of the deep lymphatic system of the leg. Br J Rad 1973;46:120-124.

SUGGESTED GENERAL READING ON VASCULAR ANATOMY

Hollinshead WH. Anatomy for surgeons, vol 2: The thorax, abdomen, and pelvis. New York, Harper & Row, 1971.

International Anatomic Nomenclature Committee: Nomina Anatomica. Warwick R, Brookes M, eds. Angiologia. 5th ed. I.A.N.C. Baltimore: Willians & Wilkins. 1983.

Kadir S. Atlas of normal and variant angiographic anatomy. 1st ed. Philadelphia: W.B. Saunders Co. 1991;1-529.

Netter FH. Atlas of Human Anatomy. Summit, New Jersey. Ciba-Geigy Corporation, 1989.

Pansky B, House EL. Review of Gross Anatomy. 2nd ed. London: The Macmillan Co. 1971;1-493.

Willians PL, Warwick R, Dyson M, Bannister LH. Angiology, Chapter 6. Gray's Anatomy. 37th edition. Edinburgh: Churchill Livingstone. 1989;661-858.

Willians PL, Warwick R, Dyson M, Bannister LH. Splanchnology, Chapter 7. Gray's Anatomy. 37th edition. Edinburgh: Churchill Livingstone. 1989;1245-1475.

INDEX

Numerals in *italics* indicate a figure.